# TEXT-BOOK OF THE SCIENCE, ART AND PHILOSOPHY

OF

# CHIROPRACTIC

FOR STUDENTS AND PRACTITIONERS

BY

D. D. PALMER

THE ONE WHO DISCOVERED THE BASIC PRINCIPLE OF CHIROPRACTIC, DEVELOPED ITS PHILOSOPHY, ORIGINATED AND FOUNDED THE SCIENCE AND ART OF CORRECTING ABNORMAL FUNCTIONS BY HAND ADJUSTING, USING THE VERTEBRAL PROCESSES AS LEVERS

---

FOUNDED
ON
TONE

---

Published in 2019 by Echo Point Books & Media
Brattleboro, Vermont
www.EchoPointBooks.com

Originally published in 1910 by Portland Printing House Company,
Portland, Oregon

Textbook of the Science, Art and Philosophy of Chiropractic
ISBN: 978-1-63561-724-5 (casebound)
Cover design by Kaitlyn Whitaker

With my kindest regards, I present you with No. 1 of the 1st issue of the first book ever published on Chiropractic.

From Son

B. J. Palmer, D.C.

to

Father,

Dr. D. D. Palmer.

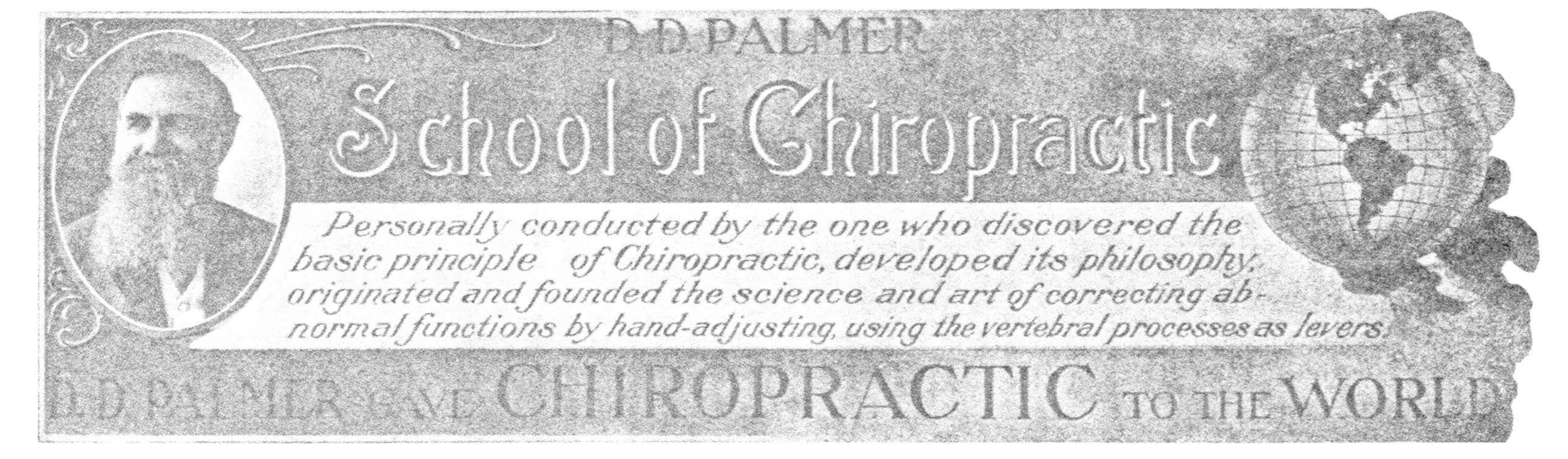


With my kindest regards, I present to B. J. Palmer, my only Son, No. 1 of the first issue of the first book ever published on the Science, Art and Philosophy of Chiropractic by the Founder of the only system which adjusts the cause of disease.

Trusting that he may again become a student of the Science, Art and Philosophy of Chiropractic; that he may seek its truth for truth's sake; that he may read and be instructed for his and other's benefit; that he may honestly and uprightly teach Chiropractic as delivered to him by its originator, is the sincere wish of his Father.

D D Palmer

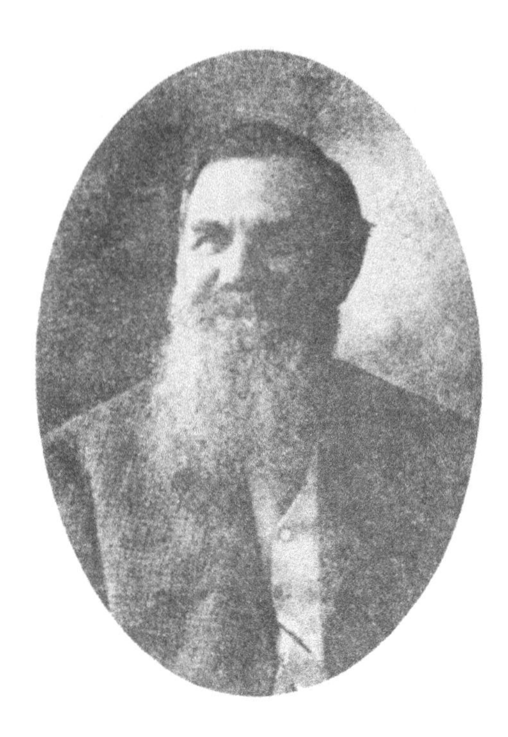

T. J. Owens, D. C., President of The Universal Chiropractor's Association, also President of The Palmer School of Chiropractic, founded by D. D. Palmer, says on page 23 of the August and September number of The Chiropractor, 1908: "The cause of disease remained an impenetrable mystery, until the month of September, 1895, when D. D. Palmer, a humble citizen of Davenport, Iowa, a man of no medical education whatever, made the most important discovery of this or any other century, viz.: the cause of any and all disease and the way to remove that cause, using nothing whatever but his hands.

"Dr. D. D. Palmer, with the assistance of the Rev. Samuel H. Weed of Monmouth, Ill., culled from the Greek language the two words Chiro and Practos, the combination of which made Chiropractic, meaning hand-done.

"The child (Chiropractic) being born and christened, it became the duty of its father to enter upon a course of training and development which would prepare the child for the duties and demands that might be made upon it.

"Some there are, I am sorry to say, who have vilely attempted to disparage the parentage of this child, but the records of his birth are too well authenticated to admit of any success of such vile traducing by the ungrateful beings who have profited most by reason of his birth. They have not even stopped at this, but have given additional evidence of their base ingratitude to their benefactor by attempting to kidnap the youngster, re-christen him and raise him as their own. Failing in this, they have tried to claim relationship with him, when the facts are, they hardly have a speaking acquaintance with him."

To all who long to elevate the human race by freeing it from ignorance, traditional prejudice, superstition and the pernicious delusions of the superiority of drug medication and the necessity of surgical mutilation, and especially to those who desire to know the best method of removing the unnatural and unnecessary condition called disease—conditions which not only cause great suffering, shorten life and lessen natural and intellectual progress, but prevent that proper acquirement of metaphysical knowledge so necessary for the next stage of existence, this book is most earnestly dedicated.

---

Life is the expression of tone. In that sentence is the basic principle of Chiropractic. Tone is the normal degree of nerve tension. Tone is expressed in functions by normal elasticity, activity, strength and excitability of the various organs, as observed in a state of health. Consequently, the cause of disease is any variation of tone—nerves too tense or too slack.

## THE SCIENCE, ART AND PHILOSOPHY OF CHIROPRACTIC.

Science is knowledge reduced to law and embodied in a system. Art relates to something to be done. Science teaches us to know and art to do. The philosophy of a science is the understanding of its principles.

Science is accepted, accumulated knowledge, systematized and formulated with reference to the discovery of general facts—the operation of general laws. Knowledge makes the principles of a science available by classification. Science is a systematized, paged index to the successive sense impressions. I created a science of principles which have existed as long as has the vertebrata.

Philosophy is the knowledge of phenomena, explained by and resolved into causes, reasons, powers and laws.

Chiropractic is the name of a systematized knowledge of the science of life—biology, and a methodical comprehension and application of adjusting anatomical displacements, the cause of biological abnormalities; also an explanation of the methods used to relieve humanity of suffering and the prolonging of life, thereby making this stage of existence much more efficient in its preparation for the next step—the life beyond.

In this volume I have systematized the knowledge acquired during the last twenty-five years, of the laws relating to life and as far as possible, explained the art of adjusting vertebral displacements, together with an extensive philosophical explanation of the laws of life and the causes of disease.

Knowing that our physical health and intellectual progress of this world and the next depends largely upon the proper alignment of our skeletal frames; therefore, I feel it my bounden duty to not only replace displaced bones, but also teach others, so that the physical and spiritual may enjoy health, happiness and the full fruition of our earthly lives.

## PREFACE.

The first volume on Chiropractic ever published was copyrighted and issued by my son, Bartlett Joshua Palmer, aged 24, in 1906, altho the most of its contents, which gave the principles of the science and somewhat of the art of adjusting vertebrae, were from my pen.

I objected to its being published at that time, because I then thot and now know, that the science had not been sufficiently developed. But in spite of my objections, the book was printed and its many readers found in it something, at least, pertaining to the science, art and philosophy of Chiropractic which never before had been made public.

The present volume has been written, compiled and copyrighted by myself. It contains valuable information which I have been 25 years in collecting. To every liberal-minded student it will appeal with more than ordinary interest, as it discourses and explains many biological and physiological problems which heretofore have been age-long secrets of Nature. In addition to other matters of great interest it answers the time-worn question, "What is life?" And points out the cause of deformity, disease and death.

Two urgent considerations have impelled me to write this book. The first is a desire, in response to numerous requests from Chiropractors and others engaged in various non-medical methods of healing, to place Chiropractic in its true light, by presenting to the world, in a logical and scientific manner, the facts and principles upon which it is founded. None the less important, consideration is the necessity of preserving my discoveries, in the original purity and integrity, by pointing out the errors which, thru stolid ignorance, have been taught and accepted as integral and necessary parts of Chiropractic.

How well I have succeeded in meeting the requirements of the first consideration, I am content to let the readers of the following pages decide. As to the subject matter of this volume it is only fair to state that it does not contain all that is or can be known concerning Chiropractic. There are still many problems for which it will be the province of this comprehensive science to furnish a correct solution. In fact, the explanation of some of these is already far advanced. These, with perhaps others of equal importance, will probably be completed by the time a second edition of this book is demanded.

The many topics discussed, however, are those of the most practical interest, and my readers may rest assured that all statements in regard to adjustments for the removal of morbid conditions have been repeatedly verified by clinical experience. I feel confident that however erroneous and untenable my views may, at first, appear, the sincere and unprejudiced reader will find in them nothing which is incompatible with the well-attested facts of biology and physiology. For this reason and the added one, that the discovery of truth should be the sole object of all investigation and discussion, I especially invite the attention and criticism of physicians and others whose medical education has been different from my own.

In regard to the manner in which I have met the second consideration, I ask no indulgence from and make no apology to my readers. After having devoted 25 years of the best of my life in study, research and experiment in developing my discoveries into an exact science, in obtaining the skill and knack of adjusting and the reason, causes and laws governing this knowledge, I cannot remain silent when teachers and self-styled "professors" in certain schools in which Chiropractic is claimed to be taught, are so obstruce, by an overwhelming ambition to be known and heralded as authors and original thinkers that they not only teach as a part of Chiropractic science and philosophy, doctrines and theories which are as absurd as they are erroneous, some of whom go so far as to deny the use, if not the existence, of important organs and functions of the body, and make startling physiological discoveries, simply by boldly giving another name to functions whose existence and duties have been known by all physiologists for generations.

Although, in some instances, my criticisms may seem personal, I can assure my readers that they are devoid of malice. My only object is to correct the errors, but I have done this in a manner which should supply its author with so much knowledge of his subject that he will have no excuse, even should he have the audacity to repeat his misrepresentations.

Exercises will be found scattered thruout the book. They are copied from books, booklets and leaflets of Chiropractors. I trust my criticisms may be beneficial to their authors as well as others; if so we are benefitted. These can be utilized as black-board exercises; if so, I would suggest that the books should not be opened during recitation, unless on rare occasions to settle doubtful or disputed points. Above all, the teacher should make a thorough study of the terms used, consulting medical and other works of reference. The teacher should make such study of the lesson, so as to be distinctly in advance of the class—prepared beforehand. These correcting exercises may be made intensely interesting, fascinating and instructive.

There are, today, about 2000 Chiropractors of various grades of attainment and efficiency, each of whom, it is presumed, desires all the knowledge of Chiropractic that can be obtained. All Chiropractors cannot, for various reasons, take a course of instruction under my personal supervision, but every one who is deprived of this privilege can purchase this book, from which can be gathered much valuable information not to be found in any other publication. The practical knowledge thus acquired will not only make each student of Chiropractic a more skillful practitioner, but will enable those in all future reading of what purports to be Chiropractic literature to discriminate between statements that are and those that are not in conformity with the basic principles of this important science. I have less than 37 years in which to direct the development of Chiropractic, and therefore I desire to see every Chiropractor an earnest student of the science and thoroughly equipped to practice this art in a manner that will at once bring credit upon himself and honor and renown upon the science he represents.

The principles and philosophy of Chiropractic include so much that is new and wonderful, beneficial, and withal so far-reaching, that several persons have tried to make fame and reputation for themselves by an endeavor to wrest from me the honor and distinction due me as the discoverer and developer of Chiropractic. But their efforts have been fruitless because they knew neither how or where to search for the lost and hidden lore which contained the essential elements of this grand science.

The basic principle, and the principles of Chiropractic which have been developed from it, are not new. They are as old as the vertebrata. I have, both in print and by word of mouth repeatedly stated, and now most emphatically repeat the statement, that I am not the first person to replace subluxated vertebrae, for this art has been practiced for thousands of years. I do claim, however, to be the first to replace displaced vertebrae by using the spinous and transverse processes as levers wherewith to rack subluxated vertebrae into normal position, and from this basic fact, to create a science which is destined to revolutionize the theory and practice of the healing art.

As much curiosity has been expressed in regard to the discovery and development of the basic principle and others which have been derived from it, a brief mention of the manner in which I became acquainted with the underlying principles of Chiropractic may be of interest. My first knowledge of this old-new doctrine was received from Dr. Jim Atkinson who, about fifty years ago, lived in Davenport, Iowa, and who tried during his life-time to promulgate the principles now known as Chiropractic. He failed, not because the principles were erroneous, but on account of the intellectuality of that time was not ready for this advancement.

Dr. Atkinson has frequently informed me that the replacing of displaced vertebrae for the relief of human ills had been known and practiced by the ancient Egyptians for at least 3000 years.

Recently I had the honor and pleasure of entertaining my old friend W. J. Colville, the well-known traveler, author and inspirational speaker, who gave me the following type-written information concerning the history of the principles which had been given to me by Dr. Atkinson. These axioms, rediscovered and known as Chiropractic, were also known and practiced by Aesculapius and his followers 420 years before the Christian era. Aesculapius was a noted physician of his time who, later, was known as the God of Medicine and Healing. In Greece his doctrines were amalgamated with those of the cult of an older Serpent-God whose function was that of healing the sick with medicine.

In mythology Aesculapius is represented as a bearded man with an attending serpent. In honor and remembrance of the fact that the principles revealed to me by Dr. Atkinson were direct from the Greeks, Rev. Samuel H. Weed, at my request selected two Greek words, cheir and praxis, meaning when combined, done by hand. From which I coined the word Chiropractic.

Mr. W. J. Colville's letter is as follows: "During my visit to Paris, in 1895, as the guest of Lady Gaithness, the famous author of 'the Mystery of the Ages' and many valuable works, it was my privilege to meet many peculiar and distinguished persons, among whom, and the most interesting of all, were some members of an Occult Society which made a specialty of Healing Ministrations. Among the methods employed by these extraordinary representatives of a very ancient cult of Aesculapius was one closely resembling Chiropractic. One case in particular which came under my direct notice was extremely thought-provoking and aroused within me an ardent desire to know much more of this wonderful system which restored a boy about 13 years of age from a condition of great suffering and pitiable decrepitude to a normal and happy state. Curvature of the spine was the malady from which this child had suffered for 11 years. The affliction dated to a fall, when he was two years of age, from which he had not in any way recovered. As the parents were of considerable means and devoted to their only son, no expense had been spared in procuring the best of medical and surgical aid obtainable. But all these efforts were to no purpose, for though operations had been performed, some of them extremely painful, and all kinds of treatments had been tested, no improvement was perceptible; the boy seemed doomed to chronic invalidism. I cannot attempt to give an accurate medical diagnosis of the case, but judging from observation and the testimony of his friends, I should pronounce the boy's condition extremely serious and seemingly incurable. When I first saw this boy in Paris, he could not walk at all, but had to be carried from the sofa, on which he spent his days, to the carrige which conveyed him to the apartment occupied by the two young men, who agreed, at the earnest request of his parents, to employ their skill in his behalf. I was permitted to accompany them to the place where the treatment was to be administered and allowed to witness the operation. The treatment struck me as quite novel, as I had not then become familiar with Chiropractic terminology or its methods. I there heard of 'luxations and subluxations of the spinal column,' and of 'adjustments' thereof, and I witnessed what appeared to me to be a very strange performance. One of the young men made a brief examination of the boy and then placed him, face downward, on a soft luxurious couch while he (the operator) placed one hand in a position covering a portion of the spine crosswise and with the other manipulated the spinal column with the thumb and finger. I occasionally heard a faint, sharp, clicking sound as the treatment proceeded and, when the operation was over, the boy declared he was entirely free from pain and feeling unusually vigorous, exclaiming, 'I am sure I shall soon be able to walk.' At the end of a week I saw the boy again. He was looking very much stronger and was positively jubilant with anticipation of complete recovery, and once more I was permitted to watch the singular treatment, which the boy seemed evidently to enjoy greatly, though it appeared to me quite heroic. Two years later I met the same boy in London, at the time of Queen Victoria's Jubilee, and I have never seen a lad of 15 years of age in finer appearance or more erect in carriage.

"The occultists who practice this method declare that, in these wondrous times of re-discovery, many of the methods employed in ancient Greece and older Egypt are being restored, and they claim that the modern practice of adjustment, as carried on by Chiropractors, was known many centuries before the beginning of the present era. Be this is it may, I saw the beneficent effects of the system as put in operation by these stalwart representatives of a cult which declares that no maladies are actually incurable, and which, without recourse to injections or mutilations of the person in any manner, accomplishes marvels of healing in strict accord with confidence in natural, scientific methods. Whether the mode of treatment here referred to is identical with what is now known as Chiropractic, I am not prepared to say, but as I have witnessed the work of both schools, they appear to me very similar and closely allied, and what is to the point of points, they actually do the work of restoring cripples to a normal condition. If we discover that ancient and modern knowledge are well-nigh identical, it can but strengthen our confidence in the immutability of universal order and encourage us to study, with ever-increasing diligence, those benign Laws of Being which, when known and honored, will secure to all freedom from the many ailments with which the fruits of ignorance still afflict our race. (Signed) W. J. Colville."

This Occult Society, referred to by W. J. Colville, had a shrine consecrated to Apollo, one of the Olympian gods. Apollo was the mythological god of healing and of ceremonial purification, the sender and stayer of plagues and the giver of sudden death. Apollo was the first Greek god to find place in the Roman religion, where he was worshipped as the god of healing. He is said to have slain a monstrous serpent which arose from the mud left after the deluge and which dwelt in the caves of Mount Parnassus. W. J. Colville was relieved of pleuropneumonia by one treatment of these Occult Scientists. In addition to the adjusting of the spine, he was commanded to bathe in water in which one of the consecrated brethren had washed his body. The father of the boy referred to by Mr. Colville, altho quite wealthy, had to kneel before and face the god Apollo during his son's treatment.

Mr. Colville kindly showed me on the person of Dr. F. H. Armstrong, the method employed by the two young men of Paris. The left hand was laid, flat and crosswise, on the back and with the right hand the spine was manipulated with the thumb and fingers. This method of proceedure is quite different from that which I employ, altho both are identical in purpose, namely, to replace osseous tissue with a view of removing pressure conditions that are the cause of disease. While the Paris gentlemen used "a soft luxurious couch," I use a hard table. A Chiropractor, to make his adjustments successful, requires upon his part firmness of the table, hand and arm, and upon the part of the patient perfect relaxation, whereas the Paris doctors, like many Chiropractors, manipulate the entire spine for the relief of curvature; I do not manipulate any portion of it. I adjust the twelfth dorsal vertebra, headward, by one move, using the spinous process as a lever. This removes the pressure which induced more than normal nerve tension, restores normal tone, circulation and by creating normal temperature the proper percentage of red and white corpuscles are restored, the tendency being restoration to normal when normal functionating is reinstated. Subluxated vertebra caused tension, tension excessive heat, hyperthermia an excess of erythrocytes and a deficiency of leukocytes, consequently softened vertebrae and curvature is the result. For further explanation, see rachitis.

Instead of using the thumb and finger when making an adjustment, I use both hands combined. The Paris doctors give the back bone a general overhauling, very similar to the Osteopaths, whereas I adjust only one vertebra, making the adjustment direct and specific, the difference being that one move adjusts, while the other manipulates, the dissimilarity indicates that one of the methods must be an improvement upon the other.

It is true that, 13 or 14 years ago, I knew but little of the science or its philosophy of the method I was about to launch upon the mentalities of the earth. It took time to absorb, develop and clothe new ideas with suitable language. No disgrace, was it? I gave credit where due. There was nothing wrong in so doing, and this I shall continue to do, trusting that I may be the recipient of yet more and greater favors.

As a means of relieving suffering and disease, Allopathy, Homeopathy, Osteopathy and now Chiropractic, have each, in turn, improved upon its predecessor. The latter, of all the others, is entitled to the seat of honor and distinction. But, as soon as the human mind is capable of absorbing a still more refined and advanced method and human aspiration demands it, it will be forthcoming and I hope to be the medium thru which it will be delivered to the denizens of the earth. A few years ago, it was thought impossible to send a telegram without using a stretched wire from post to post to convey it from one point to another. Today, by proper adjusting, messages are sent thousands of miles over land and sea without the need of posts or wire. Is it too much to expect a similar development, along Chiropractic lines, to be awaiting our beck and call?

I observe with much pleasure and satisfaction that Chiropractors are arriving at a better understanding of the essential features of the science and philosophy of Chiropractic as is evidenced by their literature. One significant indication of this change is seen in the fact that, recently, many writers and teachers correctly state that nerves are impinged upon instead of "pinched" or "squeezed." Another prognostic sign is in the attempt to explain how vital energy is conveyed by the nerves, instead of it being claimed to be similar to the manner in which sap circulates in a tree, or water passing thru a hose, or steam operating an engine, or man a machine shop filled with machines, or the electric current traveling over a wire. They are beginning to comprehend that inorganic objects and inanimate power do not illustrate or explain intellectual organic vital forces.

I am more than pleased to know that our cousins, the Osteopaths, are adopting Chiropractic methods and advancing along scientific and philosophical lines. They no longer assert (see The Philosophy and Mechanical Principles of Osteopathy, by A. T. Still, page 52) that wounded corpuscles congregate in mucous membranes causing all abnormal flesh growths. Advance we must; intellectuality, the pass-key of this age, is opening up new lines of thot; medical locks will no longer clog the wheels of progress. I trust they will find much in these pages to aid them in their progress.

It is also a pleasure for me to observe that the medical profession are absorbing Chiropractic ideas, using its methods, as shown by their books and practice.

In conclusion I desire to state that the larger part of what is "new" in this book has been derived from others, for there is "Nothing new under the sun." I am especially indebted to "another" for many, very many, new-old valuable ideas, also to those who have assisted me with advice and proof-reading and, lastly, to my faithful and ever-devoted wife for her encouragement during the many months it has taken me to write these pages.

D. D. Palmer.

---

The Chiropractor Adjuster is going to give its readers information on the science which its editor founded. It will give advanced education along this line in condensed language. It will advance Chiropractic by healthy impulses. It will adjust bent axles, wheels which do not track and luxated trolleys.

---

The Adjuster will be the mouth-piece of the original adjuster. It will present Chiropractic normally just as it should be; as it was originally intended to be by the discoverer. It will adjust all abnormalities found in Chiropractic literature; that right is inherent. This adjusting will be done on crippled literature, with the same pleasure, satisfaction and good feeling as we would that of an injured person.

As the grandson of the author, and president of the institution he founded, I feel it a personal privilege to present to our profession "THE SCIENCE, ART AND PHILOSOPHY of CHIROPRACTIC"—also named "THE CHIROPRACTOR'S ADJUSTER"—the one and only book written and published by D. D. Palmer. In doing so I accede to many hundreds of requests and letters to republish his original 1910 edition.

This long evident desire of our professional graduates to own a copy of D.D.'s own book is recognition of the fact that it is an historical document of the first importance. Page by page, it reveals the intensity of his convictions. Daniel David Palmer was dominated by a force—a brilliant mind—driving him through hardships and persecutions until his thoughts were completed and recorded in permanent form within the pages of this book, so that it might stand as his written legacy for our profession.

I have long recognized my grandfather's writing as basic to a full understanding and appreciation of our Chiropractic Philosophy; but the reader may share with me a certain reluctance to call attention to the occasionally unhappy relationship between father and son as noted here and there in these pages. I could not, of course, edit any of these portions and still present this limited reissue as a facsimile. A note of explanation concerning the two dedications of father and son, facing one another on pages 4 and 5, is in order. B.J.'s handwritten dedication appeared in the 1906 edition of his first book, and was reproduced by his father who then, in his turn, presented his first book to B.J. So you hold in your hand an exact photocopy of D.D.'s original book published in 1910.

In studying these pages it should at all times be remembered that they were written some fifty-five years ago. While the material in them clearly sets forth the unmistakable cornerstone of our Philosophy and Science, a considerable amount of additional research has, unquestionably, further developed and confirmed the scientific proof of D.D.'s original concept of the cause of disease. Starting with his own pen and thought processes, in 1895, we see, many years later, his premise today accepted and recognized, to such a position of acceptance that Chiropractors now constitute the largest of all the non-medical healing professions, and his science is practiced throughout the world.

My grandfather's work ranks as a most unique and important contribution to the many volumes of literature concerned with the health of humanity. It reveals quite clearly the source and strength of our present Profession and in strong tones it says that this incomparable science must never be dissipated or neglected or lost.

No man could have left a finer legacy or a greater challenge to the college he founded and the Palmer College of Chiropractic takes pride in remaining faithful to his inspired principles of Philosophy, Science and Art. We urge and inspire each and every student to emulate his life's work.

Of all the great truths pertaining to the welfare of humanity, none is more radiant with lasting promise than Daniel David Palmer's Philosophy. It is my fervent wish that this edition will help to unify and strengthen our profession, as well as perpetuate my grandfather's brilliant and original study of the cause and mystery of disease.

I believe this book will be a treasured and inspiring memory, reminding us of the marvelous heritage that lies within our hands.

January, 1966 David D. Palmer

## A BRIEF HISTORY OF THE AUTHOR AND CHIROPRACTIC.

**The Life of One and the Existence of the Other Are Inseparable.**

I was born on March 7, 1845, a few miles east of Toronto, Canada. My ancestors were Scotch and Irish on my maternal and English and German on my paternal side.

When my grandparents settled near the now beautiful city of Toronto, there was but one log house, the beginning of that great city. That region was then known as "away out west."

I came within one of never having a mamma. My mother was one of a pair of twins one of which died. The one which lived only weighed one and a half pounds.

When a baby I was cradled in a piece of hemlock bark. My mother was as full of superstition as an egg is full of meat, but my father was disposed to reason on the subjects pertaining to life.

I was a magnetic healer for nine years previous to discovering the principles which comprise the method known as Chiropractic. During this period much of that which was necessary to complete the science was worked out. I had discovered that many diseases were associated with derangements of the stomach, kidneys and other organs.

In the dim ages of the past when man lived in rude huts and rocky caves, even up to the present time, he resorted to charms, necromancy and witchcraft for the relief of mental and physical suffering. His whole object was to find an antidote, a specific for each and every ailment which could and would drive out the intruder, as though the disorder was a creature of intelligence. In his desire to free himself from affliction and prolong his existence, he has searched the heavens above, he has gone into the deep blue sea, the bowels of the earth and every portion thereof. He has tried animal and mineral poisons, penetrated the dark forest with superstitious rite and with incantations, has gathered herbs, barks and roots for medicinal use. In his frenzy for relief, trusting that he might find a panacea, or at least a specific, he has slaughtered man, beast and bird, making use of their various parts alive and dead. He has made powders. ointments, pills, elixirs, decoctions, tinctures and lotions of all known vegetables and crawling creatures which could be found, giving therefor his reasons according to his knowledge.

One question was always uppermost in my mind in my search for the cause of disease. I desired to know why one person was ailing and his associate, eating at the same table, working in the same shop, at the same bench, was not. **Why?** What difference was there in the two persons that caused one to have pneumonia, catarrh, typhoid or rheumatism, while his partner, similarly situated, escaped? **Why?** This question had worried thousands for centuries and was answered in September, 1895.

Harvey Lillard, a janitor, in the Ryan Block, where I had my office, had been so deaf for 17 years that he could not hear the racket of a wagon on the street or the ticking of a watch. I made inquiry as to the cause of his deafness and was informed that when he was exerting himself in a cramped, stooping position, he felt something give way in his back and immediately became deaf. An examination showed a vertebra racked from its normal position. I reasoned that if that vertebra was replaced, the man's hearing should be restored. With this object in view, a half-hour's talk persuaded Mr. Lillard to allow me to replace it. I racked it into position by using the spinous process as a lever and soon the man could hear as before. There was nothing "accidental" about this, as it was accomplished with an object in view, and the result expected was obtained. There was nothing "crude" about this adjustment; it was specific, so much so that no Chiropractor has equaled it.

If no other discovery had been made, this, of itself, should have been hailed with delight. It was the key which has ultimately unlocked the secrets of functional metabolism; it is the entering wedge destined to split the therapeutical log of superstition wide open, revealing its irrational and ignorant construction.

Shortly after this relief from deafness, I had a case of heart trouble which was not improving. I examined the spine and found a displaced vertebra pressing against the nerves which innervate the heart. I adjusted the vertebra and gave immediate relief—nothing "accidental" or "crude" about this. Then I began to reason if two diseases, so dissimilar as deafness and heart trouble, came from impingement, a pressure on nerves, were not other disease due to a similar cause? Thus the science (knowledge) and art (adjusting) of Chiropractic were formed at that time. I then began a systematic investigation for the cause of all diseases and have been amply rewarded.

I founded Chiropractic on Osteology, Neurology and Functions—bones, nerves and the manifestations of impulses. I originated the art of adjusting vertebrae and the knowledge of every principle which is included in the construction of the science of Chiropractic.

The amount of nerve tension determines health or disease. In health there is normal tension, known as tone, the normal activity, strength and excitability of the various organs and functions as observed in a state of health. The kind of disease depends upon what nerves are too tense or too slack.

Functions performed in a normal manner and amount result in health. Diseases are conditions resulting from either an excess or deficiency of functionating.

The dualistic system—spirit and body—united by intellectual life—the soul—is the basis of this science of biology, and nerve tension is the basis of functional activity in health and disease.

Spirit soul and body compose the being, the source of mentality. Innate and Educated, two mentalities, look after the welfare of the body physically and its surrounding environments.

Chiropractors correct abnormalities of the intellect as well as those of the body.

These discoveries and their development into a well-defined science are worth more to the student, practitioner and those desiring health, than all the therapeutical methods combined.

I am the originator, the Fountain Head of the essential principle that disease is the result of too much or not enough functionating. I created the art of adjusting vertebrae, using the spinous and transverse processes as levers, and named the mental act of accumulating knowledge, the cumulative function, corresponding to the physical vegetative function—growth of intellectual and physical—together, with the science, art and philosophy—Chiropractic. It is now being followed, more or less, by 2,000 Chiropractors, and its use is being attempted by several other methods. It was I who combined the science and art and developed the principles thereof. I have answered the time-worn question—what is life?

## NERVE FUNCTION

The nerves which ramify every portion of the body are composed of nerve-fibers. These are arranged in bundles. They constitute the larger share of the brain and spinal cord. These nerve-fibers are the passage-ways for conducting impulses from the center to all parts of the body, and sensations from the peripheral endings to the nerve-center.

Physiologists divide nerve-fibers, which form the nerves, into two classes, afferent and efferent. Impressions are made on the peripheral afferent fiber-endings; these create sensations which are transmitted to the center of the nervous system. Efferent nerve-fibers carry impulses out from the center to their endings. Most of these go to muscles and are therefore called motor impulses; some are secretory and enter glands; a portion are inhibitory, their function being to restrain secretion. Thus, nerves carry impulses outward and sensations inward. The activity of these nerves, or rather their fibers, may become excited or allayed by impingement, the result being a modification of functiönating—too much or not enough action—which is disease.

Spondylotherapy states under the head line of Chiropractic: "This system was founded in 1885. The theory sustaining this system presumes that, in consequence of displaced vertebrae, the intervertebral foramina are occluded through which the spinal nerves pass."

"In this way the nerves are pinched, and Chiropractors assume that such pinching is responsible for 95 per cent of all diseases. Chiropractic concerns itself with an 'adjustment' of the subluxations, thus removing pressure on the nerves."

"What the Chiropractor calls 'nerve tracing,' consists of following a sensitive nerve from its vertebral exit to and from the affected organs."

Chiropractic was discovered by me in 1895, not in 1885, as claimed by the pseudo founder, who was but three years of age at the date mentioned.

Friend Abrams has been misinformed in regard to the cause of disease as understood by Chiropractors. For correct information upon this point see various portions of this book by the founder of Chiropractic.

In regard to nerve-tracing, Friend Abrams is correct. I am the originator of nerve-tracing, as many of my old students know, for they took instruction under me when B. J. was a lad.

## CHIROPRACTIC.

The Chiropractic system, revised on earth to-day,
Was known in ancient ages, in regions far away.
Sages and seers proclaimed it of origin Divine
And practiced it in secret, at many a hollowed shrine.

The great, new light that's breaking o'er all the widespread
earth,
Is calling mystic knowledge to wider, further birth.
So, 'mid the great revival of truth among mankind,
This truth, contained in Nature, must wide acceptance find.

We know that mind is potent, that thoughts are mighty things
That soar and widely travel, as on expanded wings.
But 'tho these thoughts are able to banish ev'ry grief,
We wish a perfect method by which to give relief.

Our minds are the directors, they should our actions sway,
Sub-consciously and consciously, thought must direct our way.
But, mind doth act through matter, a vehicle it needs;
And this we need to regulate to drive out noxious weeds.

The spinal column holds, we know, a most important place.
When normal, it is beauteous, a form of wondrous grace.
But when distorted, it becomes the seat of many ills,
Which are, frequently, mistreated with ineffective pills.

Adjust the subluxations till crooked spines grow straight.
Take off from nerves the pressure which induce an evil state.
Thus many ailments vanish and health appears for all
Who, wisely, on Dame Nature for real assistance call.

No nauseous drugs or lancets we need to bring to view,
For Chiropractic action is always mild and true.
Our hands are wisely given to remedy the wrong,
So, let these useful members be praised in poet's song.

Dame Nature is beneficent, her laws are wise and true.
To learn and then obey them, is all we have to do.
And when we wisely work and plan the better way to learn
No illness will exist, because its only when we turn

Away from Nature's guidance we into error stray;
This is the only reason that you are ill to-day.
The body is an entity, although its members share
The daily work it needs must do with faithfulness and care.

When all abide together and in harmony fulfill
Respectively, their duties, they reveal God's holy will.
Should any member suffer, the other bear their part
Until the burden is removed by Chiropractic Art.

The Chiropractor teaches that all organs must agree,
That all must work together in most perfect harmony.
Thus, when all regulate the spine its functions to fulfill,
All other parts experiences alike responsive thrill.

The kidneys, lungs and liver and the spleen and heart and brain
Are organs linked together by the sympathetic chain
And from a common center, they one and all obtain
A regulative, guiding free that makes their duty plain.

Adjustment, regulation is all that we require.
It lifts the baneful pressure that smothers vital fire,
Gives freedom to the muscles that they may freely act,
And the body perfect liberty to functionate intact.

Away with drugs which poison and instruments that kill.
Let us use, in wisdom's way, of mental, manual skill.
The hands, by mind directed, can drive our ills away
And bring us advantageous health for which we all shall pray.

No cruelty, nor torturing of animals we need
To point the way to conquest over ills of any breed.
Along the gracious pathway where justice kindly rules
We learn life's useful lessons in the Chiropractic schools.

The happy day is dawning, it cometh on apace,
When wisdom linked with kindness, will all wrongs and ills
 efface.
And whatsoe'r assists to bring about that blessed day
Will drive all hateful error to oblivion straightaway.

Set free the trammeled spirit, take off the binding shroud.
Deliverance preach to captives by binding fetters bowed.
Let mind and body act as one, though each of them be free,
For only thus can we attain to perfect liberty.

Hail to the noble workers who firm and faithful stand
To bless earth's suffering millions with heart, brain and hand.
Hail to the modern system which takes the ancient rule
And well adapts its practice to the needs of modern school.

'Twas in the land of freedom where the eagle soars on high,
That Chiropractic knowledge was brought to humans nigh.
And now to every continent and island of the sea
The welcome news is spreading to banish misery.

Life more and more abundant, is what we all require,
We then, can lift the barriers that interrupt the fire.
Give Nature perfect freedom, this only do we need,
Then she, kind nurse and mother, will all requirements heed.

Arouse the latent energy! Innervate the frame!
Then no more enervation will put our hopes to shame.
Let's keep our thots directed to all that's pure and wise,
Then no ensnaring tempter will rob us of our prize.

Let all honor, then, be given unto that kindly man,
Our teacher, D. D. Palmer, whose Chiropractic plan
Has lifted many burdens, set many captives free
And whose very wise instructions are fruits from Wisdom's
 tree.

As years glide swiftly onward, with added zeal and might,
Will this new school of doctors work zealousy for right,
Till knowledge conquors folly, till reason on her throne
Dispenses boundless blessings and claims all for her own.
September 24, 1910. W. J. COLVILLE.

## THE BARBER POLE.

The barber of ye olden time practiced some of the offices of a surgeon, especially those of bleeding and pulling teeth. He was then known as a barber-chirurgian. He bled his customers to let out the impure, bad, fermented, poisoned, diseased blood. It was supposed to become stagnant, detained, obstructed, stopped in its circulation. In anemic persons the blood was thot to be lacking, owing to a shortage or insufficiency of drainage or to perverted circulation. These notions were quite prevalent when I was a boy. Indeed, we do not need to go back so far, for all I have said about them will be found in Dr. A. T. Still's book on Osteopathy, dated Jan. 1, 1902.

It was supposed that by letting out the old, worn-out blood, new, fresh, pure, bright, red blood would be supplied. On this theory Osteopathy was founded. Thanks to Chiropractic, the practitioners of Osteopathy have accepted so much of Chiropractic principles that hardly one of them now believes in that bloody delusion.

King Edward IV., of England, instituted a corporation of barber-chirurgians. Barbers and surgeons were made into separate professions by King George II. at the beginning of the nineteenth century.

The barber pole had its origin thru jealousy. A nobleman chanced to be a patient of a certain barber who had an eye open for business. He took the blood of the nobleman and striped a white pole with it. This so aroused the jealousy of his professional neighbors that they also set up poles, striping them with bright red paint which retained its color, whereas the pole colored with the nobleman's blood soon became dim and unsightly.

When the American flag of red, white and blue was unfurled, the barber, to be patriotic, added the blue; he Americanized the English barber pole.

---

Friend Carver says:—"The term abnormality is applied to every form of deviation from the usual conduct of the parts of an organism instead of the term disease. Abnormalities which therapeutists have designated as being diseases." He does not like the term disease; therefore uses "abnormality" 41 times on 4 pages, 8 times on 7 lines.

Abnormal and abnormality are not synonymous with disease. To be abnormal does not of necessity mean morbid; it refers to that which is unusual, not regular.

## INFLAMMATION.

Inflammation is a morbid condition distinguished by pain, heat, redness, swelling and impaired nutrition. Acute inflammation is one in which the process is active. Chronic inflammation is one in which the changes occur with less rapidity.

"Baron van Swieten, Counfellor and Firft Phyfician To their Majefties the Emperor and Emprefs of Germany; Perpetual Prefident of the College of Phyficians of Vienna; Member of the Royal Academy of Sciences and Surgery at Paris; Fellow of the Royal College of Phyficians at Edinburgh, etc., etc., etc.," states under date 1776: "Inflammation terminates either in health, in other difeafes, or in death. It ends in health, either by the helps of nature, or of art. By nature, the malady is carried off either by a mild refolution, or by a concoction and excretion of the matter of the diftemper. Lastly, an inflammation terminates fuddenly in death, if the caufes of the inflammation are fo violent as to deny all pafsage to the humours, while a very intenfe fever is urgent at the fame time."

James Copland, M. D., F. R. S., date 1844, states: "The true seat of inflammation is always the ganglionic nervous system and the capillary vessels of the part affected; the primary change, originating with the former, but more fully expressed in the latter, constituent of the organization.

"The temperature of an inflamed part upon, or near the surface, is usually several degrees higher than that of parts at some distance from it; and even the deep-seated viscera experience a rise of two or three degrees, and often much more, above the healthy temperature of 98 degrees.

"The functions of an inflamed organ, tissue, or part, is one of the earliest phenomena or constituents of the morbid action, being nearly coetaneous with the change in the organic nervous power, on which this action depends. The disturbance of the functions is generally in proportion to the violence to the disease. If the inflamed part performs a secreting function, the secretion is either diminished, increased, or altered in character."

McFarland states that "heat is the elevation of temperature characteristic of acute inflammation, depending upon active hyperemia, by which an increase of hot arterial blood reaches the part, and possibly in part to increased combustion taking place in it."

Arterial blood is of the same temperature thruout the body and of the same quantity and quality; therefore, the blood could not heat one portion more than another. Metabolic combustion must of necessity furnish an equal amount of heat for each and every portion.

John E. Erichsen under date 1860 says: "Inflammation is Nature's means of repairing the effects of an injury."

Gould says:—"A term applied to those tissue-changes by which irritants are eliminated and which include overfilling of the blood vessels, alterations in the blood-vessel walls, outwandering of leukocytes, exudation of plasma and multiplication of the cells of the surrounding connective tissue."

Bacteria are the medical man's irritant; they excite the phenomena known as inflammation—vascular activity, degeneration, exudation and proliferation; the blood flows more rapidly, degenerative putrefaction is expelled.

"Reactive inflammation is set up around a focus of degeneration to limit the spread of the degenerative process."

This reactive inflammation is thot to be physiologic—functional activity for the purpose of freeing the body by way of degenerative liquifaction—necrosis—liberating substances capable of producing the phenomena.

There are various forms or effects of inflammation attending each and every disease. **Disease depends upon, and is never present without, a variation of heat from the normal.**

Stengel says:—"Disturbances of circulation, innervation or metabolism may so alter cellular processes as to occasion the production of irritating and chemotactic products."

Chiropractic:—Nerve irritation creates heat by increasing molecular vibration. An excess of heat disturbs circulation, innervation and the cellular processes of metabolism.

Stengel further says:—"Inflammation represents increased and altered activity of tissues as a result of irritation; its primary object is the removal of the irritant. It is a pathological and destructive process **per se,** but considered from the point of view of its result (the removal or confinement of the irritant and the resulting tissue destruction) inflammation is essentially conservative and useful."

**Inflammation, excessive heat, is the result of nerve irritation. An increase in temperature means increased activity of bodily tissue, an exorbitant amount of functionating.** Instead of inflammation having for its primary object the removal of the irritant, the lesion, whether in the form of a poison or displaced osseous tissue, is the cause of the inflammation. Inflammation, heat in excess, is pathologic; it changes both structure and to its possessor, but he would prefer that some one else should experience it.

In defense of the theory that inflammation or fever is a body cleanser, Stengel says:—"The cellular destruction is an accentuation of the ordinary death of cells resulting from wear and tear, though the form of the cell-destruction is more violent and probably different; the post-inflammatory regeneration is effected by karyokinetic multiplication of cells, as in normal tissues."

Health is that condition of the body in which all the functions are performed in a normal degree. If they are executed in a too great or too little measure, just in that proportion will there be disease. If the cellular destruction is greater than the normal wear and tear of tissue, it is an excess—disease—and cannot be "regenerative," health restoring. Inflammatory cell destruction is not that of destructive metabolism. Inflammation destroys by necrosis, softening of tissue; is death in mass, dissolution of an aggregation of cells; while necrobiosos is death of individual cells, molecular death of tissue. Coagulation necrosis, liquefactive necrosis, cheesy necrosis, dental necrosis, dry or moist necrosis, is not that of destructive metabolism. The former is the result of an abnormal amount of heat; the latter includes a normal quantity, that which is congenial to health—normal destructive metabolism.

There are many forms of necrosis, among which are the half-dozen mentioned above. Many of these are known by one or more names. The different kinds depend largely upon the tissue involved. We do not find dental necrosis in the blood; coagulation necrosis in the lungs, nor cheesy necrosis in the nerves or muscles.

The medical idea of inflammation is that it is "conservative in tendency, benign in disposition and evidently the result of a carefully-adjusted, protective mechanism"; that hyperemia (excessive blood in a part) associated with edema (infiltration of serum) act as a diluting solvent, tending to remove and scatter the irritant; that suppuration, colliquation, burrowing abscesses and centers of necrosis are but preliminary actions for the purpose of ejecting the intruder; that degeneration, disintegration, colliquation and supperation are caused by invading bacteria which surround the lesion, causing the tissue to necrose—melt, liquify; that the tubercle, gumma, necrotic ulcers and caseous necrosis are but masses of leukocytes.

While medical men look upon inflammation as pathologic-physiologic function, they think it has a recuperative influence—a tendency toward health. The medical fraternity allow a fever to run its course (because they cannot do otherwise) to cleanse the body of impurities. They assist all inflammatory processes to suppurate in order to eliminate all putrescent matter.

The "post-inflammatory regeneration effected by karyo-kinetic multiplication of cells, as in normal tissues": The "karyo-kinetic multiplication of cells" is the common mode of cell production—functions physiologically performed. There can be inflammatory **degeneration**, but inflammatory **regeneration, never.** Inflammation increases functional activity above normal, resulting in a pathologic condition named disease. Regeneration which restores diseased tissue and abnormal functions to normal, must be physiologic.

Chiropractors look upon inflammation and fever as the result of abnormal tissue; a change of tissue causes a difference in molecular vibration; the degree of vibratory motion corresponds to the amount of heat, increased molecular action, caused by irritation, pressure on nerves, the lines distributing the function of heat. They look for and find the impingement which is causing an increase of functionating which produces heat. By removing the pressure from the channels of communication, they cease to carry an excess of heat. By doing this, Chiropractors are able to cut short all local, inflammatory conditions, as well as general fevers.

Chiropractic principles. Nerves heat the body; normal heat is health; heat in a more or less degree is disease; pressure on nerves cause an excess of heat named inflammation. Metabolism is normal when heat is natural; health is the result. These principles have been reduced to law, a formula expressing a rule of successive action of certain phenomena. They have been formulated into a system—a science.

The practical part of Chiropractic is the art of adjusting subluxations of vertebrae with the hands. Chiropractic is both a science and an art.

Chiropractic is a science, not a building: it was created, not built. Its foundation is not that of principles. It is founded on anatomy—osteology, neurology and functions. It is not built out of principles as a mason would build a house out of brick. Chiropractic is a science—a knowledge of health and disease reduced to law and embodied into a system.

Delafield says, "Inflammation is the local attempt at the repair of injury." Inflammation tends to create morbid conditions, instead of repairing them. The greater the inflammation, the greater the disturbance of functions and the morbid change of tissue. The destruction of tissue—necrosis—is because of excessive heat. All morbid growth are due to excitation—too much functionating. Heat in excess is disease creating, not health restoring.

The physician viewing "inflammation as an emergency measure incited by injury, in which the body adapts to unusual ends, as best it can, mechanisms and powers normally maintained for other purposes," takes pleasure in noting the rise of temperature, the increased pulse rate and respiration of his patient, for the greater these are the greater will be the reparation. (?). The Chiropractor finds that local inflammation and general fever injure the tissue of the patient; that high temperature softens the hard as well as the soft tissue. Heat in excess is pathological, never physiological.

We are told by books on pathology that, "Inflammation is a modification of physiological processes." That is true. Whenever physiological processes are changed from normal, in a greater or less degree, they are morbid, disease producing, pathological. All inflammatory processes, whether hemorrhagic, fibrinous, serous or suppurative are abnormal, pathological, disease creating in functions and tissue; they are in no sense health producing.

Delafield speaks of inflammation of nerves as follows:—"In the nerves, as in the brain and cord, degenerative changes commonly accompany inflammation and a distinction is often difficult. The difficulty in sharp differentiation lies in the fact that degenerative changes in nerves, when intense or long continued, often lead to inflammation, and that inflammatory conditions in nerves often determine secondary degenerative changes in the nerve fibres."

Degenerative changes always accompany inflammation in proportion to the intensity of the heat. It is not difficult to distinguish between inflammation and degenerative changes. The former being the cause, while the latter is the effect. The never lead to inflammation, but on the contrary, inflammation (excessive heat) softens nerve and other tissues. **Sure.** Inflammatory conditions of nerves determine conditions in their difference between cause and effect. Degenerative changes Chiropractor should be a close observer; he should realize the filaments. Degenerative changes in nerve tissue, necrosis, softening, modifies the transmitting force of impulses and functions thru its fibers.

Meningitis—inflammation of the meninges of the brain and cord, may occur in connection with diseases of other portions of the body. An impingement which presses against the recurrent nerve, which innervates the meninges of the cord and brain, excites its fibers and the membranes which it involves.

The following four quoted paragraphs are from Stengel's pathology.

"The alkaloids possess marked power in the production of necrosis. Acids, alkalies, metallic salts and innumerable other chemical substances may produce direct necrosis, or indirect necrosis by the preliminary production of degenerations. The same substances often cause both circulatory and mechanical disturbances, which augment their direct effects. Heat and cold act like chemicals; heat alters the properties of proteids."

Inflammation, because of traumatism or chemical substances, causes firm tissue to become softened, necrosed. Necrosis is death of tissue, degeneration. Its molecular atoms are run together; they cease to be rigid, are not suitable for the transmission of energy which supplies vital action. If the nerves, which transmit vital force, are softened, become liquified, greasy, instead of having their natural firmness, the functions which constitute life cease, the result being death.

Necrosis may be caused by direct contact of chemical substances or of direct heat, as a burn or of X-rays, as concentrated heat, or indirectly by exciting the molecular action of nerves; the result being an over amount of heat which tends to liquifaction.

It was hoped that the X-rays—concentrated light (heat)—because of its caustic action upon the tissues of the animal body would have an affinity for diseased tissue **only.** But it has been found that an over amount of heat, whether traumatic, chemical or concentrated on the surface by a sun-glass or transmitted to the deeper tissue by X-rays, causes liquifaction—necrosis.

Mechanical disturbances include those functions which are irregular because of displaced bones which press against sensitive nerves; this includes disturbed circulation as well as change of tissue. Inflammation (surplus heat), whether traumatic or chemical, alters animal tissue.

"All forms of necrosis are accompanied to a greater or less extent by the various degenerations."

Tissue necrosis cannot do otherwise than change the texture of tissue from normal to that which is not normal; thereby, changing its carrying capacity of impulses.

"At the present day inflammation is generally regarded as purely reactive in nature, the irritation causing sometimes one and sometimes another primary lesion."

Inflammation is not reactive, it is destructive. It causes morbid change in the exercise of functions and the tissue upon which it acts. The inflammatory action caused by innoculating the system with virus, a disease producer, a disturber of functions, an augmenter of necrosis to the extent, sometimes, of causing the loss of an arm or a leg, is considered a cleansing process.

The introduction of the virus of a disease into the body by a physician is legitimate; but, if it occurs by accident, it is all wrong, even if the same febrile conditions are produced.

"Inflammation, whatever its original conception, may become so extreme as to lead to necrosis. Necrosis, on the other hand, often leads to inflammation, the dead cells constituting the primary irritation."

Extreme inflammation, an undue amount of heat, will liquify any tissue with which it comes in contact, will cause tissue to soften; but necrosed tissue never leads to or causes inflammation. Dead cells never irritate, they do not become excited, they do not get inflamed. Irritation is because of tissue having too much life—not death.

The normal temperature of the body, that which is suitable for normal functionating, is 98.6 degrees. That amount of heat creates the desired firmness, the proper tonicity of tissue for the accomplishment of bodily acts, the normal performance of functions. Less or more than normal disturbs functions by changing the texture of the transmitting tissue. A temperature below 92.3 is nearly always fatal, but subnormal temperatures above this degree are not necessarily followed by death. A temperature of 95 is spoken of as one of moderate collapse.

Stengel says:—"Exposure of healthy or unhealthy tissues to X-rays causes cellular degenerations and necroses with secondary inflammatory reaction. The skin—being most immediately exposed—is the most susceptible of normal tissues; but diseased tissues and new growths are still more readily affected, probably because of their less stable condition. The epithelial cells of the skin suffer first and most intensely, the glandular cells of the skin are less prone to degeneration. Swelling and degeneration of the endothelial and other cells of the blood-vessels and thromboses may in part account for some of the results of X-ray exposures."

"Secondary inflammatory reaction" in diseased tissue is because of the added X-ray heat. "Diseased tissues and new growths are still more readily affected," because of the superadded heat.

The American Text-Book of Surgery. "Inflammation is a disturbance of the mechanism of nutrition and affects the structures concerned in this function. It is the response of living tissue to injury."

"Inflammation causes a disturbance"—it is not the disturbance. Mechanism is the arrangement, or relation of the parts of a machine. Nutrition is a metabolic function. Inflammation is the response of living tissue, because of injury to the nerves ramifying that portion or of the peripheral endings; the injury of either causes hyperthermia. Tissue damaged exhibits symptoms we name inflammation. A slight increase in temperature may be physiological. For example, in the repairing of fracture, there is a rise of temperature during the preparation of callus.

---

The nervous system is the channel thru and by which life-force—the energy which gives innervation to the essential functions of respiration and circulation—is transmitted. The two latter are the functions upon which life depends. They are carried on in proportion to the innervating force which, as we have noticed, may be either excessive or deficient, either condition causing disease and even death.

The involuntary portion of the nervous system and muscles which contract by nerve stimuli must be in normal tône in order to execute the normal amount of functionating for a healthy existence.

Innervation—the nervous influence necessary for the maintenance of life and the various functions required to be performed to produce action, is regulated by the amount of heat which may be furnished in a too great or too little degree. An entire absence of or too much innervation means death. Nerve and muscle tonicity is dependent upon, and modified by, the amount of heat. Excessive tonicity causes erethism, an abnormal increase of nervous irritability, an augmentation of vital phenomena in organs or tissue. Deficient tonicity causes atony or weakness, a lack or vitality. Heat may become so intense as to soften, necrose the tissue of nerves and muscles, thereby causing a diminution of vibratory motion by which vital energy is transmitted.

It will be seen, according to Chiropractic pathology, that death is caused by disease and disease by impingement, and the latter by poison and accidents. The Chiropractor adjusts for one as readily as for the other.

## "NERVE FORCE IS LIFE.

"**The energy that gives life to the body is now known to be nerve force**—this explains why a strong, active body, overflowing with energy, may, in a moment, become a lifeless form.

"Although no visible change has taken place, the heart has ceased to beat; the blood no longer flows through the veins to nourish, develop and sustain; the brain is dormant, the eyes sightless, the ears deaf; the lungs, stomach, liver, kidneys and other organs have ceased their labors.

"What is this marvelous change? What is the element in the living that is absent in the dead?

"There is no secret in the frame-work of bone, held together by sinews, fibers and muscles; nor in its covering of flesh; nor in the system of organs located within this framework, or in the several duties they perform.

"But the energy, the something that gives them life; the something that has been taken away—what is that?

"The answer is—**nerve force.** It is an indefinable substance which is generated in the cells of the brain and spinal cord and sent out through the system of nerves to give power to the organs, as electricity is sent out through wires to furnish light, power and heat.

"With plenty of nerve force, there is life and health; with little nerve force the body is weak and sick, and without it there is no life at all."

**There are two systems of nerves**—the outer and inner. **Through the inner nerves is conveyed the energy that gives life and motion** to the lungs, heart, liver, stomach and other organs of the body. Through the outer nerves impressions (feeling) are conveyed to the brain.

These nerves are more numerous than the blood vessels, and, in a great measure control their size, or in other words, the circulation of the blood, as well as the action of the muscles. No portion of the body, whether brain, bones, ligaments, fat, blood vessels or muscles is without its system of minute nerves. The condition of these depends upon the influence conveyed to them from the brain and spinal cord.

**If this nerve influence,** or as we prefer to call it, nerve-force, which is supposed to be similar to electricity, **is weakened, the** part supplied by it becomes feeble; if too much fluid goes to a part, **it is irritated, causing pain, congestion, spasms, inflammation and various other forms of disease.** Should there be some disease or derangement of the brain or spinal cord, or of the nerve itself, so that no nerve-force is given off, paralysis (or death) is the inevitable result.

**A multitude of diseases known by other names are due to an impairment to the whole or part of the nervous system.**

Each portion of the body is under the control of "Nerve Centers" located in the brain and spinal cord. **Disease of every organ or portion of the body may,** and very frequently do, **arise from defect in the nerve centers rather than in the organ itself.** Thus a weakness or irritability in the nerve centers of the brain causes dizziness, dullness, headache, neuralgia, etc.

A weakness of the nerve centers of the stomach produces indigestion, dyspepsia, neuralgia, wind in the stomach, etc. Weakness of the nerves of the heart results in fluttering or palpitation of the heart, etc.

Nervine allays irritation, assists the nerve cells to generate nerve-force, strengthens the nerves and through them gives renewed life and vigor to all the organs of the body.

Pains in all parts of the body are also caused by an irritated condition of the nervous system, so that headache, stomach-ache, neuralgia, rheumatism, etc., **are nervous disorders and will be relieved when the nervous system is restored to its normal condition.**

**It is the nerves that are affected**—they are weak and out of harmony, and as they control the action of all the organs, they, too, must of necessity suffer.

**All feeling is in the nerves.** Therefore, anything that weakens, or destroys the nerves, such as over-exertion, heat, accident mental effort, cold, indigestion, congestion, causes pain.

In headache it is the brain nerves that are involved. In neuralgia it is the more prominent nerve branches in some part of the head or body. Stomach pains come from a disturbance or weakness of the stomach nerves, and **in rheumatism and sciatica there is a pressure** or strain **upon certain nerves.**

**Pain is therefore relieved when the irritation or pressure is overcome.**

Cathartics and purgatives do more harm than good, as they operate by irritating the lining of the stomach and bowels, thus weakening, rather than strengthening the nerves."

The above is copied from an almanac of 1910. It reads quite like Chiropractic. I would like to see all Chiropractic literature read as well. Medicine dispensers are noting the mental pulse of the public—the trend is toward the belief that nerve disturbance, rather than impure blood, is the cause of disease.

Altho in a medical almanac, the above statements are quite refreshing when compared to some of the advertising literature of Chiropractors. The medical world is advancing. Only a very few years ago blood purifiers were the only remedies advertised—now it is nervines for the nerves. By the way, why did not some monopolistic hog get that word "nervine" copyrighted so that he alone could use it as a trade mark? The public mind is undergoing a rapid change. Instead of blood purifiers, they demand something to soothe, strengthen, tone up, relieve the tension and irritated condition of the nervous system. "Nervine assists nerve cells to generate nerve force."

Life is that vital force which some regard as physical and others as spiritual. It is manifested by the employment of the senses and voluntary movements.

Living beings are endowed with life, that is, certain powers and functions not associated with inorganic matter. Life is uncircumscribed; it is a relative term. We have live and dead rock. It is, however, usually referred to as a peculiar stimulus of organized matter which endows an individual with power to make spontaneous movements under the direction of the senses. Life is that state of an animal or plant by virtue of which any or all of its organs are capable of performing their functions.

"A strong, active body, overflowing with energy, may, in a moment, become a lifeless form." The author grasps the idea, that too much energy—too much function, may cause death—he might also have included disease.

Disease (using a medical term), abnormal functionating (using Dr. Carver's), may consist of too much energy as well as of not enough; may be overflowing or deficient in amount. Variations from the normal may cause the exhibition of either **too much or not enough life**; we may live too fast or too slow. All life is dependent upon heat, some forms requiring more and others less.

All beings which possess life, exercise certain functions requiring energy. Molecular alterations, tissue change, accomplished by an intelligent vital force, constitute a living being. To live, necessitates the possession of life. Life possesses an intelligence which pervades the universe and is expressed in accordance with the environment and the quality of the material in which it manifests itself.

What is that which is present in the living body and absent in the dead? It is not inherent; it is not in any of the organs which are essential to life. An intelligent force which I saw fit to name Innate, usually known as Spirit, creates and continues life when vital organs are in a condition to be acted upon by it. That intelligent life-force uses the material of the universe just in proportion as it is in a condition to be utilized.

The almanac referred to, recognizes two systems of nerves, the "outer," which takes cognizance of our environments, and the "inner" which runs the bodily functions.

In the tenth paragraph, we find the author is undetermined as to the nature of this energy. He considers it nerve influence, nerve force or a fluid. But he grasps the idea, that, if there is not enough, the part lacking is enfeebled; if too much, irritation and the various forms of fever and inflammatory diseases result. I wish that all Chiropractors could take in this basic principle of our science—**that too much or not enough energy is disease.**

Do not forget, that disturbance of functions, either more or less action than normal, is disease. Also that any change in structure because of too much or too little heat is disease. There must be a normal amount of energy and heat to create and maintain normal functions and structure.

In the twelfth paragraph he does not fully grasp the Chiropractic idea. "Weakness or irritability" is because of nerve abnormality and not from "defect" of the nerve centers of the brain.

Sixteenth paragraph: "It is the nerves that are affected—they are weak and out of harmony, and as they control the action of all the organs, they, too, must of necessity suffer."

Nerves are affected. Instead of their tissue being out of harmony, their condition creates inharmony. Their "suffering," or being abnormal, creates unusual functionating of the organs in which they end. Abnormality of nerve tissue may cause disease of the brain or its covering, but nerves are not abnormal because of the "nerve centers of the brain" being affected.

"All feeling is in the nerves." "Pain is therefore relieved when the irritation or pressure is overcome."

There would be no irritation without pressure. Pressure is not "overcome," subdued, conquered; it is relieved, the impinging bone is replaced, pressure removed.

"It is the brain nerves that are involved." All nerves are brain nerves, that is, they all originate in the deep substance of the brain tissue.

---

"Dr. H. A. Foster, the originator of the combined systems of Chiropractic, Electrical, Hydropathic and Neuropathic treatments."

This virtually says, that Dr. Foster is the originator of these four methods: but, I understand he means to say that he is the **originator of combining them.**

## CHIROPRACTIC ANALYSIS.

I have found it better to give regional locations for adjusting, rather than the number of the vertebra.

The nerves of innervation which go to the organs and various parts of the body do not always emerge from the same foramina in all persons. Remember that there are no two of us alike in our osseous or nervous makeup. The filaments of nerves vary in number and quality. Some are composed of fibers from the cranial, spinal or sympathetic. The spinal accessory, the eleventh cerebral nerve, has fibers from each segment of the cervical spinal cord and also from the medulla oblongata of the cranial cavity immediately above the foramen magnum. Knowing the region of dislocation, it is easy **for the Chiropractor who comprehends Chiropractic as a science,** to locate the displacement and the affected nerve by the contour of the spinous processes and nerve palpation.

The counting of vertebrae is uncertain, especially in fleshy persons. Knowing the locality, the vertebra—not vertebrae—is easily located by the Chiropractor who has learned it as a science, and the adjusting is easily accomplished by the one who has acquired it as an art. Counting vertebrae is unreliable and a waste of time.

Accumulated, established knowledge of the laws and principles regarding the functions of living tissue in health and disease, systematized and comprehended from ascertained facts, has developed a science which is serviceable and known as Chiropractic.

"**Paralysis** is caused by occlusion of nerve stimulus resulting from displacement of vertebrae in the spinal column. The gravest points of occlusion are usually upon the third, twelfth, eleventh and seventh dorsal nerves; the first, fifth and eighth cervical nerves; and the second and fifth nerves. However, in general paralysis, or **hemiplegia,** there will be occlusions thruout the length of the vertebral column; those mentioned, however, being primary."

"Nerve stimulus" is noticed elsewhere.

To say that hemiplegia is because of every vertebrae in the spine being displaced, is not specific, not scientific, does not represent Chiropractic as a science.

Upon either side of the vertebral column are gangliated nerve chains for the distribution of nerves and their impulses. These reach from the occiput to the coccyx. Nerves are distributed from them to all parts of the body, even into the brain cavity and the brain itself.

I discovered in 1888 that hemiplegia could be relieved by adjusting the fifth dorsal vertebra, relieving the fifth spinal nerve on the side affected. Bear in mind, that hemiplegia takes in one-half of the body laterally and the half of the brain opposite the side affected. Usually there can be found on the opposite side from that which is paralyzed, a depression over the organ of hope, in which the end of the finger fits. This portion of the frontal bone will be found sensitive if scratched or pressed upon. The inner and outer tables are thinned, the diploe absent; sometimes so much so that the thinned portion may be quite springy.

I have relieved many cases of hemiplegia by adjusting, replacing, the fifth dorsal vertebra. This is specific, scientific, making Chiropractic a science. Why not learn Chiropractic as a science. Why adjust thruout the whole spinal column?

Dr. C. tells us, there is, in **meningitis,** "occlusion of all of the trunk nerves of the vertebral column, resulting from reaction and construction."

Meningitis is inflammation of the meninges of the brain and spinal cord. The spinal nerve, immediately after its exit from the intervertebral foramen, gives off a recurrent branch which returns thru the intervertebral foramen. This nerve innervates the meninges of the spinal cord and brain. If this nerve is impinged upon, it becomes inflamed; meningitis being one of the resulting diseases. As each spinal nerve has a recurrent branch, it becomes necessary to examine and find the one impinged on by bone pressure. This may be known by the contour of the spinous processes and the tenderness at the place of exit and inlet. Adjusting this one vertebra will take the pressure from this nerve and relieve the inflammation.

The displacement of one vertebra, whether by accident or poison, does not react on other vertebrae, so as to occlude their foramina, thereby constricting the nerves emanating therefrom. The distribution is made thru the vertebral, gangliated nerve chain and not thru the vertebrarium.

Why should the Chiropractor "adjust to remove the occlusions at all brain and heart places"? The patient has met with an injury, a displaced vertebra. Why not locate that one and replace it? Why should he "carefully examine" for "other occlusions"? The displaced vertebra should be replaced at the first adjustment, as this is an acute disease. Affects the nerves, whose peripheral endings ramify the tissues thru which it finds entrance. I say, why is it that "frequent adjusting will be necessary for a few hours; at the beginning as often as every fifteen minutes"?

We are told by this same author that **syphilis** is caused **by** occlusions of the twelfth dorsal, first and second lumbar vertebrae; that the spread of the virus thruout the system causes constriction of the entire vertebral column.

The occlusion, closing of the vertebral foramina, is not the cause of syphilis. The poison, acting on certain nerves, irritates their structure. They, in turn, contract muscles which draw vertebrae out of alignment, thereby impinging upon nerves which go to and affect certain portions of the body.

Inocculation caused by sexual contact affects the first lumbar nerves. Then, why not replace the vertebra which is drawn out of alignment by contraction of those nerves and muscles?

"Occlusion of nerves at each foramen." Occlusion is the transient **(not continued)** approximation of the edges of a natural opening. I presume that Friend Carver means the shutting up of the intervertebral foramen, which is rarely, if ever, closed sufficiently to squeeze the nerve which occupies one-third of its space—see cut on page —. The first pair of cervical nerves emerge above and the second below the atlas in grooves, where there is an abundance of room and no vertebral notches to slide together; they cannot be occluded. The first and second pair of cervical nerves cannot be pressed or squeezed between the occiput and atlas or in the cleft between the atlas and axis, and yet there are many diseases resulting from their displacement. Right now, get your vertebral column. Look at the formation of the three first cervical vertebrae. See the vertebraterial foramina which give passage to the vertebral artery and the ganglionic nerve chain. Slid'e, luxate, the atlas toward the left or right side. Observe the **sharp**, outward edge of the inferior articular process. See where it would impinge on, **press against**, the vertebral nerve chain. No wonder that sharp neuralgic pains of the face and head is occasioned by slight luxations of the atlas. Bunions and corns are caused by displaced joints in the toes and tarsus where it is impossible to pinch or squeeze a nerve, but the displacement of those joints press against nerves and cause these affections.

The same writer states that **pleurisy** may be caused by an impingement upon any of the twelve dorsal or the last four of the cervical nerves. "No one need suffer from pleurisy longer than two or three hours if the principles of Chiropractic be at once applied at the outset."

Pleurisy, pleuritis, inflammation of the pleura, may be acute or chronic. The acute form is known by sharp, stabbing pains in the side, which are increased by breathing or coughing; the chronic, by an exudate collected between the pleura and the lung. This affection arises from an **impingement upon one nerve**; why try to adjust sixteen vertebrae to relieve sixteen pairs of nerves? We cannot adjust, replace, that which is not displaced. To move one or more of the fifteen mentioned which are not displaced, would displace them, causing impingements on other nerves and consequently creating other diseases. This is not Chiropractic.

The side affected determines whether the left or right nerves are impinged upon. By palpation we find which one of the first three dorsal nerves needs relief. Remove the pressure by moving the vertebrae above the nerve towards the shoulder on the opposite side.

If the principles of Chiropractic are understood, there is no reason why the pleuritic patient should not be relieved at once, especially if the disease exists in the acute form.

The symptoms of **peritonitis** are moderate fever, a wiry pulse, abdominal pain, tenderness and distension of the abdomen. The patient lies on his back with the thighs flexed to relieve the contraction of nerves and muscles. There is vomiting and constipation.

The peritoneum is the largest serous membrane in the body. The nerves which supply it with innervation will be found in the lower dorsal. By an examination of the contour of the spinous processes in this region and by palpation, the nerve which is impinged upon can be located and relieved. It shows ignorance of Chiropractic analysis to adjust eleven pairs (22) of nerves when **only one pair is impinged upon.**

**Typhoid fever** results from contaminated food or water which acts upon the system as a poison. Metabolism is disturbed. The symptoms and complications are various, for which see any pathological book.

The Analyzer tells us that if adjusting is begun at the first appearance of the disease the abnormality will reach no greater gravity; but, if delayed until the patient takes to his bed, it will require from one to five days to relieve all traces of fever.

I have relieved quite a number of typhoid fever cases, adjusting the fourth dorsal vertebra but once. The longest standing case was one of seven years, the patient was relieved immediately, as soon as the adjustment was given, in the presence of a physician who furnished the case. This case was pronounced typhoid when the patient was in bed. The same symptoms continued until the adjustment was made. The hot dry skin was changed to that of being moist and warm at once. Why adjust ten vertebrae from one to five days? Is it because of lack of knowledge of Chiropractic principles? Is it because the one so advising never studied it as a science, or is it because he does not comprehend what an adjustment is? Adjusting is an art, which should be practiced with scientific knowledge. There may be one or more of the complications referred to, but they all arise thru the sympathetic, gangliated chain which extends from the occiput to the coccyx.

In **brain fever** the Analyzer tells us to adjust every fifteen minutes during the first few hours.

Brain fever is an acute disease; one in which the displaced vertebra has not become disfigured. It does not need to be grown back to its former, normal shape. In chronic cases, those which have been standing for many months or years, the displaced vertebra has become ill-shaped, and the adjoining vertebrae have changed their shape to accommodate themselves to their displaced and disfigured neighbor. In such cases it takes time to grow them back to normal, but it is not so with acute cases.

If the Chiropractor understands the principles of Chiropractic; if he can locate the nerve (not nerves) impinged on, and knows just what move to make in order to relieve the pressure, he should relieve it and the inflammation at once. If he is able to replace a vertebra and it remains in its normal position, why or how can he keep replacing that which is already in place? The advice given, in several diseases, to adjust every fifteen minutes for a few hours, shows that the adviser really does not comprehend just what an adjustment is. To adjust is not merely pressing on the spine, it means to move, replace, a displaced vertebra. To adjust each and every vertebrae of the spinal column is simply an impossibility; they cannot all be displaced. You cannot replace that which is not displaced.

In brain fever, the nerve impinged on will need to be located by palpation, and an examination of the spinous process. The intense motor reaction caused by the stimulus (using the Analyzer's term), is relieved as soon as the proper adjustment is made, the nerve being no longer on a tension.

To adjust every fifteen minutes, replacing a vertebra four times an hour, shows that either the suggester does not know when he has made an adjustment or does not replace the displaced vertebrae. Remember, adjustments are only made when a vertebra is returned to its normal position, and that when Chiropractors attempt to move three contiguous vertebrae or the whole spinal column as advised by the Analyzer, that, in all probability, they do not move them, or, if they do move more than one for any disease, they displace those not displaced, thereby creating diseases instead of relieving it.

**Hydrocephalus**, an abnormal accumulation of fluid within the cranium, termed external when in the meninges; internal when in the ventricles; chronic, infantile, or congenital when occurring in infants and of slow progress; and acute when it accompanies meningitis, the tubercular form of which is often termed acute hydrocephalus. The kidneys are at fault. Adjusting the twelfth dorsal vertebra will relieve the pressure, if due regard is paid to which one or both kidneys are affected, adjust accordingly. There is no need of adjusting the other eight vertebrae advised by the Analyzer—remember that you cannot adjust, replace a vertebra that is not displaced. I desire that every Chiropractor to understand and comprehent this statement. They will then be on the road toward special, specific, scientific adjusting, creating a science.

The prone condition during infancy allows gravity to place the accumulated water in the cranial cavity inside the unsutured bones which are easily spread to accommodate the fluid which the kidneys and the serous transudate membrane failed to transude.

**Paralysis agitans,** shaking palsy, is marked by a trembling of a portion or all of the body. It usually begins in one hand. It may affect just one arm and leg, and, possibly, the head. During sleep the tremor is absent. The gait is that of festination; the body is bent forward. The center of gravity is too far forward; the patient runs to keep up with the forward action of gravity.

There is no necessity of trying to adjust nine places as directed by the Analyzer. We are told to adjust the first, sixth, seventh and eighth cervical vertebrae. We may jump on, we may press against, those four and the other five suggested, but we cannot adjust, replace these adjoining vertebrae. A vertebra displaced is not in apposition to those adjoining above and below. When the displaced vertebra is adjusted, replaced, so that its articular surfaces are in conjunction with their mates, why adjust the adjoining vertebrae—an impossibility. Such statements by a Chiropractor expose his ignorance in regard to adjusting.

In all cases of shaking palsy, the kidneys will be found abnormal in their functions; not that the kidney affection causes other affections. The nerves emanating below and next to the twelfth dorsal vertebra will be found impinged upon; their fibers reach the kidneys and the portions of the body involved. Correcting the displaced twelfth dorsal vertebra will relieve the pressure so that Innate can transmit impulses in a normal manner.

A paroxysmal affection of the bronchial tubes, with difficult and labored breathing, cough and a feeling of constriction and suffocation, is named **asthma.**

Why adjust eight vertebrae; I mean why try to adjust eight vertebrae when only one is displaced which is the cause of asthma? Sometimes one adjustment gives relief; in other cases, weeks and months may be required.

We are told that asthma is caused by errors in diet. A full stomach presses upon the lungs and helps to close the bronchial tubes; therefore, emptying the stomach removes pressure and gives relief.

**Diphtheria** is a disease of childhood. The Analyzer tells us that it is a constitutional abnormality.

Diphtheria is a result of poison taken in the system. In all probability, it is taken in the food or drink, for we find the sixth pair of dorsal nerves affected; those on the left side going to the stomach, those on the right reaching the throat.

Instead of adjusting four cervical and four dorsal vertebrae, as advised by the Analyzer, adjust the fifth dorsal, moving it in the direction indicated by palpation. If the displaced vertebra is adjusted properly, once, there will be no necessity for another, except in those rare cases in which the subluxation has existed for some time. In one case of this kind I had to adjust once a day for three days. Upon inquiry I found the patient had been subject to croup. If the adjustment is done just right there will be no need of adjusting "at periods of from a quarter to a half hour." If we replace the displaced vertebra, how can we do more? Why try every few minutes?

**Apoplexy** is supposed to result from effusion and extravasation of blood or serum into the brain or spinal cord. The Analyzer accepts this theory. The effects just mentioned are the result not the primary cause.

Pressure upon a nerve whose fibers innervate the meninges, of brain and spinal cord, causes them to be excited and inflamed. This hyperthermia softens the walls of the blood vessels and increases the tension—the strain upon an artery at full pulse.

High tension of an artery may be normal or pathological. Tonicity may be raised to a point above normal by exercise or excitement. Such a natural response is physiological. Intravenous tension is accompanied by a physiological response in the elevation of temperature during the repair of the osseous frame-work.

Inflamed vascular tissue exposed to hypertension is liable to rupture because of the softened walls. We, therefore, view pathological hemorrhage as pertaining to disease, an effect, not a cause.

**Chorea, St. Vitus Dance,** was so named because, in the epidemic of chorea in Strasburg, in 1488, those who were afflicted (using the term of superstition) were sent on a pilgrimage to the chapel of St. Vitus, at Zaburn. It is recognized by involuntary irregular, nervous, jerking movements.

The Analyzer gives seven vertebrae to adjust in order to relieve seven pair of nerves. The primary occlusion being the third dorsal, and the other six the result of motor reaction.

Palpation and the outward line of the spinous processes will reveal the displacement and the sensitive nerve impinged on. The time required to relieve the patient will depend upon the length of time the disease has been standing, resulting in a more or less ill-shaped vertebra. Daily adjusting, with an hour's rest immediately after, will gradually return the vertebra to its normal shape. If a patient with this or other diseases, goes out walking or riding, immediately after an adjustment, the exercise returns the vertebra to its abnormal position, requiring much more time to effect a cure than if he or she had rested a half-hour or more after each adjustment.

"**Gout** is but the result of sciatica and articular rheumatism together."

There are cases of gout which do not show, and have not shown, any symptoms of sciatica or articular rheumatism except such as are manifested in this disease. I have just relieved a case of gout of the right big toe, in less than a week, by adjusting one lumbar vertebra. The Analyzer is in the same dilemma as are medical men. "The cause of gout is not definitely known, but is connected with an excess of uric acid or urates in the blood."

Gout is no more nor less than articular rheumatism confined to the small joints of the hands and feet, more especially to those of the big toe. It is readily relieved by spinal adjusting. The Analyzer advises adjusting seven places, seven vertebrae as "indicated." The **science** of Chiropractic **indicates one vertebra,** depending upon whether the disease is manifested in the fingers or toes, and this can be determined by an examination of the spinous processes and palpation.

**Epilepsy.** "No case of epilepsy has ever been found that did not present a very grave subluxation at stomach place."

So far, I have had but one occasion to adjust other than the atlas for epilepsy. To adjust six vertebrae is not scientific, neither does it display a knowledge of the art of adjusting. Give one adjustment a day, for the six days of each week, until the deformed vertebra has been restored to its normal shape. Then it will remain in its normal position. Remember, when the osseous skeleton is in proper position, in all of its parts, there will be no pressure on nerves or muscles, and all will be well.

"**Consumption,** or tuberculosis of the lungs, as the process exists today, is caused specifically by occlusion of the first, second, third and fourth dorsal, and sometimes the eighth, seventh and sixth nerves."

Notwithstanding, Dr. Carver, under date of March 1, 1910, wrote me, "The only thing I want distinctly understood between you and me is, that you are not permitted to publish my letters to you or any part of them." I quote from his of Feb. 17th, 1910, "In answering your question, 'Why not be specific in Adjusting?' I simply say, that is what I teach." Giving seven pair of nerves (14 nerve trunks), the occlusion of which causes consumption is not precise, definite nor specific.

Dr. Carver states on page 4 of his Chiropractic Analysis, that he "received the very crude application of its principles from the founder."

Those "very crude" adjustments relieved him of consumption and are yet used by the founder in that "very crude application" of adjusting one vertebra for the "white plague."

I used a specific adjustment in adjusting Willard Carver. Altho it was "very crude," he was relieved by adjusting one vertebra—the one displaced and none other.

My adjusting of one vertebra for the relief of consumption in the case of Willard Carver he thinks "very crude," but the adjusting of three pair of cervical and four pair of dorsal nerves is considered by him to be precise, definite and specific. This is the specific, scientific analysis of Chiropractic by Carver.

In order to give specific adjustments, we must possess a knowledge of the disease in question and be able to trace it to its origin; not to seven pair of nerves, nor to one pair, but to the one single nerve trunk impinged upon, and sometimes even to that of one filament of a nerve.

For both **pleurisy** and **pneumonia** we are told to adjust six different vertebrae. In each affection there is only one subluxated vertebra impinging upon one nerve. Replacing this relieves the impingement. If done just right, one adjustment is sufficient.

**Adenoids** are soft polypoid tumors, consisting of loose, succulent, connective tissue, situated in the nasopharynx. They may become hypertrophied because of inflammation, but not as a result of catarrh. The mucus covering the pharynx and enlarged tonsils represent two different conditions. While either is not the result of the other, yet, they both result from inflammation caused by a nerve impingement, by a displaced vertebra, at stomach place, on the right side of the spine. Replacing this vertebra, removing the pressure from the nerve which goes to and ramifies the region of the throat and pharynx, will relieve the inflammation of those parts.

To adjust five vertebrae where only one is displaced, is not scientific, is not Chiropractic.

In **diabetes**, the "occlusion" is not at kidney place, the twelfth dorsal. (See article on diabetes.) Look for displacement at seventh dorsal, as diabetes is due to abnormal functionating of the pancreas; the kidneys acting only as excretory organs.

There is no need of adjusting five vertebrae, four of which, at least, are not displaced. Why displace those which are in their normal position? It should be the Chiropractor's business to relieve impingements, not to create them.

**Endocarditis**—inflammation of the lining membrane of the heart. The Analyzer tells us the cause is "on account of certain irritants in the circulating fluids, also by an occlusion of the fifth, seventh and eighth cervical nerves." Why not be specific? If you do not know just where the impingement is, make yourself acquainted with Chiropractic as a science, and by a knowledge of neurology, locate the nerve which innervates the heart. If the nervous influence be too great, the stimulation excessive, find what nerve is irritated, overexcited, and relieve the condition by adjusting the displaced vertebra which has caused it.

The Analyzer names four places to adjust to relieve locomotor ataxia, namely, the 11th and 12th dorsal and the 1st and 2d lumbar. "The twelfth dorsal vertebra and first lumbar are, however, anteriorly displaced about equally." Dr. Carver is right in adjusting the first lumbar. The other three are not at fault, are not displaced, consequently if moved at all they would be disarranged instead of replaced. "Anteriorly displaced.'' No vertebra can be displaced anterior of those above or below without a fracture of the oblique processes. One examination of any of the vertebrae and their articulating processes should satisfy any person that such is an impossibility.

The following is the Analyzer's analysis of **rheumatism.** ''**Rheumatism is always chronic abnormality. In other words,** rheumatism never becomes apparent at its incipiency, and only presents rheumatic symptoms when it becomes chronic. The reason for this truth lies in the fact that the active symptoms called rheumatism are always the result of an irritating substance at the periphery of sensory nerves caused by long occlusion, producing a motor-reaction and consequent widespread constriction and occlusion.''

''The **irritating substance** is an excessive and abnormal uric acid, accompanied by lime and calcareous substances in solution. These enter the area of stasis, where the **circulatory fluids** are substantially without movement as a result of occlusion and there precipitate, or, to use a common term, settle into the tissues. As this sediment continues to increase, the stasis becomes wider by reaction and occlusion, and the sediment graver. When it reaches a sufficient volume, it results in the reaction and symptoms called rheumatism.''

Rheumatism may be acute or chronic. The symptoms may be pronounced from the first and run a short, definite course, or they may be of long duration. The onset may be sudden and severe, or it may develop gradually.

Instead of rheumatism being the result of an irritating substance at the periphery of sensory nerves, we find it exists because of impingements at or near their emergence from the spinal column. The truth of this statement can be demonstrated to the satisfaction of any skeptic by the fact that a Chiropractor can promptly cause rheumatism by purposely subluxating a vertebra and afford relief as readily by replacing it. Therefore the Chiropractor should know which vertebrae are subluxated and move these only. The reason for the Analyzer's belief in this ''apparent truth'' lies in the fact that he is yet floundering in the delusions of chemical analysis; he has not outgrown his medical education.

Motor reaction, widespread restriction, uric acid and occlusion do not enter into rheumatism or any other disease, as Chiropractic causes or effects. Uric acid is not always found by chemical analysis in rheumatic patients.

''These enter the area of **stasis,** where the **circulatory** fluids are without movement.''

Dr. Carver ought to know that blood is the only fluid of the body which is said to circulate as it moves in a circuit. The passage of fluids through membranes is known as diffusion—not circulation. When liquids cease to transude they are said to be in a state of stasis—dropsy is a form of stasis. Diffusion is a physiological function; stasis is pathological, because of inflammation which thickens the membranes.

When we find the patient affected with rheumatism in upper and lower limbs, look to center dorsal. If in lower limbs only, the lumbar region; if in feet, the lower lumbar. It will be seen that the advice to adjust five places,'' together with the occlusions of heart and brain places,'' is superfluous and need not be followed. Instead of ''acid irritation producing reaction, constriction and occlusion,'' impingements will be observed by the practitioner who has learned the principles of Chiropractic.

**Smallpox** and **chicken pox,** although bearing different names, are one and the same disease, differing only in the degree of severity. Physicians are often undetermined as to which of the two diseases a case under observation belongs.

The Analyzer states that for these diseases we should adjust for liver and kidney nerves and repeat every half hour until complete relaxation has been obtained. He advises adjusting the fifth, sixth, seventh, eleventh and twelfth dorsal nerves. Why he skips those beween the seventh and eleventh I am unable to say.

I have relieved several well-marked cases of the above mentioned diseases by one adjustment of the fifth cervical. I have never needed to give the second. These diseases are acute—vertebrae have not become ill-shaped; therefore they only need replacing. Why not learn to be specific? Why not learn Chiropractic as a science?

In **malaria** and **intermittent fever** the Analyzer advises adjusting five vertebrae every ten minutes until relaxation is apparent, then twice a day. In addition, he says, ''watch carefully the heart and brain places.'' In malaria and intermittent fever there is a portion of the time during which the patient is relaxed. The relaxation period would determine the number of Carver's adjustments. The Analyzer evidently believes in sticking to his job and not allowing the other fellow to get in between adjusting periods or an opportunity to beat him out of the case. This reminds me of an undertaker who hired a man to sit up with a sick man, night after night, for a month so that the night-watch might secure for him the order for a casket. The sick man beat the undertaker out of that order by getting well.

If a vertebra is adjusted, replaced, why keep replacing it

every ten minutes? Does the vertebra become displaced in so short a time, or does the practitioner displace it while trying to replace the other four mentioned? Or is it possible that the adviser does not comprehend what an adjustment is, or when he makes one?

**Insanity.** "It is usual to find occlusion of the third, sixth, seventh, eleventh and twelfth dorsal nerves."

Why not locate the vertebra which causes the impingement, the cause of mental derangement?

Analyzer says to adjust four places for **Dyspepsia** and **sick headache.** As I have said, elsewhere, the nerves which innervate the stomach emerge on the left side of the spine, while those from the opposite side go to the throat, eyes and head. Therefore, because of a displacement of the fifth dorsal, there may be, at one and the same time, dyspepsia and sick headacre. If the stomach only is affected, stand on the left of the patient and adjust toward the right shoulder. For diseases of the throat, eyeball, or headache, stand on the right side and throw toward the left shoulder. If there be diseases which show impingements on both sides, then head the adjustment.

The Analyzer tells us that dyspepsia or indigestion, "is usually the result of the grossest and most extravagant errors in eating and diet conceivable. However, it may be caused by occlusions produced by direct injury to the vertebral column." He advises "the most rigid dieting of the patient."

I have known people who lived in dirt and filth from one year's end to the other, and yet illness was seldom heard of in their home. Usually they are tough and hearty. I have also visited homes where they were so excrutiatingly neat that hardly a speck of dust or dirt was seen inside of their doors. The children (if they had any) were kept spic and span and not allowed to sit down for fear they would get their clothing soiled. Invariably in such homes some one was complaining of being ill. If dirt is so unhealthy and cleanliness so healthful, why is the clean home such a sickly one and the dirty one so salubrious? There is a happy medium between these two extremes. We can be so filthy as to be offensive, or so neat that we are uncomfortable to ourselves and those who come near us.

Fastidious, rigid dieting has produced dyspepsia in thousands. Those who are the "grossest and most extravagant in eating" are generally free from indigestion. Obey the scriptural injunction: "Take thine ease, eat, drink and be merry."

**Bronchitis.** "The occlusion causing this process is usually of the seventh and eighth cervical and first and second dorsal nerves."

We have a process of law, chemical processes and the process of decomposition, but no bronchial process.

Bronchitis is a throat affection due to an impingement of the right, sixth dorsal nerve. Why adjust four vertebrae for four pairs (eight nerves), when only one pair is impinged? Why try to adjust those which are not adjustable: those which are already in their normal position? Why? We cannot replace, adjust, those which are already in place.

When visiting a Chiropractic clinic, recently, I observed that the number of the vertebra to be adjusted, in each patient, was recorded in a book. Of the twelve patients two were adjusted in three places, one in four, three in five, four in six, one in seven and one in eleven places.

From only three of the patients did I learn the name of the disease from which each of them was suffering. One was adjusted in four places for bladder trouble, another in three places for gall stones, and the third in eleven places for colonitis—eleven vertebrae adjusted for one disease.

The explanation for this general treatment was: "the doctor asks the patient no questions, but makes his diagnosis through the direct examination of the vertebrae." Regardless of the ailment, he adjusts any or all vertebrae that are thot to be out of alignment. A knowledge of the contour of the spinous processes is considered very essential, so that all abnormalities found in the outline of the spinous processes can be adjusted. The vertebrae were not corrected for a special disease; the whole spine is looked over and all irregularities corrected.

A knowledge of diseases is not necessary; it is not essential to know the ailments for which adjustments are given. Months of study on physiology, pathology, neurology, osetology, myology, and all the other ologies are unnecessary. This mode of procedure is what might be appropriately called general Chiropractic adjusting; analogous to the osteopath's "general treatment" which consists of manipulations and Swedish movements covering the entire body. As the osteopath learns that special moves give specific results, so the Chiropractor will in time learn to be specific in his work, making Chiropractic a science.

The "hit the high places" method would be all right if all vertebral columns were alike, in health, in the outline of the distal ends of the spinous processes. But on the contrary, we find no two of them alike; so, that, to depend upon the configuration of the spinous processes, alone, is often misleading. It is well to know the locality of the special ailment we are expected to relieve. Knowing the locality, we should be specific in determining, by palpation, the nerve impinged upon, the vertebra displaced, and the direction it should be moved in order to rack it into its normal position, and then act accordingly.

A clinic is for the purpose of instruction. Each case should be studied and information given thereon. In a Chiropractic clinic the diseased condition should be noted and the subluxated vertebra, or, at least the region in which the impingement causing the disease exists, should be pointed out. The bladder trouble was not caused by the displacement of four vertebrae; gall stones were not the result of three displaced vertebrae, and colonitis was not the result of eleven displacements. Why not learn to be specific? Why not learn Chiropractic as a science and an art?

If we adjust six, seven or more vertebrae, or adjust the whole spinal column, as Friend Carver states in his Analysis of hemiplegia—paralysis of a lateral half of the body—"There will be occlusion throughout the length of the vertebral column." In meningitis he says, "There will be occlusion of all the trunk nerves of the vertebral column." In syphilis he tells us, "There are constrictions of the entire vertebral column, with occlusion of nerves at each foramen." That is not definite, not specific, not scientific.

The entire column has 31 pairs of nerves, 62 spinal nerve trunks; these, he says, are all occluded, closed or shut up. To adjust every vertebra for a definite form of disease betrays a lack of Chiropractic knowledge. Such adjustments are neither specific nor scientific. If the clinic is for the purpose of practice, why not adopt Dr. Arnold's method of loosening up every vertebrae, from the coccyx to the occiput, and then replacing each and every one separately? That would be Chiro-prac-tice.

This book has been written for the purpose of teaching Chiropractic as a science, making the art of adjusting specific, giving a special location and adjustment for each disease so far as we know.

Any person can learn to hit the high places, replace and displace vertebrae, relieve one disease and cause others. Let us, as Chiropractors, show the world that Chiropractic is a science; that hemiplegia is caused by a displaced vertebra, the sixth dorsal; that relief is given by replacing that vertebra and none other. Why not be specific in typhoid fever. Why not learn which vertebra is drawn out of alignment, the one which causes the symptoms collectively known as typhoid? No matter if the evidence of a certain disease is manifested in various parts of the body—remember that there are two ganglionic chains of the sympathetic nervous system reaching from the occiput to the coccyx; its plexus of nerves extending into the cranium, and that these vertebral cords are distributing agencies. Why not combine the science of Chiropractic with the art of adjusting?

I am pleased to state that many Chiropractors have outgrown, and have no further use for medicine, magnetic treatment, vibrators or osteopathy. They practice Chiropractic unmixed. Now, why not take another step forward by giving only specific adjustments?

---

Vaccination and inoculation are pathological; Chiropractic is physiological.

---

"The only place where the transmission of life force as a nerve impulse from the brain to any organ or part can be interfered with is where the nerves extend out through the spinal windows between bones where they may become impinged, thus interfering with their power of transmission.

"A nerve impulse."

An impulse is a sudden, spontaneous emotion, originated by Innate, the spirit, and directed upon the mind with a certain amount of determination or force and transmitted thru the nerves to their peripheral endings; these are motor impulses. A sensational impulse is a consciousness produced by an external object or from an internal condition of some portion of the body and transmitted thru the sensory nerves to the originator of functions. An impulse is not a "nerve impulse" originating in the nerves. **The apparent origin** is in the brain, not nerves. **The real origin** is back of and behind the brain.

"Life force."

Life is never used as an adjective, it is always a noun; the name of a quality, state, or existence.

The intervertebral foramina are in nowise "spinal windows"; openings in the walls of buildings, containing transparent material, as glass, for the admission of light and to be opened at will for the circulation of air.

Nerves cannot be "become impinged between bones." Impinge is an intransitive verb, followed by, on, upon or against, as, the second pair of spinal nerves are impinged on, or upon, by the displacement of the atlas.

Impingement is a noun; it refers to the act or condition of being impinged against, as, a nerve is impinged upon by the impingement of a displaced bone.

A pressure exerted between two bones on opposite sides is known as a pinch or squeeze.

## ADJUSTMENT.

If your marriage seems a failure,
And your wife is always cross,
And the pleasure of your life,
Don't even up with the loss,
It needs an adjustment.

If your religion is out of fix,
Does not bring the joy it should;
It's twice as easy to do wrong,
As to do your neighbor good,
You need an adjustment.

If your business is on the bum,
And nothing seems to pay,
If expenses more than double
Your income, day by day.
It needs an adjustment.

If you're not feeling as you should,
Your digestion out of whack,
With cold and clammy feelings
Crawling up and down your back,
You need an adjustment.

Then consult a Chiropractor,
If you would be free from chills:
If you'd have health and happiness,
Quit taking quinine pills.
Take adjustments.

DR. ELISABETH HELFRICH.

---

## PROUD FLESH.

A fungus growth in an ulcer, or a sluggish wound; one slow to heal because of inflammation. Commonly applied to any redundant growth of granulations.

There are physiological and pathological tissue granulation; the latter occasionally forms in ulcers or wounds. It is the result of two much functionating, an overgrowth. It can be removed by the surgeon with the knife or an application of caustic.

Chiropractors can trace the inflamed, sensitive nerve from the wound or sore to the spinal foramen from which it emerges, and relieve the impingement by adjusting.

## NEURALGIA.

"How can I clear my system of neuralgia?"

Neuralgia, neuritis, is inflammation of a nerve. The pain is sharp and paroxysmal, the nerve sensitive to the touch. It is generally known as a nerve disease. The kind of neuralgia is determined by the location, also by the supposed cause.

Christian Science and mind curers advise the possessor (victim?) to "Forget it, don't think of your ailments." It is easy for the one who has never had neuralgia to give this advice, but sharp, shooting, cutting, stabbing pains are remindful.

The above question was addressed to one who believes that disease is largely due to errors in diet; therefore prescribes fasting or a milk diet. It is thot by some that neuralgia is caused either by over-eating or by a depleted system. Therefore, a supply of pure blood is needed; rules are given for health-building. Their idea is that when the body is diseased it is below par, the blood is impoverished; it, therefore, needs certain nutritious food to build up and restore lost vitality. They aim to cleanse and purify the body by fasting; to clear the system by starving this something known as neuralgia.

A great many remedies are used to rid the system of this painful disease.

Strange, indeed, that some one had not long ago discovered that neuralgia was an inflammatory condition of nerves, caused by pressure, an impingement—tension.

This item was inspired by reading the above text and the next minute relieving a case of facial neuralgia by adjusting the atlas, releasing the impingement. This relief was accomplished in an instant, no mind cure, no change of diet, no purifying the blood, no adjusting of several places; but, there was time enough for a specific adjustment which relieved an impinged nerve by replacing a displaced bone.

---

"We have hundreds of sworn testimonials on file at our office, as to the efficacy of our work, from patients who have been cured of Bright's disease, appendicitis, rheumatism, insanity, all kinds of fevers, and others too numerous to mention."

"We" have but one sworn testimonial, and that has no affidavit attached to it, but "Yours very truly." There are over 100 kinds of fevers, a very few of which "we" have seen.

## SOME QUESTIONS ANSWERED.

Dr. D. D. Palmer:—

Your view-point, in some instances, is difficult to understand. You state that a subluxated bone is the cause of 95 per cent of all diseases, but omit to mention the cause of the remaining 5 per cent. I am not able to formulate, in a sentence, your ideas of the soul—what it is, where it resides, of what it consists, or the exact time it takes possession of the body.

Your statements regarding the cause and nature of disease seem confusing. No. 8 Adjuster, "Disease is the liberating or the retarding of impulses, which excite, sway or modify the orderly transformation of energy." While in No. 7, "In disease, mental impulses are not impeded, hindered, stopped, obstructed or 'cut off.'" In No. 7, "High temperature—fever—is the cause of many, perhaps all, disorders." While in No. 8, "Heat, cold and parasites constitute a very small factor in the causation of disease."

Is it not a mistake to say, that the cause of disease, in any case, is a subluxated bone? Strictly speaking, is not the cause of disease that which causes the subluxation?

What is your definition of the real, primary cause of disease? Improper food may irritate nerves. How is it that a subluxation interferes with the carrying power of a nerve? How does a stronger impulse, or one greater than normal, get past the impingement? Is not pathology only modified physiology? How is it possible to restore normal function, when, so far as we can determine, we do not change the position of the vertebrae, which is supposed to be the cause of disease?

I think you are wrong in stating that the expression **per cent** can only be applied to substances which are divisible. Why not call the normal amount of mental impulse 100 per cent?

You have established the fact, beyond all controversy, that you are the discoverer, originator and the best qualified teacher of Chiropractic.

Dr. P., you are a thinker and investigator. I wish all Chiropractors were thus.

I do not think it strange that the Adjuster class are not able to take in mentally and comprehensively all found in the Adjuster. The three pages on biology made five lessons for my class taught in person. Of the Adjuster class, but few did more than read it, and that without using an anatomy or dictionary. How about those teachers of Chiropractic who tell me that they have not looked into The Chiropractor or Adjuster for many months, altho they take both?

"A subluxated bone is the cause of 95 per cent of all diseases." A subluxated vertebra, a vertebral bone, is the cause of 95 per cent of all diseases. I think in every instance in which I have made mention of the above fact, I used the word vertebra.

"You omit to mention the cause of the remaining 5 per cent." The other five per cent is caused by displaced bones, other than those of the vertebral column, more especially those of the tarsus, metatarsus and phalanges, which, by their displacement, are the cause of bunions and corns. For further information see other pages of this book, The Chiropractor, when I was its editor, the Chiropractor Adjuster and manuscript cared for by B. J. which was written five years before he discovered that he was the "Daddy of Chiro."

The soul is the intelligent life—life guided by intelligence. It resides thruout the body wherever there is life. It consists of expressed functional energy. Function is the action of any part of a living animal or plant, and is the result of volition.

Spirit, soul, mind and body are separate and distinct entities. An entity is a being, whether in thot or in fact. Spirit. Universal, is the sum total of the conscious intelligent element or factor manifested in the universe. Individualized spirit is the segmented portion embodied in each individual. The body, as an entity, is the organized substance which we recognize as a human being. The mind is the intellectual part, that which is conscious, that which understands, reasons, wills and thinks. The soul is intelligent life—life guided by intelligence. It resides thruout the body wherever life is manifested. The "breath of life" gives it possession with the first breath. "For whosoever will save his life shall lose it: and whoever will lose his life, for my sake, shall find it. For what is a man profited if he shall gain the whole world and lose his own soul, or what shall a man give in exchange for his own soul?" Please read and reread this portion of scripture over and over again, changing back and forth, soul for life and life for soul, until you can comprehend that soul means life and life means soul; that these two terms, life and soul, are synonymous. Now one step more. Life is the sum total of functions. It is that which distinguishes a living, organized animal from a dead animal and inorganic bodies. Intelligent life maintains the performance of functions. All vital activities are guided by intelligent life. Animal existence is dependent upon the soul—intelligent life. Intelligent life—the soul—is the bond of union which holds spirit and body together as one. Mind is the product of. soul and body—of a living body. Thru the mind Innate (spirit) conducts the functions which control the body, and looks after its external welfare. If the reader will turn to all the places where soul is mentioned, I think that thon will get a satisfactory comprehension of what I understand the soul consists.

Disease is the result of liberating too much energy, or the retarding—lessening—of Innate stimulus. The former excites, the latter depresses vital force. The ordinary transformation of energy is health. The modifying, or swaying, either way, above or below normal, is disease—augmentation or lessening of impulses, and morbidity of tissue. It is impossible to separate modified functions and morbid tissue; either does not exist without the other. As soon as nerves are made taut by pressure, just so soon they become tense; tensity changes the temperature; tensity modifies functions; abnormal temperature modifies tissue.

In disease, mental impulses are not impeded, hindered, stopped or cut off—they **are modified.** An impingement does not obstruct; it is either an excitor or a depressor. All diseases are accompanied by temperature above or below normal. Heat, cold (the temperature surrounding us, not that of the body) and parasites are small factors in the production of disease. To state, exactly and specifically, the primal cause, the abnormal condition which was the very first to set the ball rolling, that eventually made the subluxation which caused the impingement, which produced the irritation, which modified the animal temperature, which augmented or decreased the force of the impulse that changed normal functions to abnormal, is but repeating the story of "The house that Jack built."

The real, primary cause of disease is tension; the cause of tension is pressure; the cause of pressure in 95 per cent of diseased conditions, is luxated vertebrae. The cause of the remaining 5 per cent is the luxation of other bones than those of the vertebral column.

Food never irritates nerves. In proportion as the ingesta induces irritation, it becomes a poison and ceases to be food. That which is food to one may be poison to another. When that which is food for one person impairs the functions of another. it becomes a poison to that other. "Improper food" is not a food, it is a poison. Honey is food when placed in my stomach. For many years I ate a pound of honey a day—365 pounds a year. That was my table allowance and did not include the sweet morsels nibbled while handling honey. One ounce of honey will almost kill some persons—it is a poison to them—not food.

"How is it that a subluxation interferes with the carrying power of a nerve?"

Luxated bones press against nerves. By their displacement and pressure they elongate the pathway of the nerve in a manner similar to that by which an impingement upon a wire of a musical instrument induces it to become taut by displacing it from a direct line. This pressure upon a nerve creates greater tension, increased vibration, and consequently an increased amount of heat. Heat alters tissue; altered tissue modifies the transmission of impulses; modified impulses cause functions to be performed abnormally.

"How does a greater impulse than normal get past the impingement?"

You could with the same propriety ask, How does the sound (vibration) get past the bridge of a musical instrument, or why does a wire vibrate in proportion to its tensity? Nerves and wires vibrate according to their tenseness, ragardless of the bone or bridge impingement, except that a displacement of the bone or bar causes derangement in the one and discordance in the other. Vibration is a periodic motion of the particles of an elastic body or medium in alternate opposite directions from the position of equilibrium, when that equilibrium has been disturbed. An illustration is noted when a stretched cord, wire or other body produces musical tones, when particles of air transmit sounds to the ear, or when a nerve transmits an impulse—a command to perform a function. The path of the vibrated particles may be in a straight line, in any arc or curve, or in the zig zag direction of some nerves.

Impulses are not composed of substance, they are not matter passing thru tubes. They are not impeded, hindered, obstructed or interfered with by the placing of a bone in their path-way; they are transmitted by vibration. The arch or bar which is set at right angles with the strings of a violin, guitar or other stringed instrument and which serves to make them taut by elongating them, does not prevent the passage of vibration; neither does the impingement of nerves by bone-pressure obstruct the course of impulses which are but vibrations. It simply modifies normal vibratory movements.

"Is not pathology only modified physiology?"

Physiological functions modified by augmentation or diminution and morbid tissue are pathological. The amount and quality of function is determined by tension, tension from pressure and pressure from displaced bones.

"How is it possible to restore normal function, when, so far as we can determine, we do not change the position of the vertebra where displacement is supposed to be the cause of disease?"

You have assumed wrong premises. The proposition being false, you have arrived at a wrong conclusion. It is not possible to restore normal function without returning the transmitting tissue to its natural tonicity.

"I think you are wrong in stating that the expression 'per cent' can only be applied to substances which are capable of being divided into one hundred parts. Why not call the normal amount of mental impulse 100 per cent?"

Because no one can per cent it; it is not per centable. Per cent means by the hundred. Eight per cent means eight of every one hundred parts. Mental impulse has no parts to base percentage upon.

The essential elements of percentage are the base, the rate and the percentage. The base is the number upon which the percentage is computed. The rate is the number of hundredths of the base to be taken. The percentage is the result obtained by taking a certain per cent of the base. The amount obtained is the base plus or minus the percentage. You cannot take a per cent of mental impulse. Mental impulse does not possess the essential elements of percentage, namely, a base upon which to figure the percentage. A percental rate can not be computed. No amount as a result to be added or taken from can be derived by any rule in percentage.

Percentile is a term used to indicate any series of values that indicate the distribution of a large group of measurements. If the result obtained be arranged in order of magnitude and divided into equal groups, then a value lying just above the first group is the first percentile; one just above the second, the second percentile, etc. This, like all percentage is based upon a hundred parts.

Per cent is used to proportion ingredients in chemistry; to rate interest on money; to levy duty on goods. If there were a hundred impulses, or if an impulse was composed of a hundred parts or segments, we might take away a per cent, make an allowance, add a per cent, proportion it with other ingredients and make a compound. It cannot be resolved or decomposed into elements. It has no parts; it is not even composed of ingredients. We cannot charge a rate of interest, levy a duty—why continue to talk nonsense?

## VARIATION OF THE VASCULAR SYSTEM.

In botany, vascular pertains to ducts or tubes for the circulation of sap. Yes, plant fluids circulate; their juices ascend and descend—make a circuit.

In biology, vascular, in its broadest sense, has reference to the arterial, venous and lymphatic channels for the conveyance of blood, chyle, lymph and serum.

Blood is an animal fluid that circulates thru the heart, arteries and veins. It enters every organ and nearly all tissues. It supplies nutritive material to all parts of the body and removes the waste products thru metabolism. The blood is white in the mollusca and the lower forms of animals; in the mammals, birds, reptiles and fishes, in those with a backbone, it is red.

Chyle is the milk-white nutritive fluid, extracted by intestinal absorption from food which has been subjected to the action of the digestive organs.

Lymph is the fluid contained in the lymphatic vessels and thoracic duct, the result of the filtration of the liquid portion of the blood thru the walls of the capillaries.

Serum is the yellow fluid, the most watery portion of animal fluids, exhaled by serous membranes.

The blood maintains itself within the heart, arteries and veins in an uninterrupted circulating movement. It passes from the heart into and thru the largest arterial trunks and onward to the furthermost branches, collected by a system of capillary vessels, and from thence to the venous channels.

The chyle, lymph and serum are conducted thru channels and transude thru membranes by muscular pressure.

In order to have normal diffusion, endosmosis and diapedesis, it is necessary that the ducts, capillaries and membranes should be normal in size and quality; their tissues are only modified by heat variation.

---

Before arresting a Chiropractor for practicing medicine or osteopathy, it is customary for the prosecuting attorney to hire two sneaks to call upon him for the purpose of getting such information as they desire.

C. R. Webster, of Indianapolis, Ind., 850 College Ave., has a printed blank, which every patient is required to sign. This can be brot into court to offset any misstatements made by the sneakers.

This statement will need to be modified to suit the laws of the state where you practice.

The idea and blank cost Dr. Webster $25, but I am sure that a self-addressed envelope will get you a blank for the asking.

## CHEMICAL.

"Morbid, fluid solids increase the abnormal chemical compound."

Who ever saw a "fluid solid" or a solid fluid? When a solid becomes a fluid, it is no longer a solid. Fluid and solid are antonyms, words of opposite meaning. "Morbid fluid solids," three words, no two of which are concomitant or companionable, cannot be associated together. A fluid or a solid cannot become morbid, diseased, cannot express symptoms. Symptoms are morbid conditions of living bodies. A "chemical compound" is a substance made up of two or more elements.

"The deposit of an abnormal chemical in the gland."

Chemical pertains to chemistry. A chemical substance is one used in a chemical laboratory to produce a chemical effect. It will be readily seen that "a deposit of an abnormal chemical in the gland" is incongruous. Chemicals are never abnormal, neither are they deposited in a gland. Chemicals are handled by chemists, pray tell me how you could deposit them in the glands. Certain chemicals, when united in the same quantities, always produce the same, identical compound. There is nothing abnormal about it.

"Abnormal chemical substance."

A chemical substance is only used in a chemical laboratory. It is always conformable with natural laws; could not be otherwise, could not be abnormal. It must correspond with nature, with the general rule.

"Physiologists have professed to analyze saliva."

A physiologist is one versed in the science of physiology; one who has a knowledge of the properties and functions of the organs and tissue of animals and vegetables. A chemist is one versed in chemistry, one whose business it is to chemically analyze substances; one who sells chemicals and drugs. A chemist is one whose object is to investigate the nature and properties of bodies, simple or complex, organic or inorganic. The one who analyzes organic or inorganic substances is a chemist. A physiologist looks after the functions of saliva as a part of the living body; a chemist may analyze it separate and apart from the body.

"A biliary substance containing normal chemicals."

A biliary substance, is one relating to bile. Bile does not contain any chemicals. A chemical substance is one which has been produced by analysis. Solutions, decoctions or infusions are not chemicals. An element, in chemistry, is a primary part of anything which cannot be resolved into simpler component parts. The "chemical elements of bile" are, as "found by chemical analysis, water, 82 to 90 per cent; salts of the biliary acids, from 6 to 11 per cent; fats and soaps, 2 per cent; cholesterine, 4 per cent; lecithin, 5 per cent; mucin, from 1 to 3 per cent; ash, 6 per cent."

"Bile is a highly reactive chemical substance."

Bile is not a reactive agent. It does not counteract, it has no opposite action, is not interactive. Reaction in chemistry is an interaction of two or more substances when brot in contact, as, for example, acid and alkaline reaction in forming new compounds.

"Bile is a chemical substance."

A chemical substance is one used by a chemist to produce a chemical effect; a reagent; a substance used as a test to detect the presence of other substances. Chemists analyze bile into its constituents; they do not produce it by the forces, operations, or processes of chemistry; or at least they never have been able to do so.

"The consensus of supposed authority gives the chemical composition of bile."

There is no author, except Dr. Carver, who gives a "chemical composition of bile." Bile is not a chemical compound; it has not been produced by chemistry.

"Chemicals entering into its (bile) composition."

There is not, neither can there be, any chemical added to bile while it is in the living body. If chemicals were introduced into the body, they would not enter into the composition of bile.

"Grape sugar as found by chemical analysis in the urine."

The above expression is correct in construction and in fact.

"The fourteen chemicals of which the body is composed."

"The human body is composed of about fourteen original elemental chemicals."

The body is composed of sixteen chemic elements, not "elemental chemicals." An element in chemistry is a body which cannot be resolved into simpler substances. A compound is reduced to its elements by chemistry—chemical analysis. These elements are called chemic elements, because compounds are reduced to elements by chemistry. Friend Carver does not know the difference between a chemical and an element; he is as far astray on them as he is on specific adjusting. A chemical is used to reduce a compound to its elements. The physiological compounds found in the body are organic and mineral. By chemistry—using chemicals—these compounds are subdivided into sixteen elements, not chemicals.

"Uncongenial, or antagonistic chemicals."

There is nothing abnormal, uncongenial or antagonistic about a chemical. A chemical substance is one used as a **reagent**, a substance employed to produce a chemic reaction, a chemical effect. A chemical cannot be said to be abnormal, uncongenial or antagonistic. Carver's chemic analysis exposes his ignorance of chemistry, as much so as does his analysis of Chiropractic.

"In all forms of venereal abnormality, the diet should be very abstemious, and so far as possible, of the fourteen chemicals of which the body is composed."

I find by referring to a medical dictionary, that chemical always pertains to chemistry. We have chemical medicines; those formed by the aid of chemistry. Analytic chemistry deals with the analysis of substances. Chemistry is a science which treats of the elements and atomic relations of matter and of the various compounds which they form. If a compound could not be reduced to its elements and elements united to form compounds, there would be no such a science as chemistry. Chemicals are used in the various processes of chemistry. Why feed those chemicals to one who is affected with venereal diseases?

By chemical analysis the tissue of the body has been reduced to elements, not chemicals. By chemical analysis water is reduced to elements, oxygen and hydrogen. The number of chemic elements (not chemicals) known to exist is ninety-four; this is determined by chemical analysis.

"Chemicals manufactured in the laboratory of the human body."

Chemicals are never manufactured by hand or machinery. Chemicals are substances used to produce a chemical effect. Chemical medicines are those formed by the aid of chemistry.

"Where the liver is producing an abnormal uric acid."

The function of the liver is to produce bile, not uric acid. It never produces normal or abnormal uric acid. There are two biliary conjugate acids of bile. These are obtained by chemical analysis. "The bile is evaporated to one-fourth its volume, triturated to a pasty mass with animal charcoal to remove the coloring matter and dried at 100 degrees C. (212 F.). The black mass is extracted with absolute alcohol, which passes colorless through the filter. After a portion of the alcohol has been driven off by evaporation, the addition of an excess of ether causes at first a resinoid precipitate of salts of the biliary acids, which later pass over into a crystalline mass of brilliant needles (crystallized bile). The alkaline salts of the biliary acids obtained in this way are readily soluble in water or alcohol, but are insoluble in ether." Thus the chemical process is continued until the free acid is obtained.

It will be seen that the liver does not produce uric acid. It is obtained by a laborious chemical process, and when procured cannot be otherwise than normal uric acid.

Galen was a noted physician. His remedies consisted of infusions and decoctions of herbs and drugs that were not chemically prepared. Chemical remedies are those arranged according to chemical principles by chemical processes.

"Abnormal chemical combination," is often repeated; five times in sixteen lines. Synthetic chemistry deals with the building up of compounds by chemicals. A chemical compound, or a chemical combination, could not be abnormal; when combined they comply with the law of chemistry.

"The abnormal chemical result" by nerve occlusion. Nerves, whether "occluded" or not, have nothing to do with chemistry.

A chemical result could not be otherwise, than normal.

"Nutrient chemicals."

Chemical—pertaining to chemistry. Chemistry is a science. A chemical is a substance used for producing a chemical effect —not for nutrition. The words, nutrient and chemical, are not concomitant, they are diverse in their meaning; they are not relative; they are unconnectable. Nutrition embraces digestion, absorption, circulation and assimilation. A chemical is a substance which is capable of producing, with another, a reaction.

"Abnormal uric acid."

Uric acid is found, by chemical analysis, in the urine of man and animals; it is a product of nuclein metabolism. It is one of the essential constituents of all living cells.

Normal urine when kept in a cool place exhibits a formation of newly developed acid—acid urinary formation.

Uric acid is not produced by the kidneys. When the kidneys are removed uric acid continues to be formed and accumulated in the organs, more especially in the liver and spleen.

Chemical elements, including uric acid, cannot be abnormal —they must conform to the general rule of chemistry.

"Chemicals of every part of the body."

There are no chemicals in the body; you will find them in the drug store and chemical laboratory. A chemical is used to produce a chemical effect. Chemical medicines are those formed by the aid of chemistry.

"The substances taken from the chyle should comprise the original elemental chemicals of which the organism is composed."

Who ever heard of an animal or vegetable—of an organized body or a living economy, whose "original elements were chemicals"?

"In dead tissue, germs are evolved as a result of chemical changes."

Germs are living organisms which act as scavengers. Decomposing tissue calls for filth cleaners; a wise provision in nature, an act of equilibration. Germs are not evolved thru a process of evolution, no more than scavenger buzzards are evolved thru a decaying carcass. Decomposition is not a change made by chemicals—a chemical change—it is natural disintegration of a body back to its original elements.

"Powerful chemicals such as alcohol and turpentine."

The above commodities have not been produced by chemical analysis—the forces and operations of chemistry. They are compounds that have not been reduced to their component elements; they are not chemicals.

"Assimilation is the process by which chemical elements are changed or converted into living cells."

Assimilation is synthetic or constructive metabolism, anabolism—the transforming of food into a nutrient condition, so that it may form an integral part of the economy. The change is purely metabolic and not chemical.

"Improperly combined foods, result in a fermentation or in such chemical changes and combinations as to produce a poison or irritant."

Fermentation from decomposing, undigested food, is not because of its being improperly combined. Take a look at those who surround the festive board. Where do you find indigestion, fermentation? Not among those who throw into their stomachs anything and everything their eyes and nose gives assent to; but rather in the stomachs of those who are careful in regard to the amount and combination.

There is a vast difference between "Chiropractic Analysis" and that of chemical analysis.

Carver's Analysis is medical, chemic analysis; it is far from being Chiropractic physiology.

Chemical analysis is the separation of a compound substance by a chemical process into its constituents, with a view to ascertaining what elements it contains or how much of each element is present—qualitative and quantitative analysis.

There is no portion of a living body which can be reduced or returned to its chemic elements while it is alive.

The phenomena whereby organic beings transform food-stuff into complex tissue elements and convert complex substances into simple ones in the production of energy—metabolism—is quite a different process from that of chemistry; the former deals with animate, the latter with inanimate, substances.

The methods employed by chemists for analysis of tissue destroy the composition and vitality of the living body; therefore, the products obtained by chemistry are peculiar to dead rather than living material.

---

The Chiropractor defines Chiropractic: "Subluxations are corrected for the purpose of permitting the re-creation of all normal cyclic currents thru nerves that were formerly not permitted to be transmitted, thru impingement, but have now assumed their normal size and capacity for conduction as they emanate thru intervertebral foramina—the expressions of which were formerly excessive or partially lacking—named disease.

"Disease is lack of normal functions."

Energy is not a fluid, it does not flow as a current thru the nerves. It is physiologically, the potential, latent power; the action, vigor or force expended in the performance of functions.

Vital force is not cyclic, it does not move in circles. Vital energy is expended in the performance of functions at the terminal endings of nerves; it does not return in a circle or otherwise. Vital force or energy can not be transmitted in a circle.

"Permitting the re-creation."

Neither energy nor anything else can be re-created. To create, is to bring into existence something which did not previously exist. It is impossible to re-create. I created the science of Chiropractic. No one can re-create it.

"Currents that were formerly not permitted to be transmitted."

If there ever was a time when impulses were not permitted to be transmitted through the nerves of any individual, that individual would then have ceased to live.

"Transmitted thru impingement."

As I understand the principles of Chiropractic, an impingement modifies the transmission of impulses; does not transmit them.

"The expressions of which were formerly excessive or partially lacking—named disease," makes a strong contrast, a direct contradiction to the succeeding statement that "Disease is lack of normal functions."

Disease is abnormal functionating—functions performed in either an excessive or insufficient manner—not a lack of normal functions. Functions would not be normal if they were lacking. It would be better to have said, disease is a lack of functionating, although most diseases are the result ot too much functionating.

FIG. 666.—DIAGRAM SHOWING RELATIONS OF MENINGES TO SPINAL NERVE-ROOTS.

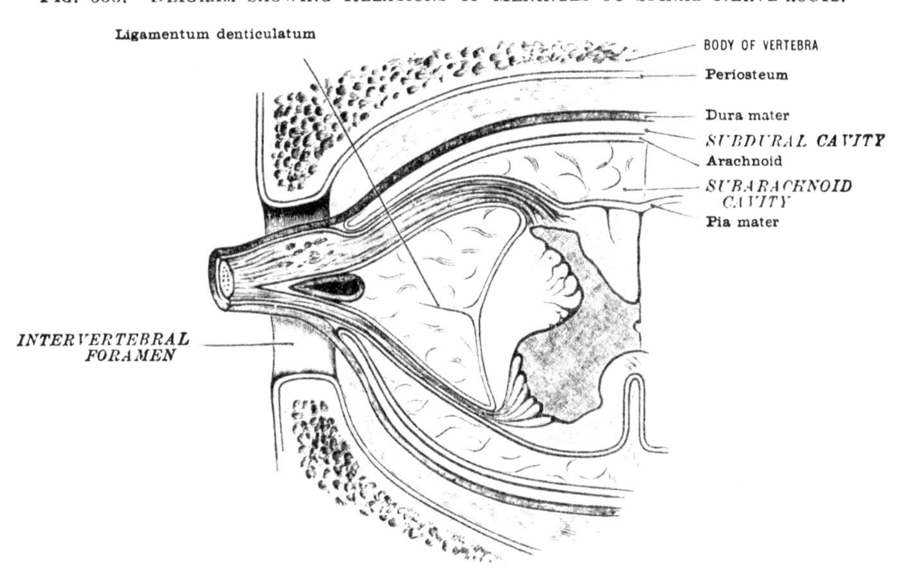


A cut from Morris Anatomy, page 895, displaying the relative size of a Spinal Nerve and the Intervertebral Foramen thru which it passes

## MUSCLE VARIATION.

We have noticed, elsewhere, the variation of the bones and nerves of the body. We find in man a deviation in the number, size and quality of the muscles. Marked deviations are noticed in their origin and insertions, the parts of the skeleton or other portion to which they are attached. They differ in their extent of fusion with each other. Some muscles, usually found, are absent in some subjects; in others they are so rarely found that, when present, they are looked upon as anomalies. Sometimes two or more ordinary muscles may be fused into one, or a common muscle may be divided lengthwise into two or more. Where muscles vary, there is a corresponding variation in the nerves which supply them.

For example, the iliococcygeus muscle is especially liable to variations. It is strongly developed in but few, is usually thin, the muscular bundles being separated by membranous intervals: it may be replaced by fibrous tissue and may even be absent.

---

Chiropractors adjust causes instead o1 treating effects.

---

A machine shop is a building where machines are made, where metal is shaped by cutting, turning and filing. Man is a living being because of metabolism, dialysis and diffusion, a group of processes whereby organs transform food-stuff into tissue elements. There is no similarity between the machine of the machine-shop and the organs of the body.

The power which runs a machine is inanimate, that of the body is intelligent. There is a vast difference between Innate, brain, nerves, organs and vital force, and the source and conduit of the power of inanimate machines. The power which runs a machine is one of expansion and contraction, that of the human body is vital energy. Expansion and contraction are laws of matter; they create the power for machines. The power that operates the human body is intelligent life, dependent upon individualized spirit. So, we know from whence vital force and the power which runs the machine are derived.

"The Chiropractor by examining the spinal column and noting the condition of the nerves and the position of the vertebrae, can accurately locate the cause of ailments and explain conditions and symptoms without asking a single question."

The above is from the pen of a D. C. who says of himself, "He stands at the head of the science of Chiropractic."

## LUXATIONS.

"The aim thruout this book has been to explain subluxations and their adjustments around six words, viz., superior, inferior, left, right, anterior and posterior. With these any combination can be elaborated upon."

I founded the science and art of Chiropractic on the plan of economy, not elaboration. The act of replacing vertebrae, is that of racking into normal position those which have been displaced by traumatism or poison.

Subluxated verterbrae are forced out of alignment by accidents and poisons. Please take your spinal column in hand. Remember: Chiropractic displacements are fixed, exaggerated lateral movements. **Vertical** displacements, when sufficient to make a complete luxation, are those known and recognized as such by the medical profession. A Chiropractic luxation is not accompanied by fracture, while those known and recognized as luxations by the medical profession usually are.

The seven cervicals and the first eleven dorsals have a lateral and vertical action of the articular processes and an axial center at the anterior of their bodies; while the last dorsal and the five lumbars have a vertical action and an axial center on the lateral line of the articular processes. The first mentioned perform an arc of a circle on a line of the articular processes; while the latter do so on the anterior of their bodies. I presume that you have your spine in hand, if so, displace a middle dorsal laterally to the left. Stand on the left side and throw toward the right shoulder. It will be found easier to get the precise movement needed by throwing the vertebra from, instead of drawing it toward yourself. A lateral displacement of the bodies of vertebrae not only impinges upon, presses against, nerves but causes a tension, a stretched, or strained condition. Study the position and the conditions imposed.

If the adjuster will try throwing a vertebra toward the shoulder indicated, with a quick energetic move, thon will find it efficacious and almost painless. Especially will it be considered so by those who have tried the "rebound" or "recoil" movement. This simple formula will save the need of a compass and its elaborated combinations as shown in the book which lies before me.

"Chiropractic is a thing of beauty, for it demonstrates the strength of a simple principle."

A thing is whatever exists, or is conceived to exist, as a separate entity; an inanimate object in distinction from a living being. Any lifeless object is a thing. Chiropractic is not a thing, is not an entity, an object, nor is it made from anything material. Chiropractic is a science, consisting of knowledge and skill concerning the art of adjusting. Beauty consists of a harmonious blending of color and figure causing delight to the beholder. Chiropractic has no form or color; is not a thing of beauty. The science of Chiropractic does not demonstrate the quality of being strong. Chiropractic is founded upon the principle that functions receive their vital force thru the nervous system. From this fundamental principle other principles are formed which assist in creating the science and are of Chiropractic.

"Fig. 2, shows the nerve immerging from the spinal canal in a healthy condition to be distributed to the different organs and tissues of the body."

Nerves emerge from the spinal canal, never immerge.

"Sooner or later the bone which is displaced will so pinch upon the nerves and so lessen the function of the organs and tissues fed by that impinged nerve that we have the so-called condition of disease."

A bone does not pinch **upon** a nerve. The condition of pressure upon a nerve is known as an impingement. Pinch and impinge are not synonymous. Tissues are not fed by nerves. To feed is to satisfy physical or mental hunger. We feed animals, not tissue. Nerves do no feeding; they do not furnish nutriment. Nourishment is furnished thru and by the fluids. Vital action thru osmosis and diffusion passes liquids saturated with nutrient substances, through the porous septa. Aqueous solutions furnish material for growth and the replacing of the wear and tear of the body.

Most diseases are the result of too much instead of too little functionating.

"The science of removing the pressure upon the spinal nerves has claims upon nearly all chronic and nervous ailments."

The science of Chiropractic has no claims upon or against any ailment, chronic, acute or nervous. Diseases do not owe it anything, therefore, it has no claims against them.

"By this movement—the vital feature of the Chiropractic system—not only are the tissues brought into proper adjustment but the dormant power of Nature in the cells is started into activity."

Physiologists know of vital functions, vital actions and vital energy, but not of "vital features." Tissues are brought into proper alignment, suitable apposition, not proper adjustment. I was not aware that it was natural for tissue cells to be dormant, non-active; that they needed awakening.

"In which event (gummata in the skull cavity or vertebral

column and calculus at points indicated) paralysis will be substantially conquered."

Think of a Chiropractor substantially conquering disease! That expression sounds Allopathic.

One of the principles of Chiropractic is that when impingements are removed vital energy performs functions normally and will, as far as possible, carry off any surplus deposit of water, gummata or calculus.

Why not, as Chiropractors, give Innate an opportunity to functionate normally instead of trying to conquer disease?

---

A teacher in a Chiropractic college says, "Dr. Gray in his great work on Anatomy has told us that these great nerve trunks carry two million filaments each." I am unable to find any such statement in Gray's anatomy.

Gray states, "Nerves are composed of numbers of nerve-fibres bound into bundles. The nerves are round or flattened cords, formed of a number of nerve-fibres. The nervous system is composed of a multitude of units called neurones. They vary greatly in shape and size. Some are so small that they become visible only under a microscope of high power; some come almost within the range of vision."

"Our combined system has proven irresistible."

As tho the disease was intelligently resisting, opposing, acting in opposition, to his system. It is difficult to root out all of superstition.

"Here is where pressure of bone cuts off life force."

Bone impingement on nerves irritate or depress their action. They do not cut off vital action.

"Luxated bones pinch nerves. Pinched nerves cause disease."

Nerves may be impinged upon, pressed against, but not pinched.

"Chiropractic is a system of manual therapeutics by which displaced tissues are brought into normal position, the vitality of the involved cells being simultaneously aroused to activity, enabling Nature to effect a cure."

Chiropractic is not a system of therapeutics; it does not use remedies. The "involved cells" may be inflamed and too active. To arouse would be to excite to action from a state of rest.

"The development of disease stopped."

Development in physiology is growth or increase; in pathology it is the same. We can say that a disease advances, increases, develops; but there is no process by which diseases are developed, except it be by vaccination and the serums.

"Health is regained when these non-active nerves are compelled to again perform their work and carry new life to the affected parts."

If nerves were non-active, the possessor would not be alive. The part of the body having non-active nerves would be dead. Non-active nerves would be devoid of life. Nerves are not driven by either moral or physical force to perform functions. Man has only one life—a life guided by intelligence. Nerves carry only impulses. The prevailing superstition is that regarding the blood; that is, that of the blood, "all life is in the blood; that there is bad blood, impure blood, poisoned blood, diseased blood."

"Systemic diseases" are those which belong to the whole body or system. Chiropractors do not know of systemic diseases, for they specifically locate the cause of all diseases; they do not look upon a disease as being constitutional.

Pressure on nerves usually excites, irritates, thereby creating various parts of the body. The Chiropractor locates this pressure, removes it, a full supply of nerve force reaches the starved and so-called diseased part of the body."

Pressure on nerves usually excites, irritates, thereby creating too much, an excess of nerve force at the peripheral nerve endings. Nerve-force is not supplied or passed thru or over the nerves; it is manifested in functional activity. Impulses which direct nerve-energy, are passed over the transmitting nerves. Pressure on nerves, or against nerves, modifies the force or momentum of impulses which cause action. The removal of pressure allows Innate to forward motor impulses (all impulses are motor) with normal force. Diseased portions of the body are not starved—where did you get that idea?

"The Howard system of physiological adjustment attacks the cause of disease, not the symptoms."

We do not adjust the physiological—the normal; it is the pathological that needs adjusting. I would prefer relieving the cause instead of attacking it; adjusting is a friendly act.

"The Chiropractor recognizes in each symptom a disease."

A physical **sign** is an evidence of disease. A **symptom** denotes the change in the patient during disease, points out its nature and location. Each symptom is not a disease.

---

Chiropractic is a science; adjusting is an art.

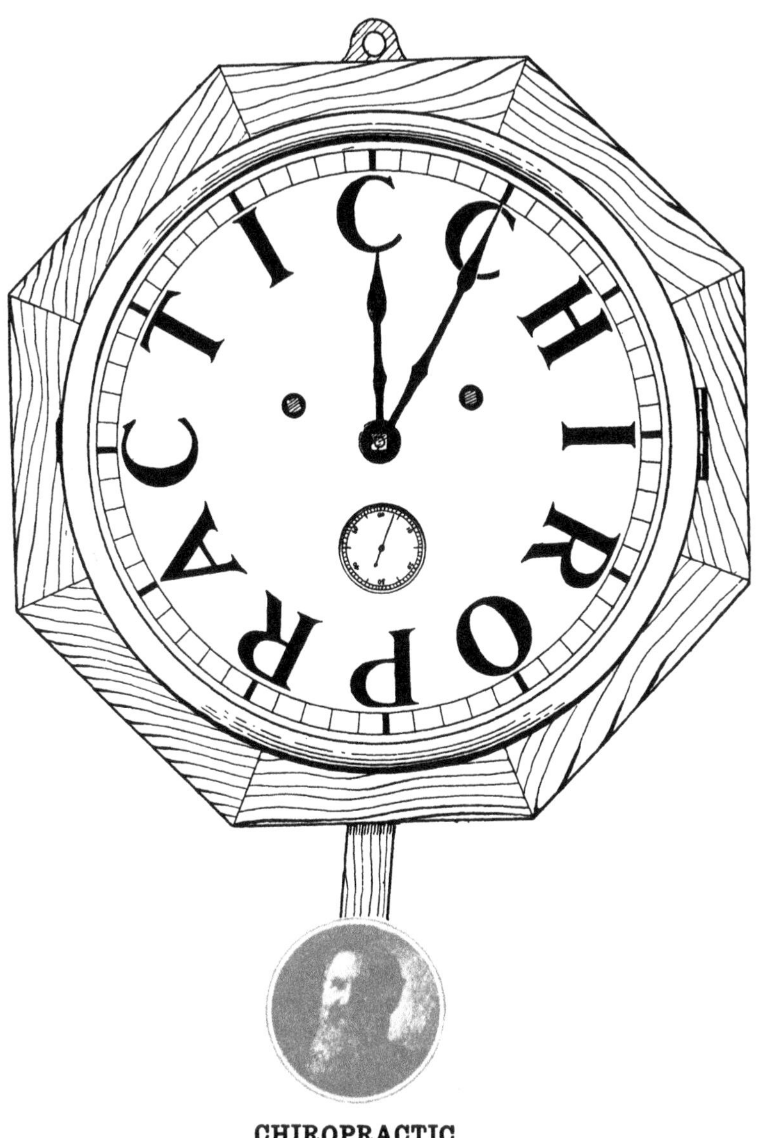


**CHIROPRACTIC**

**ON**

**TIME**

## REVOLUTION.

Chiropractic is destined to revolutionize the Old School methods of practice which have been in vogue 2,000 years. There have been, and are today many methods of treating diseases, each and every one built on the old-time notion that disease is an evil, an entity which must be driven out, made to vacate, and the system cleansed of impurities before health can be restored; that cancers, body and skin diseases are efforts on the part of Nature to rout the enemy and that inflammation and fever are purifiers.

In September, 1895, the first Chiropractic adjustment was given; for the first time, the spinous process was used as a lever, altho the way was being prepared, the principles of Chiropractic were being unfolded, during the previous nine years. Rev. Weed was my confidential friend in those days; to him I gave all new developments.

Two years after the first adjustment was given I came near being killed at Clinton Junction, Ill. I then determined to teach the science and art to some one as fast as it was unfolded. Leroy Baker, of Fulton, Ill., was my first student. He was not a graduate as represented by the "enveloper." If I had been snatched from earth-life it might have been a long time before the same combination of circumstances, combined with the same make-up of an individual, would evolve a science such as I saw in Chiropractic, therefore, I taught it as learned.

---

Spondylotherapy, by Abrams, says:—"Concussion of any of the spinous processes will **elevate the temperature**, but the best results are achieved when the spinous process of the 7th cervical vertebra is concussed."

Concussion is a shock, the shaking or jarring of a part, or the morbid condition resulting from a shock, jar or shake. The medical profession seem satisfied when they can produce disease, elevate the temperature, produce abnormal functions, morbid conditions. An agitation of the spinous processes excites the adjacent nerves, elevates their temperature.

Again Abrams states:—"In fever the author has never succeeded in **reducing the temperature** by aid of concussion of any of the spinous processes, although his efforts have been many."

Why should he expect to reduce a fever by the very means which would excite nervous action—fever?

## SUGGESTION.

Five years ago Dr. Carver was an earnest advocate of Suggestion as a therapeutic aid to Chiropractic. He was at one time a lawyer; therefore, ought to know how to present Suggestion's case. I did, then, and do now, consider Suggestion and Dr. Carver worthy of consideration. I therefore repeat my answer with some variation, as Dr. Carver has modified his mode of treating abnormality.

Dr. Carver then said: "I feel sure that where a symptom is a result of a luxated vertebra nothing but an adjustment of that displaced vertebra will cure.

"However, there are a large number of ills which affect the human body that have nothing whatever to do, per se, with the body structure and exist where there are no luxations. I refer to derangements that are the result of pernicious suggestion, such as tobacco habit, etc., and all forms of insanity."

"Suggestive Therapeutics is the natural father of Chiropractic and is all the sufficient extraneous aid it needs. It is a necessity to his practice. The operator will succeed in curing only those who accept the treatment."

"I do not know whether you give it the place in Chiropractic that it should occupy. It can be but a short time till you include a scientific suggestion as a necessary companion to the adjustments. I know that you will do this, because as the discoverer of Chiropractic you have demonstrated your intelligence and freedom from dogmas. You will see that Suggestion and adjustments are the all powerful and inseparable twins."

Willard Carver, D. C.; Dear Sir and Friend: As we investigate the field of Chiropractic, I am more and more pleasantly surprised to find that all diseased conditions are the result of bone luxations and nothing but their adjustment will give relief.

You will be interested in the Dr. Story case as it demonstrates what can be done, in a moment, by replacing a vertebra. During the doctor's mental aberrations he was treated by a very prominent healer who used Suggestive Therapeutics. He gave the doctor much more of suggestion in one of his treatments than I could have done in the short space of time used in adjusting. Suggestion, however, did not replace the displaced 4th cervical vertebra, did not relieve the pressure on sensory nerves.

You say, "There are a large number of ills which affect the human body that have nothing whatever to do with the body structure and exist where there are no luxations."

I have been a practitioner of Chiropractic, looking for osseous displacements, now 15 years. During that time I have learned that insanity, tobacco and liquor habits depend upon displaced vertebrae for their continuance. Carver's Analysis, of which you are the author, advises adjusting for insanity, hydrophobia, alcohol, gonorrhea and narcotics—the last includes nicotinism, the tobacco habit. Under the head-line of "Alcoholism and Narcotism," you state, "If the **adjustment suggested** and the rules are faithfully carried out, there will be **a complete restoration of the physical and mental condition, with the elimination of the habit.**" In the 468 pages of your book, you do not make mention of, nor suggest the use of Suggestive Therapeutics for any ailment. You now suggest diet as "a necessary companion" to the replacing of osseous tissue. In time, you will suggest replacing this with Chiropractic adjustments. The twelve pages you now devote to "human ills," had nothing whatever to do with the bony structure five years ago, and existed where there were no luxations." You, now, have learned that the bony structure has something to do with mental conditions; therefore, advise adjusting for these "physical and mental" conditions. You, now, realize that Chiropractic is able to cope with insanity, pernicious habits and other mental conditions. What has become of "Suggestive Therapeutics, the natural father of Chiropractic, the all sufficient extraneous aid it needs." Do you now think it necessary to the practice of Chiropractic? If so, why have you not so stated in your book which gives "**the principles entering into all,** with the discussion of a sufficient number to make the principles plain"? Do you yet think the Chiropractor will succeed only in those cases where suggestion is accepted by the patient? It has now been five years since you wrote, "It can be but a short time till you include a scientific suggestion as a necessary companion to the adjustments." You have evidently forgotten—I have not—about Suggestive Therapeutics being the natural father and necessary companion of Chiropractic. How about Suggestion and Adjustment being the all-powerful and inseparable twins? Have you lost one of the twins, or has suggestion killed the one who was all thot and no work? Do you miss the sufficient extraneous aid it was expected to give to the science of Chiropractic? Do you now think that suggestion is a necessary companion for Chiropractic? On a number of occasions, I have adjusted for pernicious habits of smoking and chewing tobacco and that of drink, often giving relief by one adjustment. At first, these were relieved while adjusting for other diseased conditions without a thot or expectation on the part of the patient or the adjuster that they had any controlling influence upon pernicious habits. These accidental reliefs preclude the possibility of suggestion having been used.

The constant use of narcotics causes nerves and muscles to contract and draw vertebrae out of alignment. Luxated lesions, produced by traumatism or irritation of the nervous system, excite the functions of the part wherein they are situated. This continued pressure perpetuates depraved appetites which Friend Carver calls pernicious. An inherent, habitual desire or a propensity for some personal gratification, either of the body or of the mind, may be either physiological or pathological.

By adjusting for other diseases I accidentally learned what luxations produce the constant desire for strong drink and narcotics. By scientific knowledge and practice I am able to replace these offending displacements.

Friend Carver: Chiropractic has opened up new lines of thot that Suggestive Therapeutics has never dreamed of. I am pleased to see your change along these lines, as manifested in your book, but there is much yet for you to learn.

We no longer fear zymotic epidemics. Smallpox, measles, mumps, diphtheria, croup, pneumonia, typhoid and other diseases, since, in the acute stage, they are relieved, made well, by one adjustment. In acute cases, by one adjustment, I right the wrong, replace the displaced vertebra, relieve the pressure, remove the impingement upon the nerves, allowing them to perform functions in a normal manner, and all is well; Suggestion has no more to do with fixing organized beings than it has with the correction of inorganic bodies.

Suggestion is a remedy, it is therapeutical. Chiropractors do not use remedies. Chiropractors change pathological, functional conditions into those that are physiological. Instead of suggesting to the mosquito that he should not, and shall not, bore into my cuticle with his proboscis and suck my blood, I gave him an instantaneous adjustment.

Why and how luxations of vertebrae are caused by poisons, vaccine virus, tobacco, alcohol and ptomaine poison, is taught by actual clinic work. Suggestion does not enter into this explanation. It is no more thot of by the Chiropractor than it is by the mechanic while doing his allotted work. Practitioners need to learn how, why, where and when to adjust.

Mrs. Benson took adjustments two weeks for a terrible headache. I expected to relieve her by adjusting the same vertebra as I had in others, but I failed, not because I did not use suggestion, but because her headache was due to an impingement of the 12th dorsal vertebra upon nerves which lead from that locality to the head, a fact I was not aware of previously. The failure was from lack of knowledge, not from lack of faith or suggestion. When I discovered what nerves were impinged upon, it was easy to give them ease. Such cases exclude suggestion as a factor. Of course, I cannot really say, but possibly, her husband, tiring of her long delay, had sent a suggestion that she "had better be in a hurry." An emphatic adjustment on the right vertebra, in the right direction, did the work.

I do not say that there is not as much in a suggestion as in other remedies, but I do not knowingly take time to fool with any remedy. The use of a restorative would show students that I did not know the cause of disease or where or how to adjust for it. Were I to know of a dislocation of any one of the 300 articulations which cause disease, and did not replace the dislocation, but instead used remedies for the ailment, it would show to investigators that I was not doing my duty and was criminally negligent. The physician who writes a prescription to be used externally and internally for certain symptoms, does so, because he does not know the cause of the disease for which he prescribes. I would very much dislike to own up to such ignorance which would be made manifest by my using a remedy, whether the remedy be a drug or suggestion.

Chiropractic orthopedy is clearing up one field that has been, and is yet, full of superstition. I refer to nevus or mother marks. These have their causes, but suggestion and superstition, twin sisters, will never assist us in discovering them. I have been able, in many instances, to penetrate the hidden mystery and discover causes even before birth. These are being explained to our students so that they, also, may learn to adjust for club-foot and other prenatal deformities.

So far as my experienec goes, all insanity is caused by displaced vertebrae. If so, is not the replacing of these displaced vertebrae the proper thing to do? These subluxated vertebrae may arise from traumatism or toxines.

I am ready to admit that suggestion is a valuable remedy; it is good as far as it goes. If you know what is wrong, why not adjust it? Chiropractors are not using remedies, they are adjusting causes; they are not treating effects.

In your letter to A. P. Davis, of March 2, 1910, you state, "You are a therapeutist, I am a scientist." Since when? When did you give up Suggestive Therapeutics and become a Chiropractic scientist? You logically state to Dr. Davis, "You could not expect the two (Therapeutics and science) to agree, since there is not a single basic truth in the whole of therapy and I will give you a thousand dollars to disprove that statement."

It is surprising to learn that every friend of Chiropractic thinks his method of treating diseases is just the one which ought to be used in connection with adjusting of causes. All practitioners desire to learn this science so that they may add it to their mode of healing. Each one finds that the more thon knows of Chiropractic, the less need thon has of thon's former mode of treating. The person who comprehends the philosophy and principles of the science and art of Chiropractic has no need of remedies. Herein you have my opinion of the one who uses a vibrator, electricity, massage or other remedies. What is my opinion? It is this, thon does know enough of Chiropractic to get along without remedies, or he is using it as graft.

You want to know what I mean by "thon." I have been using that word sparingly for many years. If the reader will turn to page 2147 of Webster's new International Dictionary, 1910, thon will find: "Thon, pronoun, singular. Thon, contraction of that one. A proposed genderless pronoun of the third person." In the English language we have heretofore stood in need of a third person singular pronoun.

You say, "Suggestive Therapeutics is the natural father of Chiropractic." I was present when Chiro was born. I blew the breath of life into his lungs. I am proud to say that I named him Chiropractic. He is often called Chiro in sportive familiarity or in derision. I have witnessed his frantic efforts for an existence. He has been captured, his raiment changed, his organism shorn of the cranial and sympathetic nerves. His enemies have desired his death, yet, he is developing into an intellectual giant, one destined to enlighten the whole world. During the nine years of gestation, he was formed and developed into a perfect child; his organism was perfect; but grafters and vampires have preyed upon him as parasites. I trust this book will be the means of returning to him his proper clothing and adjusting his organism so that he may look like the child I created.

His mother was known as a Magnetic Healer; Chiropractic was an outgrowth of that system. His development has been of such a sportive character that there is now but little resemblance between him and his mother. However, he has never seen fit to adopt Suggestive Therapeutics as a foster parent or allow himself to be passed as her twin, or even as a traveling companion.

You think "Suggestive Therapeutics is Chiropractic's all sufficient extraneous aid." Thus it is, each person who has a pet method, desires that we adopt it as an assistant to Chiropractic. This science, now 15 years of age. When a student takes and comprehends a course of instruction under its founder, he will not need any vibrators, orthopedic appliances or osteopathy as assistants, neither will there be any need of depriving the system of cranial or sympathetic nerves, in order to get direct mental impulse.

"The operator will succeed in curing only those who will accept the treatment." Chiropractors are not operators, neither do they give treatments. Webster says of operate, "Medical.—To take appropriate effects on the human system." Dunglison says of operation: "The application of instruments to the human body with the view of removing diseases." For the difference between treatment and adjustment, see article on Chiropractic versus Therapeutics. Come here, William, get in the front seat of the band wagon. I do not like to see you hanging on the end-gate.

Chiropractors adjust infants who are too young to comprehend suggestion, or perhaps old enough to get their backs up when we adjust their backbones. They adjust insane persons who have no comprehension of what we desire to do. They replace the luxated vertebra, take off the pressure just the same, free the nerves from impingement and allow them to perform their functions unmolested in a natural manner.

"I do not know whether you give Suggestive Therapeutics the place in Chiropractic that it should and must occupy." Such suggestions do not suggest to a Chiropractor. They are like the tinkling of an empty tin can. He does not give it, or any other therapeutical method, a place in Chiropractic. To do so would be only a hindrance to the wheels of progress. Advocates of other methods are just as much in earnest and equally as anxious that I should use their favorite mode of treatment. I have looked the Chiropractic adjustment rooms over and cannot find room for any other method; nothing more is needed. Any remedy would be badly in the way, stumbling blocks to our students' advancement. No, thank you, I do not mix, I give Chiropractic straight. If it were mixed with all the methods offered, it would soon lose its identity.

Students who think that suggestion is or ought to be a part

of Chiropractic, have as much trouble to rid themselves of the treating incubus as those who believe in drugs or any other form of healing. As they learn Chiropractic, they unlearn the treating of symptoms, as do other students who believe in Homeopathy or other methods which use remedies for effect. Whenever a practitioner, whether he be a Chiropractor or not, uses a remedy instead of hand adjusting, he does not know the cause of disease, or, knowing it, is not able to adjust the displacements. Do not forget that Chiropractors do not treat diseases; they adjust causes, whether acquired, spontaneous, or the result of accident.

Many have written me, others have personally insisted, that their "scientific system" is a necessary companion to adjusting, and ought to be taken in as a part of Chiropractic. Now, Friend Carver, you need not spend any time trying to get up any matrimonial alliance either for Chiropractic or Adjusting. They are only 15 years of age, and, while I am their guardian, they shall not take any foreigner as a partner, for they are wholly different in their natures. Such a copartnership would be incongruous, inharmonious, incompatible; would result in retrogression instead of advancement. I have no idea of allowing Chiropractic or Adjusting to give up their individuality. Chiropractic has no room or use for Miss Treatment, neither has Adjustment any need of being hampered by Miss Remedy. These girls of fashion change their clothing to suit every suitor; they would only annoy my kids. Chiropractic and Adjustment are inseparable; they desire no other company.

Yes, sir: "The discoverer and developer of Chiropractic has demonstrated that he has freedom and intelligence" enough to find his way out of therapeutics and has no longing for any of its remedies. My time is being used in discovering the cause of disease and developing a method for relief. Causes of disease and then adjusting therefor has been neglected far too long in the vain hope of discovering an antidote, a remedy, for the disorders of mankind. Please excuse me, I am in a hurry; I do not want to be delayed by any method that treats disease either mentally or physically. I am searching for causes and their adjustment. I have no time to waste on parasites.

You seem to think that Chiropractic and Suggestion are "inseparable twins." Such a coalition would be incongruous. It would be the uniting of two opposites; two adverse methods which are antagonistic; two contradictories; two propositions which are diametrically opposed to each other in thot and action. They would be antithical in contrast. Suggestion would be the counter-irritant to adjusting. Either would be repugnant to the other. The uniting of two opposites could not help but be discordant. Their characters are heterogeneous. Suggestion was born of superstition in the antique past. She is antiquated, uncouth, would be an unsuitable partner for the American juvenile, who was born in a modern, philosophical age.

Suggestion exists only as an imaginary, mythical delusion. Chiropractic is a veritable fact, yet in its teens. The idea of trying to unite, in monogamous wedlock, this American youth with an antiquated myth, or the notion that suggestion is a twin of this modern prodigy, is preposterous. Suggestion—where everything may be anything; where nature has no laws and imagination no limits.

A few months after receiving the above letter I received the following. In Carver's last letter, he suggested that I use suggestion. He now affirms that I do use it and desires an acknowledgement to that effect. I give his plea entire. Our readers can pass on his demurrer. In order to economize space and avoid repetition I will give his letter in paragraphs and answer accordingly.

"Yours received and read carefully. Permit me to answer, notwithstanding the tone of your letter clearly indicates that you leave nothing for me to say."

"The crime of being a young man, I will not attempt to palliate or deny. But I will call your attention to the fact, that about the time you brought into existence 'Chiropractic,' the science of suggestion was formulated, and wonderful development followed, with which you could not be expected to be familiar, because in those years, you were deeply absorbed in developing one of the most far reaching sciences of the world."

Friend Carver: I did not say, nor intimate, that it was a crime to be a young man. I am just as busy today developing the science of which I am the founder, as I was in years gone by. However, I am not now, nor have I been in the past, too busy to watch the evolution of suggestion.

"I used the word therapeutic with relation to suggestion, for the same purpose as I would in an argument, or plea in a lawsuit—to draw the fire of the other side, thus getting the benefit of knowing their position and strength, so as to use the same against them in the further progress of the case."

You had no trouble in locating my fortification; you felt the force of my artillery—go on with your suggestion and argument.

"Now, to my surprise, what you said on the subject of suggestive therapeutics is most profoundly conclusive that you know practically nothing of the science. You should learn that hypnosis is but an incident to suggestion and the best results are made without it."

The conspicuous absence of therapeutics in your recent work on analysis of abnormalities "is most profoundly conclusive that you (now) know practically nothing of the science" of suggestion; that you consider it useless, not a suitable companion for Chiropractic.

"You write purely of mechanics; the reader would be excusable if he concluded that you are a materialist. I, however, refuse to believe such; if I thought it were true I would write you a very different letter, because only a few years ago I was wandering in that hopeless field."

You have taken my reply just right. When I attempt to explain the cause of disease, I use bones to illustrate material joints, which by their displacement impinge on nerves, causing functions to be deranged, the results being abnormal functioning and morbid tissue—conditions which we name disease. When I go into the spiritual realm which cannot be demonstrated by material, I talk of spirits. Chiropractic links the spiritual with the material. Never mind writing me on religion—go on with your "suggestion."

"Having thus in short preface swept aside intervening obstacles, let us at once get to the 'meat in the cocoanut' of the whole matter."

That is right; get down to something real, that which we can see, feel, chew, eat and digest—the "meat of the cocoanut."

"A perfect system for the reduction of disease will not discard any agent or means which never does harm but always good, and has been known by itself or themselves to entirely remove disease."

Reduction in surgery is the replacing of a dislocated bone, hernia or other displaced parts to their normal position. Disease has no normal position—you cannot reduce disease.

Such sophistry is used by the champions of every mode of healing. Should we therefore adopt every agent used to correct abnormalities? "A perfect system" does not need to be encumbered with adjuncts. If it is a fact that disease is the result of malposition, why not correct the position of the displaced portion?

"The world has struggled in darkness, pain and misery for ages, because of the pre-disposition of those who have been able to take a step in advance of their fellows to arrogate to their discovery all the virtues, and see in it alone the solution of every difficulty. I say this, not in a fault-finding vein, but simply as referring to a very regretable human weakness known to all in a greater or less degree. I would not raise my voice to detract from the glory of Chiro in any event and certainly would not suggest an aid for it if I were not absolutely certain that it is inadequate to cover the field of cure, used in the sense of the destruction of disease. It shocks my natural prejudice even then."

Where would this science be today, how much would have been developed, of how many diseased conditions would I have located the cause, if, when I did not succeed in removing the cause by the first effort, I had resorted to some one of the many therapeutical remedies which do no harm, to treat the effects known as disease? I would have made but one step forward and that would have been retraced backward to some one of the many systems which treat disease instead of adjusting causes. "The world has struggled in darkness, pain and mysery for ages, because" every method treated the effects instead of adjusting the cause thereof. Yes, I have taken a step in advance. Why not get in step with the developer and continue to go forward. Why detract my attention from my scientific investigation by introducing antiquated remedies? By my unceasing efforts—discovering and developing—this science does not stand in need of any aid from those methods which treat disease. When you use other methods as an aid to Chiropractic, whether an assistant or not, you "raise your voice to detract from the glory of Chiro." Were you familiar with the principles of Chiropractic, you would not write of "reducing and destroying disease"; for such an idea is Allopathic. Chiropractors do not reduce or destroy; instead, they repair, make right that which is the cause of wrong-doing. It shocks your "natural prejudice" to allow me the full honor of discovering and developing the grandest science on earth.

"If I were an enemy of 'Chiro,' or even a luke-warm friend, I would just keep still and concede that your very good letter had convinced and silenced me and I had allowed the giant to go his way, deprived by prejudice of more than half his strength. But not so, for I am a Chiro enthusiast and never permit an opportunity to pass without taking up the cudgel in his behalf."

As your book of 486 pages is silent in regard to Suggestive Therapeutics, I infer that you do not now consider that Chiro is deprived of "more than half his strength" by not accepting suggestion as a daily companion. Therefore I conclude that you have been convinced, deprived of your prejudice and have become willing to allow the giant to go his way unaccompanied by Suggestive Therapeutics.

"I say 'Chiro' is inadequate to cover the field of cure. I would not make such a statement without a logical reason and one which, to me, is entirely satisfactory. Let me see if I can demonstrate its reliability."

"Chiro" would have always remained inadequate, if its developer had continued to use therapeutical methods, as many have done, instead of using the principles of Chiropractic to locate and adjust causes.

"You say Chiropractic is purely a mechanical science and consists wholly in the adjustment of luxations. It has to do simply with keeping all of the articulatory processes of the organism in proper position. In other words, it consists of and finds its ideal condition in a living body in which all the joints are in their normal position; it is based on the rule, that if all parts of a machine are in their proper place, it will operate perfectly. Is it not so?"

You are right in all your premises, except that the rules of inanimate machinery, propelled by external applied force, will not apply to organic bodies, which are functionated by internal intelligent, vital force. If you would approach my fortifications direct without so much circumlocution, much time might be saved.

"I grant you, this would be true if the basic principle were a law of nature, but therein lies the great difficulty. Let us examine this under the proper test and see what it is. If it has one exception, then it is not a law of nature, for such—it is self evident—must be universal in its application. Solely from a mechanical standpoint I grant that the rule is universal; but whenever we touch the human body and, perhaps, any animate being, we are dealing with that which is not mechanical. The law will not universally apply, unless it may be said, the mechanical always governs that which is not."

All laws are of nature—natural. All phenomena are the result of certain law conditions, an extrinsic necessity; like causes produce like results. There are laws which are general, to which there are exceptions; these exceptions are the result of conditions—laws—just as much so as the phenomena are natural—the results corresponding to fixed laws. All laws are self existent. All phenomena, of necessity conform to nature's law—there is no other. Uniformity of coexistence and succession exist as natural phenomena. The same conditions will universally produce the same effect. The phenomena may be abnormal—unusual—but they are the result of certain conditions—laws—just as surely. There are general laws which govern normal functions, for example, bodily heat at 98 to 99 degrees. Certain conditions—laws—may change the temperature to that of supernormal or subnormal. Phenomena, usual or unusual, general or exceptional, normal or abnormal, are governed by fixed laws. The Chiropractor should study these laws and by a scientific knowledge use them to advantage.

Right, you are, in saying that when we consider the human body or an animate being, we are dealing with that which is not mechanical, and yet you state in your Analysis that "the human organism is a very complete machine; a machine with all its elemental parts." The mechanical does not govern the power. Physical force governs the mechanical; the latter is subservient to the former.

"With this thought in mind, let us examine a locomotive. There it stands on the track; every bolt, tap, lever and journal is perfect. The water in the gauge stands at the proper height. The coal is plentiful and properly distributed over the grate, yet the ponderous monster does not move. The articulative parts are perfect; there is no work for the machinist. What is needed? Something not mechanical—combustion, life. This is supplied; the engine is alive, but it burns coal too fast, klinkers the grate, the gauges show low water and a high pressure of steam, which is blowing off; fuel is being wasted; its wheels slip on the rails; it cannot pull a normal load."

You have, in your mind, given us a perfect machine. Viewed as a dead piece of mechanism it is perfect, but as an active machine it is faulty. There is too much draught, the coal contains mineral which vitrifies; the injectors do not supply sufficient water; there is a waste of steam—but—what has all this to do with Suggestive Therapeutics? Are you trying to draw the attention of the jury from your out-of-date, antiquated hag?

"You say, the engineer does not understand his machine."

Why not talk about living organic bodies possessed of vital life, instead of inorganic machines run by the physical force of steam; is it because you know more of the latter than of the former?

"But I am helpless; there is nothing out of place with this engine."

Supposing you knew all about the machine in question, it would not enhance you intellectually in regard to Chiropractic or the organic beings you should be studying. But, I will say, if I had a machinist who claimed to understand his business and who could not find and adjust the displaced portions which cause the irregularities mentioned, I would dismiss him. His suggestions might suit you, but I would desire a man who understood his vocation, and knew where and how to adjust the displaced parts.

"The whole trouble lies with the things not mechanical. The intelligence, combustion and steam, which are back of and superior—so far as this engine is concerned—to the mechanical. Teach your engineer and fireman their business and normal work at once results."

The whole trouble lies with the inanimate material, that which cannot think, or reason, that which is not possessed of organic life.

"Look at this human babe. It is mechanically perfect. It is the engine with the properly filled boiler and lighted furnace."

The human babe is not a machine, is not mechanical, is not a piece of mechanism; it has not the counterparts of the engine. You might as well try to illustrate the working of a babe by that of a potato. Both have eyes and skin; they live and grow; there is far more resemblance between the functions of the babe and the potato than between the babe and the engine. The main difference lies in the fact that we are accustomed to make the foolish comparison of the engine and not the potato.

"It is mechanically prepared to do normal service, but its mother restrains it and constantly mentions that it has very delicate health, will not live long and cannot play like other children."

The babe can no more be mechanical than the engine can be organic. The latter exhibits animal characteristics, the former is inert and lifeless. The mother may restrain the child's appetite, if so it suffers. But the lying suggestions are discovered to be false and deceptive sooner than the mother expects. The child steals away and satisfies its physical and mental desires. What has suggestion done?

"Its body becomes emaciated, but it suffers no luxations. It accepts all its mother's statements, believes them to be true and, in consequence, becomes pale, weak and emaciated. The difficulty is not mechanical, but, is in the intelligence department, as with the engine, per se. Chiropractic has nothing to do. Can Chiropractors reach such cases?"

You can bet your last dollar on the Chiropractor reaching such a case. If he was a graduate of the originator of the science he would at once recognize that the emaciation, the whiteness around the mouth, the flushed cheek and the weakened condition were due to lack of digestion. Upon inquiry, he would find that the child had a capricious appetite, sometimes eating voraciously, and at other times evincing an aversion to food; that often it would be very thirsty; that the stools were changeable in appearance and consistency; that there was almost continued itching of the nose and rectum, bloating of and distress in the abdomen. These signs and symptoms suggest the presence of intestinal worms. Scavengers living upon decaying food because of indigestion—a wise provision of nature. There is one sign of worms more reliable and satisfactory than all of the above. This is a number of red papillae on the inside of the lower lip, plainly to be seen by turning the lip outward. Their number will be proportionate to the number of worms and the degree of indigestion.

The walls of the stomach consist of the serous, muscular, submucous and mucous coats together with blood-vessels and nerves. The mucous or intestinal coat, when not distended, has a rugose (rough or wrinkled) appearance. It is covered with columnar epithelium—a lens will show the openings of numerous glands. The stomach is innervated from the brain, spinal cord and the sympathetic system.

The sign of worms on the under lip, referred to, is the result of inflamed nerve fibres which cause too much innervation. Of the 5th thoracic pair of nerves, those on the left go to the stomach, those on the right to the throat, mouth, etc.

As may be seen from the above, worms are scavengers; they live upon decayed food. The nerves of stomach innervation are impinged upon by a displacement of the 5th dorsal vertebra. This luxation may have occurred at birth, by the careless handling of the nurse or from poisonous drugs. The Chiropractor replaces the displaced vertebra, takes off the pressure so that innervation may be normal in amount, and digestion then becomes perfect leaving no decayed food for scavengers. The walls of the stomach being normal, assimilation perfect, the stomach can convert food into an absorbable form. Chiropractors reach just such cases. Suggestion is but little or no benefit in restraining or promoting functions of the human body or the engine on the track.

"The child's mental attitude must be corrected. The adverse suggestion printed on the life-mind by the mother must be removed. This can only be accomplished by suggestion.

The Chiropractor may accomplish this by saying to the child at the proper psychic moment, 'I can make you well and strong.' Chiropractors never can correct the child's condition."

If, as Analysis states, dyspepsia is responsible for bad temper; that melancholia is dependent upon abnormality of the spleen and liver; that grave occlusions of any of the spinal trunks will cause abnormality in brain tissue, causing some degree of insanity; that the author has known occlusions of the sub-occipital, 3d, 6th, 7th, 11th and 12th dorsals, 2d and 5th lumbars, to cause insanity; it affirms that it is the duty of the Chiropractor to locate the principal occlusion causing insanity no matter under what name it may be classified. This being the case, why not correct the mental aberrations of children by adjusting displaced vertebrae? Why state "This can only be accomplished by suggestion"? Why not adjust the kid?

"With the firebox and the functional relations of the fire, the mechanic has nothing to do. In the realm of the machine he is supreme. True, he can adapt his machine to the results flowing from it, within certain well defined, fixed limits, but otherwise, he is helpless in its presence."

A function consists of a duty to perform or an office to fill. Official acts, the performance of duties, are functions. A function is the performance of an order of a mental command. Fire has no duty to perform, no office to fill.

The mechanic has to do with the construction of the machine; the fireman looks after the fire and fire-box; the engineer runs the engine. These laborers have nothing to do with suggestion —their work is with material substances.

"So it is with the intelligence department. If a luxation impinges upon a nerve or blood vessel going to that part of the human machine, called the brain, causing it to act abnormally, named insanity, the mechanic—the Chiropractor—is the man for the crisis."

A human being is not a machine. A crisis is that change in disease which indicates whether the result will be recovery or death. The turning-point in a disease is not the time for a Chiropractor to take the case. If thon has made a change for recovery, he would not be treating the other fellow fairly to take the case. It would make him feel sore and be no real credit to himself. If the change is for death, the Chiropractor should not be the man for the crisis.

"But if the same or another form of insanity existed, arising from pernicious and perverse suggestion and not impingement, the Chiropractor would be helpless, because he has nothing to do with that intelligence force, named the mind or soul, lying back of the mechanical and controlling it. That, which causes the heart to beat, the nerves to thrill, the lungs to perform their functions, the warm blood to continue its circuit of the entire body; that mind that never sleeps, or fails to hear the cries of distress when in need of intellectual help; that never tires standing guard over the organism as long as it remains animate; that intelligence which is not mechanical, does not depend upon its existence and yet is peculiarly its servant."

I do not know of such a function as nerve-thrilling. How about the mind needing intellectual help and never sleeping? Sleep is a condition of apathy of the organs of sense; it is a diminution of sensation, feeling and thot; it is almost a complete cessation of conscious life.

"That intelligence which, when in control, can respond to a suggestion with such power as to set up the condition of a high fever almost instantly in a perfectly well person and in as short a time return normal functions."

For an intelligence to suggest a high fever would not be intelligent. It would not be an intellectual act even if it were a possibility. To create a high fever, instantly, to increase katabolism—tissue-waste, retrograde metamorphosis, would be an unwise thing to do, would be far from metaphysical reasoning.

"That living principle which can respond to a suggestion, stop action by removing life from the material body (a demonstrated fact). That mind, call it by whatever name you like, that controls the functions and operations of the entire being, to which the mechanical sustains the relation of an incident and with which the workman has no more to do than he has with the element of combustion of the coal on the grate."

A principle is a fundamental truth, a comprehensive law from which others are derived. A principle cannot respond to a suggestion, it cannot stop an action or remove life. Thus, Friend Carver, your "demonstrated facts" are built upon fallacious reasoning. Mind does not control the functions. There is an intelligence that controls the mind and its functions, as well as the functions of the body.

"To the end that man might be and maintain his free moral agency, he is endowed with the power to lodge objective impressions on the subjective, the life-mind of himself, auto-suggestion. That mind is bound to accept them as absolute facts, not being possessed of the power of reason and analysis. It therefore acts upon them as though true, carrying into effect—as far as possible—the commands, much to the detriment to the physical being, where the suggestion tends to draw away from health and strength. It is an evident fact, that within the means of self, there is no more fruitful source of health than correct auto-suggestion."

Spirit, Innate, the intelligence which gives the mind temporary, periodical rests from sensation, feeling and thot, is possessed of reason and the power of analyzing, as demonstrated by innumerable acts during the hours of sleeping and when awake. If "it is an evident fact, that within the means of self, there is no more fruitful source of health than correct auto-suggestion," why did you not make mention of it in your Analysis of abnormalities? Did my answer to your letters regarding suggestion set you thinking; if so, these pages may cause your mind to functionate properly and reason correctly on the fundamental principles of Chiropractic from which the science, art and philosophy of Chiropractic is derived.

"The life-mind is always open to suggestion; and since our environment has more of unpleasant, than pleasant; brings more forcibly to our notice, disease, pain, suffering, etc., than joy, health and exuberant life; our auto-suggestions—if we are not advised—become wrong, suggest to our life-mind weakness and lack of health. If these pernicious suggestions are not destroyed by affirmative correct ones, for the purpose of carrying out some semblance of a simile, we will say in displacement of subjective mental force, in other words, result in abnormal mental impulse which renders health just as impossible and disease just as certain as the luxation of a joint, causing some organ or set of organs to act abnormally; as in catalepsy and many others which I will leave to your ability to supply."

"The life-mind"; by this I presume you mean that which is known as sub-conscious mind. The mind of Innate or Educated, reasons, feels, wills, remembers and thinks. "Abnormal mental impulse." All impulses, whether of the motor—centrifugal nerve-fibers or the sensory, traveling toward the center from the periphery, are normal, could not be otherwise. But if the medium thru which the instruction passes, is excited above or depressed below normal, the impulses are augmented or decreased accordingly. In the preceding paragraph, you cite me to catalepsy as one of the many diseases which you claim are caused by pernicious suggestion which, by displacing this subjective mental force, results in abnormal mental impulse, and that this condition may be corrected by positive affirmation.

In your late work, I observe that, you analyze "catalepsy as a fixation of the muscles under subjective control. Just at what point the physical condition unites with the subjective cannot be clearly laid down. It will be found that adjusting at the points indicated will at once check the increase of constriction and a general tendency to relaxation will appear. Adjusting at first should be repeated at short intervals." I am pleased to observe that you are progressing toward the science of Chiropractic.

"The Chiropractor would say, 'When I find a joint displaced, I adjust it.' I have found displaced subjective mental impulse. What shall I do--adjust it? If so, how? By the most simple method in the world. As simple as a Chiro adjustment. By the subtle and wonderful power of suggestion, by lodging upon the subjective mind an impression correcting the erroneous one. I adjust the luxated joint so that the mechanical process of the body may not be interfered with. I must now adjust this incorrect abnormal subjective condition caused by pernicious auto, or external suggestion, so that the secretions and other functions under its control, will not be interfered with. This I can only do by the power of suggestion."

As has been shown by the previous quotations from your book, you have become sufficiently Chiropractorized now to adjust osseous luxations instead of subjective mentality.

"I wrote you at first only to call your attention to the fact that the science of Chiropractic and suggestion are exactly alike in their object and application and differ only in that the object is attained in the one primarily through the physical and in the other through the life or subject-mind and that they are inseparable twins, neither can be fully and successfully practiced without the other; it is impossible for the Chiropractor to practice without using suggestion."

"Chiropractic and Suggestion are exactly alike" **only they are different.** Five years ago you thot these two were "inseparable twins." I know where one of these kids are; what have you done with Suggestion? In your late work you do not make mention of Suggestion. Have you found it possible to separate the "inseparable twins"? Can you practice Chiropractic without Suggestion?

"You cannot possibly adjust a luxated joint, without leaving some impression on the life-mind. You depend, and openly say so, for success on the Innate nerves, which are but the channels through which the subjective, or life-mind, is constantly striving to perform all of its functions. If this were not true, no luxated joint could be adjusted. It would be folly to replace it, for there would be no intelligent force to hold it; yielding to the side of least resistance, it would; by the force of gravity, return to the abnormal position. You finally succeed by virtue of this subjective intelligence, speaking through the Innate nerves, commanding the adjoining tissues, regardless of pain, inflammation, etc., to have it grasp the replaced bone and hold it in its proper place. By adjusting you set on foot an impulse of subjective intelligence that does it. In other words, you remove an impediment which the subjective intelligence had not found a way to do, and it at once resumes its function."

"You cannot possibly adjust a luxated joint, without leaving some impression on the life-mind," as much so as the saw-filer does on the saw he has gummed and filed. You sum up your long dissertation by saying, "You remove an impediment (a pressure) which the subjective intelligence had not a way to do." Why did you not sum up the whole question in that sensible matter-of-fact manner in the first line of your article?

"What infinitive assistance at this grave juncture could the Chiropractor give this wonderful intelligent force, if he but understood the science of impressing it with strong and correct suggestions. What astonished power he could cause it to bring to bear on retaining the adjusted vertebra in its proper place and by its use ameliorate the distress of adjustment.

"In the cases of Nutting and Story, you used larvated suggestion, in fact, you always do. You cannot help it. How much better it would have been in the case of Story, if, after having adjusted the luxated bone, you had been able to have gone on and driven out of his mind all of those adverse and morbid impressions. How much quicker he would have returned to the normal and gone to his family, instead of remaining—as he did—an eccentric."

Immediately, instantly, Dr. Story was able to do his own "auto-suggesting" after I had adjusted the displaced cervical. He was satisfied to remain in Los Angeles, the land of sunshine and flowers, avoiding the long cold winters of Wisconsin. For him to decide thus, did not need either open or larvated suggestion. The adjustment gave him relief inside of a minute; that was specific Chiropractic.

"I do not ask you to incorporate into, or graft onto, Chiropractic any form of treatment of disease."

You don't! Is not that the object of your two letters? You ought to know by this time that I do not treat disease, even by suggestion. Therein Chiropractic differs from all other methods.

"Suggestion is not a treatment of disease, it is correcting or adjusting the cause in that part of the organism not mechanical. Suggestion goes back behind the mechanical, to the very foundation of life and has to do with an intelligence which existed before there was a bony structure to luxate."

Suggestion, if it is anything, is a treatment. There is nothing mechanical, no mechanism, no machinery; therefore, nothing to go behind.

"I beg of you to not maim a universal law of cure by confining it to mechanical adjustment; separating it into parts and taking only the smaller; thus reducing the law to a rule that has many exceptions. Adopt the adjustment of subjective luxations, as well as those of bones, so that the rule of adjustment may apply to the mental as well as the physical."

Have you not maimed your "universal law of cure" by adopting Chiropractic straight as given in your Analysis? There is nothing mechanical, no mechanism, no machinery in the human body; therefore, there is nothing to go behind. Your "Chiropractic Analysis" is conspicuously absent of Suggestive Therapeutics, which, as you state, is the larger share of your "universal law of cure." By adopting Chiropractic your "adjustments apply to the mental as well as the physical." Do you yet realize that Innate knows more of human economics than Educated ever did or will know?

Innate always existed and always will. Progression is stamped in Innate's every act—development of material by intelligence. Changes more or less experimental, in organisms are being made to suit environments. Innate has a knowledge gleaned from a life of eternity; it runs the functions of the human body as readily on the first day of its habitation as in after years. It is infinite, unlimited in time and experience. Innate comprehends human economy—Educated looks after machinery. Educated is the mechanic. You suggest that this upstart of today should dictate to its master, its projenitor, how it should run economic functions. The functions of metabolism are as perfect, usually more so, in the idiot and illiterate than in those of education and exalted birth. Why should Educated suggest to thon's superior? In very many instances I have found that Innate for special purposes has built piers and locks; made foramina and tunnels instead of grooves; elongated processes, ankylosed joints, made new joints in unusual places; in fact, made many changes in osseous tissue to accommodate its habitation to surrounding circumstances. If Educated will replace all displacements of the bony framework, Innate will care for all internal needs.

"The Chiropractor renders his patient passive for mechanical adjustment. In order to be properly equipped, he should know how to render him mentally passive to subjective adjustment, then, the two working hand in hand, as the Creator has intended, untrameled by external pernicious or adverse influence, no diseased conditions could resist this double-headed adjustment of the mental and physical."

True, the patient should be made passive during osseous adjusting. Dr. Henry has accomplished far more in this much needed requirement by having the patient place him arms parallel with and close to his body, or the hands on the buttocks, the latter act requiring much less time, than you have been able to do, or ever can do with suggestion. Chiropractors who understand the science do not need "double-headers."

"It is because I love Chiro, as ardently as a school boy does his first sweetheart, that I beg of you to bring the science of suggestion down to date and make it the working companion of Chiropractic. Please give it a trial before discarding it.

Yours truly, WILLARD CARVER."

I am pleased to learn that you have discarded Suggestive Therapeutics; that you have brot the science of Chiropractic up to date. Now make your adjustments specific, make Chiropractic a science. Chiropractic does not need aid—Chiropractors need more knowledge.

"Suggestion," observing Dr. Carver's suggestions, volunteered assistance by mailing to me a copy of "Auto Suggestion," by Parkyn.

The author says. "It is a demonstrative fact that the benefits derived from Magnetic Healing, Sacred Shrines, Divine Science, Mental Science, Absent Treatment, Christian Science and the various schools of Medicine, are due to Auto-Suggestion." I give to Auto-Suggestion much of the same credit. But, when the surgeon sets a fractured limb or a displaced joint, suggestions are not considered, in fact, they are above being suggested to. When a Chiropractor replaces a displaced vertebra or any one of the 300 articular joints of the human body or that of any of the lower vertebrates, he does not need or use suggestion as an aid or a remedy. He has no more use for suggestions from one who has no comprehension of adjusting wrenched vertebrae, than the jeweler has for his grandmother to suggest by word or thot how he should adjust the displaced parts of a watch.

I quote from Auto-Suggestion: "Auto-Suggestion is at one and the same time the worst foe and the strongest ally to be met with in treating mental and physical disorders."

Dr. Carver states: "Suggestion is not a treatment of disease." Dr. Parkyn says: "Auto-Suggestion it at one and the same time the worst foe, and the **strongest ally** to be met with **in treating mental** and physical **disorders.**" As **I do not treat** either mental or physical disorders—do not treat effects—I have no need of Auto-Suggestion as an ally, foe or adjunct.

I also quote from Auto-Suggestion, "Every physical trouble in the human body can be traced to imperfections in the blood. Blood supplies life to every cell." This etiology tastes like Allopathy. No school of therapeutics cares to deny that statement. Their theories are built upon abnormal blood as the basis of disease. Even suggestion accepts that theory of medicine. I discovered and have advocated for many years that all physical and mental derangements are functions performed in excessive or deficient amounts. Nerves transport impulses to every part of the body, even to the cells; their execution is the performance of functions. All sensations of pleasure or distress, are of nerves—not of blood.

Dr. Parkyn says, "The blood is the actual healing agent of the body."

All reparative processes are the work of Innate, whose impulses are directed thru the nervous system, not the vascular. This bloody delusion has held the world in ignorance long enough. All actions (functions) are the result of impulsive commands sent out by and thru the nervous system; such is life. The circulation of blood, the transudation of chyle, lymph and serum is controlled by nerve impulses sent out by Innate. What has formation of character, habits, breathing or business tactics to do with the setting of fractured bones or displaced joints? I am not running a kindergarten school. My time is employed in discovering what portion of the osseous frame-work impinges upon the carriers of impulses, that create disturbance of functions named disease.

Dr. Parkyn also says."Would it not seem ridiculous if we found it necessary to instruct our horses or dogs how to breathe as nature intended they should?" It seems equally as ridiculous for Educated to tell Innate how to breathe, in horses, dogs or human beings. If all parts concerned are in their normal position, performing their normal functions, there is no need of

Educated suggesting to Innate how to breathe or perform any other function.

The economic functions are performed by Innate as well or better in the infant or in the lower orders of vertebrates than in the adult who is educated in the mazy labyrinth of Suggestive Therapeutics. Educated bothers and worries Innate when trying to direct that of which Innate knows far more than Educated will ever know.

E. E. Carey, manager of Suggestion, writes me:

"Dear Friend: The law of suggestion is just as certain as the law of gravitation. A man hears bad news; he falls in a fainting condition. What caused him to fall? Suggestion. He hears better news and recovers. What caused him to recover? Suggestion. That is all there is to it. We do not oppose Chiropractic, for it has its use; but don't try to make any one believe that the mind has no influence on the body. That is all we claim; we don't claim everything as you do, for Chiropractic."

The law of suggestion is just as certain as the law of medicine. The Chiropractor who understands osteology, neurology and the principles of Chiropractic, and knows how to apply the art of adjusting displacements of the skeletal frame, has no need of either, nor is he benefited by their use, except, perhaps, as policy, and even then I prefer straight unpolished honesty. Honesty has no need of policy. Policy looks to temporary, material gain rather than any moral principle of right. Cunningly devised policy often outweighs in the scales of justice that of honesty and honor. "Honesty is the best policy." Honesty is not policy. Policy is dishonesty.

Chiropractors have no more need of suggestion when replacing a luxated bone than a lady has when adjusting her hat or collar. Suggestion and policy are business tactics, cunning devices used to sell goods to the unwary. Suggestive medicine consists of the treatment by positive assertions addressed to a more or less hypnotized patient. Any salesman can sell goods to those who want them, but it takes policy and suggestion to sell to those who do not need or desire them.

The mind has an influence over the body and so have remedies, but I have no use for either when adjusting vertebrae or other joints.

I think that there is some good in all methods; but when the Chiropractor adjusts the bony framework to its normal position; all pliable tissue will respond and resume their proper position and consequently their usual functions—health being the result. What more needs to be done?

E. E. Carey failed to get the Chiropractic idea in my answers to Willard Carver. Perhaps I was not explicit, for this reason I will answer his letter, which reads as follows:

"Dear Doctor: I have yours of the 14th enclosing copy of an article by yourself, in which you argue that smoking cigarettes will in time produce a displaced vertebra and that by adjusting the displacement, the habit will be abandoned. The article also teaches by inference that an undesirable habit will produce displacement in some portion of the body."

The smoking of cigarettes poisons the nervous system. This poison affects sensory nerves which in turn contract motor nerves, drawing bones to which they are attached, out of alignment. Displaced bones, more especially vertebrae, press against, and impinge upon nerve-fibers, deranging their actions. Continued displacement perpetuates pain, misery, paralysis, abnormal physical desires and mental aberrations. Just as surely as bones can be drawn out of their normal position, just so surely they can be corrected by the hand. The act of smoking does not fasten, or form the habit. The poison which is imposed upon the nervous system creates these special changes for its accommodation.

On this question of adaptation, immunity to disease, that condition of the body which enables it to resist morbific influences, to adapt itself to conditions imposed upon it, can not be better said than that given on page 7 of Delafield and Prudden's Text-Book on Pathology. "The human body, like other living organisms, has acquired its present form and its varied functions through gradual adaptation to its environment.

"The maintenance of normal life of the body involves a normal mechanism and impulse to start with, and a constant and successful adjustment to the conditions under which it is placed. While the continuance of the state which we call health depends upon the approximate maintenance of the external conditions to which the body has become adapted, it should be borne in mind that the adaptive capacity of the body is in many ways of unusual surroundings and adverse influences. Thus, for example, the body can adapt itself, within the limits of what we call health, to alterations, deficiencies, or excesses of nutrient material; to varying extremes of heat or cold, moisture or dryness; to electrical tension; to animal and vegetable parasites; and to various poisons, both to those which come from without and those which result from faulty metabolism. Beyond certain rather ill-defined limits, however, the adaptive capacity cannot go, and disease results.

"The adaptive capacity may vary greatly in different individuals, depending upon age, sex, race, etc., so that adverse conditions which one individual can sustain without marked functional disturbance or structural damage may induce in another more or less serious disease. For example, children are in general much more disposed to certain diseases than are adults. This disposition to disease is not, however, always fixed, but may give way to immunity under conditions in acute infections."

Drugs affect nerves; for that purpose are they given. Astringents cause contraction of tissue. Tonics and stimulants excite action. Sedatives and narcotics lower functional activity by producing stupor. Diuretics, diaphoretics and expectorants stimulate certain nerves to over-action. A continued use of any one of these causes conditions, which we name habits, to become fixed. I was the first to determine the where and how of medication—poison.

Chiropractors are able, or at least should be, to locate the vertebra displaced, the nerves impinged upon, and to replace the vertebra and release the impingement.

One of the duties of a physician is to observe the effect his prescription has upon the nerves of his patient. His remedies may be introduced by the mouth, rectum, hypodermic syringe or arm vaccination. The kind of poison and place of entrance is to be considered by the adjuster when adjusting.

A medicine is said to be physiologic when it acts as a counter-poison. On account of individual peculiarities, called idiosyncracies, a drug may be physiologic to one person and pathologic to another. A physiological medicine is one which its effects are considered physiological in functions; if it should make the patient worse, it is pathological. A physiological antidote is one which when administered to a healthy person produces effects opposite to those produced by the poison of which it is the antidote. An antidote is one that neutralizes, not by its chemical effect on the poison, but thru its effects on the system in functionating. This doctrine of physiologic, pathologic and therapeutics was promulgated by F. J. Broussais, a French physician who lived from 1772 to 1838. This system was named Broussaism, the physiological doctrine which the excitability of the gastrointestinal mucous membrane was given much prominence. An antidote originally meant any internal remedy; it is now synonymous with counter-poison, and signifies any remedy capable of combating the effects of a poison.

A chemical antidote is one which acts by changing the chemical composition of the poison and thus rendering it inert.

E. E. Carey further says: "It appears from your literature

that you attempt to prove that everything from a stub toe to yellow fever and even corns are produced by displaced vertebrae."

In all my writings, Friend Carey has not seen a statement, of my locating the cause of either a stub-toe or yellow fever, as I have not had a case of either. I presume that he would say that suggestion was all there was to it; while Dr. Carver would say that they were because of sub-luxations of the life-mind. Corns are caused by luxated joints of the toes and metatarsal bones.

I emphatically affirm, as I did thirteen years ago, that about 95 per cent of diseases are caused by displaced vertebrae; the other five per cent, including corns and bunions, come from luxated joints other than those of the backbone. Where joints are not ankylosed, they may be replaced by one move, the tenderness disappearing at once.

E. E. Carey still further says: "We think that you would have better success if you did not take such radical grounds, for you certainly must be well aware that there are diseases which can in no possible way be connected with any physical derangement."

Friend Carey, I do not know of a diseased condition which has not its cause in some derangement of the skeletal frame. A subluxation perpetuates disease.

I am well aware that Chiropractic is a new departure, that adjusting causes is a radical change from treating effects, that it is making a greater inroad in the old methods than any other method; but I care not, so long as I know I am right.

---

The "Therapeutical Idol Shatterer, Destroyer of Superstitious Ideas Regarding Creation, Transmission and Expression of Life in Any Form and Replacer of Impractical with Practical Studies" says: "Serous circulation is broadened and more thoro reasons established for its existence. To the person wanting scientific detail of a technical nature, this is complete practical, comprehensible and **what he ought to have had thousands of years ago.**"

Such ideas, developed by the "Student, Author, Lecturer and Teacher on any phase of Chiropractic Philosophy, Science or Art, anywhere, at any time, "ought to have been delivered "thousands of years ago," for they are "thousands of years" behind this day and age of advancement.

---

"The man who is the foremost developer and propagator of the humanitarian science and art of Chiropractic."—S. H. W.

## DEVELOPMENT OF CHIROPRACTIC.

Chiropractic had a beginning. The fundamental principles had to be discovered and from them other principles and the philosophy.

Osteopathy had a beginning. Dr. A. T. Still says: "I began to give reasons for my faith in April 1855." Forty-seven years later he is teaching a class of less than a score of students. When he named his science Osteopathy I am not informed. The principles had to be collected, even if they were already known. A. T. Still is the developer and founder of the system known as Osteopathy.

Chiropractic had its beginning in September, 1895. I did not wait forty-seven years before teaching it. I sometimes wish I had, or at least until I had developed the principles I discovered into a science. If I had done this it would have saved much discussion, confusion and a whole lot of falsehoods in regard to who discovered and developed the science of Chiropractic. It is of such a nature that I could have held it a secret as long as I desired.

I saw fit to date the beginning of Chiropractic with the first adjustment, although quite a portion of that which now constitutes Chiropractic I had collected during the previous nine years.

I was not the first person to replace a displaced vertebra, as shown by a long article on luxations, "Chiropractic Sunbeans"; but I was the first to use the spinous and transverse processes as levers whereby to rack into their normal position vertebra which had become displaced. I simplified the handling of vertebrae. Instead of finding a few rare cases of vertebra which had been wrenched from their natural position, I found them very common. Indeed, I found displacements were the rule instead of the exception. Surgeons and physicians admitted that vertebral luxations **might** occur and cause diseased conditions. But I was the first to assert, by word of mouth and in print, that about 95 per cent of diseases were caused by subluxated vertebrae; the remaining 5 per cent by slightly displaced joints other than those of the backbone. I was the first to describe how and why displaced vertebrae and other joints caused diseased conditions. I have created a science of vertebral adjustment.

As will be seen by a letter, of which only a copy of the most essential parts is herewith presented, as the original is too lengthy for publication, Rev. Samuel H. Weed, now of Monmouth, Ill., lived in Colona, Ill., when I discovered and formulated the fundamental principles of the science and art of Chiro-

Monmouth, Ill., March 27th, 1908.
R. F. D. No. 7.

Dr. D. D. Palmer, Discoverer, Developer and Founder of Chiropractic,
Oklahoma City, Okla.,

Dear Doctor and Friend: I was much pleased to receive your letter of March 21st, 1908, and to learn that you are still practicing, developing and teaching that boon to the sufferer which you discovered and called Chiropractic. You developed it into a science in Davenport, Iowa, where you founded and presided over the first Chiropractic school, until driven from that city by the persecution which in our sinful world is almost sure to fall on everyone who originates and gives to his fellow man something that is both good and great. But as the early Christians when chosen as the headquarters of Dr. D. D. Palmer, the true fountain head of this science I am glad to learn that you were the first to practice and teach it in the youngest sister State of our great Republic

Said "Temple" cannot be "The Fountain Head for Chiropractic." The true Fountain Head, Dr. D. D Palmer, is in your city, but in vain would you search for him in said "Temple." I have known Dr. Palmer personally for fourteen years, that is, before he discovered Chiropractic.

that hurt on his back This was the clew I knew of the fact also that by day and by night the doctor studied over that clew, that first ray of the dawning light of the science of Chiropractic. How strange it is, if the "Temple of Knowledge does not know that Dr. Palmer is the Fountain Head.

time after Dr. Palmer had named his science Chiropractic The truth is that the doctor asked him to translate "Done by hand" into Greek, and he suggested two almost synonaimous words of that meaning, of which the doctor chose one, namely, Chiropractic. "Temple" says, "renamed,

I bespeak for Oklahoma Chiropractic College abundant success in teaching and practicing your own science of Chiropractic.

With regards to yourself and lady;

I remain Your friend,

Samuel H. Weed.

It will be observed that portions of this letter are purposely left out in order to save space

Monmouth, Ill. June 13th, 1910.
R. F. D. No. 7

Dr. D. D. Palmer, Portland, Oregon,

Dear Doctor and Friend:

You hold a relation to Chiropractic which no other person can hold, for you are the originator of the scientia et ars Chiropractica; and I am very glad you are going to issue a book. The book will certainly be indispensable for every Chiropractor, and will be recognized by the world as an authority coming from the hand of him who was first in Chiropractic.

Wishing you success both in your school and in your work as author, I remain Yours truly,

Samuel H. Weed.

practic. At this time we frequently met and conversed freely on my almost daily advancement. Therefore, Rev. Weed is familiar with the origin of Chiropractic, in testimony of which see his letter, which was quite lengthy; therefore the substance only of special interest was copied. I have the original letter.

Vol. I. of the Science of Chiropractic states under the headline of "Historical," Rev. Samuel Weed first met Dr. D. D. Palmer in 1894, after his daughter had been wonderfully cured by magnetic healing by him of a sprained ankle that threatened her life. The doctor then relieved him, by magnetic treatment. of splenic trouble which incapacitated him from preaching.

Mrs. Weed and her little daughter took Chiropractic adjustments early in 1896 and were much benefited. Afterwards Mr. Weed also received adjustments for sciatica and got relief About this time I asked him to suggest a name in Greek for the science and art which I had created, one which would mean done by hand. Thus originated the word Chiropractic.

---

"Why death is caused by impinged nerves and not by disease."

The above and many other misstatements are made by Chiropractors who are not familiar with the principles of Chiropractic; therefore, they need adjusting.

Death may be physiologic—no impingement—no disease.

Accidents may eliminate circulation, respiration or innervation either one of the three functions essential to life and no impingement upon nerves.

Death may be physiologic or pathologic. The former occurs, after a length of life recognized as being normal to mankind, from general wearing out of the body and the performance of its functions. This is usually known as "death from old age." Pathologic death occurs from unnatural causes at a time when the individual is not worn out and is yet active. It is not always possible to distinguish physiologic from pathologic death.

By far the larger number of individuals cease to exist as living beings because of conditions we name disease. Nerves may be impinged upon and cause disability or ailments, and yet not cause death.

By disease is meant either an increase or decrease of normal functionating or a structural change of any organ or part of the body from the normal state. These two conditions, altho referred to separately, are always associated—either cannot be present without the other. An increase or decrease of tonicity in nerve tissue causes a corresponding change in functions.

## WHAT IS LIFE?

Organized beings possess life; substances which do not possess organs do not have life. Every organized being experiences consciousness; unorganized matter does not. Organized plants and animals have organs adapted to continue their existence. Life is the quality or character which distinguishes an animal or plant from inorganic or dead organic bodies. Every portion of creation that lives performs functions which are necessary for its existence. Life is expressed by the process of metabolism, growth, reproduction and inherent powers of adaptation to environment. Life is the result of vital force, spiritual energy, expressed in organic creation. Organized beings grow by material taken internally. After the composition of this material is suitably changed it is deposited thruout the body as needed. Animate bodies enlarge by additions of the same material. The substances of their bodies are constantly undergoing a change, old material being decomposed and passed off, and new material taken in to replace that which has served its usefulness. This change is a process of repair. Organized beings are constantly undergoing a change of material, yet remain practically the same. Repair is accomplished by the assimilation of new material which has been taken in and digested. The actions necessary to continue a living existence are known as functions. For a normal existence, it is necessary that each and every function should be performed in a natural manner. When, by any means, the organization becomes injured or deranged, the texture too soft or too hard so that its organs can no longer carry impulses and enact them into functions, life ceases.

Life is the result of the combination of intellectual spirit and unintelligible matter. Life expressions are made manifest by acts, functions performed. Chiropractors should become acquainted with that which constitutes functions—the expressions of life—and know whether they are physiological or pathological.

---

The Chiropractic idea of disease and the adjusting of vertebrae, therefor, is applicable to all animals which have vertebral back bones. When Chiropractic methods are understood by veterinarians they will cease their cruel treatment. When poultry raisers learn to adjust the backbones of their fowls for diseases they will quit using remedies.

## A CHIROPRACTOR'S CARD.

"The human body represents the actions of three laws, spiritual, mechanical and chemical, united as one triune. As long as there is perfect union of these three there is health. This machine, like all others, is run by power, called mental impulses, made in the brain and connected with the body by a system of nerves thru which this force passes in currents, inducing the highest exemplification of the intellectual power. Functions are names given to these actions, any interference to the passage of these vitalizing currents produces abnormal functions—disease.

"The competent Chiropractor instantly locates where the 'interference' is, adjusts it, by hand adjustment, thereby restores the passage of currents—a condition of ease—normal functions—health.

"Investigation costs nothing and means health and happiness."

Triune is an epithet used to express the unity of a trinity of persons in the Godhead—the makeup of the Trinity. It is considered sacrilege to use the word for any other purpose.

Spiritual is of the spirit. Spirit is not subject to physical or terrestial laws. Spirit directs matter, man, beast, bird, fish and plants; it creates law, is not a law itself.

Chemical laws are confined to chemistry. Chemical pertains to the changes made by chemical analysis and the compounding of elements.

Mechanical relates to mechanics. It deals with the quantitative relations of force and matter, as distiguished from those which are mental, vital and chemical. It is impossible to unite an individualized portion of the Allwise with two laws which have no affinity for, or relation with, each other. They are inconcinnous.

The living body is subject to vital force, the expenditure of which is known as energy. It is not feasible to unite a spiritual entity to chemical action; the laws of chemistry and kinematics are incongruous.

Man is not a machine—a mechanical contrivance run by mechanical power. The bodily functions are carried on by an energy known as vital force. Mental impulses are not power; they do not run the body. They are a production of Innate, spirit. Power and mental impulses are not synonymous. Man is not a machine—he is not subject to the laws which govern inanimate matter. Vital force furnishes the energy—impulses direct them. Impulses are not made, they are created. Things which are made, are artificially produced. Energy and impulses are not connected with the body—are not joined or fastened by an intervening substance. Energy—force, is not a fluid—it does not flow as a current. Chemical laws are confined to chemistry—not to the body. The laws of mechanics are distinguished from those which are mental, vital and chemical. The human body is subject to the laws of vital force. The laws which govern mechanics and chemistry do not govern the human economy.

To entertain a thot of uniting spirit and mechanical and chemical entities shows a lack of comprehension of terms. It is impossible to make a union of a spiritual being, a mechanical machine and a chemical laboratory.

Functions are not names given to actions. "Vitalizing currents" might refer to the flow of blood or serum, but not to actions which produce abnormal functions.

"Restores the passage of currents."

There may be too much flow of the fluids of the body; if so, they do not need restoring.

Whenever a Chiropractor states that he **instantly** locates where the cause of a certain disease is, you may put him down as an incompetent Chiropractor—that he is a grafter, getting money by false pretenses. While I am writing this article a Chiropractor from Davenport, called and said, "I can tell what ails anyone as far away as San Francisco, without asking a question. I used to know him as a 'blow-hard'."

The writer of the above card is an M. D. and a D. C.; a bad combination if the above card is a sample.

"Man is a wonderfully made machine."

A machine is a more or less complex combination of mechanical parts, as levers, cogs, and sprocket wheels, pulleys, shafts and spindles, ropes, chains, bands, cams and other turning and sliding pieces, springs, etc., together with the framework and fastenings supporting and connecting them. A machine is designed to operate upon material, to change it in some preconceived and definite manner, to lift or transport loads, etc.

"**All nerves** are distributed from the brain cells **through the openings of the spine.**"

The twelve pairs of cranial nerves originate in the brain and **emerge from foramina in the skull.** Spinal nerves arise from the spinal cord and emerge thru the intervertebral foramina of the vertebral column. **The fibres** of all nerves may be traced into the deep substance of the brain.

"If the life giving energy, known as mental impulse, electricity, nerve force, etc., is unhindered in its course, disease cannot exist; but should **the element** that keeps the body in health be interfered with by pressure upon nerves—by subluxated (slightly displaced) vertebrae, symptoms of disease appear in the locality to which the impinged nerves are distributed."

Energy, mental impulses and electricity are not synonymous—they do not mean one and the same thing. Electricity is an inanimate force; it is an agency to whose action are due numerous phenomena in physics—the science of matter and motion. When applied to the human body, it shocks—is death dealing—does not give vitality or life. A mental impulse is an incitement of the mind by Innate or spirit, in the form of an abrupt and vivid suggestion, prompting some unpremeditated action or leading to unforeseen knowledge or insight. Energy is manifested in various forms, as mechanical, electrical, chemical and thermal. Functional energy is due to **thermal force—the amount of heat determines the quantity and quality of action.** An element is one of the simple substances of which the physical universe is composed, as earth, air, fire and water—none of these keep the body in health; are not interfered with by pressure upon nerves.

To "hinder," is to keep back, to prevent starting, to obstruct, to shut off. The larger share of diseases are the result of **too much vital force**; consequently, energy is not hindered, kept back, prevented, obstructed or shut off, but accelerated, hastened, quickened, urged, hurried, the volume and force is augmented.

"Impinged nerves."

On the fifth page of this booklet is a cut displaying how nerves are squeezed or pinched. I have never seen a cut showing how nerves are pinched between the occiput and atlas, betwixt the atlas and axis, or between the joints of the feet. Why not have cuts of these showing how the first and second pairs of cervical nerves are pinched, also those of other joints than those of the vertebral column? Why not present cuts of these which do not pass thru intervertebral foramina? Because their nerves are impinged upon, not pinched. If so, are not other nerves also impinged upon? There is a vast difference between nerves being impinged upon—a pressure on or against one side, and being pinched between two hard substances.

"Should an impingement cause pressure on the nerve that transmits the vital force to the kidneys, we have either Bright's disease or diabetes."

Bright's disease is an affection of the kidneys, but diabetes is not:—See diabetes.

"Chiropractic, done or accomplished by the hand, fixing, hand practice."

"Hand-practice" would be a systematic exercise for instruction or disclpline—such as "Dr. Arnold's Painless Adjusting," where every vertebrae of the spine is luxated, then corrected. in order to adjust the vertebra that has been violently displaced by accident, or drawn out of alignment by a toxic substance; or for that of clinics where from two to twenty-six vertebrae are thrust upon, when only one displaced vertebra is causing the particular trouble from which the patient desires freedom.

"Instead of treating diseases by the effects, we adjust the cause."

The above sentence would be good Chiropractic if the words "by the effects" were left out. Very often Chiropractors try to say or do too much.

"When a nerve is impinged upon by pressure between two or more hard substances, as two vertebrae, the function of that nerve is decreased, or rather there is a lack of ease,. so the Chiropractor defines the term of disease as a lack of ease."

A nerve is impinged upon when pressed against. When pressed between two or more hard substances, it would be squeezed. Impinged and squeezed have two quite different meanings. We adjust vertebrae, not the lack of ease.

"It may seem strange to you. but nevertheless it has been demonstrated as a fact that all the nerves of the body may be acted upon by the hands of the Chiropractor."

Such does seem strange to me. I very much desire to know how the 24 cranial and the nerves of the sympathetic nervous system can be adjusted, acted upon by the hands. All nerves are connected with the spinal nerves by communicating fibers. These fibers become impinged upon or pressed against by the displacement of bones.

"By adjusting the cause we free the circulation both of the nerve and then of the blood, permitting the refuse to be thrown out through the body in a normal way."

Circulation is the act of circulating; there is no circulation in a nerve. The nerves are channels for motor impulses outward only, and sensations inward; neither circulate, move in a circle.

"Stimulus is not a good name to apply to the electrical force which runs our bodies."

A stimulus excites or produces a temporary increase of vital action. A sedative restrains, lessens functional activity. Any vital action, or the temporary activity of nerves, or the irritation of muscles, would be a stimulus. Stimulus is not a good substitute for vital force; neither is "electrical force."

Electrical pertains to electricity, a power in nature that is manifested in inanimate bodies. Magnetism is a similar force in animate bodies. We would not use such terms as stimulus, electricity or magnetism as synonymous for vital force.

"Chiropractic, anatomy, physiology, hygiene, hydrotherapy, dietetics, rest-cure and massage. We consider all these modes of drugless healing are an evolution from medicine to Chiropractic. We have studied and practiced, with success, all these methods of relief, but, we have left them all, knowing that Chiropractic is the climax."

Anatomy and physiology are not modes of healing.

Chiropractic was not evolved from medicine or any other method, except that of magnetic. For nine years previous to the discovery of adjusting vertebrae, I was practicing magnetic healing. During that time I had developed much which afterwards became a part of the science of Chiropractic. For example, I treated (as I supposed) the spleen for cancer of the breast, effecting a cure. Now I see that I relieved the nerves in that region of inflammation. There was "nerve tracing" in its infancy. While Chiropractic is an outgrowth of magnetic healing, it is not magnetic healing advanced, is not the climax of magnetism or any other method.

"If one knew nothing of Chiropractic and had to choose between **manufactured chemical** to assimilate with **natural chemical.**"

Chemical pertains to chemistry. Chemistry is a science which treats of the elements, the atomic relations of matter and of the various compounds which are formed by elementary substances.

The science (knowledge) of chemistry consists in reducing a compound body to its elements and the uniting of elements to make a compound. For example, lye and grease are elements, which, when united, form a compound known as soap. Soap is produced by combining fats or oils with alkalies or alkaline earths, usually by boiling. The science or knowledge of making soap, so far as it goes, is chemistry. Soap is a compound. To reduce it back to its elements from which it was made is a chemical act. That is chemistry in a nut shell. A chemist knows, when a man talks about a manufactured chemical or a natural chemical, that he is not acquainted with chemistry; that he is using terms which do not apply to the science of chemistry.

A Chiropractor wrote me, "It is just as natural for me to handle diseases as to breathe."

"I tell you, I have six misplaced vertebrae. Maybe I don't suffer a little. Can't get out of my chair today."

Why not learn to handle vertebrae instead of diseases?

Objects are displaced when moved out of the place where they belong. They are misplaced when mislaid. One may know where to find what he has displaced, but he cannot find what he has misplaced. Vertebrae are displaced, not misplaced.

Chiropractic is not a method of treatment or a process of treating diseases. Instead, Chiropractors replace the parts which are not in apposition into their normal relative position

---

D. D. Palmer's thoughts continue to be ahead of the times, as will be evidenced by a persual of The Chiropractor's Adjuster. He today holds that same honored position, envied by a few of his students, who advertise themselves as fountain heads and developers of the science. There is but one fountain head and developer, there never can be but one, and that one is D. D. Palmer. There are those who try to ape that "peculiar sort of a crank," but they only succeed in making a ludicrous show of themselves; better try "to reach his intellectual level" rather than to falsify and slander their superior, hoping thereby to lower his standard so that they may then be able to attain his level of intellectuality.

It is true that D. D. Palmer always detested policy. While others said "Honesty is the best policy" he thought that honesty did not need policy, that in proportion as we use policy, we covered up honesty with deceit; therefore, his stick-to-itiveness to principle and honor made him some enemies, who could but "respect and reverence" him for being truthful and upright. While D. D. Palmer has been the means of restoring health to thousands; placing hundreds on the "road to wealth, a very few for avaricious greed and mercenary gain, have, childlike, tried to undermine his honor." These would-be fountain heads and developers "are cowards and kleptomaniacs, failing at every turn of the road."

---

"Philosophical physiology."

The above expression is incorrect. Philosophical means pertaining to, or in accordance with, philosophy. The expression the philosophy of functions or of physiology is correct.

Degree refers to a division, a space or interval.

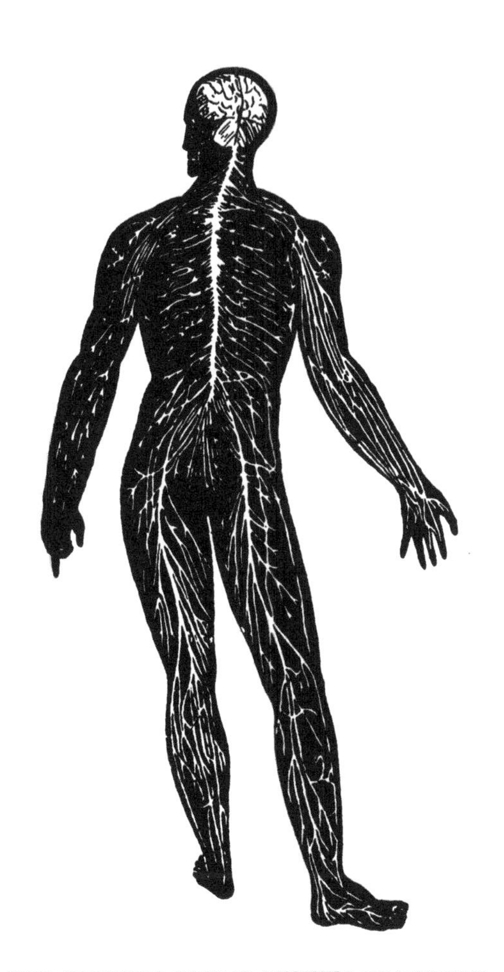

THE CEREBRO-SPINAL SYSTEM OF NERVES

The nervous system consists of the cerebro-spinal nervous system and the sympathetic nervous system

The cerebro-spinal nervous system is composed of the spinal cord and brain and of nerves joined to the brain and cord

## WHAT IS REST?

Physiologists are agreed that one day's rest in seven—a day's relief and relaxation from the monotony and strain of either physical or mental labor—is essential to health, strength and sanity.

When John Robinson, pastor of the flock that came to our shore in the Mayflower, landed at Plymouth, the day of rest was as severe, austere and solemn an occasion as a funeral.

On these same shores we have now another pastor, Dr. P. S. Grant, of New York, who would open theaters, parks and seashore places for the work-worried on their day off. His opinions, right or wrong, demonstrate the change a few generations have made.

Dr. Grant may be haunted by the menacing spirit of John Robinson, but he declares that the day will never come when everybody will go to church; hence, for those who will not go, other forms of entertainment must be provided so that they will not engage in other and worse pursuits because of idleness.

It seems to be a growing sentiment, that the day of rest should be one of recreation, a change of action and scenery; that the man or woman who is busy six days of a week should enjoy for one day the good things which those of us, who are not so busy, enjoy on week-days.

---

On the next page we give a cut of the nervous system as presented by a traveling lecturer on Chiropractic. This is some of his "specific, pure and unadulterated Chiropractic. Don't you quite agree" that "he is an original thinker, has not lived the lives of other men, has developed what came to him? He schemed" the cut on the opposite page. "He had an original way of presenting it. He is the one man of a million; he thinks out a problem. He will do in a day what others will take months or years to accomplish. Such a man of such huge, immense proportional success" does not object to such "trash, nonsense and stuff that wasn't Chiropractic. He has progressive ideas to give to his school. Where you will find one mental drone you will find others. You and we are in the work of Chiropractic." This cut was "schemed by the honored developer of Chiropractic."

The cut speaks for itself. It is in a strange contrast to that made by anatomists and Chiropractors who follow nerves in every conceivable zigzag direction. I only wish to add, that his ideas are not Chiropractic as taught by the originator and developer of this science and art.

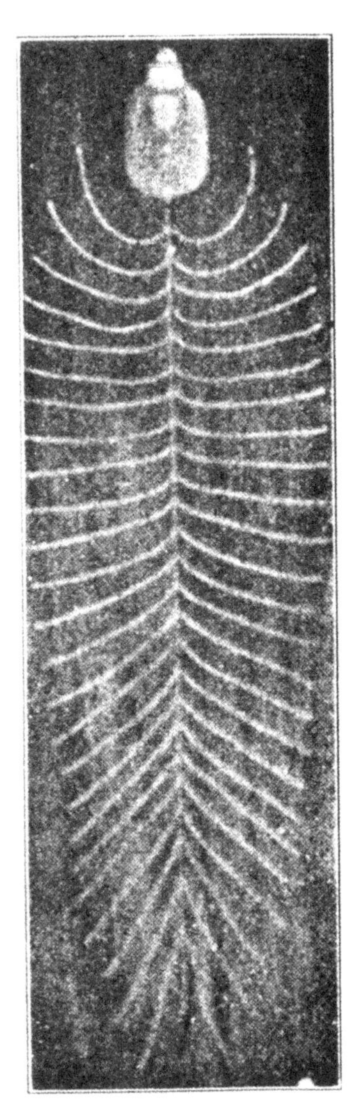

The above illustration is used to explain **"The Direct Brain System."**

"B. J. Palmer, in one of his addresses to his class in Portland this summer, aptly quoted, **'that he who tears down must rebuild greater,'** and said 'when I saw there was **no use for a Sympathetic Nervous System, I threw it out,** and then just had to put something better in its place, so **I discovered Direct Mental Impulse.'** "

## POISONS.

Poisons are substances which, when introduced into the body, either impair the function of one or more of its organs or destroy life. All poisons lead to a disturbance of the nervous system, no matter by what avenue it is introduced.

The lesions due to poisons may be local, as those from corrosives or caustics. In others the place of entrace is not affected, the pathological manifestations being due to nervous disturbance. Various forms of degeneration of necrosis may occur. The effect of a poison depends upon the nature of the substance, the amount and the individual.

---

The world's trouble is not in its badness, that which is seemingly bad is within us, that which is good should be developed instead of the bad. Wisdom is what is needed. Educators instead of hangmen will improve society. As it is with the sick in body, so it is with the sick in spirit. It is not by fear, punishment or threats that the sick are made whole; it is not by cruelty that the bad are made good. When a member of society has fallen, send for an educator to enlighten and remove the stumbling block, so that others may not fall.

---

Science is knowledge reduced to law and embodied in a system.

Philosophy is the knowledge of phenomena as explained by, and resolved into, causes, reasons, powers and laws.

Philosophy is the science of things divine and human, and the causes in which they are contained; the science of effects by their causes; the science of sufficient reasons; the science of things possible, inasmuch as they are possible; the science of things evidently deduced from first principles; the science of truths sensible and extract; the application of reason to its legitimate objects; the science of the relations of all knowledge to the necessary ends of human reason.

"Since normal nerve supply to any part of the body insures the existence of the **auto-protective power** necessary to **resist the invasion of disease**, to stop pathological processes, and to promote recovery of health—because, in short, an abnormal nerve supply means abnormal function and disease, while the existence of a normal nerve supply means normal function or health and the continuation of the same, except when **outside invasion** of etiological factors **overcome** the normal auto-protective powers."

The above does not look well in a book on Chiropractic; it savors more of suggestive therapeutics and medicine.

## SPINAL ADJUSTMENT.

"Spinal Adjustment" was written as an "important therapeutic auxiliary to the present methods of the healing art, for those who have prepared themselves for a life-work of combating the inroads of disease."

Spinal adjusting is not therapeutical—is not a **remedy** for the disturbed performance of vital functions. It does not remedy, it adjusts causes, so that Innate may correct abnormal functions and change morbid into normal structures.

Spinal adjusting is not an auxiliary to any method. To relieve an impingement in acute diseases by one adjustment in less than a minute, so Innate can transmit functions in a normal amount, is not an auxiliary to any method, neither does Chiropractic need any method as an auxiliary. Those who expect to put in a life-time combating disease, fighting the entrance of disease, as tho it was an enemy with hostile intent, should not learn Chiropractic. It is very difficult to change a medical fighter into a peaceful Chiropractor.

The author of Spinal Adjustment was a student of mine for four months. He tells us that, approximation (coming tc gether) of the vertebrae narrows the intervertebral foramina, thereby impinging upon nerves. The author makes no distinction between impinging upon and squeezing. The reader will please examine the cut on page 119. Now take your spinal column in hand as the developer of Chiropractic has done a thousand times. Observe that there are two articulations between the occiput and the atlas and two corresponding articulations between the atlas and axis. There is no intervertebral cartilage between them, as we find between vertebrae farther down the column. These articulations are covered with thin, hyaline (glass) cartilage which cannot pathologically be made any thinner, consequently, they cannot unduly approximate each other, narrowing the clefts or grooves between the occiput and atlas and the atlas and axis. The nerves cannot be pinched by their closure. I am well aware that the reader never attempts to show an investigator how a nerve can be squeezed between the occiput and atlas, or between the atlas and axis. However, we well know that there are many diseases arising from their luxation, not "approximation." "The first cervical vertebra, the one that articulates with the occipital bone, is very often subluxated. The atlas may be forcibly slipped to one side—to either the right or left—a lesion which constitutes a lateral subluxation.

"This pair of sub-occipital nerves are interfered with by lesions of the occipito-atlantal articulation, which lesions are called subluxations, and they are of quite frequent occurrence and an almost universal condition of advanced age."

This brings us to another step in the development of Chiropractic. The above statement being positively correct, then it is a fact that nerves are not pinched or squeezed in the grooves or clefts (not foramina) but, are **impinged against** by luxated, displaced, vertebrae.

The author of Spinal Adjustment says, "Practically all impingement of nerves is produced by subluxation or approximation of adjacent vertebrae, causing an alteration and narrowing of intervertebral foramina."

The author has two propositions mixed; viz., subluxation of vertebrae and the approximation of vertebrae. Subluxated vertebrae impinge upon nerves; vertebrae drawn together—an impossibility—would not impinge upon but squeeze nerves.

The author presents a cut, on page 147, of four dorsal vertebrae "showing compressed intervertebral discs and an impinged nerve from narrowing of the foramina." Why did he not select the atlas and axis? A close examination will disclose that the foramina are not narrowed because of the compressed intervertebral discs (cartilage), but because the bodies of the second and third are anterior to the first and second, a circumstance which cannot occur.

The author continually uses the term "impingement," for the condition of being pinched or squeezed. A condition of two bones that would pinch or squeeze a nerve would not impinge upon it, and vice versa. Contraction of muscles and ligaments might draw or rack a vertebra out of alignment by lateral displacement; but, "approximation" never. Furthermore, do you not see that there are no intervertebral cartilages or discs to be "thinned" between the atlas articulations above and below? For any vertebra to be displaced anterior or posterior to its neighbors, the intervertebral cartilage would have to be lacerated, which would be very improbable, either above or below, as represented in Fig. 33.

Another consideration. Cartilage may be diminished or totally destroyed by excessive heat, but as it is supplied with no nerves or blood vessels, it cannot be rebuilt; it can, however, be repaired by bands and straps of callus.

The author is away off on the proposition set forth, as he is also in his conclusion. As we have just said above, there is not

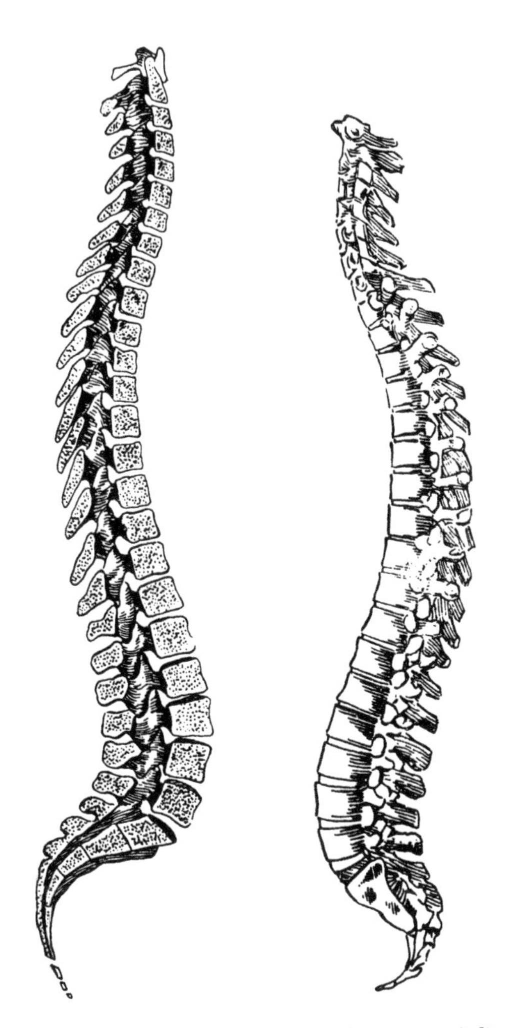

Spinal Columns, minus the intervertebral cartilage. The left one is sawn vertical, exhibiting the spinal canal

nor can there be any "approximation" of the atlas to the occipital bone; therefore, the loss of memory and mental activity will have to be sought for elsewhere. It is a well-known fact that age changes the quality of bones, muscles and nerves; also that the transmission of functions and its production is dependent upon the condition of nerves and muscles. "Slight pressure or impingement upon nerves will stimulate them to over action," but will not cause "lack of mental activity and loss of memory."

"Spinal windows partly closed."

I wonder where that boy got that idea of the spinal foramina being windows to be opened and closed at our pleasure for light and air. That must be of Bohemian origin, transferred from Oakley Smith, for I never saw anything like that in America. I was the author's teacher for four months and I am sure that I never referred to the foramina of the spine as being windows.

The author says, "Over-heat production is due to an undue excitability of the nervous system."

"In fever some stimulus acts upon the nerves, increasing their excitability, thus deranging the heat-production by causing the heat to generate faster than the same can be eliminated.

"Fever is a very common ailment, and from a very careful study of it the author has arrived at the conclusion that **the excessive heat-production,** causing a rise of temperature, **is due to an over-excitability of the nerves which is caused by the action of toxins** upon the thermogenic centers. The toxins may be produced by pathogenic bacteria, or may, in rare cases, be the result of an auto-intoxication, as in sunstroke or hysteria.

"**In all** infections and contagious **fevers the rise of temperature is due solely to the action of toxins of bacterial origin,** and their production in all cases follows a period of incubation.

"**If an infection is local, the fever caused will also be local** and will follow the development of toxins; however, we may have a general fever as the result of local infection, but in such cases there is absorption and dissemination of the toxic substance, produced locally, into the general circulation.

"**In no other case can we have fever except as a result of the action of toxins, and more commonly and almost universally as the result of toxins of bacterial generation.**

"**To stop any fever,** it is only necessary to **stop the production of the toxic poisoning** or to stop its absorption into the circulation."

How is that for Chiropractic? Is this placing Chiropractic "on a scientific basis"? ? ?

The author relates his case of mumps and that of his daughter, thirteen years of age. He does not tell his readers that I gave him that "special spinal adjustment" which so effectually relieved him. Neither does he give me the credit for that "single treatment which caused the symptoms to entirely disappear and the soreness to leave the parotid glands, nor for the complete recovery from mumps" of his daughter.

How did the adjustment stop the fever of mumps? What became of the bacteria which disappeared so quickly?

The author tries to describe a case. As I was the doctor I will correct the mistakes as related; the corrections are in parenthesis.

"At one time (the afternoon of July 12, 1903, in suite 15, Aiken Block, Santa Barbara, Cal.), a doctor (myself) was adjusting a subluxated vertebra that was interfering with (impinging upon) the spinal nerve supply (there was too much "supply") into one arm (A. R. Renwick's left hand, arm, shoulder and on up to spine was intensely hot). As a result of an impingement upon this nerve the arm was cold (intensely hot), numb (it was hypersensitive) and unnourished (being above normal heat there was too much functional activity). When the adjustment was made, in the presence of three or four persons (there were eight persons all told), for the relief of the nerve, this arm quickly became warm (it instantly became warm, being then of the same temperature as the rest of the body.) The thermic action set up (heat was lowered to normal) and the warmth that ensued (instead of dry and hot were so marked as to excite the immediate attention (before adjusting I had called the attention of the class of six) of the patient, of the doctor, and of the witnesses that were present.

"But another phenomena to be remembered in connection with this is, that the other arm became cold (became intensely hot), which had, previous to this time, been of a normal temperature. The subluxated vertebra had been thrown laterally a little too far, and while this relieved the impingement of the nerve that supplied the trophic (thermic) supply and functions of the one arm that had been cold (hot), the doctor thereby had impinged the nerve supply to the other arm ("Over-heat production is due to an undue excitability of the nervous system"), decreasing (increasing) at once the specific and thermic function in that one arm (to an abnormal degree).

"The doctor thought for a few minutes (I immediately asked, "was the body heated by blood or by nerves?" And was answered, "By nerves," by all), and asked the persons present what caused the production of heat."

The author of the above prevarication had to make the misstatement; the truth would spoil his bacterial premises and give me credit for discovering and announcing to the world that heat production is from the nerves and not from the blood.

The author says, "Such to you would appear quite foreign, especially when we consider the fact that this man (myself) was entirely ignorant of how the nerves make connection, through the sympathetic cord and through the superior cervical ganglion, with the auditory nerves."

It is surprisingly strange that the much belied man, who discovered every principle of Chiropractic, should be considered ignorant. It is to be regretted that some others are not blessed with some of that same kind of ignorance.

In the case of Roy Renwick, alluded to above, there was no "period of incubation," there were no "toxins of bacterial origin." The author says, "In no case can we have fever except as a result of the action of toxins," and this case alluded to had to be misrepresented in order to uphold the bacterial origin of inflammation and fever. I can at any time, and on any person, displace a vertebra and produce fever, the result of local inflammation. The discovery made by me, that the body is heated by nerves instead of by blood, is of vastly more importance than the discovery of the circulation of the blood by Harvey. I presume that he was lied about as much as I have been. Never mind, proper credit will be mine when I and my lying traducers have passed to the great beyond.

This discovery made by me that heat is from nerve functionating and not of the blood will, in time, knock the bacterial origin of fever into oblivion. It is difficult—impossible—to mix medical etiology and the causation of disease as known by Chiropractors.

The author says, "without auto-protection we would all succumb to the many pathogenic bacteria all about us and within us every day. Impingement interferes with auto-protection." Is that placing Chiropractic" on a scientific basis?" His pathogenic bacteria auto-protection is equaled by two cuts on pages 130 and 131 of the blind man whose sight was restored by B. J. Palmer—appropriating the other's man's credit is auto-protection. The author holds—see page 153—that heat is because of bodily combustion, a chemic action; therefore his distortion of the discovery of heat production.

The ideas presented by the author is only a belief. "We believe that within the tissues of the human body, or within the chemical laboratory of the human organism, there is produced an antidote against the invasion of practically all forms of bacterial or animal parasitic life.

"The best we can do in the case of endophytic parasites (one living within the body) is to restore the normal resistence, or auto-protection, that Nature may fight her own battles."

Just think of a chemist having a workroom, where he resolves compounds to their elements by analysis, and combines elements to make compounds. Within the tissues of the body is a very unsuitable place for a chemical laboratory. Think of an invasion of an army of bacteria; think of the antidotal fortifications nature erects for auto-protection; think of the resistence and the battles to be fought—in the minds of the author. If such be the case, is life worth living?

"Any interference with normal nerve force and energy in this (cervical) region will permit the entrance of disease germs and consequently pathological processes."

On several occasions I have relieved smallpox by one adjustment of the fifth cervical. How did a luxated fifth cervical allow disease germs to enter? Where did they find ingress and how did adjustment force them to decamp, and to what place did the invading hosts go? If the ignorant, magnetic healer had known as much about bacteria as the author of Spinal Adjustment, the science and art of Chiropractic would probably have been yet unknown.

"One hundred per cent nerve impulse necessary."

Per cent, per centum, by the hundred. Per cent is used to denote the proportion one ingredient bears to another—impulse is not composed of ingredients. We cannot per cent it by the hundred, as there is not a hundred of them. As an impulse is a sudden mental feeling that may urge an action, it would be talking nonsense to say ninety-nine per cent. An impulse is an impulse wholly or not at all; if it exists at all it cannot be in a per cent; it is either a mental force or it is not.

"I had, by giving him an adjustment, stimulated his central nervous system and re-established the normal processes of metabolism, thereby restoring ample heat-production."

By adjusting, removing an impingement, we do not stimulate or inhibit; we only make conditions favorable for Innate to restore vital force to normal; normal energy produces normal heat and normal physiological metabolism.

"**Each** special **nerve,** as it makes its exit from the spinal cord, **is surrounded by a sheath; included in this sheath is the artery** which supplies that segment of the cord from which the nerve originates, and **this sheath also contains the vein** which drains that same segment of the spinal cord."

Above this quoted paragraph is an "illustration showing the **Nerve Sheath containing Nerve, Artery and Vein,** passing unimpinged from the Neural Canal."

The nerve sheath, is known as the epineurium and is composed of the piameter and dura mater—see cut on page 67. This nerve sheath is only a covering for bundles of fibers which constitute the nerve. It in no wise covers, jointly or separately an artery or vein, altho the enveloping membrane is supplied with nerves and capillaries are to be seen arranged in long meshes between the fibers.

---

Life is action. Intelligent life is the soul.

Death is natural, whether physiological or pathological—natural change.

Disintegration, or decomposition, is not guided by intelligence.

The laws governing chemical changes and those guided by intelligence are dissimilar.

Poison destroys that which intelligent life has accomplished; changes physiological to pathological action.

Nerves are supplied with blood-vessels and nervi nervorum—small nerves which are distributed to the nerve-sheath—the covering. Each nerve, large or small, has within it the qualification of heat production—when in excess, it is known as inflammation.

A sensory nerve is one which carries sensation inward. A motor nerve transmits motor impulses—all impulses are motor—outward. If a sensory nerve be severed or injured at a designated point, the inflammatory and degenerative changes which may follow will be from the place of injury toward the spine. If a motor nerve be cut or injured, inflammation and degeneration will extend from the place damaged to the periphery. **Disease is too much or not enough functionating.** There may be atrophy of the nerve instead of inflammation. Degeneration, as a result of either extreme—atrophy or destruction—may extend not only to the spinal cord, but into it and upward to the brain; this can only exist in a sensory nerve.

Neuritis is inflammation of a nerve. As Chiropractors understand pathology, all inflammatory diseases—those in which the heat is supernormal, have neuritis, which may follow wounds or injuries. Neuritis may be acute or chronic. After inflammation subsides, the temperature may fall below normal. If so, the nerves will become sclerosed—hardened.

The first symptom of neuritis—inflammation of a nerve—is an aching pain which follows the course of the nerve affected. Pain is caused by pressure on an overly sensitive nerve. Pain is not as severe in soft tissue as in that which is hard and unyielding; for example, a felon is very painful because of the surrounding tissue being firm and unyielding and presses against the inflamed swollen nerve.

If the nerve be superficial it can be traced as a thick, hard cord. Its course may be marked by a red line, because of its condition.

In rheumatism we have more or less fever, while in neuralgia but little or none; in the former the sensation is that of an ache, while in the latter the pain is sharp. Why this difference? Take your spinal column in hand and be observant. The nerves are sensitive to pressure in either case. If you are not already acquainted with the pathway of the ganglionic nerve chain better look it up.

The cervical portion of the sympathetic, ganglionic, vertebral nerve chain is a prolongation upward of the primitive sympathetic. It obtains its spinal fibers from the upper dorsal nerves. The cervical ganglia supply fibers to the veins and arteries of the head, neck and upper limbs and to the skin of the head and neck, secretory fibers to the salivary glands and fibers to the heart.

In the neck the gangliated cord courses thru the foramina of the transverse processes of the cervical vertebrae, being continuous below with the thoracic gangliated cord and ending above in the brain cavity in the carotid plexus. Now, observe that the cervical portion passes thru openings, while the dorsal and lumbar lie against the bodies of the vertebrae and the heads of the ribs. In the latter, they, by a displacement, are pressed against; while in the cervical they are not only impinged upon but are elongated, made tense by displacement. Slip a cervical vertebra laterally and observe how it will press against the nerve, causing tensions. Be mindful of the sharpness of the impingement in the cervical; no longer wonder why neuralgia of the upper portion of the body should be of such a different character than that of rheumatism in the lower portion.

---

There is a vast difference between treating effects and adjusting causes. I was the first to adjust the cause of disease.

## WHY?

"If the subluxation theory is correct, what holds a vertebra in the abnormal position of subluxation in the acute stage? As the center of motion is so slightly changed, why does it fail to return to its normal position?"

Surgeons, anatomists and pathologists of the past have not considered subluxations only in the complete form. Therefore, this question has not come under consideration.

It will be observed that the lumbar vertebrae can be luxated only by a lateral movement of their bodies; while those of the cervical and dorsal are moved laterally by displacement of their articular processes. The axis of the abnormal movements (physiologically made pathological) of the lumbar is at the center of the articulating processes; while that of the cervical and dorsal is anterior to their bodies. Therefore, the bodies of the lumbar vertebrae impinge upon the outside edges of their superior and inferior articular processes. In the cervical, the displaced vertebra causes a tension on the sympathetic ganglionated chain.

Many subluxated vertebrae return of their own account, others do so by suitable accidents, while poisons acting as antidotes should be credited with a portion. But these forces do not return all displaced, wrenched vertebrae (the M. D.'s sprains) to their normal position. Why?

When movements are made more than normal, ligatures and muscles are unduly strained and stretched, the intervertebral cartilage is lacerated and torn from their bodies. **This violence causes them to lose, in a measure, their tonicity.**

---

"In fifteen cases wherein the stomach alone seemed involved, the most extensive group of spinal lesions in a given case was the fourth dorsal to the first lumbar inclusive; the highest was the third to the fifth dorsal; the lowest, the sixth dorsal to the second lumbar."

The writer of the above tells us that he finds, in stomach troubles, from three to ten vertebral lesions (subluxations); that the region where he looks for the cause of diseases of the stomach, covers from the third dorsal to the second lumbar—twelve vertebrae—half of the vertebral column. There is nothing definite, specific or scientific in this statement. It was made by an Osteopath and is, therefore, excusable.

If a displacement of the spine ever occurred causing impingement of the innervating nerves of the stomach, it could not cover the region named.

## REGENERATION OF TISSUE.

In biology, tissue is any one of the anatomical elements of which animals are composed, having a uniform structure and a special function. We have adipose tissue, a fatty tissue; areolar tissue, a fibrous connective tissue, one of the most generally distributed, for it is continuous thruout the body; cancelous tissue, the interior spongy part of bones; cartilaginous tissue, the gristle, which is of a medium consistency between bone and ligament. In the fetus it is a substitute for bone; in the adult it exists only in the joints and a few other places; connective tissue, that which connects and supports the frame, namely, cartilage, bone and fibrous connective tissue; dental tissue, the bony structure of the teeth; muscular tissue, voluntary and involuntary, both of which have the property of contracting and returning to their original shape; nervous tissue, tubular cords, which contain fibers, the function of which is to convey impulses and sensations from and to the brain, the brain being a part of the nervous tissue. Newly developed nervous tissue is less capable of functionating than that of older formation. Osseous tissue includes the bones; vascular tissue, that which constitutes long cylindric tubes for the conveyance of fluids, blood, chyle, lymph and serum. Inflammatory tissue is formed or grown from normal tissue, such as proud flesh; animal tissue is a general name for any of the textures which form the structure of the body.

Any tissue may become degenerated by disease or accidents. The destructive effects of inflammation are frequently repaired.

The ability to regenerate tissue differs in various species and in individuals of the same species. Animals with cold, white blood have more regenerative power than those with warm, red blood. The reproductive powers of some of the lower animals is astonishing when compared with that of human beings. The capacity to replace lost parts is greater in the young than in the aged.

A rise of temperature is always present during regeneration; this may be termed physiologic inflammation. Pathologic inflammation causes abnormal enlargements accompanied with vascular growths.

Regeneration occurs readily in the blood; also the epidermal covering of the cuticle and the epithelium of the mucous membrane. The nails grow full length in from four to five months; on the big toe in about twelve months, and more slowly in extremities with fractured bones, as the uniting of the fragments require a large portion of nutrition. The eyebrows are changed in from one hundred to one hundred and fifty days. The blood vessels and lymphatics are subject to extensive regeneration. The contractile quality of muscles may be regenerated if destroyed by necrosis. In large wounds, a fibrous cicatrix is formed. Immediate reunion of several nerves do not restore their functions at once. If a portion of a nerve-trunk be excised, the gap is filled with a juicy connective tissue.

In some glands the regenerative process goes on rapidly; in others it is comparatively slow. Partial removal of the liver and spleen has been replaced by regeneration. Cartilage is not regenerative, it is repaired by straps and bands of osseous callus. Regeneration of bone is too well known to need more than mentioning. Divided blood-vessels never reunite so as to form blood channels; the area supplied by them is replaced by other arteries. Severed nerves often unite, but their physiological action does not take place at once. If a nerve trunk is crushed or necrosed, the peripheral fibers, up to the point of injury, undergo degeneration. There is no means for Innate to forward nerve function past the disconnection, as it has no nerves or blood-vessels.

---

Chiropractic is a new profession, all others are old and crowded.

---

"The human body is likened to a machine, but in reality it is a machine-shop, occupied by a number of perfectly constructed machines supplied with power from a central source, never failing in the abundance of its supply. These machines are the organs of the body; the channels through which the organs receive their power are the nerves, the place of the emination of this power is the brain. From whence the power comes, we do not know. If man is ever able to conceive and explain from whence this power comes and what it is, he will have solved the problem of the universe."

The writer of the above (date 1908) says of himself, "He has been virtually connected with the science (since D. D. Palmer relieved him of consumption) for the last ten years. He is a lecturer of great ability, and is beyond a doubt the ablest instructor in the Chiropractic world."

There is no resemblance or likeness between a machine and the human body. A machine is an unimpassioned, automatic contrivance, composed of mechanical elements. The body is a self-conscious, appreciative, animated being.

## DON'T BLAME THE DEVIL.

The darkness of night recedes before advancing day;
So, the light of science has driven the Devil away;
But, as the shadows linger long in cellar and in tomb;
So yet, remains in many minds the old Satanic gloom.

An angry God with deadly plague chastised the world of old,
And cities knelt in filth and prayed that He His wrath withhold;
The hand of science with cleansing touch has checked the fever's sway—
God punishes man no more in this old-fashioned way.

This and many other follies knowledge has banished,
We trust the good work will go on till all have vanished;
It's up to Satan to be gone—"give the Devil his due,"
While I explain in truth, what he is supposed to do.

It is well for the young to love, for Nature points the way,
But, if men hate, it is Satan who leads their feet astray.
The laws of Nature give us thirst—the Devil pours the wines,
And perhaps, you think, that he helped me to write these lines.

There is no rule, but works both ways, which your law fails to do,
For if we love by Nature, we also hate by it, too;
Yet, all who live are ruled by the universal plan,
And Nature governs body and mind, of both worm and man.

It is Nature that stirs the tempest, and dashes high the waves,
That gives the wide, wide ocean to the mariner for his grave..
When the human mind is stirred by passion's wildest mood,
It is Nature, not Demon, that excites the surging blood.

When accidents and poisons shorten the life of any one,
Or the beating heart suddenly stops—its work for ever done,
Or dread consumption's blighting touch makes pale the cheek's bright bloom,
You say that "Nature points the way unto the silent tomb."

When no ray of reason lights the idiot's feeble mind,
Or when, each thought and word and deed is noble, true and kind;
Or though, man a fraud, wicked, low and base, as he can be;
It is but perverted Nature, wherein the cause I see.

I need not say what Nature is, or who sets her laws in motion,
But, her code rules all that live, on earth, in air or ocean;
And if all the misery of the world laid on my head,
I would not blame the Devil for what I had done or said.

It is known that sin is but disease, a weakness of the mind,
All ailments, indisposition and sickness one can find,
Are but results of vertebral displacements which unhinge
The nerves which Chiropractors by adjustments find impinged.

To say "the erring ones are of the Devil" is unkind—
Those misguided ones should deep and true compassion find;
We shall be nobler, happier far, as the world goes on,
Then what you call the Devil's work will be no longer done.

---

## CHANGES OF TEMPERATURE.

Carver: "Temperature in organs even of what is called normal, is not uniform."

The temperature varies a little in different parts of the body, that of the interior being greater than that of the surface. The blood coming from the liver is warmer than that from the lungs.

The temperature of man in health varies from 98 to 99 degrees. Heat is increased by the activity of muscular exercise. There is therefore a diurnal variation, the maximum being at 4 to 5 p. m., and the minimum at 3 a. m. If, however, the habits of work and sleep are reversed, the time of the occurrence of maximum and minimum of temperature, will be also changed.

The temperature of the mouth, axilla and rectum varies slightly.

At birth the temperature of the child is slightly above that of the mother. In old age the temperature rises, as a rule. Functional activity increases the temperature. The ingestion of a hearty meal increases the temperature. In starvation the temperature declines. Cold drinks lower and hot drinks raise the temperature. These changes of temperature are physiological.

Toxic doses lower the temperature. Subnormal temperature is found after an accident, shock, crisis of fevers or an operation; also in confusional insanity, heat, stroke and hysteria.

Severe injury to the dorsal region of the spinal cord often produces quite a fall in temperature. These changes are pathologic.

Changes in temperature may be physiologic or pathologic.

**CHIROPRACTIC (Ki-ro-prak-tik) is from two Greek words χειρ hand, πρακτος done—done by the hand—a hand practitioner—one who repairs—one who adjusts.**

The practitioner who practices the science of Chiropractic is a Chiropractor. The name of the science should not be spelled with a final "e." The art of adjusting is of a peculiar nature, one which had never been used before September, 1895. In some respects it has been modified. For instance, we find on page 58 of Neuropathy the method I taught Dr. Davis in October, 1898. "Starting at the base of the brain, at the atlas, we regulate all the nervous system involved by **our particular treatment** in the adjustment of the atlas. This is done while the patient is lying down, on the side of the head, face or front side of the body turned towards the bench. Now, then, with the head turned from you, you place the hand with the fist closed and the little finger knuckle under the mastoid process, and with a sudden movement downward, right arm stiffened, we usually get a click in the neck. This must be with sufficient force to give the cervical region a spring. This separates the facets of the two bones—that is, the articulating surfaces—and lets the air in and gives the sound."

"**Our particular treatment**" in adjusting the atlas was taught A. P. Davis by me before I knew of vertebral axial centers. Some of our earlier students will recognize it. We soon learned that the tissue over the spinous processes of the atlas became very tender. We now adjust on the posterior arch. We do not now, and have not for many years, used the "fist closed" while adjusting any vertebrae.

"In the (page 65) Neuropathic department the spinal adjustment is the main treatment."

"In the Osteopathic department much is dependent upon physical manipulations."

"The bunglesome manner (page 130) in which either, and in fact both, are taught and practiced and has been of considerable criticism, until we brought about harmony and favorable results and larger satisfaction from patients, by making out of these two methods a plausible, rational, scientific, systematized method and began to apply it in the treatment of diseases. And now, as **we have evolved** an entirely new system, based upon the law of freedom of the nervous system and named it the Neuropathic System, we are ready to demonstrate its superiority over all known methods of healing."

A. P. Davis is not favorable to a one-horse-shay; he likes to drive a seven-in-hand. He desires to be a Neuropath—one who is affected with nervous diseases.

He has "evolved an entirely new system," one composed of all the different systems with which he has become familiar. He is "ready to demonstrate the superiority" of the seven horse team, which he designates Neuropathy, "over all known methods" by using the principles of each, so far as he knows.

"While both (Osteopathy and Chiropractic) these discoveries (page 129) are marvelous, so far as the treatment, as well as the results, are concerned, yet the claims of the discoverers are founded on hypotheses rather than on real anatomical and physiological facts; and yet this seems arrogant to assume and would be, but for the known ability of the writer regarding both these so-called philosophies, especially the application of them practically, scientifically. It is a demonstrated fact that the founders of **both theories** are unlearned men and have but little understanding of the real facts concerning the fundamental principles of what they accidentally discovered."

That "known ability of the writer regarding" Chiropractic as a science and an art is very limited. Dr. Davis knows nothing of Chiropractic as a science or an art; see another article. All discoveries are more or less accidental, but the purloining of the seven systems of which Neuropathy is composed, was not accidental, it was a downright steal.

"That these two sciences (page 73) are based upon the same philosophy cannot be denied; but each of the claimants of the discoveries certainly have the one and the same philosophy and only a different method of applying it, and as the difference of treatment produces, many times, a different effect, it can be truly said that they seem like entirely different sciences; for it is absolutely true that one might receive the teachings of the one and know nothing as to how to apply the treatment of the other, to accomplish an expression of the same philosophy—'that of freedom of the nervous system.' One being called an Osteopath and the other a Chiropractor."

The philosophies of Osteopathy and Chiropractic are radically and entirely different.

The practitioners of Chiropractic are never called "a Chiropractic," except by those who are ignorant regarding its nomenclature. The practitioner of Chiropractic is a Chiropractor. A musician is one who plays music.

"Neuropathy (page vii.) is the discovery (?) of the author of this volume, 'Neuropathy.' "

**"Neuropathy is applied in the treatment of all conditions wherein the nervous system is involved."**

"When **Neuropathy** (page liii.) **is thoroughly comprehended it will be found that** the manipulations will be **much better adapted to the** accomplishment of the **purpose than any other known.**"

"**We lay much stress** (page 15) **upon the spinal treatment** in the Neuropathic department of this book."

"**Neuropathy** (page liv.) **has for its sphere the removal of nerve pressure and irritation of nerve filaments.**"

"**Neuropathy** (page 8) **is the name of the method used for all that is to be done to relieve conditions called disease,** but the terms Osteopathy, Chiropractic, Ophthalmology, Suggestion or Magnetism, designates the how it is applied."

In the last six paragraphs, replace Neuropathic treatment with Chiropractic adjustment, as the change of the word Chiropractic for the word Neuropathy constitutes the discovery of Dr. Davis.

Neuropathy is composed of Osteopathy, Chiropractic, Ophthalmology, Suggestion, Magnetic, Phrenology and Medicine. These names "designate the how it is applied."

Neuropathy is like a modern crazy quilt, or Joseph's coat of many colors.

Dr. A. P. Davis is the discoverer of Neuropathy, **a system of systems,** an inharmonious medley, of which the principles of no two agree.

Osteopathy and Chiropractic "are really (page liii.) for the same purpose—freeing of the nervous system—and they being of my own improvising (?), may as well be classed under the name Neuropathy as not."

The "improvising" consists of adopting these two sciences as his own, on the spur of the moment, without due consideration.

"It will be understood (page liv.) that Osteopathy is more especially applied to restore the circulation of the fluids of the body than for any other purpose."

"The spinous processes (page 39) will be noticed to vary as to contour in many conditions, which it is well to know about, the cause and why we aim to regulate them in our treatments."

"We recognize (page 258) the fact that the best means of restoring health and maintaining it in all climates, is **right living.**"

If so, why study the contour of the spinous processes?

If your medical prescriptions will cure by one application, afford speedy relief, will be found efficacious, will arrest and cure, are excellent remedies, cure in twenty-four hours, as you state, why is it well to know about the spinous processes?

If the Homeopathic remedies supply the elements needed to harmonize the body with itself, why spend time in regulating the spinous processes?

If a knowledge of Phrenology furnishes the means essential to harmonize the body, why take special notice of the contour of the spinous processes?

If the influence of magnetism can be directed to the cure of all diseases, why observe the variations of the spinous processes?

If disease is a migratory, mental ideality, an imaginary something, that may be eliminated, driven out by intense thinking, why waste time noticing the abnormal position of the spinous processes?

If it is a fact that all diseases are due to nerve waste, as you state, that as soon as nerve waste is stopped health is restored, why regulate the spinous processes.

If it is a well-known fact, as stated on page 329, that disease is caused by interrupted circulation, that the application of Osteopathy will almost miraculously change the tissue from disease to that of health, why use spinal adjustments?

If Neuropathy is the method used by you for all conditions called disease, and there is nothing else which so effectually accomplishes the purpose, why use any other method? If other methods were not utilized to construct a system for Neuropathy, would it not be a phantasma of the human mind?

If the secret of spinal adjustments in curing disease is the uniting of the two forces, why observe the various positions of the spinous processes?

If it is a fact that, no matter what means are used, the object accomplished is through Neuropathy, why learn any other method?

"We mean (page 47) something by this spinal adjustment treatment and no one is properly a scientific manipulator who does not understand how to adjust the spine, even if all taught by Osteopaths has been applied; for **there is nothing comparable in osteopathic manipulations which so effectually accomplishes the purpose as this does**; for no one in Osteopathy has ever known how to apply these treatments but those who have taken special instructions therein."

Dr. A. P. Davis took "special instructions therein" when Chiropractic was three years of age. Were he to take a course now under the same instructor, he would find an advancement of eleven years and a course of ten months instead of two weeks.

A study of Neuropathy shows its author is not a "scientific manipulator" of "spinal adjustment treatment." For proof of this statement see another article.

"Whether, therefore, (page 8) we use Osteopathy to free the circulation of the blood, or Ophthalmology to arrest nerve waste, or Chiropractic adjustments to remove nerve pressure, or Suggestion to stimulate mental energy, or Magnetism to concentrate mentality and change molecular polarization, the object is accomplished through the one means—Neuropathy."

What magnetism has to do with, or how it changes, "molecular polarization," I am unable to say as I do not comprehend the polarization of bodily molecules, or what change in or upon the body can be affected by polarization. Does not this portion of the harness belong to the center horse—Ophthalmology—of the lead team? Rays of light or heat may be polarized, but molecules of the body—never. I understand that the heptagonal team—Neuropathy—is composed of Osteopathy, Ophthalmology, Chiropractic, Suggestive Therapeutics and Magnetism, also, the old reliable Broncho, Medicine, and the handy pony, Phrenology; that, whatever relief or cure is accomplished by any one of this heptahexahedral team, is credited to Neuropathy.

The driver of a Neuropathic team is known as a Neuropath—a person of a nervous organization, one who has, or is liable to be affected with, nerve diseases.

---

In the preface of Carver's Chiropractic Analysis we find, "The Chiropractic Principles herein stated are those which have been demonstrated by the author to be accurate."

If Dr. Carver has given in his book of 486 pages one Chiropractic principle, I have failed to find it.

The last sentence of the preface reads, "For the present, however, it is hoped that this book will serve the student and practitioner in his advancement along Chiropractic lines, I

Chiropractors do not, or at least should not use tools with which to adjust. They do not use instruments, such as hammers, chisels, saws, planes or files; they are not using implements to perform mechanical operations.

How a book can be made to serve as a tool, utensil, implement, machine or instrument is past my comprehension. To the first person directing my attention to the page and paragraph wherein there is a thot or a hint which will serve the student or practitioner as a necessary and efficient working tool."
will present a copy of The Chiropractor's Adjuster.

## ORGANOTHERAPY.

Organotherapy is the treatment of diseases by the internal administration of animal organs or their extracts. In medical books, hundreds of years old, of which I have several, every portion of an animal, bird, snake, fish, insect and of man himself, was recommended and used as medicine for diseases. A less variety is in use today, but they are used in a similar manner and for the same purpose.

The thyroid gland, desicated, or extracts from it, are given for myxedema, cretinism, skin diseases, obesity, colloid and exophthalmic goiter. Testicular extract is used for various nervous affections. From testicular juice, spermin has been isolated and its use advised in nervous depression, debility and asthma. The extract of pancreas is used for diabetes mellitus. The dessicated suprarenal bodies—glands adjoining the kidneys —or an extract from them, are used in Addison's disease and for the suppression of catarrhal secretion. Bone marrow is used for anemias. Other extracts are made from the brain, spinal marrow, muscles, ovary, testes, heart-muscle, spleen, thymus gland and stomach.

Homologous organotherapy is founded upon the notion that the extracts of organs of animals corresponding to the diseased organ of the patient should assist in its recuperation and regeneration. This superstitious ignorance is born of the barbaric notion of the uncivilized, that the eating of the heart of your enemy will make one strong, brave and fearless.

Heterologous organotherapy consists in the use of those substances of animal organs which have no relation whatever to the disease of the patient.

In the above methods, we have physiological Allopathy and Homeopathy. Is it not time that we, as an enlightened nation, should lay aside all superstitious notions and correct the cause of disease?

---

The movements devised and perfected by D. D. Palmer are unique, unlike any used by any other school; they are direct as desired by a Chiropractor who should make a specific move for a certain purpose with an aim in view.

---

A Chiropractor who comprehends the principles of this science will have no use for adjuncts. Just in proportion as he lacks knowledge and confidence (the two go together) he will use remedies, become a mixer. The more he mixes the less use he has for Chiropractic.

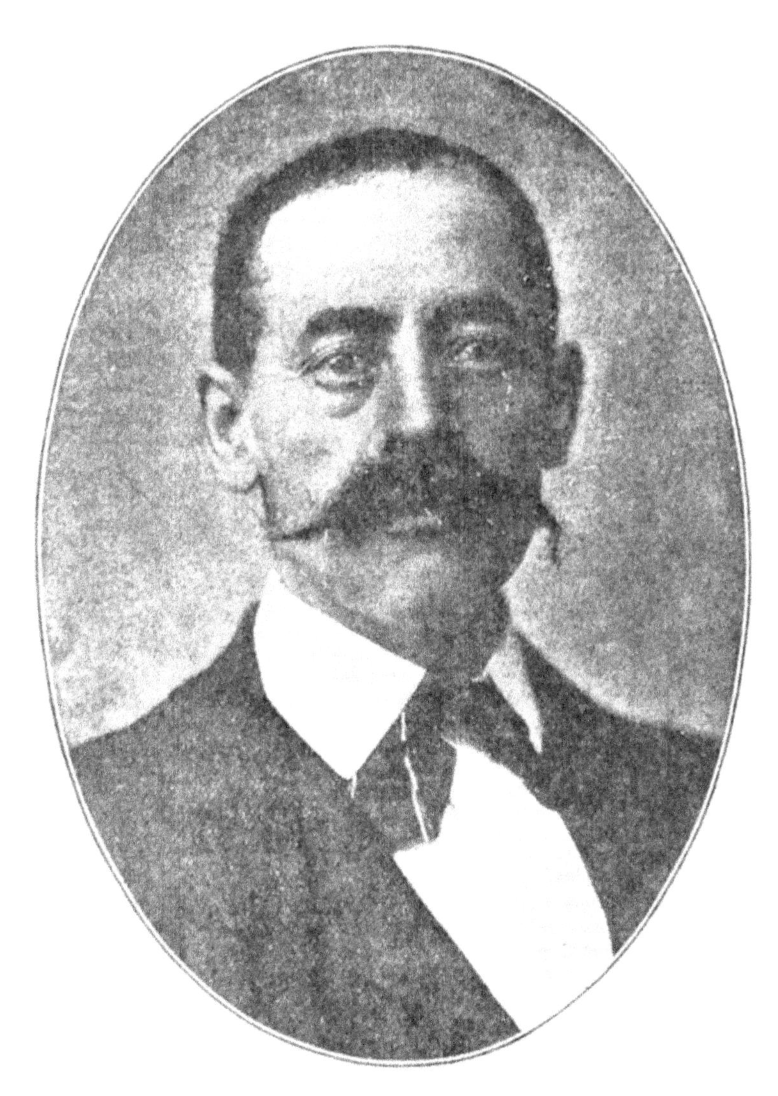

The above is a likeness of Harvey Lillard, the first person who received a Chiropractic adjustment from the hands of D. D. Palmer.

On Sept. 18, 1895, Harvey Lillard called upon me. He was so deaf for seventeen years that he could not hear the noises on the street. Mr. Lillard informed me that he was in a cramped position and felt something give in his back. I replaced the displaced 4th dorsal vertebrae by one move, which restored his hearing fully.

"Whether obstructions occur (page 377) as a result of changes in the weather, direct cold, or to continuous exposure of the body, or any part of it, to a lower temperature than normal, or to direct pressure, such as bandages, tight lacing, overcrowded vessels, impediment due to lack of fluidity of the blood, paralysis of nerves controlling the circulation in any or many parts of the body, any one or all of these causes may be and are the cause or causes of the pathological conditions that afflict mankind. Our whole theory has its origin, support, conclusion on this idea, this fundamental and unheard-of cause of disease, and perhaps unthought-of by other diagnosticians. And while we would not desire to appear dogmatic in this regard, we firmly believe that all pathological conditions are traceable to obstructed circulation somewhere in the system, and that removed, the patient has a better opportunity of recovery than from the possible influence of medication. It surely seems more rational to take off the pressure producing the pain of a morbid condition, than to impose more labor, to care for some other foreign substance that has no earthly relationship with the system, and cannot possibly have, with the idea of the necessity involved in the premises."

The above paragraph will require close study in order to comprehend the author's meaning, as it is troubled with imperspicuity, unintelligibility. I think the doctor means to say: —He has a **theory as to the cause of disease,** one unheard-of, and perhaps unthought-of, by other diagnosticians. His whole theory has its origin, support and conclusion in the fundamental idea that pathological conditions are caused by obstructed circulation somewhere in the system, as the result of some one of the six causes mentioned in the forepart of the above paragraph, which cause pressure.

He does not desire to appear dogmatic, but it is **his theory** (to which he has a right), that, if the obstruction were removed the patient would have a better opportunity of recovery than from the possible influence of medication; that it would be more rational to **take off the pressure which produced the morbid condition**; that medication, instead of relieving the system, imposes more labor upon it.

The idea of **taking off the pressure** remaining a theory with Dr. Davis; that "our whole theory" was unheard-of and perhaps unthought-of by any other than Dr. Davis! I have good reason to believe that he has been taught by Dr. Still and myself to take off the pressure. To be sure, the Osteopath's idea of taking off the pressure is different from that of Chiropractors, but he is well acquainted with both.

## CHIROPRACTIC NOT OSTEOPATHY.

Chiropractic is unlike any therapeutic method, in fact it is not therapeutical. Osteopathy is the only system which has similar features, and they, as promulgated by the founders, are as different as day is from night. A. P. Davis, a graduate under the founders of both systems, said: "The methods of Chiropractic and Osteopathy differ in application and results, as well as in name. There is no resemblance in the treatment and but little in any way except the philosophy. The application of the two is so different that learning either one gives no clue to the other."

In 1874 A. T. Still stated his observations as follows: "A disturbed artery marks the period to an hour and minute, when disease begins to sow its seeds of destruction in the human body. That in no case could it be done without a broken or suspended current of arterial blood, which by nature, is intended to supply and nourish all nerves, ligaments, muscles, skin, bones and the artery itself. The rule of the artery must be absolute, universal and unobstructed, or disease will be the result. All nerves depend wholly upon the arterial system for their qualities, such as sensation, nutrition and motion, even though by the law of reciprosity they furnish force, nutrition and sensation to the artery itself."

"Disease sowing seeds of destruction" does not affiliate with Chiropractic philosophy. "A disturbed artery." What disturbs the action of the vascular system? The science of Chiropractic says: The carrier of impulses, the nervous system, is modified in its structure, conformably modifying the impulsive force and actions of functions.

It will be observed that Osteopathy is founded on the circulation of the blood, whereas, Chiropractic is founded upon the quality of nerve tissues and its ability to transmit functionating impulses. Instead of nerves depending upon the arterial system for their quality of sensation, nutrition and motion, it is a fact, established by Chiropractic, that the arterial system depends upon the nervous system for the incentive stimulus which the latter possesses.

From the **Journal of Osteopathy** I quote: "How Osteopathy Treats the Blood. It is well known that pure blood is an absolute essential for health. The blood is the medium whereby all organs and parts of the body are supplied with nourishment for repair and growth.

"There are five ways, at least, in which the blood is influenced and treated by Osteopathy.

"The general Osteopathic treatment is something more than

a modified combination of massage and Swedish movements. Simply something more by virtue of additional manual spinal column stretching and rib separating."

Osteopathy in its treatment consists of massage, Swedish movement, rib-separating, manual and mechanical spinal column stretching. Chiropractors use none of these.

That the investigator may see the difference between the two methods, I append Osteopathy defined by Dr. William H. Cobble, an Osteopath:

"Osteopathy is a science of drugless healing, based upon the principle that the body has been endowed by Nature with all the fluids and forces necessary for the preservation of health and recovery from disease, providing the mechanism which produces and distributes these fluids and forces is in perfect mechanical adjustment."

Dr. A. P. Davis, a student of the first class in Osteopathy under A. T. Still, the Founder, states in his masterly work of 851 pages:

"Diseases are recognized as only the result of the interruption of the onward flow of the fluids of the body, in their various rounds to build up and tear down the various tissues in itself, and that when these tissues are normally built up and the waste material properly eliminated, health is the inevitable result."

In Osteopathy, pure blood is physiological; the result is health. Impure, bad, poisoned, stagnant, obstructed, diseased blood is pathological. In Chiropractic, health depends upon the proper performance of functions. Disease is the result of functions performed in an abnormal manner. Whether functions are physiologically or pathologically performed depends upon the amount of force manifested at the peripheral endings of nerves, where functional impulses are received. Osteopathy treats the blood. Chiropractors do not treat the blood—do not treat any portion of the body or any of its ailments.

The general treatment of Osteopathy: They do have specific treatment. At present Chiropractors almost invariably use a general treatment. The Chiropractic world does not yet seem ready for scientific, specific adjusting. I have had four partners, during the last fourteen years, not one of whom ever learned special, specific, scientific adjusting. Is it possible that the intelligence of the world has not yet arisen to the acceptation of Chiropractic as a science? Is specific adjusting, in advance of this age? This book aims to teach specific adjusting, making Chiropractic a science—any one can learn to give general adjusting.

Quoting yet farther from the **Journal of Osteopathy**: "Osteopathy also offers much along the line of treatment of rendering and keeping the blood germicidal."

The above characteristics are not those of Chiropractic.

**Osteopathic Health** says: "Altered blood flow means disease, the body is such a machine."

The body a machine! Altered blood flow causes the machine to be erratic in its movements! Such is Osteopathy and I am sorry to know that many, very many Chiropractors have absorbed so much of Osteopathy which they try to palm off as Chiropractic.

I, as the developer of Chiropractic, have always maintained, that when a nerve is interfered with by pressure or other injury, sooner or later, its expression becomes abnormal, manifesting conditions named disease. The vital force which controls all actions of the ligaments, muscles, bones, skin, membranes and arteries, also regulates the circulation and transudation of the bodily fluids. The vital force of Innate, communicated thru the nervous system, produces functional activity, regulates the force and amount of blood by contracting and relaxing the muscular tissue of the vascular walls, produces, by excitation, the characteristic amount, quality of force and observed in health and disease. Because of this supervision thru the nervous system, I hold that the variation of functions is also co-ordinate with the amount of heat—local inflammation and general fever. Hence, it necessarily follows that this body is functionated by nerves—not by blood as has been taught by all schools of medicine, including that of Osteopathy.

**The Pacific School of Osteopathy** says: "The legal definition of Osteopathy is a system, method or science of treating human diseases." Chiropractors do not treat diseases. They adjust, put to rights, that which is creating disease. I discovered that all parts of the human body are functionated by and thru nerves. If impulses were normally transmitted, their functions would not be augmented nor decreased.

Dr. A. T. Still defined Osteopathy as follows: "Dr. Still reasoned that a natural flow of blood is health, and disease is the effect of local or general disturbance of blood; that to excite the nerves causes muscles to contract and compress venous flow of blood to the heart; and the bones could be used as levers to relieve pressure of nerves, veins and arteries."

This pressure is referred to on Page 174 of **The Philosophy and Principles of Osteopathy** by Dr. A. T. Still. "We feel we have proven the frequent and even common occurrence of 'wreckage' of the bowels, bladder and womb, held down by contracture of the abdominal wall, the weight of the bowels with their contents, the womb and its congested body and all attached membranes and fascia, with the added weight of **congestion caused by detained venous blood.** Further wreckage continues by **interference with the arterial blood,** which is stopped from reaching its natural landings. Another consequence is a great enlargement of veins, lymphcells, cysts and tubes of receipt and distribution. The excretory channels also become shocked and confused as effects of the first pelvic wreck. From that confused pile of wreckage, we can easily account for the formation of tumors on the uterus, bladder, rectum, and for all diseases of the abdominal viscera, such as tuberculosis of the bowels, kidneys, liver, pancreas and spleen. All these effects are possible, all are reasonable and **all are indisputable effects that follow wreckage of the organs of the abdomen.**''

Please read the above explanation once more, and see what the founder of Osteopathy considers the cause of a large share of diseases. The above is Osteopathy by the founder who ought to know what constitutes Osteopathy. I fail to see any resemblance between it and Chiropractic.

**The Des Moines Osteopath** says of rheumatism: ''It is highly probable that the exciting cause is a micro-organism. Out of the laboratories of the body appear antidotes for the toxins and poisons for the invaders.''

Chiropractors consider the micro-organism a scavenger—not a cause. The Osteopath drops into the time-worn ruts of the Allopaths—antidotes, disease is an invader, a fight on hand. The body a laboratory, it manufactures antidotes to combat disease; poison for poison. This is not Chiropractic.

**The Journal of Osteopathy** says: ''Bony lesions, such as hip dislocation, vertebral and innominate deviations, as a rule, draw the softer tissues out of line, and this disarrangement or the tension of the ligaments and muscles causes an abnormal pressue on associated blood-vessels and nerves.''

There is a vast difference between drawing the softer tissues (the viscera) out of line and the drawing of hard tissue (bones) out of alignment.

Dr. George A. Still says in **The Journal of Osteopathy**: ''The continued source of energy and, in fact, the nourishment of the entire system, I found to be a dark red fluid called blood. An unobstructed, healthy flow of arterial blood is life.''

Osteopathy states: The source of energy, the vital force, which furnishes life, functional activity, is from the dark red fluid called blood. Chiropractors affirm that the primal source of energy, vital force, is Innate, spirit, directed thru the nervous system. The fundamental principles as well as the philosophy of Osteopathy and Chiropractic, differ very much.

Dr. George A. Still further says: "In our schools we teach all that the best men of other systems of therapeutics study."

Therapeutics is that branch of medical science which considers the application of remedies as a means of cure. As Chiropractors do not use medicine and have no need of remedies, therefore Chiropractic is not therapeutical; has no resemblance to any therapeutic system.

G. S. Archer, D. O., of Davenport, Ia., says in his circular: "Osteopathy has nothing in common with Chiropractic."

E. H. Laughlin, D. O., in his **Practice of Osteopathy,** gives the following for whooping cough: "Relax all tissues involved, remove the lesion, free the circulation about the larynx and whole respiratory tract, stimulate the lungs, raise the clavicles and ribs and remove all sources of irritation to the laryngeal innervation. To relieve the cough, treat down along the larynx and trachea and about the angle of the jaw. A general treatment should be given to avoid the complications and sequelae that may arise. The patient should be carefully protected from changes of temperature. During the catarrhal or febrile stage the patient should be confined to the bed. The diet should be light and nutritious. Hygiene is an important factor."

The above Osteopathic treatment takes an hour or more. The Chiropractor who is specific in his work, adjusts one vertebra giving relief at once.

Dr. A. T. Still says: "A lesion may and does appear on a part or all of the person which may appear as a growth or withering away of a limb in all its muscles, nerves and blood supply."

A lesion is an injury, hurt or wound. In pathology, any morbid change in the exercise of functions or the texture of organs is a lesion. A lesion may be the cause of morbidity or may consist of morbid change in function or tissue. It may be the receiver, or the cause, of an injury. There are many kinds of lesions. Central lesion: one affecting the central nervous system. A diffused lesion: one involving all the tissues of an organ. A focal lesion is one limited in its area. An irritative lesion is one in the nervous system which excites the functions of the part wherein it is situated. An organic lesion is a morbid structural change in the tissues of an organ. Initial lesion, the chancre, the initial lesion of syphilis, which is followed by a pathological condition of the whole system. Traumatic lesion: one due to an injury. A toxic lesion is one due to poison.

The Osteopathic treatment for diphtheria consists of more

than 200 different movements, consisting of what is called general and specific treatment, such as pulling, stretching, rotating, raising clavicles and ribs, kneading muscles; in fact, a general overhauling of the whole body, to do which takes a good operator one and a half hours. This is to be repeated every six to eight hours. The object of these manipulations is to prevent stagnation and fermentation and to equalize the circulation of the bodily fluids.

The Osteopath manipulates; the Chiropractor does not. The former uses many movements with the hands, which amounts to manipulation; the latter does his work by one movement, does not manipulate. I here refer to a Chiropractor who is specific, one who adjusts one vertebra with a special purpose. A Chiropractor who adjusts "all up and down the spine" is a manipulator. Dr. Arnold's adjusting, referred to in another part of this book, is manipulation.

The Osteopathic treatment for typhoid fever as given by E. H. Laughlin in his **Practice of Osteopathy** is as follows: "Relax all tissues involved, remove any spinal, rib, vertebral or muscular lesion present; give a careful cervical treatment (do not fatigue the patient); stimulate the lungs and heart; most of the treatment should be directed to the spine; quiet the nervous system; keep the kidneys active; gently spring the spine; in giving the spinal treatment pay much attention to the lower dorsal and lumbar regions. Treat the diarrhea in the usual way. (As given on page 41.) Relax the tissues along the spine, remove the lesion, inhibit the spine from the sixth dorsal to the coccyx, raise the ribs, free the general circulation and treat the liver. Have the patient lie on his face, place one hand over the lower lumbar region and the other beneath his knees; then press down with the hand on the lumbar region and at the same time lift up with the other hand, being careful not to lift too high and hurt the patient. Treat the liver and spleen, raise the ribs and the intestines with great care. Treat the superior cervical ganglion for the fever. This regulates the systemic circulation by affecting the general vaso-motor center in the medulla. Inhibition of peristalsis should be done by work from the ninth dorsal down along the lumbar region."

The Chiropractic adjustment for typhoid consists of one move, one displaced vertebra to be replaced, and that is adjusted by one thrust. How different to that given above—where is the resemblance—where the similarity—where any likeness? Osteopathic treatment and Chiropractic adjustment have no corresponding features. Osteopathic treatment and Chiropractic adjustment have nothing in common.

The Allopath and Osteopath agree on etiology and diagnosis; the only difference being that the latter tries to do with the hands what the former aims to do with drugs. These two systems contend that diphtheria is an enemy, a disturber of the peace; that it is caused by an invasion of bacteria; that there are good and bad bacteria, friends and foes. It is the business of the bacteriologist to devise ways and means whereby he can assist the friendly microbes to drive out or destroy the disease-provoking microorganisms.

Chiropractors look upon bacteria as scavengers who live upon dead and decaying matter. Their existence is as much a natural result as is the mold found in decaying cheese. We understand that necrosed mucous membranes are the result of excessive heat, local inflammation; that deleterious substances act upon sensory nerves, causing them to be unduly excited, inflamed. If these affected nerves end in the throat, in persons of a certain age, we have conditions known as diphtheritis. The Chiropractor replaces the luxated vertebra by one move which does not amount to a manipulation. The patient is usually relieved by one adjustment. Wherein is there any resemblance between Chiropractic and Osteopathy?

Some Osteopaths are advancing toward Chiropractic; while others are retreating back into Allopathy. Dr. Geo. A. Still makes mention of A. T. Still, saying: "At these foramina we find the seat of ninety-five per cent or more of the lesions." In all of A. T. Still's writings, he does not make mention of ninety-five per cent of diseases being connected with spinal foramina. Instead, I find in A. T. Still's book on Osteopathy of 319 pages, only seven lines which refer to vertebral displacements, and these are called **twisted vertebrae.** He frequently refers to colds, sudden changes in temperature, electrical shocks, poisons, bacteria, germs and pressure on blood vessels as being causes of disease. It abounds in such expressions as bad, impure, poisoned, obstructed, stagnant, detained, stoppage, a lack of, shortage of, lack of drainage, fermentation and diseased blood as being disease producing. He also gives fecal impaction, retention of lymph and chyle, a lack of or too much gas, constricted organs piling on each other, deposits in veins, dried ear wax and displaced ribs as causes of disease.

Why should Dr. Still give, as causes, those mentioned in the above paragraph and in the "wreckage" section, if he believed that "ninety-five per cent or more of lesions" were to be found at the spinal foramina?

Is Chiropractic Osteopathy? Wherein is there any resemblance?

## WHAT DO YOU THINK OF THAT?

I have a styloid process four inches in length and, in no portion, less than a quarter of an inch in diameter. It articulated with the hyoid bone at the junction of its body and the great cornu; also with the temporal bone in a fossa similar to that of the glenoid or mandibular fossa. Its mate is of the same size, but has an articulation midway. The hyoid bone is usually an inch in length and not more than three-eighths of an inch in diameter. The hyoid is normally supported by muscles from the styloid processes. In this instance it is supported by long bones instead of muscles, and the styloid is not a process but a separate bone. The hyoid bone is the only bone in the body which normally does not articulate with other bones, but in this instance, it articulates with two bones.

---

"When you have impulses that are tied up as in a cramp; then you feel pain. Those impulses are coming to the subluxation normally and from that on they are doubled up."

An impulse is an abrupt vivid suggestion of the mind or spirit which prompts an immediate action. Impulses are carried over the nerves by the waves of vibration.

---

A Chiropractic college announces:—"We are agents for the Twentieth Century Appliances. Besides the Solar Therapeutic Lamp and the Electric Light Bath Cabinet, we sell the Arc Lamp, Centrifugal Vibrator, Diet Indicator, Kellog Douche, Home Douche, Dynometer, Hand Photophore, Kneading Apparatus, Massage Table, Sinusoidal Apparatus, Thermophore and Vibratory Chair.

"We are also agents for the Ampliathrill, the greatest auxiliary for use in Spinal Treatment of the Twentieth Century."

He further adds:—"The Solar Therapeutic Lamp is the greatest, most powerful and most helpful light ever invented. Absolutely relieves pain. Stimulates circulation and vivifies the nerve filaments. It's a success while others are failures.

"Nothing superior, and we know of none as good. This is a sensible therapeutic agent that can be used by any one. Most powerful effects and accomplishes so much with so many diseases."

Who would have ever thot that Chiropractic would have got in such a mixup? The above appliances are hereditary—come from his paternal sire, Old Allopathy.

## NEUROLOGY A COMBINATION.

Preface: "This book embraces three of the greatest modern sciences."

Osteopathy, Chiropractic and Ophthalmology constitute Neuropathy, the combining of which is the discovery of Dr. Davis.

Introduction: "This science deserves the closest scrutiny and the most searching investigation, for it is surely worthy and will be the leading science at no distant day."

As Neuropathy is to be the leading science in the near future, we should give it the closest scrutiny and the most searching investigation. Our object in this section will be to discover of what it is composed.

Page 3: "This book includes the **best of every scientific, rational, natural method of cure for human ills ever presented to the human family.**

"**Suggests every known means to remove causes of conditions called disease.**"

LIII: "When the Neuropathic department is thoroughly comprehended, it will be found that the manipulations will be much better adapted to the accomplishment of the purpose —free the nervous system—and they being of my own improvising (?) may as well be classed under the name Neuropathy as not."

The manipulations of Neuropathy are those of Osteopathy —Chiropractors do not manipulate; they do not use the process of manipulating; they adjust.

"Every Osteopathic treatment should be accompanied with a Neuropathic treatment."

The Neuropathic treatment, referred to, is Chiropractic adjustment.

"The freeing of the nerves involved and uniting the forces will be enough usually."

Nerves and muscles have the peculiar property of contractility, manifested by shortening and synchronous thickening, whenever irritated. Neuromuscular relates to normal tension, normal response to a normal nervous stimulus; ideomotor or ideomuscular, a muscular movement resulting from complete engrossment by an idea which is automatic, as in hysteria, altho originating in the cerebrum. Tonicity is the condition of tone, or normal tension. The abnormal is known as tension or atony, a stretched or strained condition. This prerequisite to disease is due to pressure, poison or a lack of control of the emotions and acts of the patient, a morbid self-consciousness. To free the nerves of these conditions, returns the nerves to normal tonicity—normal function—health.

Page 1: This work, though not large, contains the kernel of **the sciences** which have to do in the treatment of diseases **without the use of drugs or medicines.**

Page 2: "**Foreign substances, in the way of medicines, are not needed.**"

Page 11: "No wonder the world is 'tired of medicine.' No wonder the cry is for something more tangible, more certain of favorable results, less harmful and more rational."

Without the use of drugs or medicines; medicines are not needed; the world is tired of medicine and—read the next two paragraphs:

Page 663: "So far as any medicine system is concerned, we think the Burges system the most plausible. There are a few things recommended by the doctor worthy the consideration of every one who desires to use medicine in any form we feel no hesitancy in recommending."

Page 257: "**The remedy recommended is a medicine,** but homeopathic and harmless, and often the **one which meets the necessity.**"

Page 8: "**Neuropathy is the name of the method used for all that is to be done to relieve conditions called disease, but the terms Osteopathy, Chiropractic, Ophthalmology, Suggestion or Magnetism, designate the how it is applied.**

"The various methods blend together admirably."

The application of these five systems is that of Neuropathy; the blending is what constitutes Neuropathy.

Page 8: "**Whether**, therefore, **we use Osteopathy** to free the circulation of the blood, **or Ophthalmology** to arrest nerve waste, **or Chiropractic** adjustments to remove nerve pressure, **or Suggestion** to stimulate mental energy, **or Magnetism** to concentrate mentality and change molecular polarization, **the object is accomplished through** the one means—**Neuropathy.**"

Dr. Davis has a cinch on these five systems—no matter which is practiced, the object accomplished is thru Neuropathy—any one or all of these systems are Neuropathy. He is like the medical practitioner—no matter what method you practice, you are practicing medicine.

If diseased conditions in any part of the body can be easily relieved by this spinal treatment, why look further? If, as stated, "The key to the relief of all conditions, is the removal of nerve pressure," why use any other key, when **this pass-key will unlock and free all diseased conditions?**

"A knowledge (page 160) of phrenology becomes a leverage worth considering in the execution of the means essential to harmonize the body, for one can tell how the patient thinks, and as thought controls the individual, it becomes a necessity to know what he thinks, along what lines, so as to know what means to use to harmonize him."

Is that correct? Will a knowledge of phrenology enable one to tell what the patient thinks, enable the phrenologist to read the minds of others? Is it necessary to know what the patient thinks in order to harmonize him? Is it a fact that thots control the individual, regardless of poisons and injuries? If health and disease are only conditions of the mind and depend upon wrong thinking, then it may be beneficial to become acquainted with phrenology and hypnotism so that we may harmonize the physical by harmonizing the mind. If so, phrenology is a leverage in Neuropathy.

Phrenology, craniology—the physiological hypothesis, that the mental faculties and traits of character have anything to do with disease is absurd. A number of persons are caught in a railroad wreck, some are injured, their osseous frames being more or less displaced. These displacements by their effects upon nerves and muscles induce various diseased conditions. Are their bodies out of harmony because they think thots of inharmony? Being able to read their thots (mind reading) by the science of phrenology (?) will that enable the phrenologist to relieve them without correcting the displaced bones?

Do we not find the infant and the adult, the wise and ignorant, the rich and poor, the saint and sinner, suffering alike under the same conditions? Disease has no respect for character, nor for a man's thots.

"That (page 273) there is a power within man which correlates itself with his fellow man is commonly believed; we are wont to call that power magnetism.

"It is capable of being generated, multiplied, to any degree and so directed as to produce effects almost, if not absolutely, as desired—from its application through the hands of the one imparting it. It fills all space, penetrates all substances and may be used as the messenger on all errands, for weal or woe.

"The application of this mighty force may be made at any time, on all occasions and for all mental or physical conditions, and **its influence directed to the cure of all diseases.** Whatever other agencies are being used, **this** applied **outweighs them all** in satisfying results. An influence which can be felt, one which can be directed to any locality and which can be forced into the human body by the 'laying on of hands,' the pointing of the fingers to a given locality, or sent in fragile substances for hundreds of miles and have the potency to relieve pain, should not be ignored."

The author tells us that magnetism can be used for the cure of all diseases, regardless of what other agency is being used.

Magnetic healing by personal contact, or at a distance, produces a mental effect on nerves. It is also a fact that, if the nervous system is being treated by drugs, their influence is antagonistic to the mental effect of the healer, or the one aimed to be benefited.

Magnetism, also, constitutes a part of Neuropathy.

"It would be foolish (page 163) on the part of any one to ignore the fact that through the application of Christian Science methods many cures are effected."

"We wish it distinctly understood that the term Neuropathy embraces and includes all means which aid in relieving the nervous system."

Thus, we find that Dr. Davis is indebted to Christian Science as well as Magnetic Healing and Phrenology for a portion of Neuropathy; he aims to give credit where it is due.

"If all men (page 165) who have diseases have strong enough faith in their inherent recuperative powers to persist in the thought, and do the things necessary to carry out the thought, all functional human ills would get out of the body."

"Diseases of all kinds (page 154) seem to be influenced by the **suggestions** of, and if repeated often enough so as to become fixed and a part of the life thought of the individual, the results will be as desired by the suggester, so that diseases seem to resolve themselves into a mental ideality which may be eliminated by intense thought in the direction indicating such a desideratum. **Many diseases have been permanently dispelled by this means.**"

"The fixed thought (page 165) on any assertion, if believed, brings corresponding results. It is the mind which controls the body and as 'we think we are,' and no argument can change us until we give up the thought or exchange it for another one. How the mind cures, we do not presume to state."

Suggestions are made to persons, who are in a more or less negative, hypnotic condition, for the purpose of imparting an idea which is contrary to facts. Dr. Davis tells us that many diseases have been eliminated, dispelled from the body, as tho they were entities, intelligent, imaginary beings who can be bidden to vacate. This is, also, a part of Neurology.

For fear that you might look to the wrong author, look to Neuropathy for the two paragraphs above.

"The ophthalmological department (page 698) is also invaluable and will fit in, in many a case, where nothing else will."

"It is a fact (page 201) that all diseases are due to nerve waste."

"Just as soon (page 202) as the nerve waste is stopped and the nerve pressure is removed, nature has an opportunity to resume her accustomed course, so that harmony, health, becomes established."

"The nerve strain (page 202), then, means overused. Overuse results in exhaustion, and this results in what is denominated disease. Disease anywhere in the body is a result of loss of nerve power. It may be overuse of the eyes, the spine, or any other part of the system and thereby produce exhaustion, a general weakness, and thus furnish sufficient cause for disease."

"**Nerve strain** (page 202) **of the eyes causes all functional diseases.**"

If nerve strain of the eyes is the cause of all functional diseases, disease being either abnormal functionating, or the result thereof, why look after any other system of healing or any other organ than the eyes?

"The Ophthalmologist (page 206) knows how to take off the strain, 'stop the leak' and 'fill the tank,' so that nature is free to perform her natural functions. The facts are, all functional disturbances are the legitimate result of nerve strain."

Ophthalmology is, also, hitched up with this medley of healers, in order to make a successful pull. It gives the practitioner one more method to choose from, and an entirely different analysis of disease.

Dr. Davis, as a teacher of all these methods and more yet to follow, should be a phrenologist, so he may be able to decipher the student's thots, for I am sure that the recipient of these various methods would become so confused that he would not know his own thots.

"The almost miraculous (page 234) change produced in the tissues through the application of the principles of Osteopathy, place it in the front ranks as the most stupendous fact of the nineteenth century."

"Osteopathy (page 558) is applicable to all pathological conditions, and that, too, with more certainty of relief than any other treatment—properly and intelligently applied."

"We do say (page 306) that, **more than any other system now in vogue, known or practiced by anybody to cure disease, Osteopathy is nearer a universal means of relief and cure of the ills of the flesh than any other ever tried, used or employed.**"

"That **disease** (page 329) should be **caused by interrupted circulation has been a known fact** for long years. The principles of this science are couched in the 'freedom of the circulation of the blood and other fluids of the body.' "

"It is the greatest boon (page 333) that has ever been offered to the human race for relief and cure of physical ills—acute or chronic—and all people must know it."

"'Pressure (page 373) anywhere impeding the normal flow of fluids,' is the motto of Osteopathy."

"Osteopaths (page 397) claim that when all of the fluids are freely, normally circulating through their proper channels, all of the muscles are in their normal condition and all of the nerves are free from pressure, health is the condition experienced."

"The Osteopath regards disease (page 476) as the result of obstruction, and the obstruction removed, removes the cause, whatever the name of the pathological condition may be."

"The whole cause (page 480) of disease in every part of the body being obstructed circulation, the treatment rationally resolves itself into a restoration of the circulation to a normal condition."

"The Osteopath has but one remedy (page 509)—that is, Take Off the Pressure. This cures all manner of diseases."

I think Dr. Davis has very definitely defined Osteopathy. In his Neuropathic team, he places Osteopathy, Chiropractic and Ophthalmology in the lead, using the latter as the center horse. The other four mentioned compose the wheel-team.

That the reader may comprehend this combination-team which has been named Neuropathy by "its discoverer," I will quote from page 149. "The word Chiropractic practice is simply hand practice of a peculiar character to relieve nerve pressure from the spinal nerves. Having taken full courses of instruction in Chiropractic science, and having six years' experience in its application, and having evolved from the Chiropractic, the Osteopathic and Ophthalmic sciences a system we name Neuropathy, we hesitate not to state that **our system** of practice embraces all there is known in Chiropractic science as taught by its originator and all there is in Osteopathy, and all there is in Ophthalmology."

"Neuropathy (page vii.) is the discovery of the author (A. P. Davis) of this volume (Neuropathy)."

---

Stages relate to a period of growth or space.

Degree and stages are used to express progression.

Per cent is always applied to that which is contained in 100 parts. Per cent is not an imaginary part; it is a real tangible rate per hundred, a certain portion of a hundred.

Functions may be spoken of either comparatively or relatively, but not in a positive or absolute amount.

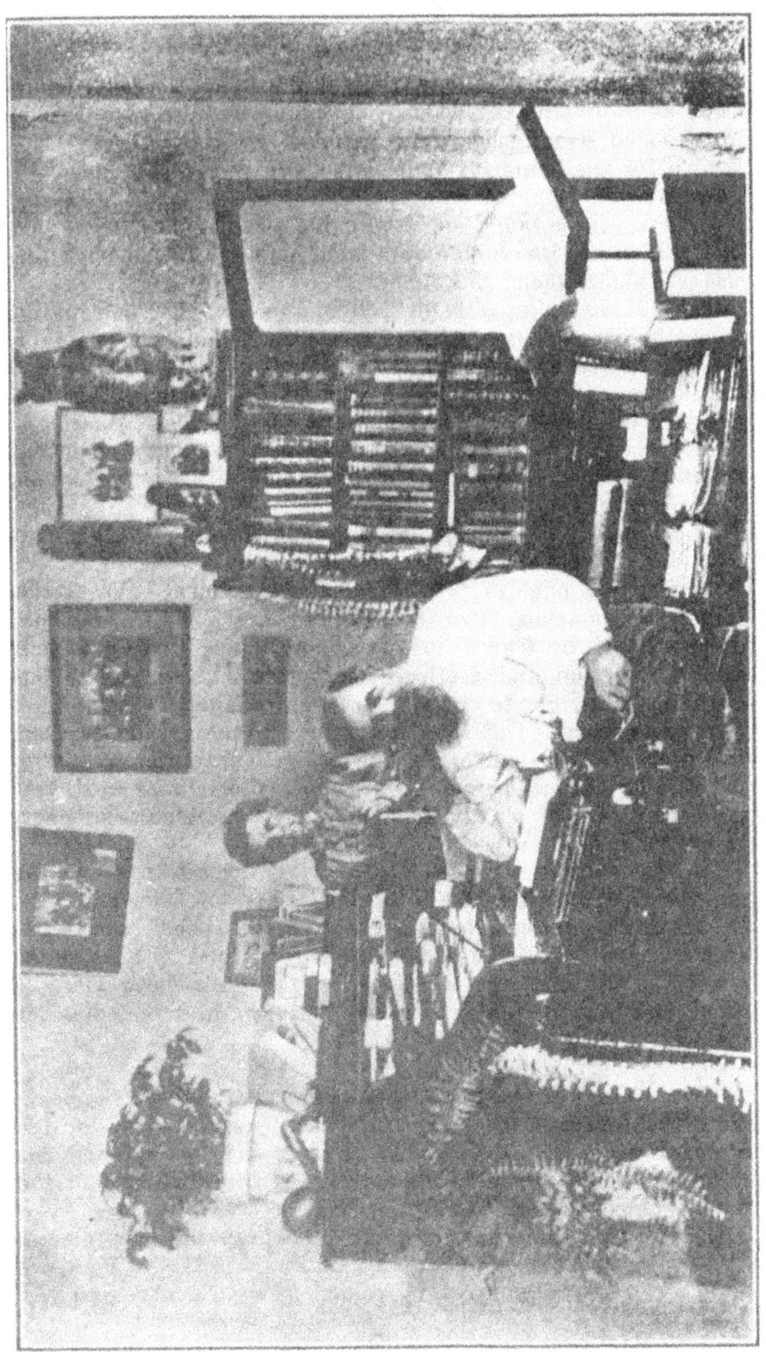

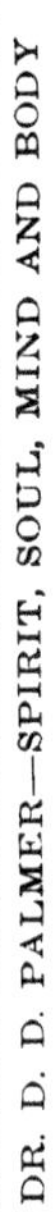

DR. D. D. PALMER—SPIRIT, SOUL, MIND AND BODY

## NEUROPATHY, BY A. P. DAVIS.

"The recipes, given for various diseases, are useful in many cases as adjuvants to the physical manipulations, and will be appreciated greatly by many people, for they are the best known for the things recommended and will suffice most admirably.

"There will be found many valuable receipts and instructions in it which are invaluable and come in the way when nothing else will suffice them." Page 8.

The "Medical Department" (this is part of the Neuropathic science?) has 43 pages which gives over a hundred "valuable receipts" for the treatment of 70 ailments. Did I hear you say that these remedies are not a part of the science of Neuropathy? We have A. P. Davis' word for it that they are.

Dr. Davis says: "It includes the best of **every scientific, rational, natural method** of cure for human ills ever presented to the human family."

"Neuropathy is the name of the method used for all that is to be done to relieve conditions called disease."

On the first page of the "Medical Department," Dr. Davis forgets all about his "two forces," and says, "We learned that disease could be traced to three conditions: first, invasion; second, retention, and the third, enervation." Next page, "The medicines get right to the work of neutralizing the toxins, removing the retained poisons and toning up the nervous system. It will be an 'eye opener' to the medical practitioners everywhere." He traces disease to three conditions, invasion of bacteria, retention of matter that should be excreted, and enervation, lack of energy.

The language used in the Medical Department, praising the remedies, reminds me of the medical books of 200 years ago. Dr. Davis says, these remedies give "speedy relief," are "efficacious"; a most "excellent remedy"; there is no "better remedy"; they are "almost a specific"; a "sovereign remedy"; they give "sure relief"; these are Nature's best remedies for disease.

Quite a contrast to—

"We would urge that the Neuropathic treatment in the back, from the fourth to the eighth dorsal, be given also; for the union of the two forces assists greatly in neutralizing the poison or excess of either the acidity or the alkalinity of the fluids—blood as well." Page 667.

Medical men cannot forget their dope, bugs and bug juice.

---

Health is better than wealth.

## WHAT IT COSTS TO DIE.

We heard of a man who was so stingy and mean that, just to save funeral expenses, he lived long after his neighbors thot he ought to be buried. But there are persons who can't afford to die, as the following case illustrates:

A young married man, the father of two promising children, earning the ordinary wages of a clerk, by strict economy had saved and laid by in the bank $85.

One night his little girl was taken ill. The physician made ten professional visits, prescribing several remedies which were supplied by the druggist. At last the doctor advised an operation which necessitated her removal to the hospital. The operation was performed with the usual success, but the child died, from no fault of the surgeon, however, as blood poisoning set in.

As soon after the funeral as the creditors thot the parent's grief had subsided somewhat, the doctor, the hospital, the undertaker, the liveryman, and the manager of the cemetery presented their bills, the sum total amounting to $268, which was a low price indeed for a funeral. The $85 was applied toward the liquidation of the incurred indebtedness, leaving $183 unpaid.

By strict economy the family had been able to lay by in the bank $5 a month. By the same frugality it will take over three years of saving to pay the cost of one death. It may be that during this three years of debt-paying that another similar expense may be added.

This bill of serial expense should not have been made. The physician, who was the first creditor, knew well the name of the disease but did not know just what caused it, and even if he had known that a vertebra, displaced by a fall from a swing, pressed against and impinged upon a nerve, creating an excited condition known as inflammation which, in turn, by transudation of heat from the inflamed portion, created the fever, the temperature of which he was very mindful to register several times each day—I repeat, even if he had known that her ailment dated back to, and was caused by, her fall from a swing, his medical education would not permit him to consider for a moment that a vertebra might have been subluxated sufficiently to impinge upon nerves or muscles, and that such a displacement could have been returned to its normal position by hand. Instead, he looked for an antidote, a something which would down that fever or at least check it until nature could overcome it.

How long will we continue to fight disease, look upon it as

an enemy, something which must be driven in or out, instead of adjusting the cause thereof? It is cheaper and much more satisfactory to engage a Chiropractor to adjust the cause of disease than to have a second-class funeral.

---

Medical and osteopathic laws are expensive to place on the statute book and very expensive to keep there. It is said, the average expense for each state for the osteopaths to keep a mount, so that they may ride, has cost them $15,000. I for one would rather walk, be independent, even if I have to fight for my privilege of using the public highway.

I am not opposed to any Chiropractor, whether he be good or bad. The poorest can accomplish more good than a medical man with his bugs and dope. Yet, I would much rather know that each Chiropractor was proficient in all that pertains toward making him or her competent in everything that goes to make an intelligent, up-to-date Chiropractor; but there are those who are not financially able to acquire this knowledge, and others who do not care to know more than the bare rudiments. The discerning public will choose those whom they think the most proficient.

---

Medical Brief says, "It is the experience of every practitioner that drugs do not have the same effect on all individuals. These idiosyncrasies are not only peculiar to the individual, but run through whole families. Just why certain drugs do not act as well in all cases is not known, but the fact must be taken into consideration."

No two persons are alike in the quality or makeup of the nervous system. That is why sensory nerves of different individuals do not sense alike and their motor nerves do not transmit the same identical motor impulse. These sensations and impulses are modified, individually, by disease—pathological physiological activity.

Drugs are foreign substances. They are poisonous, they impair one or more functions. They are given for that purpose. Innate Intelligence recognizes this fact and acts accordingly upon all intruders. All drugs change functions or tissue, therefore are pathological in their tendency. Why not adjust causes instead of treating effects? Did you ever know of a symptom or an ailment being adjusted? An ailment cannot be adjusted; you cannot fix a disease. Physicians prescribe for ailments; they do not adjust causes. If a physician knew the cause of a disease he would adjust it instead of writing a prescription to remove its effects.

## MECHANICAL CHEMISTRY?

"The mechanical and its study, human or otherwise, is complete because it takes mechanical principles exemplified to make its product—chemical. The human body is based upon both of these principles. The chemical is the product of the mechanical."

The language of the above and the ignorance it expresses in regard to mechanics and chemism will locate the author if you know him; if you are not acquainted with his characteristics well and good.

The two sciences—mechanical and chemical—are not and cannot be associated; they are separate and distinct from each other; they are not related, they are not correlative.

That which is mechanical is performed by a machine uninfluenced by the will or emotion. It is accomplished automatically. Mechanism is a term applied to machinery by which certain movements, formerly done by hand, are executed by a mechanical device. Mechanical pertains to mechanics—the science of physical force. Physical force may be mechanical, of a machine; thermal, of heat; chemical, produced and operated by the force of chemistry; electrical, executed by electricity; magnetic, animal or mineral. There are, also, the force of gravitation, the force of cohesion, the centripetal and centrifugal forces.

Animal force may be muscular or metabolic—vital. These are inherent in living organisms—not in inorganic substances.

Physical force and vital force are not correlative: as terms they are contradistinctive; the former is inanimate, the latter animate.

The science of mechanics is that of material, not vital, force. Mechanical force is not human; it pertains to inanimate machinery, it lacks spontaneity; it is physical force, it acts from the external, it is non-vital; whereas the acts of animal organisms are from the interior, an energy, a vital force from within.

Chemistry does not pertain to machinery. Chemicals are not products of machinery. Chemistry is the science which treats of the composition of substances and of the transformation which they may undergo. Chemistry is an outgrowth of alchemy. Alchemy was the medieval chemical science. Its objects were the discovery of the universal cure for disease and the means for indefinitely prolonging life. The progress of alchemy as a science was impeded by the nature of its aims and by much mystification; but, important discoveries were made incidentally. Alchemists hoped to find a panacea, a universal remedy for all diseases. Alchemistry led the way to modern chemistry. Chemistry was originally used for extracting the juices of plants for medical purposes. There are no "mechanical principles exemplified" in extracting juices from plants. Alchemy was supposed to possess the miraculous power of transmuting—changing— ordinary substances into precious ones by **transmuting** to the drug an intelligence, so that it would know where and how to go, and what to do in the part of the body diseased, in order to dispossess the intruder. Nothing mechanical—no machinery about that. Modern chemistry is the development of this chimerical dream. From the alchemical period, chemistry passed to that of iatrochemistry, in which it was joined to medicine, and not until the time of Robert Boyle (1626-91) did it become an independent science. The field of chemistry has long been divided into organic and inorganic chemistry from the belief, once current, that compounds are produced in living organisms by some vital force and are essentially different from those made in the laboratory and in organic nature. Physical chemistry studies quantitatively the relations between chemical and physical properties and phenomena; it includes thermochemistry, electrochemistry and photochemistry. Physiological chemistry deals with the chemical processes which take place in plants and animals, more especially the latter.

Analytic chemistry deals with the analysis of substances. Synthetic chemistry has to do with the building up of substances from their constituents.

Chemistry is the science of molecular and atomic structure of bodies.

The changes and combinations known as chemistry do not pertain to mechanics. Chemicals are produced by the forces and operations known as chemistry—not mechanics. Chemistry is a process—not a product. Chemical changes and combinations have nothing to do with machinery. Chemistry deals with the changes in the composition and constitution of molecules. Chemistry, as a science, investigates the nature and properties of bodies, and studies the force or power by virtue of which every combination of molecules is effected; nothing mechanical about that. Mechanical, chemical and vital are not related, are in no wise associated. Why try to mix these three separate and distinct forces that have no sociability?

Reaction in chemistry is the result of introducing a reagent or test. The phenomena caused by the action of chemic agents.

Gould's Medical Dictionary uses 38 pages to give 748 tests, or reagents. A test in chemistry is a characteristic reaction which distinguishes any one body from all others. For instance, a test paper is impregnated with a chemic reagent, as litmus. It is used for detecting the presence of certain substances or conditions which cause a change in the color of paper. A chemic reagent is that which is used to produce a reaction or to test for the presence of an element. Any substance employed to produce a chemic reaction. A test meal, is one given in order to test the action of the gastric juices, by means of which the digestive power of the stomach is accurately tested; it may be a test breakfast or a test dinner. Ewald's breakfast test for motor activity of the stomach consists of one roll and one glass of water or a cup of tea, without milk or sugar. Test types, are letters or figures of different sizes to test the acuteness of vision. While this is a test, it is not chemical. Each of the 748 tests are known by a certain name, usually the name of the person who originated it. Each are used for a certain purpose. The name of the chemical, or reagent is given, the reaction and the application.

It will be observed that chemicals are employed in the process of chemistry, to make chemical combinations and chemical changes; that to consider chemicals as the production of mechanical principles—machine made—is incongruous and incompatible; an expression characterized by inconsistency and an unsuitable connection.

---

"Do you realize that The Palmer School of Chiropractic has been doing business in Davenport for 23 years?"

Let me see; D. D. Palmer began practice in Davenport as a magnetic healer in 1886. He was then 41 years of age and B. J. was 4 years old.

The first Chiropractic adjustment was given in 1895 when D. D. Palmer was 50 years of age and B. J. was 13 years old.

A. P. Davis was my second graduate in Chiropractic in 1898. During the next five years we had one, two or three students at a time, often none. If we fix the date of the Palmer School of Chiropractic at the time we had our first student, Wm. A. Seeley, January, 1898, it would make the existence of The P. S. C. just 11 years instead of 23.

Why misrepresent? "Do you realize that The P. S. C. has been doing business in Davenport 23 years." No one who stops to figure thinks so. Would it not be just as easy to tell the truth? That depends upon who is making the statement. I feel like repeating the language of a P. S. C. graduate, who saw the family record, which stated that Bartlett Joshua Palmer was born Sept. 10, 1882. "I detest a liar."

## MAN A MACHINE.

"The three functions, so far as demonstration represents the ultimates of all leading up to one or more of these functions. That is to say, all of the machinery which enters into the preparation of substances for absorption is simply accessory to that function, which is itself accessory to circulation, aeration and assimilation. All of the machinery which takes part in the function of depuration is accessory to it and also to assimilation.

"The human organism, when looked at as a whole, is seen to constitute a very complete machine.

"Machinery of circulation.

"The human machine.

"It is a remarkable physiological fact that the machinery and operation at the point of function, no matter at what place or in what relation, or of what character, are without description and are unknown."

A machine is a mechanical contrivance used to shape, dress or combine material. There is no similarity between living bodies which possess functions and machines by which goods are manufactured. Functions are vital acts for accomplishing vital phenomena. A machine is used to manufacture materials. Functions are the result of vital force; machinery is run by the laws and properties of matter, such as gravitation, heat, light, magnetism and electricity.

To attempt to demonstrate the vital acts of the human body by the working of machinery is futile. Machinery manufactures, shapes or combines materials. Is the body one superb machine, or is it composed of an innumerable number of machines? Can any one sort out and name each of these machines?

Is it physiological to assert there is a machine at the point of each function, as stated, at the peripheral ending of each nerve; if so, there are millions of machines in the body.

The digestive juices are secreted and excreted. Secretion is an organic function executed in the glands and consists of a separation and combination of certain materials, the structure of each gland and the composition of the prepared fluids differing. Hence the formation of different fluids, as bile, saliva, urine, milk, etc. Secretions, when discharged, are known as excretions. The fluids of the body are combinations of the ingredients of food and water taken in the body; they are not manufactured by hand or machine.

Function in physiology is a term applied only to the action of an organ or a part of an animal or vegetable having vital force.

To represent the body as a mill filled with, and composed in all its parts by, machines, shows a lack of comprehension of language and the principles of Chiropractic.

The circulation in animals and plants is controlled by vital force, not by a system of machinery or machines, as Friend Carver states.

To consider the body a "human machine," would necessitate considering all animals, birds, reptiles, insects, trees and vegetables, not only as machines but each filled with machines.

"It is a physiological fact that" the secreting and excreting of the various fluids of the body, considered as the result and output of machinery "are without description and unknown."

G. H. Patchen, M. D., a logical writer on Chiropractic, falls into the above pit which has been dug by pseudo-Chiropractors. He says, "If, as we must admit, the normal body is a perfect machine, it is evident that so long as each part sustains a proper mechanical relation to every other part and is supplied with abundant power, the result of its activities, however numerous and varied, cannot be other than that of health. As the Intelligent Energy that operates the human machine is derived from an Infinite Source, the Universal Intelligence, and is, therefore, limited only by the capacity of the brain to transform and individualize it, it is evident that any excess, deficiency or irregularity of action, either of which is a form of disease, must be due to some mechanical obstruction which prevents its normal transmission."

"Each part (of a machine) sustains a proper mechanical relation to every other part, "made and operated by interaction of forces without a directing intelligence, can be truly said of any mechanical contrivance, but not of a human being.

A "mechanical obstruction which prevents the normal transmission" of "any excess, deficiency or irregularity" of "abundant power."

If the power or energy is in "excess, deficient or irregular," it causes functions to be abnormal, which is denominated disease.

An impingement, a pressure against a nerve is never a mechanical obstruction.

An impingement does not obstruct. It irritates in a large share of diseases, and excites functional activity beyond a normal degree.

The discoverer of every principle of Chiropractic, he who first put those principles into practice and was the first to teach them to others, does not admit that living bodies, controlled by functions, guided by intelligence, are inanimate mechanical machines run by and in accordance with the laws of mechanics. The terrestrial, quantitative relations of force and matter are vastly different from those pertaining to those which are mental, vital or spiritual, and should not be considered as one and the same in force or material.

"As the intelligent energy that operates the human machine is derived from an Infinite Source, the Universal Intelligence."

Energy is manifested in various forms, as mechanical, electric, thermal, or chemical. In biology, it is the internal, inherent power, the capacity of acting, producing or doing work of an organ or organism, whether exerted or not. Energy does not possess intelligence, it is not intellectual. In biology, intelligence directs the performance of functions. Energy is the sum total of the force expended in the performance of functions. Individualized Intelligence is a segment of Universal Intelligence, the Infinite Source of all intelligence.

---

Use paper napkins for spreads on your adjusting tables. They cost 85 cents a 1,000, are clean, handy and save laundry bills.

---

Daybreak of the Christian era found Medical science (?) a mixture of arrogance and superstition, of which there is still too much today. Modern intelligence laughs at the prescriptions of 2,000 years ago, which continued in general use up to fifty years ago and today. The Chinese doctors give these same remedies, and many Americans "take their medicine."

Medical education then, as now, was behind other forms of intellectual progress. Medical practice is founded on superstition.

One of the popular remedies was the brain of an owl; another the heads of mice. The eyes of a crab and the fat of vipers were two valuable remedies. Bats and grasshoppers were freely used. If a man had a cold, his physician ordered him to kiss a mule. Cuttings from four-year-old grape vines, burned in seven ditches, contained special therapeutic virtues, provided that the patient sat in the smoke from the seven ditches, each in its turn. Epileptics were possessed of the devil. All unpleasant nervous symptoms were the work of demons, a neighbor, witch, or low, degraded spirits. Doctors had to cast these out or lose their job.

There are many remedies of the superstitious past yet used.

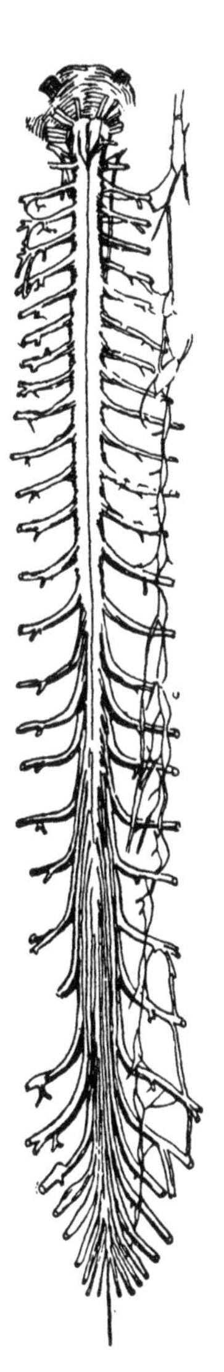

Cut showing the brain, spinal cord and the sympathetic ganglionic chain; the latter is connected with the spinal nerves and reaches from the coccyx to and into the cranial cavity.

## COMPULSORY VACÇINATION.

A Los Angeles county correspondent thus writes in regard to a boy who is kept out of school because of the compulsory vaccination law:

"The California schools are free to lousy, diseased children; but a clean boy, free from disease, must be poisoned before he is allowed to enter school. This boy is an orphan; his parents died when he was a babe; now 14 years old, weight only fifty-five pounds, was always a nervous, weakly child. From poor health and distance from schools he has had no schooling; has not attended school more than nine months altogether in his life. He now has a good school convenient for him to attend. He is old enough to know the need of an education, and has been attending school since the present term opened. He is in love with the school and the teacher is anxious to have him come. She says he is one of her brightest pupils. Much against her will, she had to tell him to take his books and go home. He is not lousy nor scabby nor has he any contagious disease nor has he been exposed to any. His weakness is constitutional. Now while he is gaining strength and his vitality is so that it would be safe to send him to school, the school door is closed against him. Why? Because he has never been poisoned by vaccine virus.

This should be a land of free schools. It is (and should be considered) a great crime to deny a child the benefit of the schools."

It is over twenty years since the British Parliament, after an exhaustive investigation, lasting several months, abolished compulsory vaccination throughout the British empire. Many Americans think it is about time for this enlightened country to follow suit.—The Columbus Medical Journal.

---

A subscriber asks some questions, which I think worthy an answer.

(1) "You state that you cured a case of typhoid fever of seven years' standing. The age needs an explanation, as seven weeks is supposed to be the limit of typhoid fever.

(2) "How do you account for real, genuine cures of diseases by other means than those of Chiropractic, as made by Homeopathy, magnetism, baths and faith cures?

(3) "If, as you state, displaced vertebrae are the cause of all diseased conditions and a cure is possible only by their replacement, are there not other ways of reducing luxations than by the thrust given by Chiropractors?

(4) "If poisons cause muscular contraction, may they not also replace as well as displace vertebrae? Are Chiropractic adjustments the only means of removing the cause of disease?"

(5) "Can you explain the periodicity of disease?

(6) "If Innate is prevented from sending a less than normal amount of impulse to a certain organ, how and why does the administration of a tonic, cathartic or a hot bath enable, for a time, at least, normal function?"

The typhoid fever case referred to, was pronounced typhoid when the patient was in bed. There was no period of convalescence. During the seven years the patient continued to manifest the same symptoms. If, on any day during this time a physician had been called to diagnose the case he would not have hesitated to pronounce it typhoid fever.

If an impingement, a pressure on a nerve, causes conditions we name disease, it is not strange that symptoms remain as long as pressure continues. Do you ask why the fever increases daily, for one, two or three weeks, then remains at this stage for one or two more, attaining a maximum of 104 or 105 degrees, then sinking by lysis? Why the change at the crisis? Why the fever continues to rise till the maximum is reached before there is a change? The excessive heat causes a softening of nerve tissue, the means of heat transferrence. Nerves softened, lose their tonicity, their ability to transfer heat, the temperature falls below normal; low enough to often cause death. The probability is that temperature in this seven-year-old typhoid case did not, at any time, reach 104 degrees, the degree at which necrosis occurs; therefore the fever continued. Fever (diffused inflammation) at 107 to 108 degrees usually proves fatal, because of necrosis.

I think all methods of treatment should be credited with making cures, relieving diseased conditions. At least patients become convalescent, get well, or some chronic ailment follows as a sequel under all. The so-called, self-limited run of fevers is about the same under all methods; they get well or die; morbid phenomena follow about the same with all methods. **Chiropractic is the only method which releases the pressure, takes off the brake, frees the nervous system from irritation** by one adjustment, inside of—shall I say one minute?—why not, when I have never taken a longer time?

I am using typhoid fever as an illustration to answer your question; could have used any other, as the same conditions accompany and follow all fevers.

Typhoid fever (diffused inflammation) causes many varied lesions. We find local necroses of the bowels, spleen and liver; degenerative changes in the kidneys and muscles; inflammatory changes in the periosteum, bones, glandular organs, connective tissue; hemorrhages from the bowels, nose and gums; all the direct result of excessive heat.

Typhoid fever has a run of from four to seven weeks. Chiropractors at any stage, remove the pressure, and free the nervous system from irritation; therefore, there remains no excess of heat.

There is a tendency for Innate to adjust itself to conditions, remove pressure, reinstate functions normally, but yet many, very many abnormal conditions remain for months, years or a life-time; whereas, an adjustment relieves the pressure, allows Innate to restore the normal amount of functionating. Magnetic treatment acts as a tonic in atony and as a relaxer of tension. Mustard plasters draw heat from the focal point inflamed to the surface—diffuses inflammation. Heat, whether that from a room or that of a bath, relieves tension. Faith, mind cures and charms affect nerves, work wonders—sometimes. Thus, each changes nerve conditions; but, is it not better to remove the cause than to treat the effects, as all other methods do?

Many vertebrae are returned to their normal position by an accident—accidental Chiropractic—during our waking or sleeping hours. Drugs, as the M. D. would say, act as an antidote, draw vertebrae into or out of alignment—sometimes. Please look to the case of snake bite (see index).

I would say that Chiropractic is the only method which intelligently adjusts displaced osseous tissue, removes the pressure, relieves irritation, thereby allowing Innate to have its impulses functionated properly.

I cannot yet explain the periodicity of disease, nor of the monthly periods, nor why it takes less power, steam or water to run stationary machinery, that of a train or boat at night, than in the day time.

Innate forwards the same impulses in disease as in health; the change—too much or not enough—is made by the condition of the transmitting nervous system; the hyperthermic condition is one of irritation, excitation, too much functionating. Or the power of transmission may be decreased, in which case functional activity will be lessened—the actions of involved organs increased or decreased accordingly.

---

If you feel bad—forget it. If you feel good—say so. Thus says Christian Science.

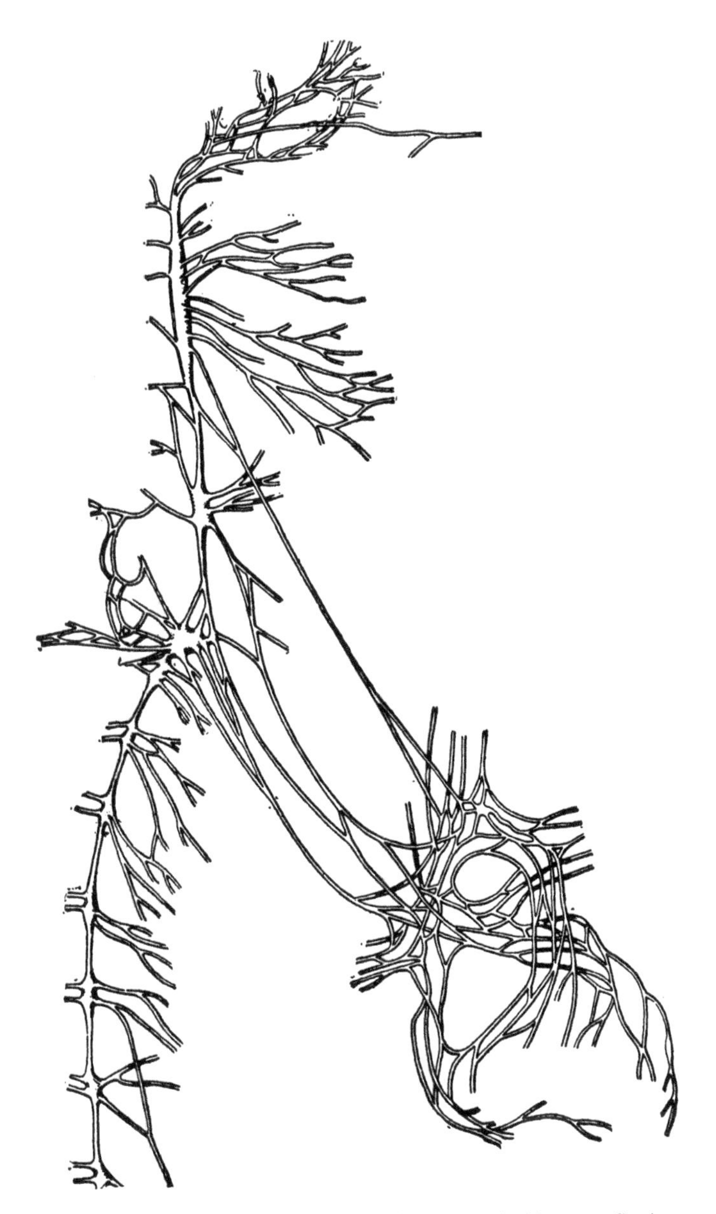

Showing the cervical portion of the Sympathetic Nervous System.

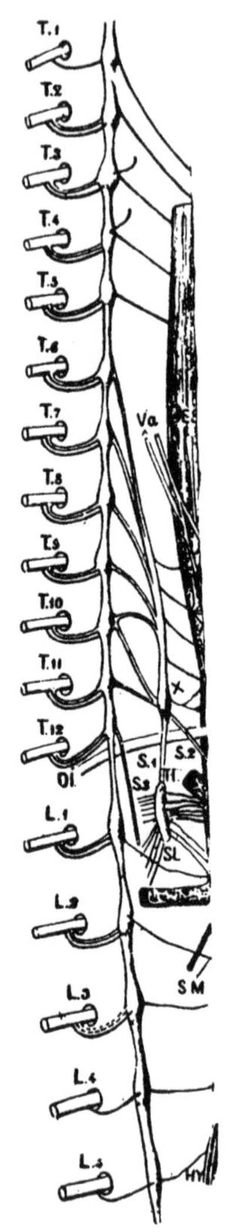


Showing the thoracic anl lumbar portion of the Sympathetic Nervous System.

## VITAL FORCE.

In all diseases we find either an excessive or a diminished amount of energy expended.

Death may be physiologic or pathologic. There are many functions essential to health; circulation, transudation, respiration and innervation are indispensable to life.

Circulation may be increased by an excess of nervous force or diminished by a lack of it. An excess of heat may soften the walls of the blood vessels so that their contents escape or it may thicken the membranes so that fluids are only partially transmitted, in which case death, the cessation of life, occurs. Similar pathological conditions prevent breathing and the transmission of normal innervation.

Observe the excessive growth of parts in acromegaly and in the giant because of over-functionating. Notice atrophied parts and dwarfs, both the result of a lack of proper nutrition —insufficient vital force. Consider wry neck in which one-half of the face is not fully developed, also, observe infantile paralysis, resulting in the unequal length of the limbs. See the Missouri giantess, observe her unusual height of eight feet due to the excessive length of the lower limbs, the arms being correspondingly lengthy.

Disease is either too much or not enough functionating. Functions depend upon stimulus, energy, vital force for their ability to act. If too great a supply, there is too much action, too much heat, too much growth, a condition productive of tumors and cancers, or the Manchnow giant, who is ten feet high and rides in a van.

If the quantity of vital force is below normal, we have a hardening of bone, or other tissue, and a lack of action and sensation—life is abnormally active.

Vitality and intellect are at their maximum—at their greatest activity—when the nervous system is free and unimpinged. Vital action is too great in fever, because of nerve-pressure.

The formation of the embryo, the growth of the fetus, may exhibit too much or not enough functional activity. The embryo is normally formed in all its parts, when functional activity is normal.

"If diseases occur because of an excess of stimulus, or over-amount of functionating, how do you account for the growth of the impregnated ovum up to the mature, normal adult? How do you account for death as a result of disease or abnormal activity?"

Disease is due to a departure from normal functional activity. Deviation either way from the normal is pathological. The growth of the impregnated ovum we have noticed elsewhere. It is at first that of a parasite. It fastens itself upon its host, draws sustenance therefrom, whether agreeable to its foster parent or not, and eventually, the entertainer adopts it. From birth to maturity, growth is made thru metabolism.

Innate, spirit, vital force, runs the material body as long as it is habitable—as long as its structure is capable of transmitting impulses and placing them in action. When, by any means, the channels of communication become useless, because of necrosis (softening), or sclerosis (hardening), functions cease and death ensues.

## HYPERTROPHY AND ATROPHY.

Hypertrophy is the result of increased nutrition. Atrophy is caused by a lack of nourishment. Either may be physiological or pathological.

When a portion, or all, of the body acquires an unusual size by an increase in bulk from pre-existing normal elements, it is said to be hypertrophied. When a part is increased by an addition of new elements it is said to be hyperplastic—affected with hyperplasia. Atrophy is a diminution in bulk, a wasting away of tissue. It may be general, affecting the entire body, or partial, affecting only a portion of it.

Normal or abnormal increase or decrease may be congenital (occurring before birth) or acquired (occurring after birth).

Increase or decrease in size depends upon the force of impulses carried over the lines (nerve-fibers) of communication. Thus abnormal growth of the whole or a portion of the body, or dwarfed conditions, are readily accounted for.

I have said these changes may be physiological (pertaining to health), or pathological (belonging to disease); the impulses (mental communicated force) may be normal—uninterrupted. If so, the enlargement or diminution is natural; but, if the vital force is increased or decreased from pressure on nerves, because of luxated joints, displacement of bones, then occur changes in the amount of impulses conveyed—functions are pathologically increased or decreased—resulting in conditions we name disease.

Exercise of any portion of the body demands an expenditure of energy in proportion to the exertion put forth. When any part of the body is super-exercised, the substance thereof is increased accordingly and vice versa. The moving energy is supplied by the vital functions; the growth or decrease is due to inaction of the vegetative function. All action, whether physiological or pathological, is functional.

Atrophy may be physiological or pathological.

Physiological atrophy depends upon normal inactivity, non-use. Tissues, when exercised, enlarge, become hypertrophied; when not in use, their substance is decreased. True hypertrophy is seen when they enlarge in response to normal stimuli. For example, after conception, the mammary glands enlarge to meet the expected demands of lactation.

Acromegaly and micromegaly are respectively abnormalities of enlargement and diminishment of the extremities or face.

Gigantism and acromegaly are forms of hypertrophy. The former is excessive in whole or in part during adolescence; the latter is an excessive growth of parts in adult life. The zone of growth during youth is between the ossified shaft and the cartilaginous epiphysis. After calcification of the cartilage, union between the shaft and epiphysis, is established, extension of growth longitudinally is impossible.

Dwarfishness and micromelia are forms of atrophy. The former is insufficiency of nutrition, in whole or in part, during the growing period; the latter is a congenital lack of development of the extremities.

In all abnormal functions concerned in the growth of the whole or of parts of the body, there will be found associated therewith either hyperthermia or subnormal temperature as the result of pressure on the same part of the nervous system.

---

"Do you think it possible, or probable, that a patient suffering from constipation of the K. P. variety and piles, could be relieved by adjusting K. P. only?"

Constipation does not come from a K. P. luxation. Costiveness does. We, as Chiropractors, have need of making a special distinction between constipation and costiveness, two entirely different conditions.

Constipation is due to functional inactivity of the intestinal canal, or from a lack of pancreatic, biliary or other secretions, or mechanical obstruction of the intestinal canal or paresis of the intestinal walls, or the use of certain food or drugs, or a general depression of vital activity. Each of these will suggest to a Chiropractor the remedy or adjustment.

Costiveness is due to a too active condition of the kidneys, which rob the intestinal tract of its proper share of moisture, leaving the stool dry and hard. Adjust the luxated vertebra at K. P. to reduce the amount of urine.

Piles is a prolapsed condition of the rectum; which may be associated with any of the forms of constipation and have a like cause.

## FEVER.

Fever is a condition in which bodily temperature is elevated above the normal. Heat production and heat dissipation are regulated in an orderly manner by the nervous system. Inflammation is an excess of local heat. Fever is heat in excess thruout the body, regardless of the surrounding temperature. A rise of bodily temperature above normal is because of nerve impingement. There are only two ways of producing abnormal, pathological pressure on nerves; toxically, by poisons, and mechanically, by pressure. Toxines (poisons) draw vertebrae out of alignment by the irritation they produce. Nerves and muscles acting in response to the stimulant, physiological acts becoming pathological ones. The quantitative relations of force and matter rack vertebrae out of alignment—out of place, they crowd against other tissue.

Heat and action are produced by irritation. A normal amount of physiological irritation, when abnormally excited, becomes pathological. Irritation of the nervous system is the only means of producing bodily heat.

Physiologists recognize that pressure or injury on the optic thalmus and corpus striatum cause a rise in temperature—greater heat production. If so, why may not similar results occur from pressure on other portions of the nervous system?

The older the patient the greater the significance of fever. A rise of two or three degrees in a man of sixty years is more alarming than that of four or five in a child of five or six years. This difference is due to a change in the texture of tissue induced by age.

Nerve tissues become firmer, not so pliable, less elastic, as age advances; it does not so readily adapt itself to heat modifications.

"Fever may be traumatic or infectious"—the result of traumatism or poison. Either causes irritation of the heat-producing nervous system. By their excitation, they cause an abnormal amount of heat.

In fever all tissues of the body suffer more or less change. The pulse in scarlatina is very rapid, but slow in typhoid. In all fevers the skin is hot and dry, the sweat suppressed and the secretions of glands and organs diminished. The urine is scanty, dark, colored and of high specific gravity. In typhoid and other slow febrile diseases, diazobenzophenosulphonic acid may be present.

The metabolic procedure in fever is greatly modified. There is loss of appetite, excessive thirst, and the functions of the various organs are more or less disturbed, as is exhibited in the excretions. These abnormal results are due to the change of temperature. Different degrees of heat correspondingly modify the texture of not only the nerve tissue, but also of the glands and membranes and the composition of the fluids of the body. Because of hyperthemia, definite morbid changes occur in various tissues of the body, notably the muscles, heart, liver and kidneys; fatty degeneration and coagulation-necrosis being prominent. These changes are the direct result of increased temperature.

**The effects of fever are destructive, not conservative.** Fever is always a disturbing element of functions and metabolic processes, it leads to various pathological consequences. It has no measure of usefulness whatever. Abnormal functions and morbid tissue are the result of fever—Heat disturbance is the cause of disease. Increased circulation and respiration are because of extra tension and firmness of the blood-vessel walls and lung tissue.

Pathologists and physiologists have been looking for a special heat-regulating nervous apparatus, which, if demonstrated, will enable them to explain the causation of fevers.

I have been successful in locating that "apparatus" and in describing its workings in health and disease. This knowledge opens to our view the cause of each and every disease. The originator of Chiropractic trusts that these pages will not only be instructive, but shed the mid-day sun-beams of an intelligent understanding concerning functions, metabolism, animal heat, transulation and circulation of the body fluids.

---

Chiropractic's Fountain Head is busy straightening luxations. The head from which all the principles of Chiropractic have originated is busy developing the science. To do this successfully it is necessary to adjust many idiosyncrasies found in Chiropractic literature.

---

"Pain may extend to neighboring nerves by reflex action, for instance, the pain in an aching tooth may extend to one on the opposite side."

The displaced vertebra may impinge upon corresponding nerves on opposite sides.

## THE FOUR FUNCTIONAL DIVISIONS OF THE NERVOUS SYSTEM.

There are four important divisions of the nervous system. First, that which relates to the origin, functionating and destination of impulses; second, that which includes the structure and relation that one part of the nervous system bears to another; third, that which concerns its ability to receive impulses and place them in action; fourth, and very important, that which deals with regeneration and degeneration—physiological and pathological action of tissue, parts or organs.

I have learned much regarding lesions—Innate's reasoning as manifested in connection with abnormalities, displacement of osseous tissue. All our acts, normal or abnormal, are dependent upon the amount of force with which functions are carried on.

Proper functionating requires a normal condition of the nervous system and a correct position of the osseous framework.

The universe is composed of matter and intelligence; the former is acted upon by the latter. All impulses of the planetary system and the animals which inhabit it, are directed by this universal intelligence which is individualized according to their needs. From this universal intelligence individualized, call it what you like, originate impulses which in the veretbrata are transmitted thru the nervous system.

We have elsewhere said that impulses are always transmitted from Innate, the originator, outward, that is, from the center to the periphery; where they affect motor nerves causing action. They are therefore efferent impulses. Are there not afferent, sensory impulses carried inward by the sensory fibers?

The office of the nervous system is to adapt activities to the conditions of life. Adaptation and correlation are perfected thru experience; this is true thruout creation. In all the vertebrata, the same general plan of organization is the measure of adaptation, being correlated with the survival of the best qualified. Animals of the greatest mental and physical types have the most highly developed nervous systems. Not only is this true in species, but it also exists in individuals of the same species.

Structure and function, normal or abnormal, go together. Function is dependent upon structure. The nervous system adapts itself to its surrounding environments. As the necessary adaptation and correlation are successfully carried out.

the organization of the nervous system is perfected, made conformable to its requirements.

In the organism of the vertebrata, there are two different factors in operation; actions in relation to the external world, our surroundings, and our internal activities and the processes of nutrition. Our acts in relation to our external surroundings consist in securing food and raiment, protecting ourselves against the elements and our enemies—those who wish to possess that which we desire. The internal activities include the processes of metabolism, the transudation of chyle, lymph and serum and the circulation of the blood.

The acts of the nervous system are two-fold. It receives sensations from the external and internal organs and directs its responses to those afferent impulses. A distinction is made between the somatic and the visceral, those which concern the welfare of the body and those which affect the internal activities.

The somatic portion of the body takes in the skin, muscles, bones, etc., by and thru which it deals with its surroundings. The viscera comprises all which is concerned in nutrition, anabolism and katabolism. A part of the soma, skin, tongue, eye and nose comes in contact with the external world and gives impulses, suggestions to the manager of the nervous system. The muscles and the skeletal frame respond to the efferent impulses which cause appropriate movements. This somatic afferent division of the nervous system consists of the peripheral nerve-fibers and the central receiver of afferent impulses and formulator of efferent impulses which affect the welfare of the animal in its surroundings. Mankind is included among the animal creation. The afferent impulses of gustatory and olfactory impulses arising from without are directed to the central where Innate takes cognizance and acts accordingly.

Modified bodily temperature causes a corresponding modification in afferent and efferent impulses and functions. Normal heat insures normal functions.

In the lives of all vertebrate animals there are four kinds of nervous activities, namely, the reception of somatic impulses and the directing of somatic movements; the reception of visceral impulses and the directing of their activities. Corresponding to these four kinds of activities, there are four distinct divisions of the nervous system, the somatic afferent and efferent, and the visceral afferent and efferent. These four kinds of activities are found in all parts of the body, each of the four functional divisions being represented in each and every portion.

Reflex movements are often the results of afferent impulses without sensation, an example being the twitching and jerking movements during sleep and the involuntary change of position to avoid danger. Actions which are unconsciously made are reflex movements,

---

Carver's Chiropractic Analysis: "Elevated temperature is the primary symptom following a new occlusion or an occlusion that is made graver by some accident or contingency. It is therefore one of the most, if not the most prominent symptom of all acute abnormalities, and has therefore received very prominent notice throughout the therapeutic world. It is, however, the evidence of an abnormal combustion resulting from the failure of equilibrium of chemical combination, which has resulted from chemicals of combustible quality being brought together in the compound in excessive quantity, or the counter of the proposition, not a sufficient quantity of chemicals of a passive nature being added to the compound to neutralize combustion. This condition, varied in the character of its expression, constitutes every form of fever possible, including inflammation."

The above is Carver's Analysis of fever and inflammation. What has luxations of vertebrae, impingements of nerves and adjusting to do with such a chemical analysis? I fail to see anything in it resembling the science or art of Chiropractic. Carver is trying to make a chemical analysis without the knowledge of chemistry or chemicals. He tries to turn vital metabolism into a chemical laboratory.

Combustion is the state of burning—the continuation of combustion, supported by combustible material, results in the production of light or heat, or both. It is a mutual chemical action and reaction of the combustibe material and the oxygen of the atmosphere whereby a new compound is made—the elements having changed their form.

"Abnormal combination." Combustion is natural—could not be otherwise—it is a chemical process—obeying certain fixed laws

Combustion from "chemical combination, **resulting from the failure** of equilibrium." Combustion could not consume without an equilibrium of chemical force and chemical elements. Combustion is not the result of failure of equilibrium; it is due to the proper combination of chemicals.

The science of Chiropractic and that of chemistry will not mix—they are heterogeneous—not even heteromerous.

## TORTICOLLIS—WRY NECK.

There are several forms, and many causes, of wry neck. We wish to confine this article to that kind, which is represented in the cuts on page 179.

Erichsen says that this form of wry neck is caused from spasm or paralysis of one of the mastoid muscles.

Whitman thinks a contraction of one or more of the muscles, with or without pain, which controls the head, is the cause, or it may be due to disease of the spine.

Debrueil affirms that there is unequal development of the cerebral hemispheres with asymmetry of the skull.

Gowers is certain that the muscular contractions depend on the over-action of the nerve cells and not on any irritation of nerve fibers. The treatment advised is manipulative, mechanical or operative.

Dunglison refers to a form of muscular rheumatism, seated in the neck, which causes the head to be held to one side. His remedy is division of the contracted muscles.

Dorland says torticollis is an unnatural position of the head due to actual and persistent organic muscular shortening.

Gould agrees with Dorland when he says wry neck is a contraction of one or more of the cervical muscles, usually of one side, resulting in an abnormal position of the head.

Moore is not backward in giving his opinion. He says wry neck may be due to muscles, **nerves** or nerve centers being **injured at birth** or **bones may be** broken or distorted. The very fact that so many medicines have been recommended, is evidence that they are all disappointing. The proper treatment, in the majority of cases, is an operation followed by mechanical treatment.

Bird's opinion: Wry neck and the asymmetry are **due to** central **nerve-lesions.**

Cooper says: **If the cervical vertebrae have grown in a distorted direction** the position of the head cannot be rectified. He advises an incision of the contracted muscles.

Knight says torticollis is caused by inflammation. He advises an extension support.

Hare says that facial asymmetry is sometimes seen as a congenital effect, and curiously enough, is often developed in children who suffer from congenital wry neck. It is due to a distinct nervous lesion.

Young thinks that the majority of wry neck cases occur at birth from injury during delivery by forceps. **Wry neck depends upon a deficiency of the cervical vertebrae.** In rare cases fracture and **dislocation of the cervical vertebrae have been**

**observed as causes.** The operative procedures employed are tenotomy, nerve stretching, nerve division and nerve-section, with plaster-of-Paris cast or mechanical appliance after operation.

Tubby gives his observations. "There are contractions of the facial muscles and **alterations in the cervical spine. The intervertebral discs, in old standing cases, are wedge-shaped.** The asymmetry of the face is due to delayed development on the affected side. On the side of contraction, the line joining the external angular process of the frontal bone with the angle of the mouth is less than on the other side. It is possible that impeded blood supply may cause retarded development on one side, but the matter is still in the region of speculation."

Anders affirms that "Wry-neck may be a congenital or an acquired condition. 'Congenital torticollis,' or 'fixed wry-neck,' is the result of an atrophy and shortening of the sterno-mastoid muscle, **brought about by some intra-uterine condition, or possibly by an injury at birth.** The right muscle is most commonly affected. The head turns slightly towards the sound side; the eye may deviate and curvature of the cervical spine may develop.

"Facial asymmetry is a usual concomitant of this condition. The face on the same side as the lesion develops less rapidly than the other side, and in time secondary contracture of the unopposed muscles takes place. The torticollis can be cured by tenotomy, but the facial asymmetry persists."

If, as Anders suspects, congenital torticollis is caused by injury, traumatism occurring at birth or intra-uterine, why not adjust such portions of the skeletal frame, which by their displacement impinge upon nerves and muscles, when by this means the facial asymmetry, as also the torticollis, can be corrected?

Moore says of torticollis: "Many cases have their origin at birth; the muscles may be torn, **bones may be** broken or **distorted, nerves may be injured.**"

Torticollis refers to a peculiar position in which the head and neck is held, when the sternomastoid muscle of one side is rigidly contracted. It may be permanent or spasmodic.

Gerdes claims that in wry-neck the **scalenus anticus** (a muscle attached to the first rib and to the **transverse processes of the 3d to the 6th vertebrae.** These muscles are **supplied by direct branches of the cervical nerves) is as frequently at fault as the sternomastoid.** This author advises resection (excision) of the scalenus anticus as well as that of the sternomastoid.

Campbell tells us that, "Permanent wry-neck is usually of congenital origin, resulting from the rupture of a muscle dur-

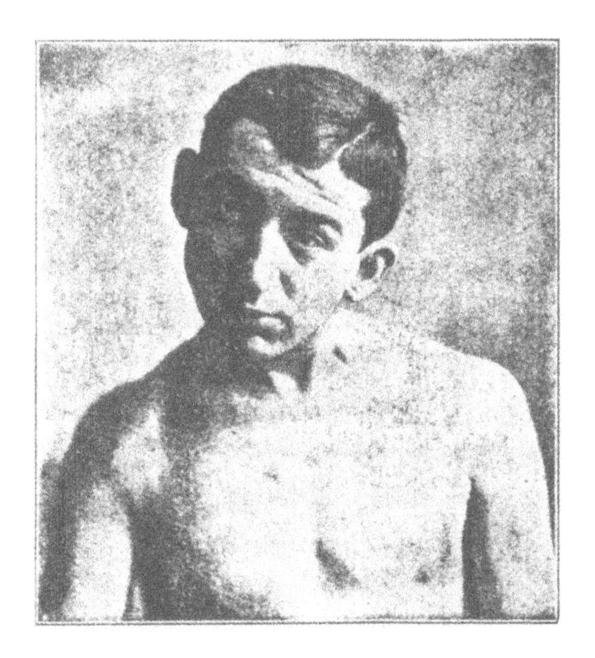

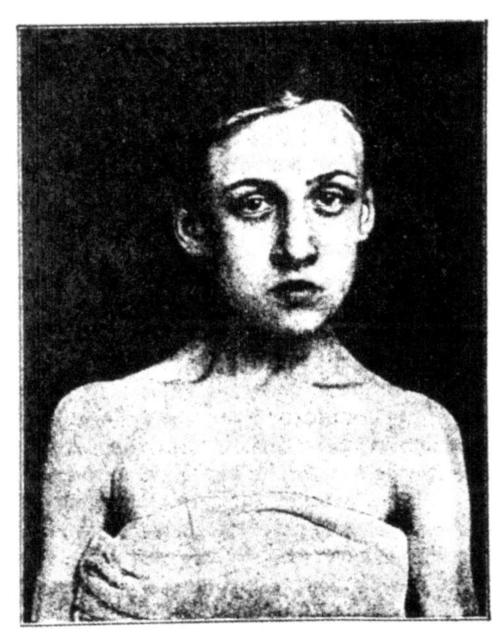

**Taken from Whitman's Orthopedic Surgery, Published by Lea & Febiger, Philadelphia.**

ing parturition. The cicatrix undergoes subsequent contraction, and malposition of the head and neck are the result.

"Spasmodic wry-neck is due to reflex **irritation which throws the muscle into a state of clonic and later, tonic contraction.** It may be relieved by resection of the spinal accessory nerve."

It is strange, indeed, that practitioners have not learned that wry-neck was the result of contraction of muscles and that the contraction of muscles is due to nerve irritation, and as Campbell asserts, may be relieved by cutting the spinal accessory nerve, which originates in the cervical vertebrae, and which as he claims is due to injury during parturition. Displaced cervical vertebrae cause nerve tension of the cervical nerves; nerve tension contracts muscles, and there you have it.

Anders considers wry-neck a form of rheumatism. He says: "Torticollis (Myalgia Cervicalis)—Here the muscles, some or all, one one side of the neck, and at times the throat, are implicated. The head is held toward the affected side, so as to relax the group of muscles involved, and on attempting to turn it the patient rotates his entire body in a pivot-like manner. The complaint is frequent in young persons."

Boyer says of wry-neck: "**Many examples have happened, in which one of the** inferior oblique, or **articular processes of a cervical vertebra has been dislocated,** so as to cause a permanent inclination of the neck towards the side opposite to that of the displacement."

Howe describes a case of torticollis, caused by cervical dislocation: "Some years ago I was called to a lady who had had her head drawn forward. **The contraction had wrenched at least three of the cervical vertebrae from their articulations,** and greatly distorted two others."

Displacement of a cervical vertebra caused the curvature and a decrease in nutrition.

Samuel Cooper with a physician's comprehension, affirms: "Spontaneous displacement of the atlas may depend upon caries and scrofulous disease of the articular surface, or upon the exostosis of its transverse process, or a similar tumor growing from a neighboring portion of the os occipital, or petrous portion of the temporal bone. By these causes, the an terior, or posterior arch, or one of the sides of the atlas, has been made to intercept a third, the half, and even two-thirds of the diameter of the foramen magnum. Notwithstanding the very remarkable constriction of the medulla spinals thus occasioned, life may be carried on, and the nutritive functions performed sufficiently well to afford time enough for the exostoses to attain a large size, or for the ankyloses, binding together the head and most of the cervical vertebrae, to acquire great solidity. The atlas is never found free and distinct, when thus displaced, but it is confounded at least with the os occipital, and mostly with five or six of the subjacent vertebrae. Another interesting fact is, that, in cases of this description, the joint between atlas and occiput is never the only one which is displaced and deformed, unless the disease be very slightly advanced; for the articulation of the processus dentatus and the occiput retain their natural position with respect to each other, and the atlas alone seems to be displaced between them. Sometimes, the second vertebrae is out of its place with respect to the os occipital in the same direction as the atlas, but in not so great a degree. Lastly, **in some instances, the two vertebrae are twisted in opposite directions,** one to the left, the other to the right; or vice versa."

Moore says but little, but says it well. "**Many traumatic cases have their origin at the time of birth, bones may be broken or distorted, nerves may be injured.**"

Ashhurst claims, "Why-neck, torticollis, or caput obstipum, arises from spasm of one of the sternomastoid muscles; the head being drawn to the affected side. On close examination in wry-neck it will be found that there is a triple displacement of the head, which is drawn downwards, rotated outwards, and inclined laterally towards the affected side. The features lose their symmetry; the half of the face, and even of the head, on the affected side, becomes less perfectly developed; the true line of the eyebrows, eyes and mouth become displaced and lowered.

"In torticollis the affected sterno - cleido - mastoid will be found hard, defined, shortened; and sometimes both divisions of the muscle are equally tense, standing out in strong relief, so as almost to look like two distinct muscles. In other cases one division, and then most usually the sternal, is chiefly affected. After a time the cervical vertebrae participate in and maintain the displacement, becoming rotated on their axes and curved. Eventually the whole spinal column participates in the displacement, and lateral curvature sets in. The deeper muscles also become shortened, and the anterior margin and clavicular attachment of the trapezius will often be found tense and preternaturally defined.

"Wry-neck occasionally appears to be congenital; more frequently it is acquired, coming on in childhood after measles or scarlatina, or as a consequence of inflamed cervical glands. It not unfrequently commences with an ordinary stiff neck from cold. In whatever way it originates, the spinal accessory nerve is probably at fault, and it is owing to the irritation of it that the sterno-mastoid and trapezius muscles take on a spasm action. In spasm of sterno-mastoids the head is thrown forwards, the muscles projecting in great relief. In these cases, the disease will usually be found to have had a rheumatic origin. Deformity in this situation may also occur from diseased cervical vertebrae, or from the traction of the cicatrix of a burn. The conditions here, however, are peculiar, depending upon causes that are irrespective of the state of the muscles, and may readily be distinguished from the true form of the disease produced by the causes above mentioned."

Wry-neck is a fixed spasm, a continuous contraction of nerves and muscles, a form of tetanus. Displaced cervical vertebrae cause tension by their impingement.

A pre-natal cervical vertebral displacement, which is possible, will cause the bilateral asymmetry, as in one of post-natal.

Ashhurst states that wry-neck may follow measles, scarlatina or inflamed crevical glands. The impingement which creates tension, inflammation, fever and other symptoms of the above mentioned diseases, also caused the sequela known as wry-neck. The fever designated as measles or scarlatina was the acute stage of the injury which bcame spastic wry-neck.

Ashhurst considers the spinal accessory nerve at fault. The 11th or spinal accessory nerve consists of two parts, different in origin and distribution, the spinal portion is formed from a series of rootlets which emerge from the lateral aspect of the cervical segment of the spinal cord and an accessory portion from the medulla; this nerve being really both spinal and cranial. This nerve is formed from the cervical sections of the spinal cord, passes upward into the cranium, thru the foramen magnum and then makes its exit downward thru the jugular foramen. Anatomsits differ in regard to the location of, and the number of cervical segments from which the spinal accessory arises; they usually state that it arises from a series, often as low as the 6th or 7th cervical nerve-roots. So far, I have found the displacement of the third cervical vertical impinging upon one of the third cervical nerves as the cause of wry-neck.

Bradford has certainly made a study of wry neck. He intended to name all the probable causes. He states: "Abnormal pressure of the uterus is accountable for the cranium and the face being smaller at birth. **Imperfections in the atlas and cervical vertebrae** have in some cases been the cause of congenital torticollis. Dislocation of the upper cervical vertebrae is usually accompanied by torticollis. This may be the result of inflammation, myositis, of the sternomastoid muscle. It may be the result of acute diseases, such as typhus, meningitis, scarlet fever, diphtheria, inflammation of the cervical lymph nodes, deep cervical abscesses, retropharyngeal abscesses, inflammation of the ear, parotitis, adenoid vegetations in the nasopharynx, tumors of the neck, cerebral lesions, cervical adenitis and neuralgia of the spinal accessory of cervico-bracial nerves. Ocular torticollis may accompany a difference in the plane of vision of the two eyes of a difference in their power. Frequently no definite cause can be found to explain the occurrence of the affection, but it is evidently the result of general malnutrition or general nervous disturbance having this as a local manifestation. It may be a congenital distortion, or of gradual development from any of the causes mentioned above or from no cause known. The changes described are to be classed as fibrous myositis, the reason for which has not yet been formulated."

I have quoted twenty authors on wry-neck so that the reader may become acquainted with its symptoms and know the different opinions which various orthopedists and medical men entertain concerning its cause and the different methods of treatment they recommend. In summing up their different methods of treating wry-neck, I am led to say of them, as did Moore of medicines: the very fact that so many methods of relief have been recommended, is evidence that they are all disappointing.

These writers state that the head is drawn awry by the contraction of cervical muscles, but they differ greatly in their conception of the cause of the contraction. They name spasms, paralysis, over-action of nerve cells, muscular rheumatism, central nerve-lesions, inflammation, impeded blood supply, abnormal pressure of the uterus, injuries at birth, no cause known and pure speculation as probable causes. These investigators who associated diseased, distorted and dislocated cervical vertebrae with the disorder came very near discovering the real, causative lesion, as now understood by Chiropractors.

The pathological conditions existing in torticollis were, ofttimes, demonstrated by autopsy. The contracted muscles were examined macroscopically and microscopically, but the cause continued to be speculative and unknown. Even the discovery, made known by post mortem examinations, that cervical bones were distorted and dislocated, was of no value because it was not used. No one thot of replacing vertebrae or would have dared to try to replace them had the thought been conceived. Neither, previous to my discovery, had the idea that, by replacing them, they would grow back to their normal shape, ever entered the mind of man. Thousands of orthopedists, anatomists and pathologists were anxious to relieve these unfortunates, but their knowledge of anatomy and orthopedy did not enable them to do so.

The substance of these contracted muscles is changed to fibrous tissue. In some instances the **muscle and sheath are fused** into one fibrous band; the change being made by inflammation. The displaced vertebra impinges upon nerves and muscles; pressure irritates, excites the nerve tubes and their fibrous contents. Excited nerve and muscle tissue contract lengthwise and expand crosswise. Nerves expand crosswise and contract lengthwise, cause and increase of all functions which they innervate. Thus we have contraction of nerves and muscles and inflammation along their pathway, more especially at their peripheral endings.

The two ears differ in size, the one on the contracted side being smaller and below the level of its mate.

The unequal development of the face, skull, ears and cerebral hemispheres, are due to delayed development of the affected side on account of malnutrition.

Many cases of wry neck show a difference of vision in the eyes and in the functionating of the auditory nerves. There may be incoordinate action of the external ocular muscles on the affected side.

Bradstreet noticed that wry neck was often a sequela of acute fevers and inflammatory diseases. It often followed cervical abscesses, tumors of the neck and the nasopharynx space.

Students of Chiropractic will understand that displacements of the fourth cervical would be very liable to impinge upon the spinal accessory and cervio-bracial nerves, causing a portion of the diseases mentioned, and that a mistake might have been made in naming the remainder.

The most positive and by far the most satisfactory proof of my assertions are found in the relief given to wry neck patients by adjusting the displaced cervical vertebrae.

Looking over the above mentioned authorities, it will be noticed in the portions I have brought out in black face type, that many have observed in wry necks that cervical vertebrae were distorted and deficient in some portions, and that the intervertebral discs were wedge-shaped.

I have presented two illustrative cuts of wry necks; one of which is extremely, the other slightly, asymmetrical. The deviation of the line of the nose from a right angle to the line of the eyes, is quite noticeable. Furthermore, the distance from the outer point of the two eyes to the outer corners of the mouth is not the same, while the cheek, on the contracted side, is less prominent and the features, on the affected side of the face, are smaller than those upon the other side. This asymmetry can be diminished and all deformity corrected and functions restored to normal if the cervical displacements are corrected in early life.

I will quote from one more author that we may the better draw the line between Surgery and Chiropractic.

The American Text-Book of Surgery, after giving a description of wry neck, says, "It has been produced by an habitual malposition of the head, assumed because of existing ocular defect. It is often congenital and causes failure of a muscle to develop proportionally. The short muscle from long-continued inaction becomes atrophied from disuse, the relative contraction increases, and the cervical vertebrae undergo changes from the unequal action of the muscles and fascia. If it first appears in adult life, instead of being spastic it is intermittent, spasmodic, and generally affects one or more of the muscles innervated by the spinal accessory nerve. When acute, it generally passes away under the influence of rest, heat and time, but it may become chronic and permanent. The spasmodic variety may disappear without treatment, often after the employment of baths, friction and massage, change of locality, etc., or it may remain until stretching, section, or removal of a portion of the spinal accessory nerve be done; and even these operations may leave the patient little or no better than before.

"Rectification of the malposition can often be effected, at least to a considerable extent, voluntarily or by manual pressure, but at once recurs when the pressure is removed. This apparent correction is caused by the alteration in the relative positions of the cervical vertebrae. There may be a question as to the existence of caries of the cervical spine, but the history of the case, the absence of bilateral rigidity, and the character of the deformity, will generally suffice to indicate the nature of the trouble.

"The deformity produced is proportionate to the degree of contracture, and ordinarily is not relieved by any treatment except surgical."

The displacement of a cervical vertebra at birth or during infancy causes it to become ill-shaped—wedge-shaped; this causes the "malposition of the head"—leaning to one side. The "ocular defect" is often seen in these cases; the vision of one eye deficient, perhaps entirely absent, altho it may appear to the observer the same as the good eye. Muscles and nerves atrophy and fail to "develop proportionately." The statement: "cervical vertebrae undergo changes from the unequal action of the muscles and fascia," should be reversed, as Chiropractors have very often proven. Displaced vertebrae become wedge-shaped, because of luxation; they impinge upon nerves and muscles, causing their contraction. Instead of stretching or removing a portion of a nerve by resection, why not relieve the pressure by adjusting the displaced, ill-shaped vertebrae, which will then assume a normal shape. Care should be taken to not overdo, for fear of leaning the head to the opposite side. "If," as the author says, an "alteration in the relative positions of the cervical vertebrae" makes an "apparent correction," why not continue to alter the vertebrae until they are corrected? Thanks to Chiropractic, there is relief for such cases outside of surgery.

From the Chicago Sunday Record-Herald of October 9, 1910, I quote the following:

**"USE HANGING AS CURE**

**"Patients in English Hospital Suspended by Neck at End of Rope—Special Apparatus Used—Subjects Respond Well to Strenuous Cure Administered Every Morning.**

"(Special Cable Dispatch to the Chicago Record-Herald.)

"(Copyright, 1910, by New York Herald Company.

"London, Oct. 8.—Hanging from the neck by a rope has become a recognized form of treatment for certain nervous diseases at the National Hospital for the paralyzed and epileptic in Bloomsbury. In wry-neck in particular, this hanging is said to have given results, certain cases totally unrelieved by other more conservative methods of treatment responding well to this strenuous cure. The apparatus used consists of a metal tripod eight feet in height, with a pulley at the top. Over this pulley is passed a rope attached to two large metal stirrups, well padded with leather, one of which fits beneath the patient's chin and the other beneath the protruding part of the head. The principle of the treatment is that the weight of the patient's body is used to stretch the contracted neck and muscles, which cause the head to be held on one side.

"'We begin the treatment,' said one of the hospital staff in explaining it, 'by gently pulling the free end of the rope until the patient is raised up on his toes. After being kept in this position for a few seconds he is given a few moment's rest. The second time he is raised a little higher, so that more strain falls on the neck's muscles. The process is continued every morning for a fortnight, the dose being gradually increased until toward the end of the treatment the patient can stand being suspended clear of the ground for twenty or thirty seconds.

"Immediately after each morning's treatment the patient is at once put back to bed, where he stays until the next morning's treatment. While this hanging cure has given good results in certain cases, it must not be understood that we treat all wry-necks in this way.' "

Suspension by the neck is orthopedical. It has been practiced many years; it is given in orthopedic books. Thomas H. Story, D. C., of Los Angeles, Cal., has been using that form of treatment for eight years.

As all the conditions of wry-neck are caused by a displaced cervical vertebra, why not adjust, replace it?

---

The following quotations are from a leaflet headed Chiropractic:

"We do not treat symptoms, but relieve the cause and Nature adjusts itself."

Nature is the power which produces existing phenomena; the agency which carries on the processes of creation; it embodies the total of all finite agencies and forces. Nature is natural. Can you think of Nature adjusting itself?

"There is no quackery attached to the Chiropractic method."

Quackery is a term which cannot be attached to or applied to a science. The practioner may be a quack; his boastful pretensions may be quackery. Quackery is a term applied to the practitioner, not to the method which he practices.

"These facts have been shown in the past, and are being demonstrated before the public eye at the present time."

Why not say, These facts are being demonstrated, using five words instead of twenty?

"It would be folly to condemn without investigation; if not at first, at least as a last resort."

The first proposition is well said, but the last sentence is ambiguous. It really says, it is folly to condemn at first, at least it is folly to condemn as a last resort.

"Perhaps at this moment you are suffering the fatal results of some dreadful disease, the cause of which may be removed by a few adjustments."

How could a person suffer the fatal results? If their disease was one of fatality, why try to remove the cause?

"If poison is taken into the system, we have an unnatural element."

An element is one of the ultimate, undecomposable constituents of any kind of matter—see article on chemical. Any one of the 94 elements could not be considered as unnatural. Poisons excite the nervous system. Poisons may be reduced by chemical analysis to their elements.

"Excites the nervous impulse."

Nerves may be excited; not the impulse.

"Take hearing as a given example. Today you hear perfectly every sound taking place—you are working with 100 per cent of current thru 100 per cent of matter. But tomorrow you have lost 10 per cent of current—you hear only thru 90 per cent of current passing thru 100 per cent of matter still."

In biology, the term tissue is preferable to "matter."

Sound is a sensation, having as its source some body which is set to vibrating in waves which pass, by means of an intervening medium to the ear and thru the mechanism of the inner ear stimulate the auditory nerve. It is a form of vibrational energy which occasions a sensation we name hearing. It is usually transmitted to the ear by the vibrations of the air. A musical sound is due to regularly recurring waves; a noise is due to irregular or confused vibratory waves. To be heard as a tone, a sound must have a vibration numbering at least 16 to 20 per second. Orchestral instruments produce from 40 to 4,750 vibrations per second.

Sound is not a fluid; it does not flow as a current; it is conducted by vibration. Teachers should think twice before they rush their thots into print.

"He is only working 50 per cent of his brain; only getting 50 per cent current."

If he was working 100 per cent of his brain—he might be capable of comprehending the nervous system.

Per cent is a rate by the hundred; one or more parts of any thing which is or can be divided into 100 divisions. A sub stance or entity which is not capable of being divided into 100 parts, cannot be percented.

Fifty per cent would be 50 parts, the half of the whole 100 divided parts. A brain has not 100 parts. It connot be fractioned into 100 parts. It is strange, indeed, that any one with a mathematical education should ever think of dividing a brain into 100 lots—no one but a pseudo Chiropractor would think of doing so. It is an impossibility.

If he is working 50 per cent (half) of his brain; which half is he not working?

Current means a continuous motion in the same direction—a flowing. Sound, light, impulses and vital energy do not flow. Current is applied to **liquids** which **seek to find their level.** Therefore, electricity is said to flow; it is analogous to the motion of a stream of water or other liquid finding its level. Motor and sensory impulses do not flow as a current; neither does sound, light, sensation, vital force, or energy; **they are transmitted by molecular vibration.**

## CHIROPRACTIC BEAMS OF LIGHT.

After discovering that vertebrae could be readily moved, displaced or replaced, by hand, using the spinous and transverse processes as levers, I was curious to know whether surgeons and anatomists were conversant therewith. When I personally questioned medical men regarding subluxations and their replacement, I was met with such answers as "You must be a knave or a fool; if a knave you should be in the penitentiary, if a fool you should be in an insane asylum." Fifteen years has modified the answers of medical men, they now think as the boy did, when he attempted to put on his boot and found a kitten in it—"There is something in it."

Before entering into the subject, it is well to notice that a luxation of a joint, which includes those of the spinal column, is a dislocation; a displacement of two or more bones whose articular surfaces have lost wholly, **or in part**, their natural connection.

A luxation is complete when the bones have entirely lost their natural connection; incomplete, when they partly preserve it.

A Chiropractic luxation **is one in which the articular surfaces are not wholly separated.** My writings were the first to announce that 95 per cent of all disease are the result of slightly displaced vertebrae which press against nerves causing impingements, the result being too much or not enough functionating, and that the other five per cent are from luxated joints elsewhere than in the spinal column; for example, those of the feet, causing corns and bunions.

I was not the first to replace the joints of the vertebral column. I, however, was the first to use the spinous and transverse processes as levers, by which to adjust, replace or rack them into their normal position. I was also the .first to create the art of adjusting and a science pertaining thereto. Many others had replaced vertebrae, but none had made a business of it; none had stated that all diseases were the result of displaced joints; none had ever affirmed that poisons drew vertebrae out of alignment.

While it is a well-known fact that I was the first to replace the joints of the toes, thereby relieving the pressure from nerves which inflamed the cuticle, by which the enlargements named corns and bunions were produced, there were those, years before me, who knew that corns and bunions were caused by luxated joints of the feet.

It is interesting as well as instructive to look over the past and see how near many surgeons and orthopedists came to answering the time-worn question, what is disease? The answer to this very important interrogation was gained by hard study during my 25 years of investigation. This period covers the nine years of magnetic practice during which I had learned much of value. In fact it opened the way which culminated in the production of the science and art which I had the pleasure of naming Chiropractic.

Be it remembered, that the teachings of the medical schools were, that it was the next thing to an impossibility and very rare to luxate or displace a vertebra; that it took great force and to attempt to replace one where the patient had survived, was extremely dangerous, almost certain death. It is no wonder the medical world looked upon the originator of vertebral adjusting as a crank, a knave, a fraud, a fake, and a grafter. In this place allow me to say that I have received less ill treatment from medical men than of our cousins the osteopaths, and less abuse from the osteopaths, who are appropriating the Chiropractic movements and somewhat of the principles of the science, than from Chiropractors who are reaping financial benefits from the 25 years of my hard study and close observation.

The luxations usually referred to by medical writers are complete luxations. They know of no other. Complete luxations rarely occur without fracture and are of very rare occurrence; whereas, those known to the medical profession as sprains of the backbone caused by strains, are of very common occurrence.

We give below many extracts, relating to luxations of the vertebral column.

Samuel Cooper, a writer of 1822, says: "Every kind of joint is not equally liable to dislocation. Experience proves, indeed, that in the greater part of the vertebral column, **luxations are absolutely impossible,** the pieces of bone being articulated by extensive, numerous surfaces, varying in their form and direction, and so tied together by many powerful, elastic means, that very little motion is allowed. Experience proves, also, that the strength of the articulations of the pelvic bones can scarcely be affected by enormous efforts, unless these bones be simultaneously fractured.

"The large surfaces, with which these bones support each other; the number and thickness of their ligaments; the strength of their muscles; the little degree of motion which each vertebra naturally has, and the vertical direction of the articular processes, **make dislocations of the dorsal and lumbar vertebrae impossible,** unless there be also a fracture of the above mentioned process. Of these cases I shall merely remark, that **they can only result from immense violence,** that the symptoms would be an irregularity in the disposition of the spinous processes, retention or continuance of the urine or feces, paralysis, or other injury, to which the spinal marrow would be subjected. Similar symptoms may also arise when the spinal marrow has merely undergone a violent concussion, without any fracture or dislocation whatever; and it is certain, that most of the cases mentioned by authors as dislocations of the lumbar and dorsal vertebrae, have only been concussions of the spinal marrow, or fracture of such bones.

"The os occipital, and first cervical vertebra are so firmly connected by ligaments that **there is no instance of their being luxated from an external cause,** and, **were the accident to happen, it would immediately prove fatal** by the unavoidable compression and injury of the spinal marrow."

If I had been familiar with and had imbibed such teachings as the above, Chiropractic would not have become known, until a duplicate of myself and my environments had been found.

Concussion consists of a severe shaking or jarring of a part; also, the morbid state resulting from such a jarring or shaking. Compression is the state of being compressed, squeezed, reduced to a less volume by pressure.

Delpech asserts, without modification, that a careful examination of the form and situation of the bones of the spine must convince the observer that accidents causing **displacement of vertebrae cannot occur.**

J. L. Petit relates an incident wherein a child was instantly killed by being lifted by the head.

C. Bell relates a similar case and adds: "Patients can hardly be expected to survive a mischief of this kind, when the transverse ligament is broken, and the process dentatus is thrown directly backward against the medulla oblongata, **the effect must be instant death.**"

Dupuytren gives a warning, which if heeded by Chiropractors, would allow thousands of sufferers to continue in their misery until an operation or death put an end to their suffering. "**The reduction of these dislocations is very dangerous,** and we have often known an individual to perish from the compression or elongation of the spinal cord **which always attends these attempts.**"

When Mesmerism was first promulgated, the medical fraternity and the priesthood cried humbug. The only difference being that the Roman clergy had a knowledge of Mesmerism, now called hypnotism, which the medical profession did not possess; but, when they discovered it was true, they wanted a law passed forbidding any one, except physicians, to practice it. Thus it is with the science of Chiropractic. It was at first tabooed; now, when known to be a fact, laws are desired for its prohibition.

Howe gives a similar warning. "**Death has occurred from attempts to effect reduction in cases of vertebral luxations.**"

If Howe could see Chiropractors reduce luxations by the thousand, he would have a good reason for changing his mind.

Cooper has been educated along the same line. "In the spine, the motion between any two bones is so small, that **dislocation hardly ever occurs,** except in the first and second vertebrae, altho the bones are often displaced by fracture."

Kirkland has the same opinion. "There are some luxations which are far worse injuries than fractures. Of this description are the dislocations of the vertebrae; cases which, indeed, **can hardly happen without fracture, and are almost always fatal.**"

Dr. Kirkland makes three statements, which have been proven erroneous. First, that luxations of vertebrae are worse than fractures. He is not aware that ordinary luxations can be reduced in less than a minute. Second, that dislocations of vertebrae can hardly happen without fracture. Today it is known that the per cent of fractures is not one in ten thousand.

Third, that they are almost always fatal. Fatality because of a luxated vertebrae is very rare indeed, unless we take into consideration the many diseases which arise from displaced vertebrae.

Anders reports under "Compression of the Spinal Cord" that "The postmortem findings will depend upon the degree and duration of the pressure. The cord will be more or less flattened and distorted at the seat of pressure, and in the early stages hyperemic, and possibly softened. Later it is hard, sclerosed, and of a grayish color, and above and below the compressed region degenerated areas will be seen on sectioning the cord. The nerve roots will be more or less damaged by compression.

"Two groups of symptoms are present and typical cases—first, those due to involvement of the roots, and, second, those dependent upon involvement of the cord itself—ascending and descending degeneration. The former gives rise to pain, neuralgic in character and radiating along the course of the nerves. The parts supplied are usually tender, and there may be paresthesis and formication. These irritative symptoms are followed sooner or later by those of paralysis, and hence the anethesia.

"The spine should be carefully examined and palpated for points of tenderness."

Anders states: that compression of the spinal cord flattens and softens and later it becomes hard and sclerosed. At first there is neuralgic pain, then paralysis. He advises palpating for tender spots.

Stimpson says: "The possibility of the occurrence of **pure dislocation** of the lumbar vertebrae, **which has long been in doubt** because of the close interlocking of the processes and the strength of the ligaments, is **proved by two cases** collected by Blasius and also by two others, in which there was present associated, but unimportant, fracture of some of the processes.

"Dislocation forward or backward is possible only after fracture of the odontoid process or rupture of the transverse ligament, or by the slipping of the **process** beneath the ligament."

Stimpson informs us that dislocation of the lumbar vertebrae, altho doubtful, has occurred in four cases, but the displacing of the atlas, he states, cannot occur without fracture. Were he to witness the work of Chiropractors, he would no longer doubt the possibility of dislocation of the atlas and lumbar vertebrae.

Regional Anatomy by McClellan, date 1892, states: "**Dislocation of the spinal column is especially grave. A simple dislocation of any of the vertebrae can happen only in the cervical region,** as the construction of the dorsal and lumbar vertebrae is such that a dislocation necessarily involves a fracture of some part of the bone."

While Stimpson says that dislocation of the lumbar vertebrae has been proven and cites four cases, McClellan affirms that a dislocation of these vertebrae cannot occur. Each of these authors were students of the spinal column and were honest in their statements.

Gerrish sums up his investigations and agrees with McClellan. "**Simple dislocation** between two vertebrae **is,** therefore, **almost impossible,** unless perhaps in the cervical region, where the surfaces of the articular processes are more nearly horizontal."

Lawrence reiterates the statements made by other writers. "The possibility of the occurrence of **complete dislocations** of the vertebrae without fracture, has long been a disputed point among many of the first surgical writers."

The reader will observe that Lawrence refers to complete dislocations, as tho he also recognized partial or subluxated vertebrae.

Gray, in his fourteenth edition, which was in use fifteen years ago, states:—"The ligaments which unite the component parts of the vertebrae together are so strong, and these bones are so interlocked by the arrangement of their articulating processes that **dislocation is very uncommon** and, indeed, unless accompanied by fracture, **rarely occurs,** except in the upper part of the neck. Dislocations of the **occiput from the atlas has only been recorded in one or two cases**; but dislocation of the atlas from the axis, with rupture of the transverse ligament, is much more common; it is the mode in which death is produced in many cases of execution by hanging. In the lower part of the neck—that is, below the third cervical vertebrae—dislocation unattended by fracture occasionally takes place."

For some reason Gray has changed the above paragraph in his 1905 edition, as follows: "The main joints of which the spine is composed, together with the very varied movements to which it is subjected, render it liable to **sprains, which may complicate other injuries** or may exist alone; but so closely are the individual vertebrae articulated that these sprains are seldom severe, and an amount of violence sufficiently great to produce tearing of the ligaments would tend to cause a dislocation or fracture."

The reader will please reread the two statements of Gray on the surgery of the vertebral column. It will be observed that the latest is less unfavorable to the science and art of Chiropractic. Authors of anatomies are watching the educational pulse; they aim to keep abreast of advancing thot.

Eisendrath makes some pertinent remarks on the subject. "A dislocation of a vertebra is defined as an injury in which the processes of one or both sides have completely separated from each other, accompanied by more or less displacement of the vertebral body.

"True dislocations are most frequent in the cervical region, quite rare in the dorsal and rarest of all in the lumbar region. We usually speak of **the upper of the two vertebrae as the dislocated one.** Dislocations of the vertebrae are best divided into dislocations by abduction or rotation and dislocations by flexion."

Dislocation by abduction—vertebrae drawn out of alignment, out of the median line; by rotation, one rotated more than normal; by flexion, one displaced by bending. Remember, luxations of vertebrae are normal physiological acts expressed pathologically—functions performed in too great a degree.

Campbell says: "The multiple body segments of which the spine is composed and their firm ligamentous union, indicate that **fracture without dislocation of the spine, or the reverse condition, is exceedingly rare.** In the cervical region a dislocation may occur without fracture, but in other regions they do not occur separately; hence the term fracture-dislocation is appropriately applied to this form of injury."

Erichsen in his first edition remarks: "On looking at the arrangement of the articular surfaces of the vertebrae, the very limited motion of which they are susceptible and the way in which they are closely knit together by strong ligaments and short powerful muscles, it is obvious that **dislocation of these bones must be exceedingly rare.** So seldom, indeed, do they occur, that their existence has been denied by many surgeons. Yet there are a sufficient number of instances on record to prove incontestably that **these accidents may happen.** Those cases that have been met with have usually been associated with partial fracture, but **this complication is not necessary.** In all, **the displacement was incomplete,** and, indeed, **a complete dislocation cannot occur.**

"**Dislocation of the atlas from the occipital bone has been described** in two instances only.

"**Dislocation of the axis from the atlas** is of more frequent occurrence. **It may happen with or without a fracture of the odontoid process.**

"**In the dorsal region dislocation of the spine,** though excessively rare, **may** occur. The last dorsal vertebrae has been several times found dislocated from the first lumbar.

"**Dislocation of any one of the five lower cervical vertebrae may occur.** The third vertebrae is that which is less frequently dislocated; the fifth that which is more commonly displaced. Treatment of these injuries is sufficiently simple. **No attempt at reduction can of course be made.**"

Anatomists have given special attention to the study of the vertebral column, admiring its strong and apparently invulnerable qualities; its adaptability to withstand jars and strains.

I have spent many years in searching for its weak points and in determining how to adjust those which have given away. I reasoned if vertebrae could be displaced, they could be replaced. I observed the spinous and transverse processes and devised a method whereby they might be used as levers to adjust, replace or rack the articular processes into their normal position. After spending twenty-five years in accumulating scientific facts along this line and fifteen years in adjusting vertebrae, I have formulated a science and an art whereby the displaced portions of the vertebral column may be replaced and the weak spine made strong by adjusting osseous tissue.

I have found the last dorsal to be the one most frequently dis placed, as it is not as well braced as are other vertebrae; the third cervical luxated oftener than any other cervical; the atlas comes a close second and the fourth next in frequency. The axis is seldom displaced; the seventh the least frequent of any of the cervicals, owing to its being well supported by the broad, short, stout pair of ribs and the clavicles. If Dr. Erichsen had observed a Chiropractor replacing luxated vertebrae, using the transverse and spinous processes as levers, whereby to replace displaced spinal segments, he would not have said "No attempt at reduction can of course be made."

Stimson further remarks that it does not seem improbable that some of the severe sprains of the lower portion of the back which leave a more or less permanent weakness or sensitiveness of the part, may be fractures of the arch without displacement and possibly without union.

Bickham in his extensive volume states: "Dislocation of the spinal vertebrae is caused by the articular process of the higher vertebrae gliding downward and forward over the lower. If the gliding has gone far enough to cause the posterior margin of the upper articular process to pass beyond the articular margin of the lower articular process, where it becomes interlocked, dislocation is said to have occurred, the body of the upper vertebrae having glided to some extent over the body of the vertebrae below. If the gliding has been less extensive so that these margins have not passed each other, and interlocking, therefore, has not occurred, subluxation is said to have taken place."

Bickham aims to describe, first, a complete, and secondly, a partial dislocation. He should have used the word upward instead of downward. To slide one or both of the articular processes of the upper vertebrae **upward** and forward, would make the interlocked dislocation referred to. Such a complete dislocation is possible with the six lower cervical and the upper eleven dorsal vertebrae. To do so with the atlas, the last dorsal and the five lumber vertebrae is out of the question. The only possible complete dislocation of the lumbar vertebrae, wherein their articular surfaces would loose, wholly, their natural connection, would be that of the articular processes of the upper vertebra sliding upward, forward and to the right or left, thereby straddling one of the lower articular processes. Such a complete dislocation is barely possible, but must be exceedingly rare and paralysis of all nerves from the point compressed would be the only result.

The second condition referred to, is possible; but, a partial displacement, known as a subluxation, is oftener that of the articular surfaces separating laterally, instead of vertically.

Any displacement or dislocation of the supporting osseous framework, whether that be a fracture or a displaced joint, causes either **over tension or relaxation of nerve tissue.** As I have said elsewhere, functions are dependent upon nerve vibration, and vibration, upon the amount of tension. Tension is the state or condition of being stretched or strained to stiffness. Nerves and muscles have a normal tension known as tonicity. To lessen or increase this tension is to modify vibration, accordingly. A displacement may relax or increase nerve tension.

The spinal nerve as it passes out of the intervertebral foramen, divides into a posterior, primary division for the supply of the posterior part of the body and an anterior primary division for the supply of the anterior part of the body. Each of these divisions contain fibres from both motor and sensory roots.

Before dividing, each spinal nerve gives off a small recurrent, a meningeal branch, which innervates the meninges of the spinal cord and brain. This recurrent nerve is joined by a communicating branch from the sympathetic. The anterior, primary division of certain cervical, dorsal and lumbar nerves give off nerve filaments to the sympathetic gangliated cords; these are the visceral branches of the spinal nerves.

The spinal nerves are divided into the above four branches immediately upon their exit from the spinal foramina. Any displacement, more than normal movement, of the supporting osseous framework—the vertebral column—causes a tension, a contraction of some one or more of these four branches of spinal nerves. More than normal tonicity, means a greater vibration, impulses forwarded with too great force—too much functionating, which is disease.

Normal tone or tension is that state or condition of the body or any of its organs or parts, in which the animal functions are performed with due vigor. Functions are but acts performed in response to the commands of impulses. Impulses receive their force from the transmitting medium. Force is determined by the amount of vibration, as much so as the pitch and vigor of the tone of the strings of a musical instrument is determined by the rate of their vibration. A high pitch results from a rapid, and a low tone from a slow, vibration. To pinch a nerve, in the vertebral foramen or elsewhere, would have a similar result as the pinching of a string of a musical instrument—paralysis of its function, by stopping its vibratory movement—its carrying capacity. For this reason, a vertebral luxation—a complete displacement, one which pinches—causes paralysis; whereas, an impingement increases tension, heat and functionating. To increase tension by impingement or otherwise, is to increase vibration and its carrying capacity, thereby increasing functional action.

Bickham continues: "Dislocation is most common in the cervical region (owing to the play of the vertebrae), usually between the fifth and sixth vertebrae; next, between atlas and axis. It is rare in the lumbar region, and rarest in the dorsal."

He tells us that dislocation is most common in the cervical region between the fifth and sixth, and next, that of the atlas and axis. He says in the first quoted paragraph, that a luxation consists of a **complete vertical separation** and a subluxation of a **partial vertical separation. The articulating surfaces** between the atlas and axis **are horizontal.** There is no possible show for "interlocking"; therefore, no complete luxation. The only possible displacement being laterally; that between the odontoid process and the ligamentary articulations; all told, a play of three-eighths of an inch laterally, that divided in half, allows three-sixteenths of an inch displacement of the atlas, to the left or right, which I have corrected hundreds of times by giving the thrust on either side of the posterior arch, relieving the tension, a strained or stretched condition, caused by displacement and a possible impingement.

Neurectacy—nerve-stretching—was first introduced by Nussbaum in 1872. Vogt has shown that a nerve can be stretched one-twentieth of its length and that it yields most at its spinal extremity. The nerves most commonly stretched are the facial, the spinal and the sciatic. Whether nerve-stretching produces any effect upon the spinal cord of the patient is disputed; nevertheless, there are quite a number of deaths recorded from lesions of the spinal cord **after nerve-stretching.** There are two methods, namely: that of an operation and the bloodless method. The latter can only be applied to the great sciatic nerve. The patient is etherized, the leg kept extended at the knee, the entire lower extremity is used as a straight, stiff lever and carried into a forced flexion at the hip.

Nerve-stretching is for the relief of pain and spasm. Neurectacy has been tried in wry-neck, ataxia, paralysis, myelitis, palsy, athetosis, epilepsy and tetanus, with little or no benefit. In tic-douloureux facial neuralgia, the facial nerve has been stretched; in some cases relief has continued for months, or years, but, in time, relapse follows; the patient is usually willing to submit to repeated operations for relief.

Nerve-stretching will relieve pain. Why? **Because it relieves tension.** Nerve-tension causes pain and disease. Why not find the cause of nerve-tension, nerve-excitation and relieve it? This is just what Chiropractors are doing; but, how few realize that they are relieving nerve-tension by replacing displaced bones?

Walton in a New York Medical Journal says: "Cervical dislocation occurs more frequently than is generally supposed and the results of the injury are nearly always susceptible of speedy, safe and complete amelioration.

"Three methods of treatment have been proposed: (1) Reduction by traction, with or without abduction and rotation. (2) Reduction by abduction and rotation, but without traction. (3) Reduction by dorso-lateral flexion combined, if necessary, with slight rotation. This last method, in the author's opinion, is the best. The employment of traction is a futile measure. Not infrequently **reduction takes place spontaneously, during sleep,** at other times it occurs accidentally **during the relaxation** produced by an anaesthetic. In seven cases observed by the author reduction took place as follows: **two reductions occured in sleep,** three during etherization and two were effected by operation."

Cervical dislocations are far more common than medical men have supposed. Chiropractors have no use whatever for the three methods given by Walton; neither do they need a machine for stretching the spine. Chiropractic—done by hand—is just what the author of the science meant to express and do.

Howe gives an interesting case I think worth repeating. "In 1856 I was summoned to an Irishman, who had fallen from a chamber window to the ground, head foremost. I found the patient with his head twisted to one side and rigidly held in that position. He uttered cries of distress and called lustly for relief; 'a stitch in my neck, dotchter, a stitch in my neck.' I took hold of his ears and endeavored to pull and twist his head into its natural position, but was unable to accomplish my object. By pressing my fingers into the soft structures of the neck, I could feel a bony displacement to exist between the third and fourth vertebrae, though I was unable to discover the exact nature or extent of the luxation. Perhaps another vertebrae was implicated in the displacement. By help of assistants who laid hold of the patient's head and feet, we made powerful extension and counter-extension, together with some twisting motion, and reduction, which was attended with an audible snap, was accomplished. The patient then moved his head and neck with ease and complained no more of sharp pain. He suffered from great soreness in the neck for a week or more, yet recovered without physical defect or lasting functional impairment. **I am quite sure no process of bone was broken; and that the injury was a simple luxation**, occurring between two or more of the cervical vertebrae."

Erichsen coroberates the above by giving similar cases: "**Dislocations of the articular processes of the cervical vertebrae occasionally occur.** In these cases the patient, after a sudden movement, or a fall on the head, feels much pain and stiffness in the neck, the head being fixed immovably, and turned to the opposite side to that on which the displacement has occurred.

In these cases I have known reduction affected by the surgeon placing his knees against the patient's shoulders, drawing on the head, and then turning into position, **the return being affected with a distinct snap.**"

If the one who had the following accident, should read the above cases, he would not regret being adjusted by a Chiropractor:

Frank Runge, who lives at 611 West Sixteenth Street, has enjoyed the unique distinction of having his neck dislocated and then fixed up again. One morning he did not arise from his slumbers as soon as his sister and aunt thought he ought to. So they went to his room, each taking hold of a foot and tried to pull him out of bed. He playfully resisted, and, in the melee that followed, managed to displace five bones in his neck. The bones were the atlas, axis, third, fourth and fifth cervical. The accident was a painful one. Runge's head was so turned that his face looked over his shoulder.

The young man was carried to a buggy and driven to my office. I discovered the cause of the trouble at once. After three adjustments the neck was in as good working order as ever. The cure was remarkable as the accident was peculiar.

The reduction was made by using the hands in connection with the spinous processes as levers with which to return the vertebrae to their normal position.

Vertebrae are often displaced by trivial circumstances; many times when we are unprepared to meet emergencies. Many luxations are made during sleep when we are fully relaxed. Sudden movements, superinduced by dreams, often replace as well as displace bones.

The New York Journal of Medicine, 1852, contains this account of a dislocation of a dorsal vertebra. "The injury was produced by a fall of a door, the man being under it in a stooping posture. The lower extremeties were immediately paralyzed. At the seat of the injury, which was **at the junction of the lumbar and dorsal** vertebrae, **there was a marked appearance of displacement of the parts** which seemed to arise from a fracture and dislocation or a sliding of the body of one vertebra over another. The surgeon placed the patient on his front and fastened a folded sheet under his arms and another above his hips; chloroform having been administered, extending and counter extending forces were applied by means of the sheets, and the vertebrae were reduced.

"In six or eight weeks the patient recovered the use of his limbs and normal evacuation took place. Ultimately, the recovery was complete, though a prominence remained at the seat of injury."

There are two portions of the above to which I desire to call especial attention. The prominent visible displacement of the spinous process, which the surgeon failed to fully replace, as shown by the last line. Also, the use of the folded sheets, the same as described by Dr. Langworthy, the Frank Dvorsky method. This method is not new nor confined to the Bohemians; it belongs to orthopedic surgery, therefore is not Chiropractic.

The following quotation is taken from the American Text-Book of Surgery. "Fractures of the spine, as compared with other fractures, are rare, constituting only 3.3 per cent of nearly 52,000 fractures treated in the London Hospital during thirty-five years.

"The prognosis in all cases (of fracture dislocation) is unfavorable, both as to recovery of function and as to great prolongation of life, becoming more serious in direct proportion to the higher situation of the fracture, the severity of the injury which causes it and the amount of crushing or of dislocation."

Pott mentions a case where no known violence had been observed. The first intimation was a sense of weakness, accompanied by a dull pain in the backbone. The weakness and lassitude made even a small amount of exercise result in fatigue which was followed by an unusual sense of coldness in the thighs and a partial diminution in sensibility not accountable to changes in the weather. In time his limbs were frequently convulsed by involuntary twitchings, more so in the night than during the day. He finally became unable to walk. The ability to retain or discharge his urine and feces was also lacking.

Pott continues to explain: "In the adult I will not assert that external mischief is always and totally out of the question; but I will venture to affirm, what is equal, as far as regards the true nature of the case, which is, that altho accidents and violence may in some few instances be allowed to have contributed to its more immediate appearance, yet the part in which it shows itself, must have been previously in a morbid state and thereby predisposed for the production of it. **I do not by this mean to say that a violent exertion cannot injure the spine, or produce a paralytic complaint**; that would be to say more than I know; but I will venture to assert that no degree of violence whatever is capable of producing such an appearance as I am now speaking of, unless the bodies of the vertebrae were by previous distemper disposed to give way; and that there was no supposable dislocation, caused by mere violence, done to the bones of the back, which bones were, before the receipt of the injury, in a sound state."

The previous morbid state, referred to by Pott, caused by distemper, which predisposes vertebral dislocations and paralytic conditions, is that of caries or rickets. Chiropractors find that these predisposing causes have their origin in vertebral displacements.

Ayers, in The New York Journal, reports a case of dislocation occurring between the cervical vertebrae, from some unknown cause, as the man was drunk when he received the injury. The account goes on to say that "his neck was rigid and exhibited a peculiar deformity which could not attend any lesion except **luxation of one or more of the cervical vertebrae.** There was no paralysis, but **intense pain attended the displacement.** Great difficulty was experienced in attempting to drink or swallow food. The esophagus and larynx seemed to be pressed upon by the bulging forward of several of the cervical vertebrae. The back of the neck was rendered excessively concave and the integument was thrown into folds as it is when the head is forced back against the shoulders; the front of the neck presented a corresponding convexity. **Between the spinous process of the fifth and sixth cervical vertebrae, a marked despression could be felt** and that was the point at which the greatest distress was felt by the patient." Dr. Ayers, with several assistants, who agreed with him in his diagnosis, **performed a successful reduction** while the patient was under the influence of chloroform. Extension was applied to the head and counter extension to the shoulders, and while the head was rotated and pressure made upon prominent points in the neck, **the displaced bones returned to their former position,** the neck and head resuming their natural attitude and aspect."

Chiropractors never give anesthetics to render the patient insensible to pain. To adjust a displaced vertebrae requires less time than it does for a surgeon to get ready. The poorest Chiropractor would more than equal a score of the best surgeons, when it comes to resetting the bones of the back.

That "marked depression" was the separation between the spinous processes, a lordosis, caused by a tilting of one of the vertebrae.

Samuel Cooper remarks: "I believe no modern practitioner now ever advises supporting the spine with machinery, on the supposition of there being any **dislocation; an error,** which formerly prevailed.

"**The cervical vertebrae,** however, not having such extensive articular surfaces and having more motion, **are occasionally luxated. The dislocation of the head from the first vertebrae**

**and the first vertebrae from the second, particularly the last accident, is the most common; but luxations of the cervical lower down, though very rare, are possible."**

The American Text-Book of Surgery, date 1904, containing 1363 pages, published by W. B. Saunders, Philadelphia, has on the page, from which I quote, three cuts of three pairs of cervical vertebrae displaying luxated articular processes similar to those often seen in the advertising booklets of Chiropractors. The disquisition is so instructive that I shall quote quite at length.

"Dislocations of vertebrae are commonly associated with fracture, but **a number of cases have been reported and verified by post-mortem examination in which uncomplicated dislocation has occurred.** They were nearly all of the cervical region. A few dorsal dislocations have been noted, the majority of them affecting the twelfth dorsal vertebrae. Only three or four cases of dislocation of the lumbar vertebrae without serious fracture have been recorded and confirmed by autopsy.

"**Vertebral dislocations** may be caused by forced flexion or extreme extension. When produced by such forces they will uniformly be bilateral and either forward or backward. **They may also be produced by extreme lateral motions of the spine or by excessive rotation.** In either of these cases they may be unilateral, either forward or backward and may be incomplete, that is, **the articular surface may remain in contact at their edges**; or complete, in which case the inferior process of the upper vertebra passes farther forward and sinks into the notch between the body and the superior articular process of the lower vertebra.

"**It is usual** in treating of dislocations of the vertebrae **to speak of the upper one as the vertebra that has been dislocated**. Of course, there are the usual associated lesions, including rupture of ligaments, muscles and blood vessels, **injuries to nerves and often laceration of the intervertebral disks.** In the absence of deformity the symptoms will be the same as those of fracture of the vertebrae. Crepitus and preternatural mobility are not always obtainable in fracture, and indeed **cannot with propriety be sought for in the majority of such cases.** In the cervical region it may be possible to recognize the change in the relations of the transverse processes, the body of the dislocated vertebra may be felt through the pharynx, and the absence of the corresponding spinous process may be noted on the back of the neck. The rigidity and **the attitude in which the neck is held will often be very suggestive,** but may be closely simulated by the muscular contraction and pain due to contusion of muscles or to **inflammation of the intervertebral joints.** The paralysis will depend upon the extent of the displacement and the corresponding damage to the cord, and may vary from a very slight paresis to extensive paraplegia. Usually motor paralysis is more marked and extensive than sensory paralysis, and both kinds are apt to be less absolute in dislocation than in fracture. In some cases of dislocation paralysis has been entirely absent.

"Although **many surgical authorities have objected to any effort being made to reduce luxation on the ground that the attempt may cause the immediate death of the patient, especially if the luxation is in the upper cervical region,** it yet seems proper in the majority of cases in which dislocation is diagnosticated to attempt to replace the part by means of traction aided by flexion or rotation. **It is right that the patient and his friends should be informed of the risk of immediate death during this procedure, but the surgeon may conscientiously and urgently advise that the risk be accepted.** The maneuvers will depend upon the seat of the dislocation, but, **as a rule, no special method can be indicated.** If in a cervical luxation an unnatural prominence in the pharynx can be felt, reduction may be facilitated by making backward pressure with the finger through the mouth while at the same time traction is kept up from the chin and occiput. When the displacement is unilateral, rotation should be used in addition to extension and counter-extension. The head, which is apt to be inclined to one side, should be carried still farther in that direction, so as to disengage the processes of the luxated vertebra, after which it should be gently rotated and bent toward the opposite side, extension and counter-extension being kept up during the whole of this procedure. In the lower segments of the spine the methods already described for rectifying the deformity in fractures apply equally to luxations. In the majority of cases the operator will be in doubt as to whether or not a fracture co-exists.

"The prognosis is, of course, more favorable in uncomplicated luxations which have been reduced than in fracture, but **the injury in all cases must be regarded as a very serious one.** Even after reduction paralysis often persists, and death ensues on account of the injury to the cord."

This Text-Book gives advice for fracture-dislocation which is applicable to the above. "Perhaps the most important advice to be given to the general practitioner in relation to the treatment of this condition is a caution against the use of braces, corsets, jackets and other mechanical appliances which by confining the movements of the chest and supplying an artificial support in place of the muscles which it is most desirable to develop, actually do great harm to many patients instead of good."

I am pleased to see stated in one of the leading text-books, that partial dislocations do exist; that intervertebral discs may be lacerated, nerves injured and articular surfaces partially displaced. These are, in a measure, the principles for which I have been contending during the last fifteen years. The principles of Chiropractic are beginning to permeate the medical and osteopathic professions; those accepted will lead to further investigation and advancement. When it becomes a generally accepted fact among the medical profession, that vertebral luxations do exist; that they can be readily reduced; that by vertebral adjustments, acute diseases disappear as does the morning frost before the rising sun; that the one who knows how, can reduce vertebral luxations; that the red flag which has been held so long before the medical profession has faded to a pure white, they will admit the truth of the basic principles of Chiropractic, but will then ask legislators to pass laws forbidding all except those who belong to their own ranks—those who were formerly foremost in pronouncing Chiropractic a fraud—to use the hands only to adjust displaced vertebrae.

Beck recognized that vertebrae might be racked out of their normal position. "The most important sign is the traumatic kyphosis, produced by a displacement of the spinous process, whereby a prominence is caused. Sometimes more than one vertebrae is concerned."

A vertebrae displaced affects the two with which it articulates, and those only; adjusting the one displaced, corrects its relation with each of the others.

Wharton and Curtis have definite ideas regarding vertebral luxations. "Compression of the spinal cord may be caused by displaced bone (from fracture or caries), by a foreign body such as a rifle ball lodging in the canal, by bloodshot, inflammatory exudates, or tumors in the canal.

"Complete rest is the only method of treatment, except the administration of the usual tonics, hot and cold baths, massage and gentle exercise with a free outdoor life. Occasionally some counter-irritation by a thorough cauterization over the spine is of advantage.

"In the vertebral column fracture and dislocation are almost invariably combined; the interlocking of the bony processes making it difficult for a dislocation to occur without fracture and **the dislocation is usually the more important part of the injury. To distinguish between the two is often impossible. Simple dislocation is rare except in the cervical region,** but there it presents a definite clinical picture."

Dunglison allows two sunbeams to shine on the pages of his dictionary. "(1), Spinal irritation, a supposed erethistic state of the spinal cord, indicated by tenderness on pressure over the spinal process of one or more vertebrae, or over the nerves proceeding from the cord and distributed to the parts at the sides of the spine, and, (2), Spinal localization, the designation of a particular part of the spinal cord as the center of certain physiological functions or of muscular movements or reflexes."

Gould's Dictionary: "Spinal irritation, a form of neurasthenia characterized by pain in the back, tenderness along the spines of the vertebrae, fatigue on slight exertion and occasionally numbness and tingling in the limbs."

Lippincott's Medical Dictionary states: "Spinal irritation, any condition of functional derangement and nervous irritability accompanied by tenderness over the spine."

The above expressed Chiropractically would read: Nervous irritability accompanied by tenderness near either side of the spine and functional derangement indicates spinal nerve irritation.

Cunningham gives the Chiropractor some good hints. "Fracture-dislocations of the spine are commonest in the lower cervical and dorso-lumbar regions; that is to say, where the movable cervical and lumbar regions join the more fixed dorsal region. The spinal column above the injury is generally displaced forwards, so that the spinal cord is often severely lacerated or completely torn across by the upper end of the portion of the column below the fracture.

"To understand the effect of lesions of the cord, it is necessary to be familiar with the sensory and motor distributions of the various spinal segments. Transverse lesions of the cord above the fifth cervical spine (that is, above the disc between the fourth and fifth cervical vertebra) are quickly fatal from paralysis of respiration, as the phrenic nerve arises mainly from the fourth segment. In transverse lesions of the cervical enlargment the cutaneous insensibility does not extend higher than a transverse line at the level of the second intercostal space. The diagnosis of the particular segment involved is arrived at by testing the motor and sensory functions of each segment. The sensory areas corresponding to the lower four cervical and the first two dorsal segments occupy the upper extremities, and are placed in numerical order from the radial to the ulnar side of the limb. The sensory area corresponding to the second, third, and fourth cervical segments occupy the occipital region of the scalp, the back of the auricle, and the masseteric region, the whole of the neck, and the shoulders and upper part of the chest down to a horizontal line at the level of the interior end of the third intercostal space. In total transverse lesion of the cord in the dorsal region the upper limit of the anesthesia is horizontal, and reaches to the level of the terminations of the anterior primary divisions of the spinal nerves, which arise from the spinal segment opposite the vertebral injury. Hence the upper limit of the anesthesia is at a much lower level than that of the injured vertebrae. For example, a fracture-dislocation at the level of the eighth dorsal vertebrae involves the origin of the tenth dorsal nerve which ends at the level of the umbilicus. The sensory zone corresponding to the fifth dorsal segment is at the level of the ensiform cartilage, that of the tenth at the level of the umbilicus, while that of the twelfth reaches down anteriorly to the upper border of the symphysis. The sensory areas corresponding to the lumbar and sacral segments."

The above quotations need no comment. This text-book of 1388 pages is published by William Wood and Company, of New York.

Spinal irritation is the erethistic (abnormal increase of nervous irritability) state of the spinal cord, or the nerves proceeding therefrom. This sensibility can be readily determined by pressure upon the spinous processes, or upon the nerves as they pass from the foramina.

Post mortem investigations have shown that certain parts of the brain have special functions. See Dunglison's Medical Dictionary.

Localization, when applied to the brain, is the determining of the various faculties in the cerebrum that preside over certain physiologic acts; or of the seat of pathologic conditions interfering with the proper function of these centers. When applied to the spinal cord, it is the designating of a particular part as the center of certain physiological functions or muscular movements or reflexes.

Lippincott's New Medical Dictionary: "Localization, the determination of the points at which normal functions or pathological conditions originate."

Those very "points" are being determined and localized by Chiropractors. In inflammatory cases, these "points," previous to Chiropractic adjusting, are tense, cord-like; immediately after the adjusting, the nerve is flaccid, not so sensitive, the pressure and its resultant irritation has been removed.

The American Text-Book of Surgery: "Contusion of the spinal cord may result from severe pain, but usually occurs as a consequence or forced flexion of the vertebral column. It is accompanied by hemorrhage into the substance of the cord—hematomyelia—which usually occupies the gray substance, and may extend to a considerable distance. It is accompanied by motor and sensory paralysis and a diminution of the reflexes. It may be followed by acute myelitis and all the phenomena attendant upon degeneration or destruction of the substance of the cord. It is obviously difficult to diagnosticate a fracture in which no deformity exists. The prognosis is, however, more favorable, and in cases of contusion of the cord of moderate severity the improvement which occurs at the end of the first or second week will serve to show the character of the lesion.

"As to the diagnosis of these various forms of injury, the time which elapses between the accident and the development of the symptoms is one of the most important factors. If the symptoms occur instantaneously after a grave injury, the cord has probably been compressed by a displaced vertebrae, and the case has been one of fracture or luxation or of the common lesion which combines them both, the so-called fracture-dislocation. If the symptoms have not made their appearance for some time, possibly hours after the injury, the cause is probably hemorrhage, paralysis not having been produced until a sufficient amount of blood had accumulated to cause the necessary pressure. If the hemorrhage is intra-medullary, less time will elapse than if it occurs between the membranes and the walls of the canal. If the symptoms of paralysis do not appear until a period varying from a week to one or two months, they are probably due to pressure by inflammatory lymph the result of an external pachymeningitis."

In myelitis of the spinal cord, occasioned by subluxation, the location of which is determined by the contour of the spinous processes.

"The diagnosis of severe sprains" is not difficult. Learning what portion of the body is affected, knowing what nerves ramify that region, and where they emerge from the spinal canal, because of their sensitive condition they can be readily traced by palpation, and not the least of the aids to a Chiropractor's diagnostication, is the "irregularity in the line of the spinous processes."

An M. D.'s sprain is a Chiropractor's luxation. As sprains are of all degrees of severity and may be followed by a great variety of symptoms, so it is with displacements of the vertebral column.

Macdonald is aware of there being luxations of vertebrae, complete and incomplete. "Although this accident is generally a complication of fracture, there are many cases recorded of pure dislocation. The injury occurs most frequently in the cervical region, owing to the smaller size of the vertebrae and their less intimate apposition. The fifth cervical seems to be the most liable to displacement. In the dorsal region the twelfth segment is the one most frequently displaced. In the lumbar region the accident is very rare. The dislocation is generally bilateral, but a number of unilateral luxations are recorded. The causes of the injury are forced flexion or extension, extreme lateral motion or rotation."

Under diagnosis he says: "Our main reliance must be placed upon the following points: The neck is rigid and the head turned to one side in unilatral luxation; the spinous and transverse processes may be felt to be displaced. If the dislocation is in the upper cervical region, respiration is difficult, or it may even be suddenly arrested, producing death. The finger should explore the pharynx for displacement of the body of a vertebrae. For the rest, the paralytic symptoms will afford some evidence. dislocation above the bracial plexus causes paralysis of both upper and lower extremities, as well as of the trunk. Motor is more marked than sensory paralysis, and may range from slight paresis to complete paraplegia. The attitude assumed by the patient is sometimes very characteristic, as in a case reported by Ayres, in which the head was thrown back, the neck perfectly rigid, and the larynx projecting forward."

As to treatment he advises: "This dislocation is a serious injury, and the patient's friends should be warned of two dangers. If reduction is attempted, instant death may result, especially if the displacement is in the upper cervical region. On the other hand, to allow the pressure of the displaced vertebra upon the cord to continue is certain to result in destructive changes and probably death. An attempt at reduction should therefore be made. This is affected by gentle and steady traction upon the occiput and chin. If a displaced vertebra can be felt in the pharynx, the finger of the operator should make firm pressure upon it while steady traction is kept up. Should the luxation be unilateral, rotation of the neck should accompany extension."

The reader will observe that Macdonald refers to complete dislocation. The partial dislocations he places under sprains. As I have said before, the M. D.'s sprain is the subluxation of the Chiropractor. Macdonald continues:

"**Sprains of the back are very common injuries, and occur in all degrees of severity.** Violent exertion, as in lifting heavy bodies, may cause injuries of the muscles alone, resulting in a stiffness of the back and a local tenderness which will soon pass off.

"In more severe injuries the ligaments of the spine may be overstretched or torn, and in the case of the ligamenta subflava the rupture may be attended with hemorrhage, resulting in paralysis. The bones may be injured, the vertebrae separated from the intervertebral substance, and the cord itself may suffer.

"The symptoms will depend upon the extent of the injury. There is usually more or less shock, pain, tenderness. and swelling; ecchymosis is slow in making its appearance on account of the thickness of the skin. In some cases a considerable quantity of blood is poured out, forming a hematoma, which if not absorbed may require incision. In severe cases it may be a difficult point to decide whether the spine is fractured or not. The degree of paralysis will have to settle the question. In severe sprains or contusions, as when a man falls across a beam or iron bar and has his body forcibly doubled up, the lower limbs may be more or less paralyzed, but the paralysis is never so complete as that which results from fracture.

"A rigidity of the muscles is usually a prominent symptom, and in medico-legal cases plays an important part, owing to its resemblance to Pott's disease. When the injury is unilateral the rigidity will be confined to the injured side—a condition which cannot be simulated."

Under the head of treatment he advises: "Shock, if present, must be relieved by stimulants, morphine, or hot applications, after which absolute rest constitutes the principal treatment. Friction and massage are very valuable in reducing swelling and promoting absorption, and strapping the back with broad bands of adhesive plaster extending around two-thirds of the body will afford relief."

Several authors refer to vertebral subluxations as "Railway Spine," as explained by Macdonald. "Railway Spine. The peculiar circumstances attending railway accidents, and the frequency with which such injuries are the subject of litigation, give them special interest to the surgeon. A person whose back is injured in a railway accident may sustain any degree of injury from simple strain or contusion of the muscles to laceration of the ligaments or fracture of the spine, but additional elements come into the case by reason of the fright and shock which attend the accident. The passenger may be roughly awakened from sleep by the catastrophe. The screams of his fellow-passengers, the sight of dead and mangled bodies, the horrible sensation of being held down by portions of the wreck, and, to crown all, the outbreak of fire, which he feels will surely reach him before he can be extricated, produce impressions on his mind which last for weeks and months and add a neurotic element to the traumatism. Long after the injury has had time to heal the patient complains of vague pains or pains that exist only in his imagination. There are tender spots, lameness and weakness of the back, inability to incline the body from one side to the other or to move the shoulders. Numbness and tingling in the lower limbs are frequently complained of, as also is anesthesia or hyperesthesia. The skin is moist, or in some cases bathed in profuse perspiration, while the kidneys act freely, compelling the patient to get up several times in the night. The eyesight is affected, according to the patient's story, although no changes in the retina or other parts of the eye can be found to account for these subjective symptoms.

"The mental condition is more or less affected. The patient is nervous and incapable of concentrating his attention upon his business or anything that requires continuous volition. He becomes despondent and gloomy, looking forward without hope and filled with the idea that ruin stares him in the face.

"These are the cases that bring out two types of expert witnesses, one side swearing that the man is seriously injured and permanently disabled, the other side testifying that the symptoms are fraudulent and only assumed for the purpose of mulcting the railway company. The examination of such patients must be conducted with great care, and, while it is necessary to be guarded against so-called 'litigation symptoms,' fairness and justice demand that all real symptoms should carry due weight."

The above quotations are from Surgical Diagnosis and Treatment by J. W. Macdonald, M. D., published by W. B. Saunders, Philadelphia.

Physicians have been taught that dislocations of vertebrae rarely occur without fracture. This is the case with complete dislocations, such as are referred to by Macdonald in the first three quoted paragraphs consequently, if there is no sign of fracture, it is considered that the spine has been sprained.

While the fifth cervical vertebrae may be the most liable to complete displacement, I find the atlas and third cervical are much oftener subluxated—sprained. In the dorsal region, I fully agree with Macdonald that the twelfth segment is the one most frequently displaced.

Take notice: Macdonald refers to reduction of complete displacement being a dangerous operation; he does not refer thus to partial displacement—sprains. Sprains, subluxations, of the back are thot to be very common by Macdonald and no doubt most of pathologists fully agree with him. While it is generally known that the spine may be wrenched, the vertebral articulations abnormally moved too far laterally or vertically, it is thot that when not fully displaced, they return to their normal position of their own accord.

In a complete dislocation (take your spinal column) the superior articular processes of one vertebra are posterior to those of the one above. This, from the shape of the articular processes, can more readily occur in the cervical than in the dorsal, and in the dorsal region more easily than in the lumbar.

A cervical, dorsal or lumbar vertebra cannot be displaced anterior to its fellows without being completely luxated, their articular surfaces having wholly lost their connection. Consequently, cuts displaying the body of one vertebra anterior to the one above or the one below, need adjusting, as no such subluxation can exist.

The oblique processes; the dorsal and the cervical, minus the atlas, are ascending oblique, the lower the descending oblique processes, forbid the sliding forward or backward of any of the vertebrae, without fracture of these oblique processes, except it be of the atlas and even there we find a wise provision which would as certainly prevent it, because of the short, stout transverse ligament.

It will be interesting to observe the difference between future editions of pathological and surgical books and those of the past in regard to the cause, nature and effect of vertebral subluxation and the method of reducing them.

Injuries to the spine similar to those caused by railway accidents, are incident to all the avocations of life; they may occur even during sleep. "From baby in the high chair to grandma in the rocker," the axial bones are as liable to be displaced by noxious substances which enter the system in our food and drink or by inhalation as they are by accident direct.

Dorland's Dictionary has nearly a page devoted to "Localization of the functions of the segments of the spinal cord."

In a measure, spinal localization as given is correct; but, owing to variations in the arrangement of osseous tissue and the nervous system, there can be no set rules to go by.

Brodie has his opinion as to the origin of caries. He gives encouragement to those affected with it. "In many instances, caries of the spine has its origin in the body of the vertebrae themselves, which are liable to the same disease of the cancellous structure that is noticed in the articulating extremities of other bones. In some cases, rest in a horizontal posture, below ground, I believe, must soon be the patient's doom."

Caries are usually found in vertebrae; necrosis in the long bones. The cause of either is inflammation, localized, excessive heat.

Delafield and Prudden say but little about vertebral luxations. "The spinal cord may be compressed or lacerated by penetrating wounds, by fracture or **dislocation of the vertebrae**, or by concussion without injury to the vertebrae. If life continues, the nerve elements may degenerate."

Tubby sheds a ray of light on nerve impingement. "Osteo-arthritis and osteitis-deformans cause a general kyphosis; nor do they give rise to reflected pain, unless it may happen—a rare event I imagine—that the nerves are pressed upon as they issue from the spinal canal."

Of the "Bonesetters," he says: "Such cases drift about until they fall into the hands of the 'Bonesetter,' who with one jerk relieves the patient of his or her disability, and arrogates to himself the credit of putting in a dislocated bone." This remark looks strange sandwiched in between the one above and the following copied from page 81 of his Orthopedic Surgery:

"I recently **removed the breast** of a patient who, having found **a tumor** which she was afraid might be a **cancer**, kept the matter to herself for nine months. During this time the growth steadily increased, and in the last two months she had suffered from very **severe pains in the spine at the level of about the fourth dorsal vertebra and also around the sides of her chest. When the spine was examined, a well marked angular curvature was found.**"

The dorsal vertebra was sufficiently tipped to expose a spinous process and cause that "well marked angular curvature." Cancer of the breast has its cause "about the fourth dorsal." Sensitive nerves may be tracel by palpation to and from the breast. The patient will notice a difference before and after adjusting, in the sensation, by pressure, on the cancer and the nerves proceeding from the spine to the affected breast.

Carver. "A subluxation is that condition in an articulation in which, by reason of a sprain, laceration, or contusion, the **elemental parts of a joint** have lost their harmonious and normal relations. This concept of articular displacement entirely leaves out luxation, which is a condition where, as a result of some or all of the injuries indicated, the **elemental parts of the joint** have entirely lost their apposition. This is a condition classified as being 'out of joint,' and does not come within the province of the Chiropractor, but has for a long time been held to be within the scope of surgery. Luxation is therefore not a term which properly belongs to Chiropractic. A subluxation, however, is any articular displacement of the character defined less than a luxation."

A luxation is a dislocation. Either of these conditions may be defined as "a displacement of two or more bones whose articular surfaces have lost, **wholly or in part**, their natural connection." There may be present laceration of the intervertebral cartilage; or, in compound fracture, a laceration of the surrounding tissue. A sprain never produces a luxation. An M. D.'s sprain is known to a Chiropractor as a displacement, or a luxation. Elemental means pertaining to elements, to first principles, to primary ingredients. Therefore, it is a term which cannot be applied to the parts of a joint. He should have said "the articular processes have entirely or partially lost their connection." Luxation and subluxation are proper terms for Chiropractors to use when designating complete and partial displacements respectively.

A. T. Still allowed a ray of light to shine on this question when he said: "I contend that the curing comes direct from the liberation of the interspinous and costal nerves, freed from bone-pressure on the nerves of motion, sensation and nutrition.

"A wrench of the spinal column has been given with force enough to slip the vertebral articulations and inhibit nerves. We should remember that slipped or twisted vertebrae must be sought out and adjusted.

"The osteopath should let his eye rest day and night on the spinal column, to know if the bones articulate truly in all facets and other bearings, and never rest day or night until he knows the spine is true and in line from atlas to sacrum, with all the ribs in perfect union with the processes of the spine.

"Thus we see the importance of a perfectly normal spine at all points of articulation."

A. T. Still refers to the wrenching of a spinal column as tho it was an unusual accident.

A. P. Davis, M. D., D. O., describing a cervical treatment says: "This movement should be done with caution, so as not to dislocate the neck.

"It was long thought that the dislocation of a rib was responsible for all the mischief; or a dislocated hip, or a slipped vertebra, had much to do in producing disease of all kinds; but the intelligent in the ranks of Osteopathy are ready to concede the cause to other sources, and now it is a pretty well settled fact that **dislocation does not** play such a role in the **production of disease** as was formerly attributed to it."

The neck is that part of an animal which connects the head with the trunk; it cannot be dislocated. He no doubt referred to the cervical vertebrae.

Neuropathy by A. P. Davis: "**That there are impingements of nerves** along the spine we readily and freely grant, and know to be a fact but to assert that luxations, or even **partial luxations are responsible** for nerve impingements, **we most emphatically deny.** Any one who has ever examined a spinal column can very readily see that to dislocate a vertebra, absolute violence must be inflicted! When a vertebra is luxated anywhere, a paralysis immediately ensues to all parts below the luxation, in which the nerves coming out of the foramina below the luxation occur, and suspension of all functions where the nerves below the part end."

Dr. Davis recognizes impingements—pressure on nerves—but denies that luxations—partial or complete—are responsible. If displaced bones do not impinge—press against nerves and muscles, pray, tell me what does.

Joy M. Loben in The Chiropractor: "It is there (spinal foramina) and there alone that the soft nerve passes between two hard substances capable of producing a constriction."

There is quite a difference between constriction and compression. Constriction in anatomy is usually applied to orifices which are constricted in a circular direction. Compression makes more compact, reduces the volume of pressure. Two hard substances (bones) might squeeze or compress a softer substance (nerves), but do not constrict. Two hard substances are not capable of constricting—encircling—an orifice.

Stengel: "The most frequent injury of joints is that known as luxation, in which the relations of articulating bones are disturbed. In these cases the ligaments and other soft tissue around the joints are more or less torn, and in consequence become inflamed. If the luxation is reduced, this inflammation subsides quickly, and frequently normal conditions are restored. If the luxation persists, various secondary changes may occur. Ankylosis in abnormal positions may take place by the formation of fibrous adhesions, or in more favorable cases a false joint may be established.

"Ankylosis is the term applied to the condition in which the normal movability between articulating bones is prevented by interosseous attachments. Pathologically, ankylosis may be fibrous, cartilaginous, or bony."

Stengel tells us that the inflammatory conditions in luxated joints exist because the ligaments and other soft tissue are torn. But luxated joints in which there is no laceration, manifest as much heat as those lacerated. He, also, says, that if the luxation is reduced, the **inflammation subsides quickly.** The subsidence is certainly not due to the immediate healing of the torn tissue, but to the removal of impingements from sensory nerves.

C. Bell refers to the destruction of the intervertebral cartilage and the forcible separation of the spinous processes of the last cervical and first dorsal.

McMurrich incidentally makes a few remarks upon this all important subject. "**The parts of the spine most exposed to injury** are the thoraco-lumbar and cervico-thoracic, partly because here more mobile parts are joined to those which are more fixed, and also from the amount of leverage exerted on the thoraco-lumbar region; and, in the case of the upper region, because this is affected by violence exerted on the head. The chief provisions for protection of the cord are the number of bones and joints which allow of movement without serious weakening, the three curves and columns, cervical, thoracic and lumbar, ensuring bending before breaking; the large amount of cancellous tissue and the number and structure of the intervertebral discs all tending to damp vibrations; the large size of the theca vertebralis and the way in which the cord, anchored and slung by the thirty-one pairs of nerves and the ligamenta denticulata, about twenty in number, occupies neutral ground in the center of the canal as regards injury directly and indirectly applied."

The chief provision protecting vertebrae from being racked out of their normal position, is to be found in the transverse processes with the additional rib-supports acting as braces. A personal examination of hundreds of vertebral columns, usually displays a weak place at the thoraco-lumbar junction.

Helferich: "In the dorsal and lumbar regions pure dislocation is exceedingly rare. **The possibility of true dislocation in the region of the dorsal and lumbar vertebrae has been proven on the post mortem table,** but must be almost impossible to recognize in the living subject, i. e., it must be difficult to exclude fracture."

Helferich refers to true and pure dislocations, as tho there were those which were false and mixed. He thinks it almost impossible to recognize in the living subject a vertebral displacement which is not associated with fracture. A knowledge of anatomy, pathology, functions and nerve tracing, with practice, tends toward making one proficient in the science and art of Chiropractic. It is not necessary for Chiropractors to use a dissecting table to determine dislocations of vertebrae.

Erichsen's latest edition states: "Partial dislocation may exist unsuspected, the case being considered one of simple contusion."

He says that sprains, strains, **wrenches and twists of the spine are of very frequent occurrence. They may be followed by**

**every possible kind of mischief to the vertebral column, its bones, or ligaments.**

He continues to state that **sprains or wrenches of the spine will frequently lay the foundation of serious organic disease of the bones and articular structures, leading to angular curvature, abscess, paraplegia and possibly a fatal result.**

"**One of the most remarkable circumstances connected with injuries of the spine is the disproportion that exists between the apparent trifling accident that the patient has sustained, and the real and serious mischief that has in reality occurred, and which will eventually lead to the gravest consequences.**

"**Although there is often a long interval between the time of the occurrence of the accident and the supervention of the more distressing symptoms and the conviction of the serious nature of the injury that has been sustained, it will be found on close inquiry, that there has never been an interval, however short, of complete restoration to health.**"

Partial dislocation may exist unsuspected. The medical profession are hunting for antidotes, not causes. Erichsen's explanations are so plain and correct that they need no further elucidation.

Landois: "Fractures, caries and necrosis, and also inflammatory processes, which render movements of the bones painful, impair such movements or even render them wholly impossible. A similar result is caused by dislocations or inflammations of the joints, relaxation of the articular surfaces (ankylosis) or between the ligaments and soft parts surrounding the joint. Deviations from the normal function may further be caused by abnormal curvatures of the bones, enlargements (hyperostosis), or outgrowths (exostosis). Among the abnormal positions of the skeletal parts that occur frequently are to be included curvature of the spinal column laterally (scoliosis), backward (kyphosis), or forward (lordosis)."

All of the pathological conditions mentioned can be traced to luxated vertebrae. Accidents displace, and poisons draw, vertebrae out of alignment.

Howe saw the need of Chiropractic sunbeams, but because he did not know their worth or dare not proclaim them, he drew down the blinds and closed the doors.

Hare asks a question and then answers it as best he can. "The spinal lesions giving rise to paraplegia of the lower extremeties are numerous. Given a case of paraplegia, or paralysis of the lower extremeties, what may be its cause? When paraplegia occurs in a young child it is due in a great majority of cases to caries of the vertebrae, and the pressure so produced does not necessarily depend upon compression by the bones. but by the inflammatory exudate."

The vertebra displaced, the nerves impinged upon, the lesion which produces paraplegia, paralysis of the lower half of the body, will always be found in the lower dorsal or upper lumbar; the exact location depending upon the upper line of paralysis.

If Erichsen had used the word luxation instead of compression he would have voiced my sentiment. "The effects of concussion of the spine, whether arising from violence directly or indirectly applied, are occasionally slow in manifesting themselves to the full intensity, so slow, indeed, that the patient may not connect their supervention with the injury which he had sustained some length of time previously."

Foot allowed sunbeams to penetrate his sanctum sanctorum, but did not know of their usefulness: "**Dislocation of vertebrae may be due either to direct violence or to a fall. If the dislocation is complete, it is often found to be associated with fracture and to have produced fatal lesions of the cord. There are instances, however, in which dislocation is only partial** and in which the cord escapes serious injury. **This is especially true when a partial dislocation takes place between the axis and atlas. Such a patient may escape paralytic symptoms and may live with it unreduced.** If the head and body are pulled strongly apart and the neck is manipulated, **the dislocation may be reduced. This procedure is not without risk of sudden death.**

"**Dislocation of either dorsal or lumbar vertebrae without fracture** rarely occurs and when it does so, it **is a partial dislocation** in most cases. **Attempts at reduction should be made under general anesthesia with great care.**"

If Foote should see a Chiropractor adjusting vertebrae at the rate of one a minute without an anesthetic, pain or fear, he would be pleasantly surprised. To pull the "head and body strongly apart," increases the resistance to be overcome. Instead, the hands should be laid along side of the body or on the buttocks. This position of the arms causes the patient to be more relaxed than when they hang downward. The patient should be relaxed while being adjusted.

Simpson desires to know the truth regarding vertebral luxation. "Concerning the frequency of dislocation of the vertebrae widely different opinions have been held, some denying even the possibility of dislocation without fracture, others think them rare, and others, again, claiming that they are quite common."

"**The nerve trunks at their point of emergency through the intervertebral foramina may be compressed between the articu-**

**lar processes of one vertebra and the body or pedicle of the other.**

Howe sees daylight. "**In the cervical and lumbar regions,** when motion is not restrained by the vertical articular surfaces, **dislocation can occur without** the absolute necessity of a **fracture**; but **in the dorsal region,** where the processes overlap, and are closely locked, **simple dislocation seems impossible.**

"However, **there have been reported during the last few years a number of well authenticated dislocations of the vertebrae, in different regions of the column.** The case of Charles Butcher, who slipped on some steps, while carrying a heavy load on his head, in the end **proved that a vertebral luxation can occur.**"

Today, thousands of cases of vertebral luxations without fracture are attracting attention, in fact, they have become so common that they are looked upon as of ordinary occurrence.

M. Roberts reports a carpenter, who, when attempting to raise a heavy scaffolding pole, at a certain point being unable to sustain it any longer, received its weight upon his back. The accident was immediately followed by complete paralysis below the point injured. Dissection showed that the fifth was separated from the sixth dorsal vertebra. There was no fracture of any process.

Beck desires to say: "Fractures of the spinal column are rare, less than one per cent.

"**The most important sign is the traumatic kyphosis produced by displacement of the spinous process, whereby a prominence is caused.**

"In view of the fact that the brachial plexus is composed of the fifth, sixth, seventh and eighth cervical nerves as well as of the first dorsal nerve, it will be understood why paralysis of the upper extremities as well as of the abdominal and intercostal muscles is present in fracture above the third dorsal vertebra.

"**If the phrenic nerve,** which branches off between the third and fourth cervical vertebrae **is compressed** in this region, **its paralysis will be the consequence and death will follow almost instantly.**"

Bickham, 1908: "Dislocation of the spinal vertebrae is caused by the articular process of the higher vertebrae sliding downward and forward over the lower. If the gliding has gone far enough to cause the posterior margin of the upper articular process to pass beyond the articular margin of the lower articular process, where it becomes interlocked, dislocation is said to have occurred. If the gliding has been less extensive, so that these margins have not passed each other and interlocking, therefore, has not occurred, **sublaxation is said to have taken place.**

"Dislocation is most common in the cervical region (owing to the play of the vertebrae), usually between the fifth and sixth vertebrae; next, between atlas and axis. It is rare in the lumbar region and rarest in the dorsal.

"Dislocation should be reduced by non-operative measures if possible. If they cannot be so reduced, there are those who make no further effort at rectifying the lesion, provided no nervous symptoms be present. If, however, nervous symptoms be present in a case which has withstood non-operative efforts at reduction, operation is then indicated. What has been said applies to recent dislocations."

I herewith reproduce a cut from Bradford and Lovett, which.

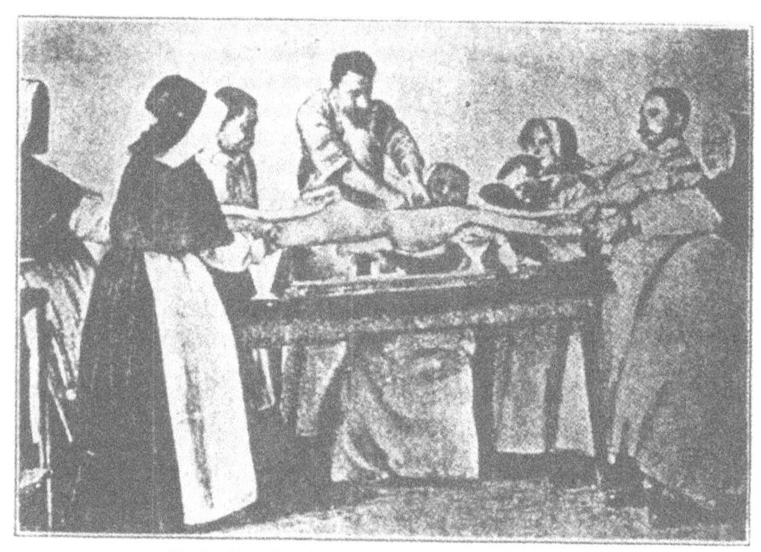

**Reduction by the Method of Calot. (Redard.)**

Copied from Orthopedic Surgery by Bradford and Lovett.

of those preceding, comes the nearest to a Chiropractic illustration I have seen.

Points of resemblance: The patient is lying face downward on a table. As can be seen, two uprights are used instead of a bifid table or heavy solid pillows.

Points of difference: Calot has eight assistants, the Chiropractor needs none. Extension, by five persons. The Chiropractor finds that forcible extension causes a resistance and muscular contraction by the patient, which is very objectionable.

The operator is using his thumbs; whereas the Chiropractor uses both hands. The operator, shown in the cut, does not assume the position of a Chiropractor. Chipault operated first in September, 1893. I made my first adjustment in September, 1895. Judging from the illustration and the following descriptive history, Calot and Chipault had not thot of using the spinous and transverse processes as levers by which to rack displaced vertebrae into their normal position. The region operated upon as shown in the cut, indicates a forcible reduction of the 9th or 10th dorsal vertebrae. If so, a bifid table is not needed.

Bradford and Lovett give the following interesting history: "Forcible correction of the deformity, with or without anaesthesia, is a method revived in recent times by Chipault, of Paris, although ordinarily identified with the name of Calot. Chipault operated first in September, 1893, reducing the deformity and wiring together the spinous processes of the affected vertebrae. He published an account of this method on March 9, 1895. On December 22, 1896, Calot published a paper on the method, in which he said that his first operation dated back only a little over a year. The priority of forcible reduction belongs clearly to Chipault. Wiring the spinous processes of the vertebrae was, however, first advocated by an American, B. E. Hadra, in a paper read and discussed before the American Orthopedic Association, at Washington, September 24, 1891. The method has been largely advocated and finds a place in modern orthopedic treatment. It has been demonstrated that, under ether, a recent deformity, even of large size, may be partially or wholly corrected. Also that much temporary improvement in the deformity may be affected by exerting traction or moderate pressure on the deformity without the use of an anesthetic. It has been shown that it is not a proceeding attended with as great risk of life, either near or remote, as would have been supposed. Many casualties, however, of various sorts have been reported. It has been shown that paralysis is often improved or cured by this manipulation, although cases of paralysis occurring after it had been reported."

The American Text-Book of Surgery: "**Sprains of the spine are of all degrees of severity.** The structure of the vertebral column is so complex and its relations are so numerous and varied that **a great variety of symptoms may follow a sprain** according to the extent of the damage which is inflicted. In the middle degree of sprain the muscles alone are involved, and then we have merely a temporary stiffening and a little local tenderness over a limited area. In more serious accidents, as those occuring during railway collisions, the ligaments may also be involved and are sometimes actually torn. When this happens in the case of the ligamenta subflava', there may be immediate and severe extradural hemorrhage, followed by temporary paraplegia. The symptoms which are never absent are pain and stiffness. Occasionally there is a little local swelling, but this it not constant. **The pain is referred to the extremities of the injured nerve, sometimes shooting down the limbs, occasionally, when the injury is at the lumbo-dorsal junction, being referred to the pubic region. The skin over the injured part is apt to be exceedingly tender.** The stiffness produces a degree of rigidity of the spine which resembles very much that seen in Pott's disease, **the patient involuntarily immobilizing the vertebral column and avoiding rotation and flexion as carefully as possible.** When the injury is unilateral this muscular rigidity is very marked on the injured side, and is a valuable means of distinguishing real from asserted injury, especially in medicolegal cases, as it cannot be simulated.

"**The diagnosis of severe sprains followed by great helplessness and by some degree of paralysis will sometimes be difficult, as** the condition may closely simulate that of fracture. In the latter, however, the paralysis is more absolute, the disability more complete, the tenderness over the spine less diffuse, and **there is often an irregularity in the line of the spinous processes which will serve at once to indicate the more serious character of the injury.**

"**The later symptoms of spinal sprains are, after all, the most serious and annoying. At the time of the accident there may be the form of general nervous depression which we know as shock, which may even deepen into its graver variety of collapse**; or in neurotic patients there may occur the more localized disturbance of cerebral origin known as acute hysteria, but this, as a rule, will disappear within a short time. **Later,** however, **two forms of sequela may occur which take a chronic character,** and which are classified by Thorburn in his excellent book on this subject **as neurasthenic and traumatic hysteria.** In the former condition **there is a general defect in the nutrition and nerve power, which when it follows a traumatism is manifested by weakness, loss of memory, mental confusion and irritability, insomnia, headache, eye-strain, photobia, irregular and frequent pulse, dyspepsia, etc.** These symptoms occur in patients who have had mild shock at the time of the accident, and they will generally pass away after rest and tonic treatment. They are very common, and are often associated with some belonging to traumatic hysteria."

From Spondylotheraphy by Abrams, of San Francisco, Cal., I quote: "In 1834 William and Daniel Griffin, physicians, respectively, of Edinburgh and London, published a work in which 148 cases were analyzed, showing the relation of certain symptoms to definite spinal regions. These symptoms were associated with spinal tenderness in fixed regions. They concluded that the tenderness in question was either primary in the spinal cord or secondary to visceral or other diseases. The Griffin Brothers queried as follows: "We should like to learn why pressure on a particular vertebra increases, or excites, the disease about which we are consulted, why it at one time excites headache or croup or sickness of the stomach. Why, in some instances, any of these complaints may be called up at will by touching a corresponding point of the spinal chain?"

At this period (1834) Swedish gymnasts, notably among them Ling, observed among cardiopaths, tenderness over the 4th or 5th dorsal nerves when this region was subjected to friction. The Swedish school recognizes definite areas of spinal tenderness identified with the various organs. Thus, in affections of the stomach, tenderness is observed in the region of the 6th, 7th and 8th dorsal nerves on the left side and manipulation of the region in question often evokes eructation. Many others have verified these observations, but it remained for me not only to locate by palpation the impingement which is the cause of the tenderness and to trace the injured, sensitive nerve from the point of its impingement from the spine to the affected part or organ, but, more than this, to devise the Chiropractic method of adjusting vertebrae by racking them in their former position, thus relieving the pressure **against** nerves, by releasing their impingement—a vast difference.

Paraplegia involving the lower half of the body is recognized by M. D.'s as a result of pressure on the spinal cord; why not, also consider hemiplegia, a lateral half, as resulting from displacement and impingment?

The expressions of pain from injured nerves, is always manifested at their peripheral endings.

Gould and Pyle state: "Injury to the spinal cord does not necessarily cause immediate death. Mills and O'Harra, both of Philadelphia, have recorded instances of recovery."

Astley Cooper says: "Dislocations are only possible when the muscles are unprepared for resistance; otherwise the greatest force would hardly produce the effect."

For this reason I desire the patient to be fully relaxed when receiving an adjustment. Bones are easily displaced or replaced when nerves and muscles are relaxed.

It has been one of the rules of my life, that what is worth doing at all is worth doing well. In Chiropractic this is especially so; particularly when laying the foundation for a coming science which is destined to be the grandest and greatest of this or any age.

I, as the originator, the fountain head, the founder, of the science and art of adjusting vertebral luxations by hand, using the spinous and transverse processes as levers, have the pleasure and satisfaction of turning on the effulgent rays of the midday sun upon this much mooted question—a question upon which the medical world ventured to shed only a few moonbeams, or an occasional ray of sun light, for fear of losing caste while enlightening suffering humanity. The world will be the wiser and better for my having lived.

In this lengthy article, full of interest, I have given the result of many examinations of anatomies, physiologies and pathologies, from which I have gleaned the various opinions regarding vertebral luxations. I have aimed to make this compilation as complete as possible, so that future authors, practitioners and students may refer to it for the various opinions regarding displacements of vertebrae up to the year 1910. The investigator for hidden lore will stop and wonder why there should have been such varied opinions, when luxations are known to be so very common and reduction so easily accomplished.

Many surgeons assert that dislocations of vertebrae are impossible; others, that complete dislocation cannot occur. Not a few state that luxations can only occur when accompanied by fracture; while others as certainly affirm that displacements can exist but only in the cervical, dorsal or lumbar, as determined by their individual experience. Again there are those who are just as sure that, in the greater part of the vertebral column, luxations are absolutely impossible and that when they do occur it is always the result of great violence. Some are more lenient, declaring that dislocations of the vertebrae may occur without fracture; that where a vertebral column is weakened by caries, luxations are possible. Others are willing to swear that displaced vertebrae are quite common; that the foramina may be narrowed and nerves compressed by their occlusion.

In regard to the luxations, there is a great difference of opinions. Many surgeons think it impossible, and that an attempt at reduction would cause instant death. Some state that dislocations may be reduced, but with great risk; others aver that wrenches occur more frequently than is generally supposed and that the injury is speedily relieved, in some instances during sleep, while the patient is fully relaxed. Some have progressed so far that they avow that not only paralysis, but a great many diseased conditions, are caused by vertebral luxations.

To review the various methods advised for reduction of luxated vertebrae, would be to create a sardonic smile on the faces of those who have learned to use the spinous and transverse processes as levers whereby to rack displaced vertebrae into their normal positions.

---

"Chiropractic is a name given to the study of the etiology of disease, and the art of restoring to normal all morbific conditions."

Chiropractic is a name I originated to designate the science and art of adjusting vertebrae. It does not relate to the study of etiology, or any branch of medicine. Chiropractic includes the science and art of adjusting vertebrae—the know how and the doing. Restoring morbid conditions to normal is the result of the art of adjusting. The study of the causation of disease—the sum of knowledge regarding the causes of disease is the science of etiology—not the art.

"Chiropractic originated in Davenport, Iowa. In the year of 1895, Dr. D. D. Palmer, who was at that time a magnetic healer, came in contact with one Harvey Lillard, a janitor, in the building where he had his office. This man was so deaf that he could not hear street noises nor the tick of a watch, for the period of 17 years. This man's hearing was restored by Dr. Palmer, by the adjustment of a vertebra that was out of position. Although the adjustment was crude and without knowledge of the result that would follow, Dr. Palmer was favored with the fact that the adjustment was given correctly, which resulted favorably. This gave Dr. D. D. Palmer the theory of displaced bones causing disease by impinging nerves."

I "came in contact" with Harvey Lillard. To come in contact is to touch. We had been in touch for many years; very many times we had come in contact.

"A vertebra which was out of position."

To be out of position, is to lose one's position, an office or employment. The vertebra did not lose a position; it was luxated.

"Although the adjustment was **crude and without knowledge** of the result that would follow, Dr. Palmer was favored with the **fact** that the adjustment was given **correctly,** which resulted favorably. This gave Dr. D. D. Palmer the **theory** of displaced bones causing disease by impinging nerves."

An adjustment "given correctly" was not so very "crude."

"This gave Dr. D. D. Palmer the theory."

From the moment that Mr. Harvey gave me the information

that 17 years previously he was in a stooped, cramped position and felt something give in his back, and at that time he became deaf, the principle of adjusting vertebrae for the relief of diseases was a theory. That theory became a demonstrated fact a half hour later, then it was no longer a theory.

"Displacements of the spinal column cause the contraction of muscles which in turn draw and impinge nerves, creating too much or not enough action—disease."

The normal or physiological stimulant of a muscle is by way of its nerve; as in voluntary movements, the motor impulse affects the nerve by excitation. Therefore, muscle contraction depends upon the stimuli transmitted to it thru its nerve. The doctor corrects the above abnormal statement on page 11 where he says, "All pathological conditions are due to their interference by impingement on nerves at some point of emergence at or near the spinal foramen."

"Nerves are the means of communication."

Sure. Correct you are—not muscles.

"Physicological" is one of the branches this "college" claims to teach. Physico relates to the science of physics—that branch of science dealing with the material universe; natural philosophy. Logical, is the science or art of reasoning. So, this science advertises to teach natural philosophy.

"Kiro-pathologically" is another branch taught by this college. "Kiro" is a nickname for Chiropractic. "Pathologically" is an adverb; therefore is not the name of any branch of learning. Pathological is of or pertaining to disease. Literally he claims to teach Chiropractic disease.

Another branch taught is "Histological"—pertaining to histology. Just think of a Chiropractic school teaching histology—the science which treats of the minute structure of animal tissue, only discernible with the aid of the microscope—and that without a microscope in sight.

"Osteology, neurology and Kiro-physiology, are taught thruout the course, as Chiropractic is founded upon these especial branches of anatomy."

Just think of an "Imperial College" advertising "Kiro-physiology" as a branch of anatomy—one of the three upon which Chiropractic is founded. Physiology is a branch of biology, which deals with the processes, activities and phenomena incidental to and characteristic of life or of living organisms. Physiology is the study of the functions of the organs and parts during life, as **distinct from anatomy** which deals with their structure.

"Anatomy physiological" is one of the branches of education taught by this college. Anatomy is the dissection of organized bodies. Physiological is an adjective, of or pertaining to physiology. It is here wrongly used as a noun, the name of something. Anatomy refers to dissection and physiology to vital phenomena, the science of functions of living bodies. The Imperial doctor has tried to make a compound word of dissection and functions, unite the dead with the living.

"Kiro-symptomatology" is another branch of instruction taught by "the master of clinic lectures." "Kiro" is a nickname for Chiropractic. Symptomatology is that branch of education which treats of symptoms. Chiropractic—symptoms—please tell us what those symptoms are.

"Hygiene" and "hygienic" are used as synonyms of pathology—health and disease as synonyms is the limit.

"Impinged nerves, the cause of pathological changes."

Pathological: pertaining to pathology. Pathology is the science of treating diseases, their nature, causes, progress, manifestations and results. What has "impinged nerves" to do with pathology?

Students are required to study "anatomy Kiropathologically" six months "to learn of the seriousness of his work."

"Orthopedic anatomy makes the student acquainted with the mechanical make-up of the human frame."

Orthopedics is the correcting and prevention of deformities—not the study of anatomy.

"By and through nerves, all of the vital elements are furnished."

An element is one of the simple substances of which the universe is composed. Vital belongs to or relates to life, as vital energies; vital functions; vital actions; vital center; vital force; vital heat; vital principle; or vital affinity.

"Kiro-regonatomy refers to regional anatomy taught chiropractically."

"Regonatomy" displays ignorance regarding regional anatomy.

"The bones are studied physiologically."

Physiology is a branch of biology, distinctly different from anatomy. The study of bones is included in anatomy, not physiology. Physiology studies their functions—their actions, not their structure.

"Peripheral nerves."

Nerves have peripheral terminations, away from the central nervous system. There are no nerves known as "peripheral nerves."

"The impingement of nerves is taught according to mathematical and philosophical laws."

I was not aware that elementary, abstract, applied, or the higher mathematics of algebra, geometry and trigonometry had anything to do with the impingement of nerves. A philosophical law is one which is invariable under given conditions. The laws of mathematics and philosophy are not related to "the impingement of nerves."

"Dr. Lavalley makes claim to the discovery as to how the nerves become impinged."

If all the statements made by Chiropractors were true, there would be left the bare fact that I gave a "crude adjustment which gave hearing to a deaf man."

"Edison did not discover electricity, but he developed it; nor did Dr. Lavalley discover Chiropractic, but he has developed it as no other man has been able to develop the science."

This 16 page booklet is largely copied; to this extent its composition and expression are good.

---

The Adjuster contains much new thot for thinkers.

---

Webster's Dictionary, 1910 edition, says: Chiropractic:—A system of healing that treats disease by manipulation of the spinal column.

Chiropractic is not a system of healing. Chiropractors do not treat disease; they do not manipulate the spinal column. Chiropractors adjust any or all of the 300 joints of the body, more particularly those of the spinal column.

---

Carver's Chiropractic Analysis states on page 411, that corns are caused by "an inactivity of the kidneys." Is this one of his Chiropractic principles he refers to in his preface? If so, it is no wonder that he has promised to give us another corrected edition of his book.

Is it possible that every person who has corns has "inactivity of the kidneys," and that when I relieve one or more corns in as many minutes, that the kidneys become active again? This may be "Carver's Chiropractic Analysis"; if so, it is far from being demonstrated.

Corns and bunions exist because of displaced joints of the feet. Replace the joint where the corn or bunion is found and the enlargement will disappear. This may require one or many adjustments, depending upon whether ankylosis is present or not.

There is no relation whatever between kidneys and corns.

## PURPURA HEMORRHAGICA.

This term refers to hemorrhage of the skin, the blood being lodged between the layers of the cutis vera and the epidermis. This effusion may have the appearance of bruises, ruptured blood vessels, papules, blebs, or blisters. These conditions may appear either independently of, or in connection with, special diseases. It is apt to follow an inflammatory condition.

Dr. Carver tells us it follows a prolonged inflammation; that it is the result of great flaccidity and relaxation of cellular structure.

In all inflammatory diseases there is an overaction of functions with corresponding tissue changes, excessive heat, swelling, an overfilling of blood vessels and overgrowth. When tissue becomes flaccid, relaxed, conditions just the opposite of those mentioned above prevail. Do not forget, for one moment, that disease is either too much or not enough functionating.

Pathological hemorrhage, whether external or internal, is the result of inflammation which softens the walls of the blood vessels and increases the rapidity, force and strain of the blood.

Dr. Carver says, "The occlusions causing this abnormality will be found to be numerous."

Not so very numerous that the scientific Chiropractor cannot, by palpation, find the nerve impinged upon and the subluxated vertebra which causes the impingement.

He further says, "Concomitant with adjusting the third, fourth, eleventh and twelfth dorsal nerves, very careful dieting and complete rest will usually result in rapid restoration."

It will be observed, that he advises the adjusting, returning to their normal position, of two contiguous vertebrae. A vertebra cannot be displaced without subluxating its articulating surfaces in connection with its adjoining vertebrae, both above and below it. If this subluxated bone be replaced, its articular connections made normal, what more do you want? What more can or should be done? Why adjust or try to replace its neighbor above or below?

If the principles of Chiropractic are correct,—if displaced bones press against nerves and muscles, thereby causing too much or not enough functionating,—I say, if the axioms of this science are correct, what has "very careful dieting" to do with the causes or the correction of displaced osseous tissue?

"The detection of a constriction, as opposed to a subluxation, often requires the most profound skill. A subluxation requires replacement until the elemental parts of the joint have had sufficient time, under restored stimulus, to return to the normal."

Constriction is a condition of being narrowed by binding. A muscle may constrict any portion of the body by contracting. A constriction cannot be opposed to a subluxation. A displacement may cause a nerve to act on a muscle in such a manner as to constrict any portion of the body with which the muscle may come in contact.

It certainly would "require most profound skill" to detect that which does not exist.

"Elemental parts of a joint."

Elemental pertains to elements, the first principles or primary ingredients. There are no primary ingredients or first principles in a joint. A vertebra, long displaced, becomes ill-shaped in all its essential parts. It will need replacing until it has grown back to its normal shape.

"To illustrate: A small boil is held to be a local condition, and, indeed, so far as we can discern, presents no general effects; yet we know that it does so. But a malignant boil of considerable size, while it comes within the classification of a local abnormality, is really general in its effects, the irritation of the same frequently being of such gravity as to produce motor reaction and consequent occlusion, involving the whole organism, sometimes resulting in a general fever."

Large or small boils are local, the result of nerve impingement which is expressed by an inflammatory condition known as boils or carbuncles.

A "malignant boil" would be one threatening life. Boils are not considered malignant, threatening life.

We are told that the irritation of the boil produces motor reaction and occlusion, involving the whole organism and resulting in general fever.

Local heat, inflammation, is disseminated by exosmosis to the neighboring tissue, and so far as organs and membranes are overheated, they are modified in their functions.

The irritation of a nerve produces, at its terminal ending, an excess of heat which is transmitted thru the tissue. The boil does not irritate other portions of the body; it does not cause motor reaction; it does not incite or repress the action of other organs after the boil has ceased to be inflamed. Neither does it involve the whole organism by occlusion—a closing or shutting up. "General fever" is the transudation of heat from the inflammation expressed in the boil.

The above quoted paragraph is not logical, consistent or analytical Chiropractic.

## PATHS OF PROGRESS.

By B. D. Stillman, Chicago, Ill.

A youth starting out in life,
Ambitious to win fame,
Decided to affix M. D.
To ornament his name.
He chose the path his father trod,
And studied night and day,
He soon was giving poisoned drugs
The same old-fashioned way —
**An Allo-path.**

If morphine pills and calomel
Were good enough for Dad,
It didn't suit his customers;
He found their action bad.
He entered a more modern school,
Which "high deglutions" taught,
Traveling on a broader path
Where many cures were wrought—
**A Homeo-path.**

Ever ready for new thots,
And losing faith in pills,
He found a more progressive path,
A sure cure for all ills.
He gave up drugs entirely, and
Is now in great demand.
He doesn't give prescriptions now,
But does it all by hand—
**An Osteo-path.**

Progression seems to be his forte,
He studied water cure,
And uses "Nature's medicines,
Sun, air and water, pure."
And all these paths have taught him thus:
The best one in the land—
That Nature is the Doctor, and
To know and understand—
**A Hygeo-path.**

H. L. Nutting thinks the following two verses should be added to bring the Paths of Progress up to Chiropractic:

Yet still he seems dissatisfied,
He wore an anxious mien;
For yet withal, his patients died
He fixed not the machine!
Ah! He learns the cause—
Luxations to adjust—
And now he deals with Nature's Laws,
In Chiro puts his trust—
**A Healthy-path.**

And evermore he is the one
That overcomes the ills,
Known now to be but accidents,
That pain the body fills.
He finds the cause, not air or sun,
But bnnes just out of place.
With Chiro hand the wórk is done,
Disease then leaves no trace—
**A Chiro-path.**

---

The following is a copy of a letter received by Dr. A. P. Davis from Dr. T. Easton Williams:

Dec. 17, 1909.

A. P. Davis, M. D., D. O., Baker City, Ore.

Dear Doctor:—I recently purchased a copy of your latest book—Neuropathy, which deals with Chiropractic and other important branches of the healing art and which sounds profusely of the language of an able therapeutist and not merely that of the modern book maker.

In the mean time, allow me to make the following statement: You are the only writer that I ever found that explained the correct principles of Chiropractic in accord with both anatomy and physiology.

All other writers (Palmer included) appear dreamy, speculative and fanciful, to say the least.

Personally, I have taken instruction in Chiropractic; but my instructor knew nothing of spinal anatomy; he knew nothing of the origin of spinal nerves or their distribution to special organs and remote parts of the body.

Therefore, it is indeed very refreshing to refer to your book, Neuropathy, before we "punch the other fellow's back," for empirical methods in any line is simply fumbling in the dark.

Please allow me to say, Neuropathy is splendid in every department and well worth the money paid for it. Long may you live. Fraternally yours,

T. EASTON WILLIAMS, M. D., M. E., D. C.

We give the above space because it has some points we wish to call special attention to. Dr. Williams says that Chiropractic is an important branch of the healing art. Dunglison defines the healing art as that of medicine. Chiropractic is not a branch of medicine. There is no more resemblance between Chiropractic and medicine than there is between a Chiropractor's office and a drug store.

The Doctor is frank in stating that he has personally taken instruction in Chiropractic from one who knew nothing of spinal anatomy, the origin of spinal nerves or their distribution. He might have added "or of Chiropractic." I am sorry to say that many would-be teachers of Chiropractic know as little of nerves and their distribution as the teacher referred to. Some publicly state that there are no cranial or sympathetic nerves; that all nerves issue from a spinal cord and go direct to their appointed places. If Dr. Williams is a reader of the Adjuster, or should attend a class recitation in the D. D. Palmer schoolroom, he will know that there is at least one exception.

It is fair to presume that his instructor knew as little of Chiropractic, as a science and art, as he did of anatomy; therefore, the Doctor's knowledge of Chiropractic is indeed very limited, altho he thinks, from what little he has learned, that "it is an important branch of the healing art."

"You (A. P. Davis) are the only writer that I ever found that explained the correct principles of Chiropractic in accord with anatomy and physiology."

The explanation referred to is, Neuropathy, which teaches how to unite the two forces—the positive and negative—the acid and alkaline secretions, whose separation cause disease, in such a manner as to remove it. This uniting is done by the operator placing (See cut in Neuropathy page 100) his right hand outside of and on the clothing (coat, vest and undergarments on) flat and crosswise of the body; the left hand also flat and crosswise on the right hand. Then by a quick downward pressure the two forces (positive and negative) which control the acid and alkaline secretions are united—how, he and I are unable to explain. Dr. Williams thinks this miserable subterfuge to be Chiropractic, and in accord with anatomy and physiology. These two M. D.'s cannot get away from chemistry, and continue "simply fumbling in the dark," as evidenced by the following quotation from Neuropathy:

"The two forces which control the body and regulate physiological action.

"What these two forces are and how they originate are far from being understood.

"That the functions of nerves should be changed by pressure would seem reasonable, but what particular change takes place in the structure which makes the difference in the product in the secretions is the most abstruse problem, perhaps, we have to do with in the way of solution.

"Why certain influences produce in one set of nerves a chemical result just the antipodes of others has not been observed outside of my own investigations, and why this is so I pretend not to explain on any hypothesis whatever, except it be to fulfill the demands of nature itself in the human economy and make it harmonize with all other things in nature."

What these two imaginary forces are and how they originate alkali and acids are not problems capable of solution; they are doubtful theorems not susceptible of proof.

That pressure on nerves changes their functions is not only reasonable, but a demonstrated fact, daily proven. How pressure causes one set of nerves to secrete an excess of alkali and another a surplus of acid is an "abstruse problem" very difficult of solution or comprehension.

Why pressure should cause one set of nerves to produce a chemical result just the opposite of others has only been observed by one investigator and he does not "pretend to explain it on any hypothesis whatever."

Why a man of more than ordinary reason should entertain such an untenable proposition is past my understanding.

Drs. Davis and Williams' idea of Chiropractic, pathology and physiology are certainly "**dreamy, speculative** and **fanciful, to say the least.**"

---

"Normal circuit to mental impulses."

**An impulse does not make a circuit.** Mental impulses go away from the central nervous system and to the terminations of nerves; these are motor impulses. Sensory impulses go to the central nervous system and away from the external. Neither motor or sensory impulses make a circuit.

---

"The only Chi-ro-paths, originator and founder of the Chi-ro-path-ic system. Regular graduates."

Pathos as a prefix means disease. What it means as an affix, I cannot say, but presume it is the same; if so, Chiropath would mean a Chiro disease. They are not only the originators and founders of this disease, but, also, regular graduates.

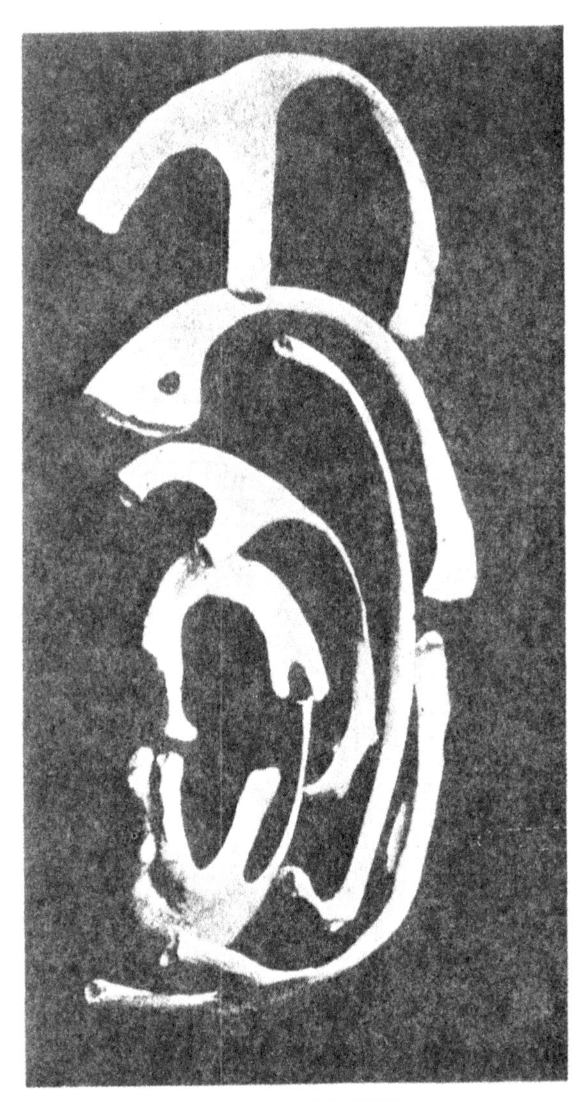

DICHOTOMOUS RIBS.

Sometimes the sternal end of a rib is cleft, appearing double; at other times the cleft may be incomplete so as to form a perforation.

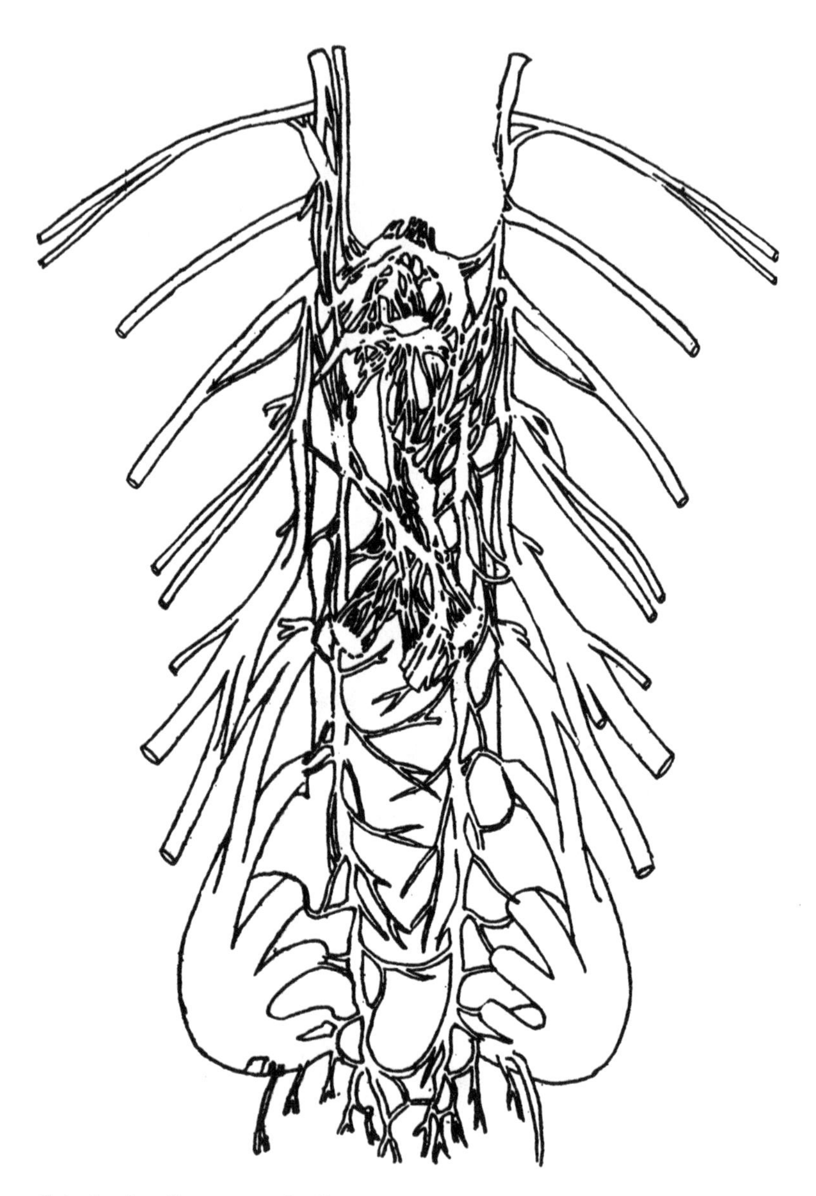

Cut showing the communicating cross-trunk nerves of the two ganglionic sympathetic nerve cords.

## RACHITIS.

Rachitis, or rickets, is an interesting disease for practitioners to study, as it includes many affections caused by **hyperthermia and seborrhea.**

Rachis means the spine, and rachitis an inflammation of the vertebral column.

Dorland's Dictionary states: "Rachitis, or rickets, is a constitutional disease of childhood, in which the bones become soft and flexible from retarded ossification, **due to deficiency of earthly salts.** The disease is marked by bending and distortion of the bones, under muscular action; by the formation of nodular enlargements on the ends and sides of the bones; by delayed closure of the fontanels; pain in the muscles; **sweating of the head,** and degeneration of the liver and spleen. There are often nervous affections, **feverishness** and convulsions."

Dunglison's Medical Dictionary says: "English disease, rickets. Disease characterized by a softened condition of the long bones, leading to curvature of their shafts and swelling of their extremeties, a crooked spine, prominent abdomen, large head and often precocity of intellect, and is accompanied by leanness, general debility and indigestion It frequently induces atrophy and hectic. Rickets occurs particularly during the first years of existence of **weakly children** brought up in damp or dark dwellings and badly nourished. Some children gradually recover their health; others become more and more deformed and ultimately die of consumption, **dropsy** or other organic disease. Pure air, a healthy situation, nourishing diet, exercise, sea or common cold bathing, tonics and eutrophics afford the best prospect of success."

Gould's Dictionary informs us: "Rachitis, the 'English disease,' a constitutional disease of infancy, characterized by impaired nutrition and changes in the bones. Rachitis was first accurately described by Glisson, in the seventeenth century. The disease comes on insidously at about the period of dentition and three general symptoms are usually present—a diffuse soreness of the body, **slight fever, and profuse sweating** about the head and neck. Coincident with these the skeletal lesions appear, the chief of which are the bending of the ribs, the arching of the long bones, with thickening at the junction of the shaft and the epiphysis and the development of hyperostosis on the frontal and parietal eminences, producing the caput quadratum. Dentition is delayed, nervous symptoms are marked, as peevishness and sleeplessness, and in some cases convulsions and laryngismus; and all the manifestations are accompanied by a state of general weakness. The cartilage between the shaft and the epiphysis of the long bones is greatly thickened, the **line of ossification is irregular and more spongy and vascular** than normal and beneath the periosteum, which strips off easily, there is spongoid tissue resembling **decalcified bone.** Kassowitz regards the hyperemia of the bone, the marrow, the cartilage and the periosteum as the primary lesion, on which all the others depend."

Lippincott's Medical Dictionary states: "Rickets. A disease of childhood, in which there is a lack of the earthy salts in the bones, with resultant curvature and deformities of them, affections of the liver, spleen, and mesenteric glands, a prominent abdomen, and a condition of general weakness. Nourishing food, fresh air, exercise, and tonics furnish the best mode of treatment."

In England rickets is accountable for more deformities than any other single affection. Thus, it is impossible to omit a short notice of the disease in considering the pathology of deformities. It is known on the Continent as the "English disease," on account of the first thorough treatise upon it being by an English writer. In 1660 Francis Glisson, Professor of Medicine at Cambridge University, described rickety deformities and suggested their treatment by mechanical support and gymnastics. In orthopedy the deformity is treated; in Chiropractic the cause is adjusted.

Rachitis is thot to be a constitutional disease, that is, one not attributable to any specific cause but depending upon an inherent, hereditary, abnormal structure of the tissue of the body; where or how, pathologists do not pretend to explain. A constitutional disease is one in which all functions are involved.

Rickets is characterized by bone softening, crooked spines and curvature of the long bones, which become ill-shaped, owing to their softness. The epiphysis, its cartilage and the adjoining portion of the shaft, are enlarged, even to the sternal ends of the ribs. This condition is known as rose-garland on account of the nodules appearing at the junction of the cartilage and ribs. There is always more or less seborrhea present.

Osteomalacia and rickets, are similar in their main characteristics. While rachitis is considered a disease of childhood, being only occasionally found in the fetus and the adult, osteomalacia is confined to adults, more especially to females, and of cases of this class the majority are those which follow childbirth. **In rachitis the lime-salts are not deposited in the usual amount; whereas, in osteomalacia the lesion consists of the softening of fully formed, hard, bone tissue by the removal of the inorganic salts** from which their natural solidity is derived.

Among the causes assigned by pathologists for osteomalacia are, lack of lactic acids, defective nutrition, pregnancy, rheumatism, infection, intoxication, changes in the trophic nerves, ovarian and uterine disorders. These are all results of a common cause rather than the causes themselves.

In rachitis the bones fail to harden, while, in osteomalacia there is a progressive softening, which results in all sorts of deformities. In osteomalcia, as in rachitis, the marrow adjoining the **epiphyseal tissue is congested and red,** the fat is absorbed or assumes a gelatinous appearance. While there is usually an affection of the bones, the changes may be confined to single bones of hard tissue.

McFarland wisely says: "The ordinary form of osteomalacia begins in the spinal column and thorax and spreads to the bones of the limbs and head."

A Chiropractor acquainted with the pathological conditions and principles of Chiropractic recognizes that **continued, excessively high temperature**, hyperthermia, **is the cause of all conditions known as rachitis and osteomalacia. Temperature above normal softens bones by furnishing a superabundance of red corpuscles and a lack of leukocytes.** In all cases of death by fever, superinduced by traumatic or toxic injury, the bones and their marrow will be found of a **reddish color, owing to an excess of red corpuscles and a lack of the white.** When bones are eburnated, ivory-like in color and texture, there has been, in the recent state, following the heat period, a lack of the red and an excess of the white corpuscles. In health there is an equilibrium in the number of the erythrocytes and leukocytes.

The kinetic force, also known as vital energy, depends upon and is modified by the amount of heat which imparts an oscillating motion to the molecules or particles of matter. Varying degrees of temperature, therefore, represent corresponding intensity of oscillation. Normal temperature—normal functions—health.

In rachitis, malacia and all diseases wherein there is an excess of heat, there will be found an activity of the nervous system in proportion to the amount of temperature. Heat, not only **causes nerve tension** by thickening and contracting nerve and muscle tissue, but a higher rate of vascular circulation which is increased by the tension of the nerve plexus in the walls of the vascular system. It furthermore causes a thickening of the transudating membrane, which results in abnormal metabolism in the double form of a decrease in anabolism or constructive or synthetic metabolism, and an increase in katabolism or destructive metabolism. Heat in excess retards ossification and softens bones and organic tissue.

I find in pathological physiology that subnormal bodily temperature tends to harden and ossify tissue while hyperthermia tends to soften it. The performance of functions, whether normal, in excess or subnormal, depends upon and varies with the amount of bodily temperature. The temperature will be normal if the transmitting channels possess normal tonicity.

McFarland affirms: "Rachitis is a constitutional and nutritive disorder. The disease is not infrequently congenital and seems to be hereditary. **The exciting cause is unknown. In the congenital form malnutrition probably operates through the mother. The marrow is chiefly of the red variety** and occupies greatly exagerated spaces in the rarefied bone. The nutritive disturbance depends upon other factors than starvation, for young animals, when half-starved for prolonged periods do not develop rickets."

**Excessive heat is a prominent factor in rachitis.** The exciting cause of hyperthermia is in those substances introduced into the alimentary canal for alimentation which, **instead of being nutritious, act as a poison.**

Whitman asserts that rachitis is a constitutional disease of infancy, caused by a weakness that may be inherited, or it may be the direct effect of illness or improper hygienic surroundings, as lack of sunlight, damp rooms, overcrowding or poor ventilation. **The direct cause is improper nourishment**, due to artificial food during the nursing period, improper diet after weaning, prolonged lactation, or a defective quality of the mother's milk. **The etiology of the affection is unknown.** Medical treatment is of secondary importance. It is unlikely that any drug has a very direct influence on the disease. Distortions of the softened bones are caused by atmospheric pressure, the force of gravity, habitual posture, muscular action or injuries. **Profuse perspiration,** especially about the head, and restlessness at night are common symptoms.

Whitman further advises: "The correction of the deformity may be accomplished by massage and by direct manipulation of the spine. The child is placed, face downward on a table; one hand is applied over the projection and with the other the legs are raised to throw the spine into a position of over-extension. This stretching is performed slowly and carefully over and over again at morning and night and the manipulation is followed by thorough massage of the muscles. If the deformity is marked and if the general rachitic process is still active, the infant may be kept for several months in the recumbent posture, on the frame or similar support."

Whitman never once thot that "improper nourishment" not only does not nourish, but acts as an irritant or poison to the nervous system, causing an excess of heat. Substances are poisons because of their exciting or depressing effects on nerves. "Improper hygiene" would be like "bad health." Whitman had an idea of correcting spinal curvatures, vertebral displacements by hand. But instead of manipulating, massaging, he should have adjusted, replaced the displaced vertebra by one move. He did not even dream of using the spinous processes as levers. He used over-extension, massaging and stretching the spine, and performed his work slowly and carefully. I have advised, from the first, to avoid stretching and to do adjusting **quickly**. I, in a great measure have reversed the movements of orthopedists.

Hare states: "In children who are sufferers from rickets the teeth decay very early and rapidly. The presence of other fontanelles, than the anterior, in a child's skull after it is several months old, indicates rickets, syphilis, hydrocephalus, or some intracranial growth producing pressure on the cranial bones and preventing their approximation. In severe cases of rickets the anterior fontanelle remains open until the third or fourth year, and should the rachitic tendency be developed in early life, the edges of the fontanelle may not only fail to be approximated, but may actually recede from each other."

Neuralgia, neuritis, which is but inflammation of the nerves, when of the teeth, accounts for dental necrosis and the lack of ossification of the dental membrane. **Remember, excessive heat softens and subnormal temperature hardens all tissues.**

Openheimer claims that malaria is the main cause of rickets.

Miasma is a noxious effluvium which emanates from decaying vegetation in marshy districts or in prairies when much sod is being overturned. From these sources issues an exhalation which is poisonous to human beings; it excites the nervous system and creates fever. Openheimer allowed a Chiropractic ray of intellectuality to penetrate his vision.

McDonald maintains that rachitis or rickets is a disease of infancy and childhood, having as its leading features a deficiency of lime salts in the bony framework and absorption of bone already formed. He says it is generally seen among the poor in crowded, unhealthy portions of cities, where ventilation is bad and the general **surroundings are unhealthy**. It begins about the first or second year of life, rarely after the sixth. Its starting point is the epiphyseal line, where there is found a deficiency of lime salts and at the same time an increased growth of cartilage. Hence, the bone is wider and thicker at this part. The child is loose-jointed, the ligaments being relaxed, and movements of the articulations frequently cause pain. When

**the spinal column is the seat of the disease,** one or another of the various spinal curvatures may be the result. Rachitic children are often hydrocephalic, and deformities of the cranium are not uncommon.

The spinal column seems, to pathologists, to be "the seat of the disease." Spinal curvature is a prominent characteristic of rachitic affections. Rachitic children are often hydrocephalic —dropsical. These conditions point to the 12th dorsal, the second spinal center. It is understood that when we adjust the 12th dorsal, it is to relieve an impingement upon the 12th dorsal nerves. All observing pathologists speak of the unhealthy surroundings of rachitic children. By this we understand, that there are noxious effluvia arising from putrescent meat or decaying vegetation which poison the atmosphere they breathe. Putrid meat and decaying vegetation are poisonous whether their substance is ingested or their effluvia breathed.

Bradford and Lovett assert that debility from any cause which impairs nutrition, may be the cause of rickets; that syphilis is an indirect cause; that, when the disease is left to itself, it generally runs its course, and, after a decided degree of bony deformity has occurred, the process of bone softening is spontaneously arrested and the bones hardened in their deformed condition; that drug treatment is, manifestly, secondary in importance to careful regulation of the diet and hygiene. One finds a long list of drugs which are advocated by various writers. Nothing definite is known as to the cause of osteomalacia.

Delafield and Prudden state: "The physiological growth of rachitic bones present three phases. They grow in length by the production of bone in the cartilage between the epiphyses and diaphysis; in thickness, by the growth of bone from the inner layers of the periosteum. At the same time, the medullary canal is enlarged, in proportion to the growth of bone, by the disappearance of the inner layers of bone."

**Rachitic growth** of bones is **pathological.** To change epiphyseal cartilage to bone requires a subnormal temperature which does not take place in a rachitic bone until after it has been subjected to an undue amount of heat.

Moore avers that a number of theories have been advanced as to the exact cause, but all are unproven. One thing sure, it is not hereditary.

Cooper informs us that the cause of rickets is involved in great obscurity. No medicine is known which possesses any direct efficacy in cases of rickets.

Gould and Pyle state: "There are several theories as to the causation of rachitis, one being that it is due to an abnormal development of acids. There is but little doubt that defective nutrition and bad hygienic surroundings are prominent factors in its production."

Tubby says: "Various theories have been advanced and at present (1896) there is not one which will bear searching examination. Heredity plays no part in the production of rickets, nor does syphilis. The bones in severe cases pass through three stages, that of congestion, of softening and of sclerosis."

Tubby's two periods, congestion and softening, cover the same time. There are but two conditions—malacia and sclerosis—a **preponderance of heat** with a superior **abundance of red corpuscles,** or a **diminution of heat** and an **increase of colorless** corpuscles.

Pinel avers that "rickets seem to consist of a want of firmness in the bones, in consequence of a deficiency in their structure of the phosphate of lime. **The causes of this affection are involved in great obscurity.**"

Anders says of this disease: "A constitutional disease of childhood, exhibiting gross nutritive changes, chiefly in the bones and cartillages, causing deformities, and also in the ligaments, muscles and other anatomic structures.

"Derangement of the nutritive processes which retards and otherwise modifies the growth of the bony skeleton, particularly of the skull, the ends of the ribs, and of the long bones. The latter soften or remain unduly flexible as the result either of the absorption of ossified structures or of the greatly diminished deposition of lime-salts. The periosteum is thickened and easily separable from the shaft.

"The chemist has shown us that rachitic bones may contain less than half the normal percentage of lime-salts.

"The disease is dependent largely upon improper or insufficient food, and among hand-fed children the disease is much more common than among those at the breast. It also occurs in breast-fed infants when the mother's milk is poor in quality as the result of previous ill-health, or too long continued lactation. Certain forms of diet predispose to rickets, they do so chiefly for the reason that they either are defective in certain particulars or do not supply certain necessary articles in adequate proportion.

"As faulty diet is in a great measure responsible for rachitis, proper feeding is an important factor, and if the child cannot be satisfactorily nursed by its mother and if it is under the age of six months, a wet nurse should be procured. Should this not be practicable, it must be hand-fed, and the best artificial food is cow's milk, if properly prepared.''

Erichsen affirms that ''rickets is a disease of early life, usually being met with in scrofulous children and never occurring after the age of puberty. The structure of the bones is changed, the earthy matter being deficient and the organic material in excess; so that, the bone continues to be soft, flexible and cartilaginous in structure, at an age when its tissue ought to have under-gone proper consolidation.''

Kilian makes mention of rickets always appearing first in the head, the forehead being especially protuberant.

Rokitansky declares that ''rickety children are not usually tuberculous; if they live, however, past the age of puberty, they may eventually become sufficiently powerful in frame.''

Stengel says: ''The causes of rickets are still very obscure. The disease is in some way connected with improper nourishment, though there is probably also an inherited disposition. Formerly it was supposed that the presence in the digestive tract of lactic acid in excess prevented the proper absorption of calcium; this theory, however, is generally abandoned. The process of rickets is failure of development of the normal structure, rather than absorption of existing bone. The original calcareous deposit around the cartilage cells is largely or completely absorbed, as in normal bone-formation, and, often, more rapidly. The blood is more or less profoundly altered. Decrease in the number of red corpuscles and leukocytosis are the conspicuous features. Nucleated red corpuscles may be found in more or less abundance, according to the grade of anemia, and the leukocytosis involves a special increase of mononuclear, and myelocytes may be present.''

Stengel's description is of the sclerotic stage, the anemia of rachitis in which there is subnormal temperature and **eburnation, a decrease in the red and a corresponding increase of the white corpuscles.**

Young recognizes three changes which lead to deformities, that of congestion or invasion, softening or deformity, hardening or sclerosis. He says there is no evidence that the disease is ever transmitted.

The author of the American Text Book of Surgery informs us, in regard to rachitis, that ''the most important cause of all is improper feeding. In menageries, where animals live under highly artificial conditions, the disease is frequently observed. Rachitic bones are frequently so soft that they can be cut with the knife. As a result of this softening great deformity often occurs. In older children such changes are seen in the bones of the thorax, spine, and extremities; less frequently in the skull. The ligaments are relaxed and movements of the joints are often painful. The promontory of the sacrum is depressed and the pelvis thus greatly narrowed. Curvature of the spine, as scoliosis or lateral deviation, kyphosis or curvature with convexity backward and lordosis or curvature with convexity forward, are also observed. In the skull the bones are often unnaturally thin and crackle under pressure like parchment. This condition is known as craniotabes. Dentition is often delayed and during convalescence progresses with great rapidity. It is always irregular. After the disease has run its course, calcification may take place on an increased scale and sclerosis of the bone may occur. The brain may be hypertrophied and sometimes is sclerosed; hydrocephalous may also occur."

The observations of McFarland and that of the author of the American Text Book differ regarding rachitic affections in wild animals which are kept in captivity. Improper food is that which irritates, becomes a poison and causes an excess of heat. If the young in menageries get the mother's milk there is no reason, unless the mother has fever, why they should have rickets. The full grown animals should not exhibit malacia unless they have continued fever. Craniotabes, craniomalacia, is a softening and thinning of the cranial bones in spots. This condition is usually accompanied by caries of the inner table. Gould says that the last mentioned condition is only encountered during the first months of life, up to the sixteenth month. I have seen this condition existing in adult skulls. In hemiplegia patients, in whom the paralysis is of long standing, there will be found a depression, which fits the finger-end, over the organ of hope, in the frontal bone, just forward of the coronal suture, on the opposite side to that affected. Such patients are melancholic. The thin place will be found sensitive to scratching and pressure; sometimes it is so thin that it can be bent inward by digital force. The depression and melancholia are due to inflammation in that region. "Dentition is often delayed and during convalescence progresses with great rapidity." The primary eruption of the teeth is tardy when the temperature is above normal and progresses rapidly during convalescence when the temperature is subnormal—bone formation progressing in proportion to the amount of white corpuscles in the blood.

Landois, referring to rickets in children, finds identically the same lameness in young domestic animals, both conditions being caused by the non-absorption of calcium-salts of the food on account of persistent disturbances of digestion. Persistent absence of earthy salts from the food results in a deficiency of them in the skeleton; the bones become thin, transparent and even flexible. Analogous disturbances of the motor functions develop if the fully developed bones subsequently lose their calcium-salts to the extent of one-third or one-half (halisteresis) and thus become soft—osteomalacia. A certain minor degree of fragility of the bones and halisteresis occurs in old age.

The persistent disturbance of digestion and the lack of absorption of calcium-salts is the result of too much heat. For proper assimilation it is highly necessary to have normal temperature. The fragility of bones in the aged is not on account of halisteresis, but, as a result of an increase of calcium-salts.

Knight says:—"Rachitis is the abnormal condition of the formative process in the growth of bone; it tends to great aberration of the normal form of the skeleton and as a pathological condition invites special investigation from the practitioner of medicine."

Rindfleisch states:—"The cartilage of rachitic bones expands as a broad, translucent, grey and very soft cushion between the cartilage on the one side, and the completed osseous structure upon the other.

From the statements of Knight, Rindfleisch and others, it will be observed that excessive heat tends toward growth of cartilage, and subnormal temperature to that of ossification."

Gray affirms:—"Cartilage does not contain blood-vessels except in regions of very active growth or ossification."

Beattie and Dickson claim:—"Thickening or clubbing of the growing ends of the bones is a common feature, which may persist in later life, though in many cases it may disappear. The bones are usually short and thick, but, during the active course of the disease, they bend easily and give rise to various deformities which may become permanent when the soft rickety bones become denser and firmer, as they do when the active period of the disease passes off."

In many cases, the rachitic, clubbed ends of bones, in time, assume their normal size and shape. There is a strong tendency on the part of Innate, individualized spirit, to restore to normal all abnormal deficiencies or growths, when the nerves are freed from impingements and functions are restored to normal activity.

Clark tells us:—"The condition of bones is of chief interest to the surgeon; there are many considerations that make it desirable to recall the general pathological changes as well. The disease affects the alimentary tract and the whole organism as well as the bones. The abdomen is distended, the liver and spleen may be enlarged, muscles are weak, and there is often marked nervous irritability. The disease, it is true, is often observed in breast-fed infants, but the more marked cases are nearly always in children who have been brought up on **artificial foods, which are less assimilable than the natural, raw diet proper to infants up to the age of nine months. Systematic sterilization of milk as a preventative of tuberculosis plays a part in the production of rickets.''**

Wharton and Curtis maintain that children who are fed upon the breasts rarely develop rickets unless the lactation is prolonged or the milk becomes of a poor quality from a coincident pregnancy.

I fully agree with Clark, Wharton and Curtis that artificial food is not natural or suitable for the babe during the first nine months of life up to the natural age of ablactation. **Artificial ingesta irritate the alimentary tract, acting as a poison instead of a food.** The nervous system is irritated, excited, overheated; this creates abnormal metabolism and all the diseased conditions known as rachitis.

Eisendrath says:—"The most characteristic deformity of rachitis is a backward curvature (kyphosis) of the spine, which is uniformly distributed over the entire body. **There is never any breaking down of bone in rickets, or formation of sinuses.''**

The heat conditions of rachitis and caries are quite different; in the former the heat is diffused, while in the latter it is localized. In necrosis and caries the heat is circumscribed and intensified locally, sufficient to cause death and disintegration of bone, while in rachitis and osteomalacia it is diffused thruout the body affecting the functions generally. In rachitis and osteomalacia tissue is modified thru abnormal functionating, while in necrosis and caries the result of direct heat is the death of bone. In softening of bones without disintegration, the general heat is due to an impingement upon the 12th dorsal nerves, the second central place, while in necrosis and caries the subluxation causing impingements resulting in localized hyperthermia, are upon other nerves, determined by the locality inflamed.

Stimpson claims:—"That friability, due to rachitis, is found only in childhood, for the disease is one which involves the bones only during their period of growth, and consists, essentially, in the prolongation and exaggeration of the embryonal or developmental condition of the shaft, in consequence of which its strength and the firmness of the union with the epiphyses are diminished. Union after fracture takes place rather more slowly than in normal bone and sometimes fails entirely. The callus is usually large, but, as it is composed of the same soft embryonal tissue whose excess is the pathological feature of the disease, it is lacking in firmness."

Union of fractures in rachitic persons, if at all, is slower and lack firmness, than in those of normal temperature.

Stimson explains why callus is not furnished in some cases of fracture. "The effect of the preliminary rarefaction of one or both fragments may not have been corrected by subsequent ossification and they remain soft and spongy, or atrophied and pointed, and even this process of rarefaction may be so exaggerated as to create as distinct a gap between the fragments as if a piece had been removed or even to transform the entire shaft of the bone into a fibrous cord. Certain general conditions have been deemed a cause of delay or failure of union either through a specific poison, as in syphilis, or through a deterioration of the health or a lowering of the vitality induced by them, as defective innervation, pregnancy, lactation, defective nourishment and acute diseases."

Of callus formation Beck says:—"Meanwhile the ossifying inflammation of the periosteum creates abundant bone-substance, so that enough material for thorough consolidation is furnished. Sometimes callus formation is late. The cause for this condition can seldom be elicited. Syphilis, scurvy, rickets, malignant bone-disease and paralysis are generally held responsible for it."

The callus for union of fractures, in rachitic and osteomalacial cases are largely of cartilaginous tissue; osteoid tissue being scantily supplied. The greater the heat, the more hyaline cartilage and the less of leukocytes. Often fractures, in badly nourished persons, those who have a general fever, fail to unite because the abundant callus is largely cartilaginous and not supplied with lime-salts. Similar failure of union occurs in marasmus, senility and infectious diseases. If the temperature is below normal, there will be a lack of callus which will harden quickly.

Da Costa tells us:—"The most distinctive single sign of rickets is the so-called rachitic rosary, which consists of a beaded line paralleling each sternal border and corresponding to the course of the chondrosternal articulations. This double line of prominences, due to thickening of the costal cartilage, is to be felt in almost every rickety child and in advanced cases it is also clearly recognizable on inspection."

Richerand firmly believes that rachitis is only one of the effects of scrofula in its worst form.

Morand affirms that rachitis may even take place in the fetus in utero; but, the most common period of its commencement is in children between the ages of seven or eight months.

Delpech does not approve of the use of mechanical contrivances for the improvement of rickety bones, but, where malformations are not constitutional, as in club foot, he consents to their use.

Hutchinson says:—"In cartilaginous tumors we have, apparently, an interesting illustration of Cohnheim's theory, in that by far the largest number of them appear near the epiphyseal lines of the bones, where, as has been repeatedly demonstrated, islands (blood islets) of embryonic or infantile cartilage are quite liable to persist, imbedded in the bone tissue. These islands are most common in rickety bones and chondroma is peculiarly liable to occur in those who were rickety in early life."

Stanley observes that "rachitic tibiae and fibulae become curved; they sometimes acquire increased breadth in the direction of the curve, losing a proportionate degree of thickness in the opposite direction. Hence, the bones become, as it were, newly modeled, passing from the cylindrical into the flattened form. This would seem to be designed for the purpose of enabling them to support more efficiently the weight of the body, since, by this alteration they acquire increased breadth and power of resistance in that direction, in which the greatest strength is required. The apparent enlargement of the head is not because of enlargement of the cranial bones, but in consequence of the want of development of those of the face."

Functions are the result of directions of the "Designer," the intelligent entity which superintends all actions whether in sleeping or waking hours. In rachitis, the functions are pathologically performed owing to portions of the skeletal framework being displaced. The skeleton consists of the hardened portion of an animal, for the protection, attachment and retention in proper position of the soft parts. There are three forms: bony, cartilaginous, chitinous, calcareous or silicious. Man and the higher animals have an endoskeleton, an internal framework. Many of the lower animals, for the protection and attachment of their organs, have an exoskelton, represented by an integument, modified by the disposition of chitin, lime or other hardened substances, as shells, armor plates, scales, nails, hair, horns, hoofs, teeth and feathers and the vertebrate neuro-skeleton, and the vertebrate endoskelton, so-called from its being made up of parts which serve to protect the central nervous system. It will be readily seen that any displacement of the skeleton will also displace some portion of the softer parts. The abnormal changes in bones noticed by Stanley are physiological, they were made for a purpose.

Whereas, pathological changes are aberrational, not made with an aim in view. In rachitis, functions are abnormally performed.

Wells expresses himself as follows:—"In rickets, as with osteomalacia, chemical studies of the bones have thrown little light upon the etiology, or pathogenesis of this condition. None of the various hypothesis as yet advanced to explain this defective ossification has satisfactorily explained all the observed facts."

Wilson perceives that the origin of rickets has frequently been imputed to the results of dentition. He says:—"Circumstances considered tend to prove the scheme of using internally the phosphate of lime, could present no chance of benefit because there is no proof of a deficiency of lime in the system, though the arteries of the bones do not deposit it in the natural degree."

Boyer describes the appearance of rickety bones:—"**They are lighter than natural and of a red or brown color.** They are penetrated by many enlarged blood-vessels, being porous and as it were, spongy, soft and compressible. **They are moistened by a kind of sanies, which may be pressed out of their texture,** as out of a sponge, or rather from a macerated hide after it has been tanned. The walls of the medullary cylinder of the great bones of the extremities are very thin, while the bones of the skull are considerably increased in thickness and become spongy and reticular. All the affected bones acquire a remarkable suppleness; but if they are bent beyond a certain point they break. Instead of being filled with medulla, the medullary cavities of the long bones **contain only a reddish serum,** totally devoid of the fat oily nature of the other secretion in the natural state."

Sayre affirms that "Rachitis is one cause of acquired deformities; these, however, are of constitutional origin, depending upon the mal-nutrition of the system and want of the proper inorganic or earthy deposits in the bones; thus rendering them unable to bear the weight of the body, and allowing them under this superincumbent weight, and the contraction of the stronger muscles, to assume various distortions."

McCurdy records: "Rickets is a constitutional disease, generally of children, characterized by disorders of the digestive system and manifesting itself in alterations in the shape and form of the bones.

"Malnutrition must be considered the principal factor in its production. Various theories have been advocated as causes, as the acid, mineral, vaso-nervous and inflammatory. Anatomical studies have demonstrated the fact that the blood vessels are always larger in rickets, which results in congestion of the bone. The dilatation of the blood vessels is no doubt due to the general constitutional weakness.

"As per the classification of the majority of authorities, four varieties are recognized, viz.: congenital, infantile, adolescent and senile.

"The bones during the course of the disease pass through three stages, viz.: congestion, softening and sclerosis. The dilated condition of the blood vessels formerly referred to, results in hyperemia and this interferes with the nutrition of the bone. The periosteum thickens and is red, beneath which the bone is spongy and arranged in layers, and the normal compact bone is displaced. The diaphyso-epiphyseal cartilage is now congested, or it may be transparent and enlarged and this congestion afterwards extends to a uniform tumefaction of the epiphysis. Many joints may become involved at the same time, notably the ankles and wrists."

To say that rickets is a constitutional disease, that malnutrition is the principal cause, that acids or minerals are supplied in an amount either too great or less than usual, that the vaso-nervous systems are deranged, or that inflammatory conditions are at fault, gives conditions, rather than causes. As to the four varieties—they are simply such as occur at four different periods of life. As the quality of tissue varies at different ages, the effects resulting from the same cause will differ accordingly.

Garrod and Fletcher enumerate the causes of rickets, as ill-health of the mother during pregnancy; want of fresh air and exercise during pregnancy; numerous and rapid pregnancies; multiple pregnancies; age of mother at time of birth; lactation during pregnancy; heredity and syphilis.

The above conditions exist in many mothers who have a large number of healthy children free of deformities.

Tilbury Fox says that the children of mothers who menstruate during pregnancy are more likely to have rickets.

Joukwoski informs us that more than half the children of St. Petersburg die before the age of ten years, and sixty per cent of all children under five years of age are rachitic.

Gee found that 30 per cent of all sick children under the age of two years were rickety. Ritter, of Prague, found 31 per cent, and Perry of Philadelphia, 28 per cent of children under five years old rickety.

Snow of Buffalo, N. Y., concludes from his observation, that the reason Italian and negro children are so frequently afflicted with rickets is, that there is a tendency in a Southern race to deteriorate when living in a Northern climate.

Volkmann and Heuter's theory is that pressure of muscles, etc., upon the surface of long bones causes atrophy and that the bone increases in size where no pressure is made. They say: "In case of bow-leg the pressure on the inside, or concave side of the tibia would cause atrophy, or diminution in the tissue, resulting in an increase in the curvature, and the increased pressure upon the convex side increases cell proliferation and consequent thickening of the parts, which with the diminished pressure upon the concave side would increase the curve of the bone."

Julius Wolf argues that the pressure theory, as given above, is incorrect and that the reverse is the proper explanation of rachitic deformities. He states: "Abnormal increase of tension and pressure instead of producing atrophy, as the pressure theory would have it, does just the opposite, resulting in accretions of bony material. The amount of bone thus added is proportional to the increase of burden at every point in the bone; therefore, the greater the pressure at any one place the greater is the amount of bone which must be here laid down to resist it."

Muscular contraction is due to stimulus, irritation received from Innate in normal quantity, or from traumatic pressure or toxic poisons. Atrophy or hypertrophia of long bones, are abnormal conditions brought about from increased or diminished nerve tension, causing abnormal contraction of muscles.

T. P. Pick, states: "Rickets produces a condition of the bones which disposes them to fracture, and not only this, but on account of the unsteadiness of gait of rickety children and their proneness to fall, the accidents which occasion fracture are more liable to occur in them than in healthy children. So that from the pressure exerted upon them, or even from muscular action, the bones from a rachitic child are often broken, and it is not uncommon to find several broken in the same patient, or it may be the same bone broken in more than one place."

Samuel Cooper says:—"When rachitis is general, the spine becomes shorter and is curved in various directions; the breast becomes deformed not only in consequence of the curvature of the spine, but by the depression of the ribs and projection of the sternum. The bones of the pelvis fall inward and the os pubis generally approaches the sacrum. No medicine is known which possesses any direct efficacy in osteomalacia or rickets. Tonics are indicated and should be employed. The state of the bowels must in particular be attended to. The disease appearing to consist in a deficiency of lime in the bones, proposals have been made to exhibit internally the phosphate of lime; but this chemical project has had no success. More good is generally affected by keeping children in healthy situations and in a salubrious air, than by any medicine whatever."

Rachitis, or rickets, is a disease wherein all the bodily functions are disturbed. The patient is irritable, sleepless, feverish, the abdomen is bloated and the stool movements abnormal.

Food is nutritive material taken into the body of an organism for the purpose of growth, repair and the maintenance of the vital processes. Poison is any substance which when introduced into the animal organism, destroys life, impairs functions and produces a morbid condition of tissue. In health, functions, tissue and temperature must be normal. Any deviation of the latter makes a change in the action of organs and the substance of tissue. The ingesta may become food or poison. That which is food for the mother may be poison for her babe; age modifies the tissue of the nervous system and its alimentary requirements. The mother's milk is the natural and proper food for her infant up to ablactation, the end of the nursing period; the next best is the milk of a cow whose date of calving should correspond to that of the birth of the child.

Digestion is the process of converting nutritive material into an absorbable form by the dissolving action of secretions. In man, the digestion commences in the mouth by the addition of saliva and is continued thruout the alimentary canal by the action of biliary acids, gastric, pancreatic and intestinal juices. These secretions act normally when the temperature is 98 to 99 degrees Fahrenheit. A higher or lower temperature impairs their usefulness and causes their functions to be abnormally performed. Normal heat, therefore, is absolutely necessary for normal action of the digestive juices.

The mother's milk may be poison to her babe instead of nutritious. During the first few days following delivery, the breasts secrete milk of a yellowish color and of considerable consitency, in which large cells completely filled with fat granules are present. This quality of food is adapted to the needs of the child during the first few days of the nursing period. It is well known that many substances introduced with food, drink, or as a medicine, are secreted in the milk. Odorous substances, such as anise, vermuth, garlic, flavor the milk; chloral hydrate, opium, indigo, salicylic acid, iodine, iron, zinc, mercury, lead, bismuth and antimony change its quality. They are not adapted to the needs of the child, therefore, they are poison. Any ingesta, which irritate the nerves of the digestive tract, by their exciting effects increase the temperature. Inordinate heat deranges not only metabolism but all the functions of the body.

The secretion and quality of milk is influenced by the nervous system. Emotions of joy, grief, fear, hate, awe or reverence affect the milk. Because of this excitement, the secretions are affected; they are mentally magnetized. Love or hate, joy or grief, fear or boldness, affect the secretions of glands and follicles. Excitation means an increase in temperature which is not compatible with the normal performance of functions either secretory or excretory.

"Improper food," a diet which irritates the nervous system causes inordinate heat. Heat, when exorbitant, changes the usual amount and action of secretions. Normal temperature is absolutely necessary for the "catalytic" and "hydrolytic" action of the "enzymes." Temperature above or below 30 to 35 degrees centigrade creates a corresponding amount of red and white corpuscles. Normal temperature creates one white corpuscle to 650 of the red; this number varies in health from 500 to 700. Pathologic variations either greatly exceed or fall short of the above number. The ingestion of food increases the number of the white 30 to 40 per cent. Fasting lowers the per centage of leucocytes. In the new-born babe the percentage of the white corpuscles is greater than in the adult. As age advances, functions being normal, there is a decrease in the number of the white corpuscles because there is less demand for bone material.

The blood is the nutritive fluid of the body; it carries foodstuffs to the tissues after being properly prepared by the digestive apparatus. The composition of the material transported depends upon the amount of heat, which in turn determines the quality of tissue. The leucocytes are not always the same histologically and, no doubt, their functions are as diverse as their morphology.

The "center place" of the vertebral column is the 6th dorsal vertebra which may impinge the 6th pair of thoracic nerves. This impingement causes more diseases, more especially in the line of fevers, than that of any other pair of nerves. I was the first to draw special attention to this fact. I therefore named it the center place. I now name the 12th dorsal vertebra, which, by its displacement impinges upon the 12th pair of dorsal nerves, the second center place, being midway between center place and the coccyx. Impingements on the 12th pair of dorsal nerves cause more diseases, with the one exception of the 6th dorsal, than does pressure upon any other spinal nerves. Whenever I find a person with clammy hands, feet always cold on account of perspiration, I locate the cause at the 12th thoracic vertebra. The following diseases and symptoms: Scurvy, seborrhea, cretinism, spongy gums, hemorrhagic diathesis, decalcification, eburnation, osteitis deformans, osteomalacia, lack of ossification, fragilitas ossium, large head because of hydrocephalous, profuse perspiration, nervousness, emaciation, dropsy, general weakness, indigestion, hectic fever, soreness over the body, sleeplessness, laryngismus, constant fever, and last but not the least, curvature of the spine, including, lordosis, scoliosis, and kyphosis, unmistakably point to an impingement upon the 12th pair of dorsal nerves. One case of scoliosis was straightened, while writing this article, by adjusting the 12th dorsal vertebrae. I do not hesitate to locate the impingement, the irritation which causes the symptoms known as rachitic and osteomalacia at the 12th dorsal, the second center place.

I find in McClelland's Regional Anatomy, a note made by me in 1901—nine years ago—that displacement of the 12th dorsal was the cause of spinal curvature.

Displacement of the 12th dorsal vertebra impinges upon the twelfth pair of thoracic nerves, creating an inflammation which, when diffused, is known as fever. Curvatures of the spine exist because of the softening of vertebrae and muscular contraction which draw vertebrae out of alignment. This scattered inflammation accounts for degeneration of the liver and spleen, the increased size of the cartilage and the reddened color of the bones and marrow, a condition known as hyperemia.

Having observed that unsuitable ingesta irritate the nervous system, contracting certain nerves and muscles which draw the 12th dorsal vertebra out of alignment and impinge upon the 12th pair of thoracic nerves, causing an inordinate amount of heat which modifies metabolism and creates all the symptoms collectively, known as rickets; knowing all this, what shall we do about it? Why not quit giving "improper food," undo the wrong done, replace the 12th dorsal vertebra and allow the functions of the 12th pair of thoracic nerves to functionate normally. Functions performed in a natural manner will correct abnormal tissue.

---

The doctor who has no patients loses none.

---

By the way, why is the food of restaurants and hotels tasteless, lacking the relish which we find in our homes? Because their cooks have no loving interest, nothing outside of a monetary value. They fail to magnetize it with an appetizing flavor; therefore tasteless. It is a question whether a cook cannot poison the guest by magnetizing the food with hatred.

## NEUROPATHY, BY A. P. DAVIS.

"It will be a matter of the first importance to every one who reads this book that it does not matter what the patient complains of, the **spinal treatment, from the fourth dorsal down to the twelfth,** at least, **if not clear down the entire spine,** should always be done. This unites the two forces, remember, and neutralizes the excess of acid or alkali and allows nature to begin to adjust itself harmoniously. In all Osteopathic treatments, the spinal treatment as shown under Neuropathy, should receive special attention if you wish to be successful in your treatment in the cure of disease of any and all kinds. **There is no better way to alleviate human suffering than this spinal adjustment,** as it is one of the essentials in all diseases of whatever character, nature or degree, in all ages."

Why does A. P. Davis say? "Spinal treatment from the fourth dorsal down to the twelfth?" Is it possible that he has not learned to adjust the other fifteen true vertebrae? Those mentioned by him were the only ones I was able to adjust at that date, 1898. "If not clear down the entire spine." Nothing scientific about that expression. He does not comprehend Chiropractic as a science or an art.

---

"Tightness of nerves produced by and pressure then created upon one or more sides by bone makes the same abnormal functions as, and is equivalent to, entire pressure, and is a constricting force modified."

I think the author means to say: "Bone pressure on one or more sides of nerves, creates a modified tension proportionate to the number of sides the nerves are pressed against. This constricting force causes the abnormal performance of functions." Bone pressure does not constrict. Tubes, ducts, the esophagus, urethra, the intestines are subject to stricture, a ring-like obstruction around their canals. Bones may crush or squeeze, but they never constrict.

"This form of illustrating is unique, but conveys the simplified fundamental ideas that sailing a ship on the human body thru life depends upon."

---

When Chiropractic was an infant I jealously watched its development and growth. But there came a time when unprincipled shysters tried to change its principles. There are many claiming to practice Chiropractic who know but little of it as a science.

## NEUROPATHY—LUXATION.

"Chiropractic Science (preface vii.) rationally explained and the 'Luxation Fad' eliminated, and shown why."

All right, Friend Davis. Perhaps you know more about this Science than the man who created it, or the 2,000 or more practioners who are daily adjusting, moving, vertebrae. They know by the sense of feeling that they **do move.** They know by the contour of the spine that vertebrae are not in line. By using the processes as levers they know that they rack them back and into their former position. An examination shows, by the sense of sight and feeling, that the outline of the spinous processes has been changed by adjustment. The sense of feeling thus confirms that of sight and hearing. The testimony of these senses is sufficient to convict you of ignorance or wilful misrepresentation. The patient's sense of feeling also corroborates the knowledge of the adjuster..

Gustave Noque, an anatomist, who has many years of experience in the preparation of skeletons and vertebral columns, says under date of Dec. 26th, 1909, "In my long experience in practical work, I do not recollect to have seen one spinal column without any curvature in one place or another." Dr. Davis would have a good time eliminating the "Luxation Fad" from the man who has handled a thousand vertebral columns in the recent state to his one.

On page 145 of "Neuropathy" I find: "The spinal curvatures seen everywhere **are direct results of nervous irritation, resulting in contraction of muscular fibers, and a gradual curve a consequence.** To relieve that condition, **'take off the pressure'** is all that is needed. To relieve the victim of amenorrhea or dysmenorrhea, we simply remove the pressure from the nervous system ending in the organs involved. **The same law holds good for any other functional disorder known to humanity, or to the doctors.**"

Page 66: "Every condition denominated by Chiropractors as 'luxation,' being an impossibility in the very nature of things."

Page 69: "The nervous system of the spine consists of what is termed the cerebro-spinal nervous system, as well as the sympathetic nervous system. This nervous system of the spine emerges in leashes along the sides of the spine, underneath the lamina, in thirty-one places, from the atlas to the coccyx. The bones are held together by ligamentous structure joining on from process to process, from lamina to lamina, together with the periosteum, on the posterior aspect, and laterally, with a fibrous cartilaginous substance, on the inside of the bodies of all the vertebrae; and the muscle-tissue attaches to this cartilaginous, ligamentous structure, posteriorly, in five layers. **These** five layers of **muscles are the levers of the spine. The contracting of this muscular structure is caused by irritation of the nervous system ending in the muscular structure**; because, the only property of the muscular tissue is to contract, and **never does contract unless as a result of irritation.**"

Page 107: "We are inclined to attribute the belief of spinal luxation, or sub-luxation, to a morbid mental conception, rather than to anything else. Hence luxations of the spine are not causes of disease. That is an assumption without the shadow of a possibility only in cases of positive violence."

If the above statements are true, over 2,000 Chiropractors, 5,000 osteopaths and thousands of patients are deceived; they have "**a morbid mental conception.**" Chiropractors and bony lesion Osteopaths hear that! Your mental conception of luxated vertebrae is conceived by a diseased brain. Does not Dr. Davis need an atlas adjustment?

Page 66: "The question is asked, **Why the deviation in the processes of the spine at the places from whence the nerves emanate from the cord through the foramen ending in the part diseased?** It has been shown in our previous remarks, that the muscle fiber has but one function, and that is to contract. From this fact the facets are strongly drawn together by the contraction of the **muscle fiber**, and if the muscle fiber that contracts **is attached to the ends or sides of the spinous processes, the tendency is to incline the bone in the direction of the contracted muscle, and the sudden movement in that particular locality relieves the contraction of the muscle.**"

Now, doctor, you talk Chiropractic. The spinous processes are found to deviate at the foramen from which the nerves emanate which go to the part diseased. Contracted muscles attached to the spinous processes incline the bone in the direction of contracture. A sudden movement (an adjustment) in that particular locality, relieves the contracted muscles. Now you are all right. Stay right there. Your book eliminates the "Luxation Fad."

Page 109: "We deny luxations being the causes of nerve-impingement."

Page 65: "In the Neuropathic department ('Chiropractice, really what we call Neuropathy,' Page 1), the **spinal adjustment is the main treatment** and in the Osteopathic department much is dependent upon physical manipulations."

Page 64: "The thumb placed alongside of the spinous processes and the force applied with the other arm—hand against the thumb, will be a good way to reduce the prominent projection of the processes."

Is that the way you adjust vertebrae? You surely have the "Luxation Fad" as a freak. Every Chiropractor will smile when he learns how you eliminate the "Luxation Fad."

Page 4: "Neuropathy rights a large per cent of **affections which result from spinal irritation,** and the **remedy may be found in the spinal adjustment alone.**"

Page 106: "**That there are impingements of nerves along the spine we readily and freely grant, and know to be a fact; but to assert that luxations, or even partial luxations,** as he (D. D. Palmer) is wont to assert, **are responsible for nerve impingements, we emphatically deny.**"

Page 24: "When the operator **applies these adjustments properly** and **uses the proper force** (which will be soon attained), **the treatments will be easily and quickly done, and confidence established.**"

Page 62: "There are **no special manipulations** anywhere in the body which have for their sole object any **specific effect** at particular places as such, for no **disease will succumb** to any treatment made simply by relieving any one set of filaments as such, but relief is dependent, not only upon relief of pressure of said filaments, but **because the forces are united and filaments freed** which end where disease exists."

"In case of typhoid or puerperal fever, we have to adjust the area which first unites the forces and then relieves the nerves which end in the parts affected. In puerperal or childbed fever, we usually afford relief by adjustment at the **second and third** lumbar."

Persons may succumb to disease, but disease does not succumb to treatment.

The doctor tells us that we must first unite the "two forces" by adjusting; then proceed as directed by Chiropractic. Adjusting the two forces is Neuropathic.

Dr. Davis should know that Chiropractors relieve acute diseases, usually, by one adjustment. Puerperal fever in the lumbar, typhoid and pneumonia in the dorsal and smallpox in the cervical, regardless of the Neuropathic fad. Chiropractic (Neuropathy) is specific. That one specific adjustment to unite the "two forces" is Neuropathy.

Page 27: "That a simple **movement in the spine at a particular spot,** seemingly not differing in its contour from any other along the spine, should produce such a change in all of the relationship of the entire body, seems almost incredible, and **yet such is the case.** From a racking pain, that almost drives one to insanity, come the calmness of a May morning, and the tranquility of the flowing of a gentle brook. This is not only the case in a single instance, but there are no less than thirty-one such places from the atlas to the coccyx where **adjustments may be made with astonishing results**—the cripple is made to walk and the lame man leaps as a freed slave from bondage. No wonder that such treatment has become so exceedingly popular with those who have witnessed its marvelous results."

One simple movement, known as adjusting, at the particular spot designated, replacing a displaced vertebra, often produces an entire change from a diseased condition to that of health.

Chiropractic adjusting is done regardless of uniting or separating the "two forces" of Neuropathy. Thousands of Osteopaths and Chiropractors are doing good work, who know nothing of the Neuropathic "positive and negative forces," and who are not able to designate what organs secrete acids or alkali. Chiropractors should be specific, making one "simple movement in the spine at a particular spot" and in the right direction. This is true in regard to twenty-four vertebrae, which by their displacement may impinge upon any one of the sixty-two bundles of nerves which emerge from the spinal foramina. Instead of there being "thirty-one such places," there are twenty-four. The nerves are not always paired as are the foramina. While nerves pass out of the left and right foramina of the dorsal respectively, for the left and right lungs, and also for the kidneys, the innervating nerves destined for the stomach, spleen and heart are supplied from the left side, and those for the liver and pancreas from the right. The nerves destined for the throat and eyeball proceed from the right side. The adjusting must be done accordingly. Do not forget that there are twenty-four bones from the atlas to the last lumbar, where adjustments may be made with astonishing results, providing the vertebrae are moved in the right direction to relieve the impingement.

---

"Disease and Its Cause" is the title of an eight page booklet.

"Chiropractic removes the disease when administered by the Chiropractor."

Chiropractic is a science and an art. Who would think of administering a science and an art to remove disease?

"Abnormal pressure on nerves."

Any pressure on nerves is abnormal—why say abnormal pressure? Where will we find normal pressure?

Foramen and foramina are spelled foramine, in this eight page book.

"The brain generates innate life essence."

An essence is the virtue of or the quality of a substance separated from its grosser parts. An essence is extracted instead of generated. "Innate life essence," three words which are not companionable, are not collaterally connected with each other.

"The organ ramified by such nerves becomes abnormal from lack of nerve stimuli and we are sick."

The stimulus of the body cannot be plural (stimuli). All fevers and inflammatory conditions are because of too much stimulus or energy.

"Abnormal pressure on nerves is caused by compression of the inter-vertebral-fibro-cartilage, causing abnormal function or disease."

Compare the above with, "Chiropractors find subluxated vertebra out of proper articulation."

"Pain of any kind causes contraction of muscles."

Now, what do you think of that? I have been thinking that nerve irritation caused muscles to contract. Pain is due to an excessive stimulation, an over irritation of sensory nerves.

"Most of the principal muscles have their origin, or insertion, at the spinal column."

Such ignorance is being passed off as Chiropractic knowledge, and it is copyrighted, 1910. I wonder where this D. C. acquired his knowledge of anatomy?

"Abnormal pressure on trunk nerves obstruct nerve stimuli or life essence."

This short sentence has four false, deceptive statements.

"We transgress natural laws by a lack of proper diet."

How does a lack of food cause subluxations, or compression of the inter-vertebral-fibro-cartilage?

"Nature throws off disease."

What is that you say? Disease is a something which can be handled, thrown out or off, got rid of?

The climax of absurdity is reached under the head-line of germs. "To pinch a trunk nerve between subluxated vertebrae, nerve stimuli or life essence, which is Nature's germicider in the human body, is obstructed, and the organ which it should supply becomes dormant or a favorable place for germs to thrive and rapidly multiply."

He closes his pseudo-Chiropractic by advising "When nerve stimuli is shut off, it would be wisdom to immediately consult a competent Chiropractor—the linemen of life—who has thoroughly mastered the science."

"Brain Nerves—is used to express the additional idea of the place of origin of all nerves in contradistinction to the terms 'spinal, cranial,' or 'sympathetic nerves.' The Chiropractor has no 'spinal' or 'sympathetic nerves' to worry about. All fibers expand from the brain, thus the preference for 'Brain Nerves.'"

"Brain Nerves" is not an "additional idea." There is nothing anatomically new in stating that the real origin of all nerves is in the brain, for every anatomist is aware of this fact. For convenience, the nervous system is divided into the cranial, cerebro-spinal, sympathetic, efferent and afferent systems. **Nerves do not expand,** increase in bulk, without additional substance, **they emerge** from the brain substance or spinal canal.

"Serous circulation locally confined to the neck, head and upper shoulder region also receives its mental impulses through nerves emitting at these points."

To emit is to flow out, as fire emits heat, boiling water emits steam, the sun emits light. Nerves emerge or arise from the spinal canal or the brain; they never "emit" from any substance. **Nerves never "emit" or emerge from "points."** The tapering end of any part of or portion of the body would be the last place I would expect a nerve to "emit" or emerge from.

Serous, in biology, means pertaining to, or of the nature of, serum. Serum is the yellowish fluid separated from the blood after the coagulation of the fibrin. Fibrin is a solid, white, inodorous proteid. A proteid is one of the constitutent aliments of the tissue and fluids of the body.

Shed blood, not in circulation, but outside of the body, exposed to the atmosphere, coagulates, separates into a dark-red clot and a yellowish fluid known as serum. The serous fluids are found in the cavities of the body, more especially those lined by serous membranes. Normal blood consists of 79 per cent of water and 21 per cent of solids.

Serum is the most watery portion of animal fluids **transuded** (not circulated) by serous membranes. Animal blood serum containing antitoxin is employed as a specific in the treatment of many diseases.

Serum confined locally to the neck, head, and upper shoulder region, as stated by the author, does not circulate. As stated above and verified by anatomists, serum only exists in drawn blood and in bodily cavities which are lined by serous membranes. It, therefore, does not exist in "the neck, head and upper shoulder region."

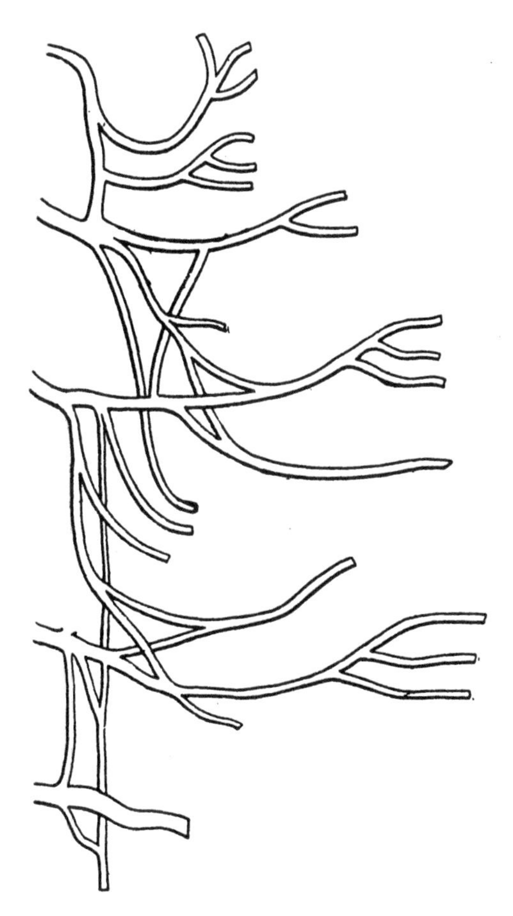

Cut of the cervical plexus, showing the communication of nerve fibers from one nerve to another.

## NEUROPATHY.

N. B.—My remarks are in parenthesis in the following:

Baker City, Ore., Feb. 6, 1910.

Dear Doctor D. D. Palmer:

I have the Chiropractor Adjuster and have read it carefully and noted what you say about my book and also scanned the criticisms concerning it.

I presumed that you would discern the difference in the divisions of the book and not jump at the conclusion that I practice medicine or Osteopathy simply because I published these sciences in the same book.

(It is presumed that you practice all you recommend, as there is nothing said to the contrary. On page 8 you tell us, "**The various methods blend together admirably.**" And "There will be found many valuable receipts and instructions in it **which are invaluable and come in the way when nothing else will suffice but them.**" On page 665 you say: "In the treatment of the various conditions called disease, it is well to have various resources to draw from in order to meet the special demands at the time so as to render the needed service for the given condition." When I read the above and many other similar statements I thot you meant just what you said. Excuse me for making the mistake; I fear others will do the same. It is self-evident that you published the book to suit the liking of each and every practitioner and patient.)

You should certainly know that all the people are not educated up to the use of Chiro, Osteopathy, Neuropathy or medicine. People when they get sick want help. Many are used to medicine—some want one thing and some another.

I have fully demonstrated the fact that Neuropathy is the best—but leave these other sciences to the judgment and the habit and desire of the owners of the book—and as Neuropathy embraces the entire nervous system, and the others do not, I leave the people to their own choice.

(If your book Neuropathy demonstrates anything, it certainly does demonstrate that each science is the very best, for which see an article on Neuropathy. "Some want one thing and some want another." Your book was written to fill each and every want. A book of policy—to please everybody. You know what I think of policy.

(What? "Neuropathy embraces the entire nervous system." You are now talking to the founder of "Chiropractice, really what we call Neuropathy."

(Neuropathy, page 73. "Whilst there is indescribable merit in both of these [Osteopathy and Chiropractic] sciences and each has an important place, and without them there is an unfilled 'niche' in the curriculum of treatment, we are not so circumscribed in our limitations and compasses of the sciences of healing as to assume that even they include all that is necessary to know how to stop all progress, or to embrace all the causes of human ills; that each may be advantageously useful and accomplish much good, relieve much suffering, take off the 'pressure' from many nerves, arrest many pathological conditions and bring joy and gladness to many afflicted mortals; yet there is some of the nervous system which these systems are inadequate to affect in any way directly, and leave them for other means to be used to wholly embrace all of the nervous system of this body of ours. So that to be panoplied with a full armamentarium for all contingencies we would most earnestly advise the consideration of a means of cure, with the others mentioned, a method of 'stopping waste'—'nerve waste'—which is not accomplished by either Osteopathic or Chiropractic. This means is found in properly applied Neuro-Ophthalmology."

(We are told on page viii., that this book embraces three of the greatest modern sciences—Osteopathy, Chiropractic and Ophthalmology. On page 73 we are informed that the two former "fill an unfilled niche," that they do not embrace all the causes of human ills; they do not reach all of the nervous system; but, Ophthalmology reaches the portion not reached by the other two systems.

(Page 698, "The ophthalmological department is also invaluable and will fit in in many a case where nothing else will.")

I shall not defend the use of medicine nor Osteopathy, but gave these as separate and distinct departments—leaving the people to make their own selection as to which to use.

Another thing that seems strange to me is that you would introduce and comment on what you absolutely know I do not practice, and take up valuable space in a journal that might be of better use to subscribers.

Of course you edit the journal, and have a right to say what you are a mind to, but to criticise me unfairly seems altogether out of place.

I shall hope to see you ere many weeks, and will talk to you face to face—friendly of course.

I cannot see why you harp on things different from what you endorse, and make up the bulk of your journal about something foreign from Chiropractic eleucidation, and which should interest subscribers. Objections to what is taught do not enhance the science we advocate, do they?

(There is no better method of teaching, than that of comparison—the examination of two or more objects, subjects, or systems, for the purpose of discovering their resemblances or differences, their relative estimates. Neuropathy is Chiropractic, only that the science and art of adjusting subluxated vertebrae is left out.

(It is the business of this journal to draw the line of distinction between Chiropractic and other systems.)

You know that I use Ophthalmology for the same reason you do Chiro—to free the nervous system—and if it does this is it not the right thing to do?

If the way I treat the spine—CURES a large per cent of my cases, what objection can you file to it?

(In your treatment of the spine, you do and do not treat the spine. You move vertebrae and you do not. You unite the two forces instead of moving vertebrae. You remove impingements and you do not. You are all things to all men. "Many are used to medicine—some want one thing and some another.")

I am sure that there will never be any improvement on the philosophy I have expressed in my book—the Neuropathic Department, and while it cures I have no objection to placing it alongside of other sciences for comparison. It is separate and distinct and when people are educated up to it, it will take the lead and be recognized as worthy of the highest consideration.

I have said the above as explanatory of the facts as they should be known—and not leave the impression that I am practicing all the series I have studied.

(Doctor, are you not egotistical in saying, "I am sure that there will never be any improvement on the philosophy of Neuropathy"?)

(I have read your book carefully and do not remember an instance wherein you mention which of the many methods therein referred to and recommended, you do or do not practice. I was led to believe from what you state that each and every one of them are the very best; that Neuropathy takes in more or less of each, therefore is not a separate and distinct science. Yes, I understand: you replace the science and art of Chiropractic, the subluxation of vertebrae, with the positive and negative forces; instead of adjusting vertebrae, you connect these two forces; instead of nerves being impinged upon, they have too much or not enough tonicity.

(From the reading of your book, Neuropathy, I fail to see where your science "is separate and distinct." Without Chiropractic there would not be, could not be, such a system as Neuropathy. Without Chiropractic, there would not be even a ghost to name Neuropathy.)

## COMPOSITION OF NERVES AND THEIR FUNCTIONS.

Carver: "A nerve is a single filament or thread."

B. J. Palmer: "**A nerve is made up of nine fibres conveying nine functions,** viz., calorific, trophic, motor, secretory, excretory, reproductive (?), circulatory, reparatory, nutritive."

Gould: "An elongated, cord-like structure made up of aggregations of nerve-fibers and having the property of transmitting nervous impulses."

Dorland: "A cord-like structure which conveys impulses from one part of the body to another. A nerve consists of a connective-tissue sheath enclosing **bundles of nerve-fibers.**"

Lippincott: "Nerve. A long medullary cord connected with the brain or spinal marrow and forming the channel or instrument by which sensation, volition, or vital influence is conveyed from the periphery to the central nervous system (afferent N.) or from the central nervous system to the periphery (efferent N.). Every nerve-fiber is directly connected with and presided over by a nerve-cell, a prolongation of whose body it really is. According to function the principal varieties of nerves are depressor, inhibitory, motor, pressor, secretory, sensory, tri-splanchnic, trophic, vasoconstrictive, vasodilator, vasomotor, vasosensory."

According to Lippincott there are a dozen or more kinds of nerves, each having its special function.

Dunglison: "Nerves extend from the nervous centres to every part of the body, communicating frequently with each other. According to their origin they are termed cranial and spinal. Each nerve is composed of several filaments. Experiments and pathological facts have proven that the anterior column of the spinal cord and the anterior roots of the spinal nerves are inservient to volition or voluntary motion; and that the posterior column and roots are destined for sensibility. Hence the **spinal nerves, which have two roots, must be the conductors both of motion and feeling,** while the **encephalic,** which, with but few exceptions, **have but one, can possess but one of these properties: they must be either sensitive or motor** according as they arise from the posterior or anterior column of the medulla."

Webster: "One of the whitish and elastic bundles of fibers, with the accompanying tissues, which transmit nervous impulses between nerve centers and various parts of the animal body."

Dutton: "Nerves are composed of one or more, sometimes nearly a hundred nerve-fibers, each fiber forming a means of communication between two parts more or less distant from each other."

Carver: "The nervous system is that class of nerve tissue

which extends from brain cells in threads and receives from brain cells that stimulus, and conducts it to the various places in the organism, where it is to be used. Of course the **number of such threads of filaments is beyond comprehension,** and they can only be said to be sufficiently numerous to supply all of the tissue cells of the body, including the brain and nerves themselves."

It will be understood that **millions of filaments** have origin, extension and ramification within the tissues of the brain, and the various adjacent tissue, which are so infinitesimal as to have entirely escaped notice, and to be practically incapable of isolation.

The demonstrative dissectionist has satisfied himself with discussing only the principal nerve trunks and the chief ramification of their branches, and has entirely failed to disclose filamentous ramification.

Filaments from the spinal trunks also return and ramify the internal substance of the neural canal, the spinal cord, the medulla oblongata, pons Variolii, and all parts of the brain. These fibers are properly termed returning filaments, and their function should be studied with much care, since their condition is responsible for so much mental as well as physical abnormality.

Cunningham: "Nerve-fibres arranged in bundles of greater or less bulk form the nerves which pervade every part of the body. They also constitute the greater part of the brain and spinal cord. Nerve-fibres are the conducting elements of the nervous system; they serve to bring the nerve-cells into relation both with each other and with the various tissues of the body."

Nerve stimulus is an original, **elemental energy.** It is not manufactured, generated or composed, but has a continuous, non-varying, eternal existence. It is an **intelligent energy, emanating directly from the central intelligence of the universe** or Creator.

Kirke: "A nerve is composed of a number of bundles of nerve fibers bound together by connective tissue. Some of the nerves conduct impulses from the nerve-centres and are called efferent; those which conduct impulses in the opposite direction are called afferent. When one wishes to move the hand, the nervous impulse starts in the brain and passes down the efferent or motor nerve-tracts to the muscles of the hand, which contract; when one feels pain in the hand, afferent or sensory nerve-tracts convey an impulse to the brain which is there interpreted as a sensation."

Davis: "That the force or power which controls this body of ours should be somewhere is self-evident; but what that is, we are as ignorant of as if such a thing did not exist."

Pressure upon a nerve, at any point of its course, from its origin to its terminus, if strong enough to interfere with the passage of impulses it conveys, will cause, at its termination, a condition called disease.

The spinal curvatures, seen everywhere, are direct results of nervous irritation, resulting in contraction of muscular fibers, with a gradual increase in the curve as a consequence.

The capacity of an organ depends altogether upon the nerve power governing it, and this fact should never be overlooked by the intelligent practitioner of this or any other system.

The Chiropractor will find much of interest in Howell's Physiology, published in 1909, by W. B. Saunders Company, Philadelphia. "The question of the **nature of the nerve impulse** has always aroused the deepest interest among physiologists. It has constituted, indeed, a central question around which have revolved various hypotheses **concerning the nature of living matter.** The importance of the **nerves as conductors of motion and sensation** was apparent to the old physiologists, and the nature of the conduction or the thing conducted was the subject of many hypotheses and was called by many different names. For many years the prevalent view was that the nerves are essentially tubes through which flows an exceeding fine matter, or the nature of air or gas, known as the animal spirits. Others conceived this fluid to be of a grosser structure like water and described it as the nerve juice. With Galvani's discovery of electricity the nerve principle, as it was called, became identified with electricity, and, indeed, this view occurs in modified form today. Du Bois-Reymond, after discovering the demarcation current and action current in muscle and nerve, formulated an hypothesis according to which the nerve fibers contain a series of electromotive particles, and by this hypothesis and the facts upon which it was based, he thought that he had established the "hundred-year-old dream" of physicists and physiologists, the identity of the nerve principle and electricity. His theory today has fallen into disrepute, but the facts upon which it was based remain, as before, of the deepest importance. In the middle of the nineteenth century those who were not convinced of the identity of the nerve principle with electricity, believed, nevertheless, that the process of conduction in the nerve is a phenomenon of an order comparable to the transmission of light or electricity, with a velocity so great as to defy measurement. But in this same period a simple but complete experiment by Helmoltz demonstrated that its velocity, as compared with light or electrical conduction through the air or through metals, is exceedingly slow—27 meters (90 feet) per second. Modern views have taken divergent directions; the movement or excitation that is conducted along the fiber has been named the **nerve principle, the nerve energy, the nerve force, the nerve impulse.**''

**The strength of the impulse and its velocity may be modified** in various ways: **by the action of temperature, narcotics, pressure,** etc. **Variations of temperature,** as stated before, **change the velocity** of propagation **of the impulse, the velocity increasing with a rise of temperature** up to a certain point. So, also, the irritability as well as the conductivity of the nerve fiber is influenced markedly by temperature. **If** a small area of **a nerve trunk be cooled or heated, the nerve impulse,** as it passes through this area **may be increased or decreased** in strength **or may be blocked entirely.**

The older conceptions of the nerve principle, while they varied in detail, were based upon the general idea that the nervous system contains a matter of a finer sort than that visible to our senses. This matter was pictured at first (animal spirits), and later as a material comparable to the luminiferous ether or to electricity. Since the discovery that the nerve impulse travels with a relatively slow velocity and is accompanied by a demonstrable change in the electrical condition of the nerve, two main views regarding its nature have been entertained. Many physiologists conceive the **nerve impulse as a progressive wave** of chemical change which is started at one end by the stimulus and is then self-propagated along the fiber.

**Whether or not the nerve impulses in various nerve fibers differ in kind is a question of great interest in physiology.** The usually accepted view is that they are identical in character in all fibers and vary only in intensity. According to this, a sensory nerve—the auditory nerve, for instance—carries impulses similar in character to those passing along a motor nerve and the reason that in one case we get a sensation of hearing and in the other a contraction of muscle is found in the manner of ending of the nerve, one terminating in a special part of the cortex of the cerebrum, the other in a muscle. From this standpoint the nerve fibers may be compared to electrical wires. The current conducted by the wires is similar in all cases, but may give rise to very different effects according to the way in which the wires terminate, whether in an explosive mixture, an arc light, or solutions of electrolytes of various kinds.

Brubaker, 1908: ''The nerve-fibers which constitute by far

the larger part of both the peripheral and central organs of the nerve system, are simply the axonic processes of neurons with their secondary investments, the myelin and neurilemma.

"The metabolism of the central organs of the nerve system is more active and extensive. Any withdrawal of blood, from compression or occlusion of blood-vessels is followed by impairment of nutrition and loss of function. Withdrawal of the blood supply is followed by a loss of irritability.

"As to the nature of the nerve impulse generated by any of the foregoing stimuli, either general or special, but little is known. It has been supposed to partake of the nature of a molecular disturbance, a combination of physical and chemic processes attended by the liberation of energy, which propagates itself from molecule to molecule."

Nerves respond to stimulation according to their habitual function. Thus, stimulation of the optic nerve, if sufficiently strong, results in the sensation of light; of a motor nerve, in contraction of the muscle to which it is distributed; of a secretory nerve, in the activity of the related gland, etc. It is, therefore, evident that peculiarity of nerve function depends neither upon any special construction or activity of the nerve itself nor upon the nature of the stimulus, but, entirely, upon the peculiarities of its central and peripheral end-organs.

The American Text-Book of Surgery: "Contusion and compression are the most frequent injuries. Wounds may be either clean-cut, incised wounds, or more or less extensive lacerated or contused wounds, such as those caused by missiles of war, those which result from railroad and machinery accidents, punctured wounds and the like.

"The old views of the dangers of sutures as applied to nerves are entirely exploded, and numerous cases in which suture of a nerve has been practiced immediately after the injury prove that recovery of function is greatly facilitated by such suture. Hence, precisely as is the case with a tendon, a nerve should always be sutured immediately if possible, even if the section of the nerve is only partial. Supposing first that the nerve is merely divided, without loss of substance, and that the ends can readily be approximated, two or three sutures should be passed not merely through the sheath of the nerve, but through its substance. These should be preferably of fine silk, and inserted by sewing needles. The part should then have absolute rest on a splint, so that the nerve-ends should not be torn asunder by motion of the limb. In one published case in which no such means were at hand an ordinary hare-lip pin was inserted obliquely through the two ends of the ulnar nerve and a loop of fine silk thrown over its point, brought out through the wound, and secured to the head of the pin. At the end of three days the pin was withdrawn, thus loosening the silk, which was easily removed. The result was in every way satisfactory. If the ends are so far separated that they cannot be readily approximated, one or both ends of the nerve may be stretched until they can be placed in contact, and the same process then carried out. Sensation will return, as a rule, before motion, and, in view of the time that elapses before the nerve will be able to carry the stimulus of volition to the muscles.

"If, after stretching, the ends of the nerve cannot be approximated, two methods are open to us; neutral infixation as above described, or the transplantation or grafting of nerves. If a nerve can be removed from an amputated limb (the two operations of nerve suture being simultaneous), a portion of human nerve can be transplanted. If it be impracticable to obtain a portion of human nerve, a suitable portion of a nerve from one of the lower animals can be removed, placed in its proper position, and satured at both ends to the cut ends of the nerve. It is probably a matter of indifference whether this nerve be a motor, sensory or mixed nerve, **the nerve tubules being simply subservient to the transmission of the nervous impulse in either direction.** Peterson has collected 20 cases of nerve-grafting. Whether the operation is done immediately or as late as several months after the injury, is not, it would seem, of great moment. Sensation returned in some cases almost entirely and motion was improved or even almost entirely restored."

"A nerve is made up of nine fibers conveying nine functions."

Gray: "Nerve-fibres serve to conduct nervous impulses and bring nerve-cells into relation with each other and into relation with other structures. **Nerves are composed of numbers of nerve-fibres** bound into bundles."

Cunningham: "Each spinal nerve is attached to the spinal cord by two roots, called respectively dorsal (posterior) and ventral (anterior). The dorsal root is larger than the ventral root; **it contains a larger number** of rootlets, and the individual rootlets are of larger size than in the ventral root."

Dutton: "Each nerve of the body is a cord, or bundle of nerves, containing, sometimes, several dozen nerve-tubes or fibers, each tube forming a distinct nerve, and running a separate and independent course to its destination."

McMurrich: "The dorsal and ventral nerve-roots are not attached to the cord as such, but are first **frayed out into numerous thread-like bundles** of axones which are distributed along their lines of entrance and exit. These bundles are the root filaments of the respective roots."

Sobotta: "All along the spinal cord and symmetrically from both halves of it, pairs of nerves arise, called spinal nerves. There are thirty-one pairs of them. The nerves of each pair have their origin from the left or right side of the cord at the same level, and each nerve arises by two separate roots which emerge at the anterior and posterior lateral sulci, and are accordingly termed the anterior and posterior roots.

"The anterior is the motor root and represents the centrifugal path entering the spinal nerves to pass to the muscles, the posterior is the sensory root, the centripetal path entering the cord and conveying impulses from the sensory end-organs. **The separate nerve bundles** which leave the cord in the anterior lateral sulcus or enter it at the posterior lateral sulcus are known as root filaments, and in the anterior root **they appear as numerous, thin threads, while in the posterior root they are** thicker, but **less numerous. The whole number of nerve fibers is much greater (almost three times as great) in the posterior root than in the anterior**, and the posterior roots are, therefore (those of the first cervical nerves excepted), always the stronger."

"A nerve is made up of nine fibres."

Gerrish: "**A number of nerve-fibres gathered into a coherent bundle** constitutes a funiculus. A **single funiculus** with its wrappings **may constitute a nerve**; but **usually a number of funiculi are grouped together in a nerve.** The epineurium is also supplied with nerves, called nervi nervorum ("the nerves of the nerves").

Landois: "The simplest form of nerve-fibers are the primitive fibrils or axis-fibrils, distinguishable only with high powers of the microscope.

Strange, indeed, that thousands of dissectors of the human body did not care to take enough time or interest in their work to count the number of fibres in a nerve! Surprising that they had not observed that the number nine were always present! But, instead, we are told that **a nerve may be composed of one fibre**, or it may be **constructed of numerous thread-like bundles of fibres**, each of which appears under a high power microscope as a **great number of thin threads.** Far more astonishing is it to learn that men of brains do not, or dare not, question the teacher's say so.

The student will comprehend that a nerve may consist of any number of filaments, from "a single filament" to a great number. Filaments are continually escaping from one nerve to join another. Consequently there is no regular number of filaments which compose a nerve.

"A nerve conveys nine functions."

Function is the normal, special action of an organ or part of the body, for accomplishing vital phenomena.

Nerves do not convey functions. Their function is to carry **sensation inward and impulses outward.**

To excite or irritate nerves causes molecular action, more action, more heat. Heat is produced, emitted by nerves, but not carried.

Dunglison tells us: "Experiments and pathological facts have proved that the anterior column of the spinal cord and the anterior roots of the spinal nerves are inservient to volition or voluntary motion; and that the posterior column and roots are destined for sensibility. Hence the spinal nerves, which have two roots, must be the conductors both of motion and feeling, while the encephalic, which, with but few exceptions, have but one, can possess but one of these properties; they must be either sensitive or motor according as they arise from the posterior or anterior column of the medulla."

"Circulatory" pertains to circulation—fluids, only, can circulate. The body manifests arterial, venous, capillary, primitive, embryo and fetal circulation.

"**The serous circulation is an original theme,**" a modern discovery (?), not one by accident, "but the outcome of months of study." The author of "serous circulation" could have saved himself from committing a serious blunder and from misleading his students by referring to any dictionary where he could have learned the meaning of circulation. To circulate is to move in a circle, to move round and return to the same point; blood circulates but **serum does not.** Serum is transudated by the laws of vital osmosis—regulated by affinity. Such discoveries (?) envelop the science of Chiropractic instead of developing it.

"Trophic" pertains to nutrition—the process by which tissue is built and waste removed—metabolism.

"Motor" nerves carry motor impulses—not motor functions. The function of motion is general thruout the body—not local.

The function of "secretion" is an organic function, chiefly executed in the glands. An excretory organ is one charged with the office of excretion.

"Reproductive" is pertaining to reproduction—generation—the generative organs are reproductive. Nerves do not carry the function of reproduction.

"Reparatory"—having the power of restoring or repairing. The quality of restoring, repairing is metabolic. Abnormal growths are reduced by destructive metabolism. Parts are reproduced by constructive metabolism.

"Nutritive" is trophic. A **mis**count—one fibre too much.

---

"Occlusion of stimulus is the cause of all abnormality."

The appended glossary tells us that abnormality means having lost the equilibrium of function. An equilibrium is an equipoise, a state of rest, a cessation from motion, a mutual counteraction of two or more forces. Of stimulus, the glossary says, the energy of force which acts through the brain and nerves, constructing and maintaining the body and controlling all of its functions. It defines occlusion: suppression, checking, hindering, retarding, stopping or lessening, as of nerve stimulus.

As a clincher, the Analyzer adds: "As a corollary to the fact that occlusion of stimulus causes all abnormality, the effect of a complete occlusion of stimulus in one nerve fibre is the death of that fibre beyond the point of occlusion."

It is not a "fact that occlusion of stimulus causes all abnormality."

It is not a fact that occlusion, imperforation, the transient approximation of the edges of a natural opening causes all abnormality—disease. A large share of disease—all inflammatory and fever cases—are because of **too much stimulus,** and not because it is shut off.

Occlusion is the closing of an orifice. It is not the suppression, checking, hindering, retarding, stopping, or lessening of a fluid, solid, stimulus or energy. The closing of an opening may suppress, check, hinder, retard, stop or lessen the passage of the nerve stimulus, but it does not excite, inflame or cause fever.

Occlusion is not the cause of disease. Nerves are impinged upon, pressed against, not squeezed or pinched.

"The equilibrium of function." To bring the action or function of any organ to an equilibrium, a state of rest, a cessation, would be death.

Abnormality means anomalous, irregular, deviating from the rule. Carver's analysis, according to the science of Chiropractic, is incorrect physiology.

"The science of function and the science of adjustment."

The adjustment of vertebrae or other joints, is the act of adjusting, the placing into proper relations those which were displaced.

Accumulated and established knowledge of the qualities and functions of living tissues, systematized and formulated with reference to general truths pertaining to the normal or special action of a part or an organ might be classed as "The science of functions."

Adjusting is an art, not a science. A person may be able to adjust vertebrae, many do so, without any scientific knowledge of the reason for doing so. They learn it as an art; they know how, but not why. The art of adjusting should be guided by scientific knowledge.

---

The following does not look well in an osteopath journal. How would it appear in Chiropractic literature?

"Bovinine gives rapid results in all blood impairments and disturbed cellular reconstruction.

"Bovinine not only builds up the blood, but tones up and normally stimulates the food-forming organs and restores by natural means the body to health.

"Medication—Convalescence, wasting diseases and wherever a food or tonic is indicated."

Bovinine is a preparation composed of ox-blood, egg-albumen, boric acid and brandy. The blood is worth no more or less than the amount of nutriment there is derived from it by digestion. If I were to use ox-blood, I would want it fresh; even then I prefer beef-steak. Egg-albumen consists of 20 per cent of the white of hen's eggs. I like my eggs fresh right from the poultry ranch. Boric acid is a crystaline mineral found in the volcanic regions of Tuscany, Italy, for which I have no use. Brandy is an alcoholic spirit distilled from the juice of fruits or potatoes. I take my brandy straight; no mixing for me; even then I prefer it fresh from the fruit.

The above three quoted paragraphs, copied from the Osteopath Journal, may be Osteopathy, but they have no representative in Chiropractic literature.

---

Before me is a booklet of 12 pages.

"Chiropractic, the archway to health." An archway is a passage under an arch. I fail to see how Chiropractic resembles an arch.

With but few exceptions it is copied from a neighbor's booklet—a human mill filled with machines. The toes and fingers are considered as 20 machines. This firm has three "D. C.'s." Not one of them has ever graduated nor had conferred upon them the degree of D. C.

## THE SKULL AND ITS APERTURES.

Man, in his physical makeup, is the highest embodiment of the vertebrata—having an internal jointed bony skeleton.

The spinal column, sternum and cranium are modified vertebrae. The flat bones in the median line, in the front of the chest, are three in number. Like sacral vertebrae (the lower expansion) and the four bones which form the cranial vault (the upper expansion of the vertebral column), they become fused in adult life. The spine has facets and demifacets for the articulation of the ribs. In like manner, the sternum has facets and demifacets for the articulation of the costal cartilages. The occipital, two parietal, frontal, two temporal and sphenoid bones form the brain case and articulate with the bones of the face which, like the sacrum, fuse in adult life.

The cranium of mammals, by a close study, permits the recognition of a systematic arrangement of vertebrae. The skull is composed of seven cranial vertebrae; the sacrum of five.

The chorda dorsalis, the notocord, the embryonic spinal cord, the axis around which the first parts of the fetus is formed, passes into, and is protected by, these cranial vertebrae, after the manner in which the spinal cord is safely lodged in the canal of the spinal column.

The transition from movable vertebrae to those that are flat and fused is more pronounced in those at the upper extremity of the vertebral column than in those of the lower extremity. The change from the cervical to those of the cranial is very marked from the third cervical upward, including the axis, atlas, the ring which forms the foramen magnum and the bones which constitute the vault of the skull.

The development of the bones of the face is intimately related to the transformation of the curves of the visceral. The clefts are analagous to the openings between the arches of the spinal vertebrae. The processes of the cranial laminae articulate with those of the facial bones and eventually fuse. Harelip is usually complicated with a cleft palate, a malformation of the superior maxillary bone due to a lack of fusion.

The olfactory and optic nerves, tho classed as cranial, are metamorphosed parts of the brain. All other cranial nerves are segmentally arranged in a manner similar to the spinal nerves. The brain and the cranial nerves are protected by the neural arches—the bones forming the cranium.

In the development of the skull, three stages are recognized: the membranous, in which the encephalon is enclosed only in a membrane—the dura mater of the adult; the chrondral, in which the base and lower parts of the sides of the braincase become cartilaginous leaving the sides and roof membranous; the osseous, in which both cartilage and membrane become ossified from a large number of ossified centers which first appear in the membrane. The primitive cranium is membranous, which, in turn, is partly converted into the bones of the cranium, while the remainder represents the dura mater of the adult, an inner lining for the skull, the periosteum of the cranial bones and a tough protective envelope to the brain. The dura mater is closely adherent over the whole of the base of the skull, where it is prolonged thru the foramina, becoming continuous with the pericranium (periosteum of the skull) and blends with the fibrous sheaths of the nerves and vessels which pass out of and into the cranium. Over the vault, its attachments are chiefly in the region of the sutures where its outer fibrous layer separates to form the venous sinuses. Elsewhere, it is comparatively loose, so that extravasation from rupture of the meningeal vessels or purulent accumulations may collect between the dura mater and the bone causing compression of the brain. Such pressure, if occurring immediately after an injury, is probably due to a depressed fragment of bone; if some time after, it is likely to be an effusion of blood or pus. The inner table may be fractured and the fragments may press on the brain with no solution of continuity externally perceptible.

In a morphological sense, the primitive cranium is the dura mater; the nerves are extra-cranial after leaving this membranous covering.

It is interesting to note that no two skulls are alike in shape or size, even the parts or openings which are paired may differ greatly. Skulls vary in their thickness, density, weight and color. Excessive heat (fever) causes the diploe to enlarge, while a temperature lower than normal will lessen the cancellous portion and condense and increase its weight. The same conditions hold good thruout the osseous skeleton. The condensing and thinning of the cranial bones may be physiologic or pathologic.

The veins of the diploe are of comparatively large size, but their walls are very thin and imperfect. They form irregular communicating apertures, which terminate in four or five main descending channels, some going outward thru the external table and others inward thru the internal. In old age the cancelous portion is reduced in proportion to the decrease of animal heat.

Physiologically, the decrease in animal heat, the cancelous diploe and the blood circulation, should diminish gradually in old age.

Before me lies a skull of a female, 27 years of age. Her bones are half the usual size. The skull is eburnated; the bones of trunk and limbs are normal in quality. The vertebral column has a curvature.

A displacement of the 12th dorsal vertebra; the second center place, caused an impingement upon the 12th pair of nerves, which resulted in the above pathological conditions.

Bones which are eburnated—ivory-like in quality, shiny, dense and hard—have been subjected to intense heat. Reaction setting in, the temperature goes below normal and they become eburnated. In this aged skull of a young person the sutures are obliterated and there is no trace, whatever, of the diploe. The bony framework, up to and including the atlas, had normal heat, while the entire skull was supplied with less than the usual amount. These changes, occurring in a person of the age of a century or more, would be physiological, but, at the age of 27, are pathological. The retention of normal temperature is conducive to long life. Excessive heat—too much functionating—softens bones causing them to become friable and the processes more or less deficient, as shown by a skull of reddish cast.

Periostitis, osteitis, caries and necrosis occur in the bones of the skull as elsewhere. These conditions may follow typhoid fever or other inflammatory diseases. For relief the Chiropractor will locate and adjust as in other portions of the body.

Hypertrophy of the bones of the skull, with sclerosis and disappearance of the diploe, is a result of osteitis, inflammation of bone, followed by subnormal temperature.

Normal skulls are as dissimilar in their makeup as are the mental and physical expressions of their owners. This difference is augmented by disease—heat modification. The variation in the shape and position of the condyles is so great that those of one skull will not fit the atlas of any except the one to which it belongs. No two skulls have nerve and blood vessel passages alike. Even those paired in the same subject often differ in size, shape; one even may be entirely lacking.

To study the skull to advantage it is necessary to have at lease three specimens. One should be bisected horizontally so that the skull-cap may be removed and the cranial cavity exposed to view; another bisected on the mesial line, dividing the skull into two lateral halves; the other, a disarticulated skeleton of the head so that each of the 22 bones which compose the body framework may be examined separately.

The skull includes the entire skeleton of the head with the mandible. The cranium is the surrounding bones which enclose the cranial cavity, the mandible excluded. The calvarium, the skull-cap, the vault of the cranium, is that part of the skull which remains after the 14 bones of the face have been removed.

The foramen magnum is an oval opening at the base of the skull. In the adult it is about one by one and a half inches in diameter. It surronds and transmits the medullary oblongata. The lower portion of the oblongata is in the foramen magnum; the remainder, less than an inch in length, is just inside of the cranial cavity. From the medulla oblongata arise the seven pairs of cranial nerves. The spinal accessory originates in the spinal cord as low as the sixth or seventh cervicals. From there it ascends, gathering fibers from each of the cervical nerves as it passes upward thru the foramen magnum, where it joins the vagus (10th) nerve, which originates in the oblongata.

The skull is furnished with many passages for nerves and blood vessels. They are known by various names according to their shape. Foramina are openings thru bones; a canal is a narrow tubular passage; a groove is a furrow or shallow depression in a bone; a suture is the line of junction between cranial or facial bones; a fissure is a narrow deep cleft or groove; a cavity is a hollow space in the skull filled with air; a notch is a deep indentation; a cleft resembles a crack; a tube is a long cylindrical hollow; a sulcus is a narrow channel, trench or furrow; a meatus is an opening or passageway; a sinus is a cavity or pocket, filled with air; an antrum is a chamber cavity in a bone; a vestibule is an interchamber; a fenestra is a window-like opening; cochlea, a spiral opening; concha, a hollow resembling a conch shell. Lacerum openings are those which have the appearance of being torn or rent.

Creation affords no greater variations than those found in the human skull. When comparing a number of them it is surprising to find so many deviations from the general rule in the size and shape of the passages for nerves and blood vessels, especially, when, as often appears, we find many of them lacking. Such nerves and blood vessels, if they do exist, must hunt other openings.

The Chiropractor often deals with the unusual, the abnormal. Therefore, such exceptions to the rule as are mentioned above are interesting to the developer of the science of Chiropractic.

---

The sick need help, not drugs, nor incantations.

## NEUROPATHY—FEVER.

On page 505, Dr. A. P. Davis thus describes fever: "This phenomena in the body (known as fever) is characterized as a rise of temperature, increased circulation of the blood, marked tissue change to a greater or less degree, disturbance in the secretions, mental excitement or depression."

All writers describe diseases alike, but, as to causes they differ materially. Neuropathy says:—"**The causes of fever are a mooted question.** Many theories are advocated, but the most plausible seems to be that of central disturbance near the corpus striatum, due to blood pressure. The cause of the **blood pressure is as much a mooted question as the cause of fever.**"

Pathologists are in the dark as to the cause of fever, a symptom accompanying most diseases. McFarland says:—"Fever may be traumatic or infectious. There is no specific microorganism of fever, which is to be looked upon as the result of irritative and usually toxic disturbance of the nervous centers concerned in heat regulation." Delafield and Prudden state: "In the great majority of cases fever is due to the presence in the body of deleterious substances, either introduced from without, or, more commonly, produced within the body." Stengel gives the etiology of fever as "Any chemical, mechanical, or bacterial injury of the tissues may liberate toxic substances, which in turn act upon the nervous system and occasion the phenomena of fever."

The production of heat is a function. Fever is always associated with a general disturbance of functions; metabolism is deranged. **Fever is dissipated heat from local inflammation.** Joints, glands or organs which exhibit heat above normal are inflamed. One of the functions performed by nerves is the production of heat. Heat is produced by molecular vibration. If normal nerve vibration is disturbed, normal heat becomes modified accordingly. If nerves are irritated they become excited—molecular vibrations are increased and the measure of heat corresponds. If nerves are free to vibrate normally, all functions are performed in a natural manner.

Investgation by pathologists has not furnished any evidence as to the existence of a heat-center in the brain. Iujuries of the caudate nucleus, optic thalmus, corpus callosum, septum lucidum and trigone cause a rise in temperature and an increased metabolism. But the same may be said of injuries to any portion of the nervous system, more especially the ganglionic centers.

Referring to fever, Dr. Davis says on page 513, "The whole nervous force has turned its attention to renovating the system of its poisons and you need not, under any circumstances, undertake to change the order of things." Under the same heading on the next page, "Remember that Nature is now master of the situation; she is asserting her prerogative and she will perform her labor, if left alone, perfectly; and if you will sit by and watch her wisdom in sweeping and garnishing her apartments, you will learn a lesson you never knew before."

The above sounds very much like Allopathy. From which Dr. Davis graduated 48 years ago. That education in a measure sticks to him and is visible in many places in Neuropathy. Hare says on page 448, "Indeed, in some cases moderate **fever probably aids the body in combating,** or rather, **conquering the disease** which has attacked it."

The Old School of medicine look upon disease as an enemy which must be conquered, subdued, vanquished, routed, driven out. They declare war, they muster their forces, arm themselves with death-dealing poisonous drugs, they have quite a combat, a great fight, and imagine they come off the battlefield victorious.

Davis and Hare think fever a body-renovator; that it renews, restores the body to its former vigor, purity and freedom from poison. Therein lies the principle of vaccination. Nature has a house-cleaning and should not be molested in her domestic work. According to this view fever is a kind of chemical combustion.

Neuropathy, page 610: "Decomposition may ensue from two causes: the one being due to disturbance of nerve centers, producing paralysis of nerve filaments all along the line to their terminals, and the other from pressure somewhere along the course of the nerve—in or on its surface, or at its terminal.

"In all fevers the friction is caused by decomposition of the elements."

The doctor mixes Allopathy and Chiropractic—the principles of which are antiopdal.

Page 57. "Remember, we have certain conditions to overcome and these conditions are the result of the two forces being separated—either the excess of the one or the deficiency of the other."

May it not as well be that the "two forces" should be separated and that by uniting they cause trouble? Is there any reason for believing that the separation or the connecting of forces causes disease? Have we any knowledge of these "two forces" which Dr. Davis has discovered?

Page 14: "That one can be so manipulated as to free the circulation of the blood, **stop fevers** and **relieve** pain and **inflam-**

**mation is a fact** which has been amply demonstrated in this country."

Page 22. "Recognizing **the fact that two forces are to be considered in all movements to adjust the spine when treating the patient for any ailment,** we should aim to unite them so that harmony of action at once begins, and this is done by the hands along the spine, so placed as to bear down suddenly at given places along the spinal column."

Page 62. "In case of typhoid or puerperal fever, we have to adjust the area which first unites the forces and then relieve the nerves which end in the parts affected. In puerperal, or child-bed fever, we universally afford relief by adjusting at the second and third lumbar."

"Pneumonia we find yields quickest by adjustment."

Page 58: "**Our adjustment** affects the pneumogastric nervous system, the phrenic nervous system, the circulation of blood and regulates the heart's action and thereby **reduces all fever in every part of the body**; it is essential that we know that the cervical area of nerves are freed from impingement and that the muscular system in that particular area be in a normal, relaxed condition."

If, as you state, **one can be so manipulated, so adjusted, as to universally afford relief and reduce in all parts of the body inflammation, pneumonia, typhoid, puerperal and all fevers, by freeing the nerves from impingement, why not do so? Why let the fever run its usual course? Do you really think fever a good thing?**

Referring to fever as being a good "**thing.**" I am using the A. T. Still idea, the man from whom you borrowed, without due credit, the idea of the "two forces."

In A. T. Still's book on Osteopathy, page 229, "As we line up to learn something of the causes of **fever,** we are met by heat, a living fact. Does that put the machinery of your mind in motion? If not, what will arouse your mental energy? You see that heat is not like cold. It is not a horse with eyes, head, neck, body, limbs and tail, but it **is** as much of a **being** as a horse. **It is a being of heat.** If cause made the horse and cause made the heat, why not devote energy in seeking the cause of both?"

"**Who says heat is not a union** of the human gases with oxygen and other substances. * * * How fast must the heart or life-current run to ignite the gases of the body and set a person on fire to fever heat? * * * We know man is the greatest engine ever produced, complete in form, an electro-magnet, a motor which would be incomplete if it could not burn its own gases." Page 233: "Fever is electric heat only." Page 83: "Let me call your attention to the fact that you should know as physiological reasoners, that phosphorous with oxygen and surface air, assisted by nerve and blood motion, aided by electricity, **produces a union** between the oxygen and phosphorous, and the addition of nitrogen, which occupies much cellular space in the body, produces the combustion known as fever heat." Page 52: "At this time we wish to call your attention to the electrical disturbance of nerve-fibers as they cross one another and produce another manifestation known as fever heat, or lower temperature."

Dr. Davis has replaced the phosphorus and the gases with acid and alkali secretions and aims to use Chiropractic adjustments as the method of exchange.

---

## WHOOPING COUGH—PERTUSSIS.

This disease is known by the peculiar paroxysm of coughing, ending with a prolonged whooping respiration. The close of the paroxysm is marked by a long drawn inspiration, due to spasmodic closure of the glottis. This disease is more often met with in children than adults. Severe cases are sometimes followed by convulsions, pneumonia, chronic bronchitis, tuberculosis or nephritis.

Delafield says: "The proof that bacilli are the excitants of this disease has not been furnished."

Stengel has no doubt of the lesion being bacilli; but he is at a loss to know which one of the many are to blame, as pathologists have found at least a half dozen kinds. Of one thing he is certain. "Decided relative excess of lymphocytes is a valuable diagnostic peculiarly of the blood."

Dunglison says of this disease: "It is rare for it to affect an individual the second time. In the treatment all that can be done is to palliate. It must be borne in mind that the disease will in time wear itself out." Another author states: "To cut short the disease, a great many remedies have been administered; the fact that these remedies are so numerous indicates that no one of them can be relied upon for all cases." Still another says: "Relative excess of lymphocytes is a valuable diagnostic peculiarity of the blood." Histology finds 15 per cent of blood-leukocytes in normal blood. It may be "a valuable diagnostic" knowledge to know all this, but I fail to see where the value comes in, judging from the encouragement (?) in regard to treatment given above. This is one of the "self-limited by inherent qualities which is said of a disease that runs a definite limited course irrespective of treatment."

The Chiropractic lesion will be found at S. P. on the right.

## THE SCHOOL-CHILD UP TO DATE.

By Elsie Duncan Yale in "Life."

Make haste to school, my little child,
Or else you will be late;
Your books are all aseptic now,
And here's your sterile slate.

Your pencil has been boiled an hour—
'Tis germless, now, I hope;
And don't forget to wash your desk
With this carbolic soap.

And lest about the schoolroom floor
Some unseen microbes lurk,
Just sprinkle formaline around
Before you set to work.

You'd better put, for safety's sake,
Bichloride in the ink;
And water that has not been boiled
You must not dare to drink.

Of course, when recess comes around,
Some food you'll want to munch;
So in this disinfected box
Is predigested lunch.

And since 'tis said that in a kiss
Bacteria may dwell,
I may not give you, as I'd like,
A mother's fond farewell.

---

## NEUROPATHY, BY A. P. DAVIS.

"The book contains matter not found elsewhere, **hence needed.**"

It does contain some ideas not found elsewhere, but that of itself is no reason why it is needed or valuable.

"The subjects presented are replete with most valuable information."

That remains for the reader to determine; the mere statement that anything is valuable does not make it so.

"Neuropathy * * * embraces the entire nervous system—its freedom from pressure, waste and irritation."

The author excepts cataractous conditions, as he told me that they were neither from, nor caused by, any abnormality of the nervous system.

"Neuropathy is the discovery of the author of this volume."

The author tries to explain what Neuropathy is—just listen.

"It includes the best of every scientific, rational, natural method of cure for human ills ever presented to the human family." Page 7.

Neuropathy is like Naturopathy and Chiropathy—a pick up of anything and everything that their authors find lying around loose. Neuropathy is a science (?) composed of such parts of various methods as A. P. Davis sees fit to purloin and claim as his own. His right and title is based on his naming this nondescript.

A science consists of a knowledge of principles and causes, mutually related, which are comprehended under one general law and embodied into a system.

"Whether, therefore, we use Osteopathy to free the circulation of the blood, or Ophthalmology to arrest nerve waste, or Chiropractic adjustments to remove nerve pressure, or Suggestion to stimulate mental energy, or Magnetism to concentrate mentality and change molecular polarization (?), the object is accomplished through the one means—Neuropathy." Page 8.

A mongrel consisting of parts of so many systems conglomerated into a heterogeneous mass, does not constitute a science.

"Neuropathy is the name of the method used for all that is to be done to relieve conditions called disease, but the terms Osteopathy, Chiropractic, Ophthalmology, Suggestion or Magnetism, designate the how it is applied." Page 8.

Neuropathy is not only a medley of the above five methods, but it employs any or all of these methods in their application. Of itself it is no science or art.

"It includes the best of every **scientific**, rational, natural method of cure for human ills ever presented to the human family." Page 7.

Neuropathy is a pick up of every system which Dr. Davis considers scientific, rational or natural. It is a mongrel of so many breeds that it would be impossible to get a correct pedigree. It is no wonder, as stated by Dr. Davis, that "the sketches sent forth through journals have scarcely indexed the meaning of the science in a manner that **brought out** anything more than **ridicule and repugnance.**"

## THE DECLINE OF THE DRUGGING PROFESSION.

### Indisputable Evidence That the Use of Medicine in the Treatment of Disease Is Being Universally Abolished.

By Charles Merriles.

The use of drugs, so far as the treatment of disease is concerned, will soon be a thing of the past. Drugs are rapidly being abandoned. The public is speedily awakening to the value of drugless methods of curing disease. They are turning from the so-called science of medicine, for the simple reason that drugs have not been achieving the results that can be secured by other methods. In fact, in many instances it is quite plain that drugs have been the cause of chronic diseases that are usually termed incurable. To the ordinary layman these statements may seem unbelievable. They will naturally be doubted by those who have put their faith in drugs in the treatment of all human ailments. Medical doctors, themselves, however, are awakening to the marvelous revolution in the healing art that is surely impending. Within the last two or three years there has been a great change in public opinion as the result of newspapers and magazines publishing articles from many sources emphatically condemning drugging in the cure of disease. The public can hardly avoid education on this point.

Some time ago "American Medicine," one of the most prominent medical publications, stated that the incomes of many medical men had been reduced nearly one-half, and that the average income of physicians in the city of New York was at that time only $1,500.00 per year. In a recent issue they state that there has been a still further reduction and that the income of the New York doctors will at present average but $1,200.00, while the average throughout the whole country was less than $600.00. They stated that the doctor's income was steadily decreasing and that their income had decreased one-half within the last two years.

Now, this statement comes from a prominent medical publication. From within the ranks of the medical profession they are admitting that the income from the practice of many physicians has decreased fifty per cent within the last two years. If the same percentage of decrease continues, it will not be long until the medical profession is entirely wiped out of existence. It will not take very much figuring to determine how long it will take at the present rate of decrease for such a result to occur. The profession of doctoring, from a medical standpoint, will soon lose its attraction to the ambitious young man. In fact, it is already time for it to lose its attraction. With thousands of doctors already hardly able to make a living, what can new and inexperienced men expect from this profession? It seems to me it is time for the medical man to wake up, and it is more than time for the medical schools to begin to see the "handwriting on the wall." I hardly think they are desirous of turning out students who will be compelled to turn to manual labor in order to secure a livelihood, and under the circumstances they will have to "break the ice" and begin to regard the healing art from a really scientific standpoint, as it is treated in the columns of this publication. The healing art of the future will not have anything in common with the science of drugging. It will abandon drugs entirely and we will have instead the use of water, diet and exercise in such a manner as to bring about the results that are desired, and they will be brought more speedily and far more safely than through the use of medicine.

Medical men can no longer afford to ignore the various methods of healing that are now taking the place of so-called medical science. For a long time the doctors have stood on their dignity. They have felt it was beneath them to recognize investigators outside of their own rank. But I am convinced that they will soon have to recognize the investigations of the so-called laymen, and begin to learn from them, or else they will have to seek employment in the corn fields, upon the street-cars or at other occupations that they consider menial.

As a student of the healing art in all its various phases, I am naturally deeply interested in every method that will promise a definite cure of any complaint. I know if a patient were under my care and I should find he was unable to secure improvement, that if he should go elsewhere and secure a definite and permanent cure, that I would be intensely interested in the methods that were used in bringing about the cure. This, it seems to me should be the policy of any intelligent, conscientious man, be he physician or student, but this is not the view of many members of the medical profession. They have been brought up in accordance with a certain code of ethics; they have been taught that there is but one way to cure disease, and their policy is not to recognize, nor even to investigate, any other methods that might be presented.

Many physicians seem to believe their profession has a monopoly of science, and that they have monopolized all the knowledge appertaining to healing, and that it is impossible for anyone outside of their ranks to know or to learn anything concerning disease and its cure. The time is not far distant when policies of this kind will begin to waver and will fall amid chaotic confusion. Either the medical men will begin to adopt the methods we are advocating and use them in their practice, or else they will cease to be regarded as exponents of the healing art. The people of today want to know: they want to be shown: they are all "from Missouri" as far as the desire to see into things is concerned, and the more you know of drugs, the less faith you will have in their value. When the medical men, themselves, call attention to the fact that their incomes have in many instances decreased by one-half in two years, you can well understand in which direction we are moving, and it is away from medicine into the light—into the truth so far as the healing art is concerned. We will leave superstition in the background. The ignorance, the bigotry that is so often in evidence in medical lore, will also have to sink into well-deserved oblivion.

In the recent issue of the medical magazine already quoted, there were various causes given for the decrease in the income of medical men. Some of the explanations for this condition will no doubt be of interest to our readers, and I quote them herewith:

"The monstrous evil of the abuse of medical charity has all but pauperized the medical profession," is the declaration of the writer under discussion.

"The future of the American medical profession would give many of us more concern if we were not well aware of the sound foundation on which the modern practice of medicine is based. Prophesy as he may, the pessimist cannot shake our confident expectation that scientific medicine will ultimately triumph over all 'pathies,' cults, and charlatanry. Logic, truth and science must sooner or later prevail.

"But however certain we may feel that the time is not far distant when medical science will be universally accepted because of its manifest accuracy and efficiency, we must ruefully admit that the situation at present is very far from satisfactory. Two great evils stand foremost as the most serious of several confronting the medical practitioners of this country. No medical man who is in touch with medical affairs as they are today, can deny that the condition of the average practitioner is far from encouraging. We are a long ways from going to the 'demnition bow-wows' as some of the 'calamity howlers' are claiming.

"Nevertheless, in many of our large cities there has been during the last two years a decline in general and family practice of over fifty per cent. In even plainer language, if it is possible, we mean that many excellent general practitioners of ten, twenty, or even more years' experience are seeing today not over one-half as many patients as they were two years ago.

New York, Brooklyn, Philadelphia are prosperous cities, but our information shows that in certain localities within their confines this decline is even greater.

"Still another will say that the trend of the profession toward organization, in the eyes of the laity, a phase of trades unionism, has made medicine a sordid business, and by eliminating the element of mysticism has removed the one factor that held—some say fifty per cent of those who seek medical treatment. Still another will state that the enormous extension of surgery has truly frightened the people and made them exceedingly chary of consulting the modern progressive physician, who, though he may not be an operator, is keen to recognize surgical needs and possibilities and advise accordingly."

---

## THE SMALLEST BABY.

Little Miss Cade weighed 13 ounces when born; she now weighs 19 pounds.

This tiny bit of humanity was born at St. Helens, Ore. She was so small that she could be placed in a small teacup and completely hid by another. Her hands and feet were the size of a rat's foot; her head as large as a bantam egg. She is perfectly formed.

Over a year ago there was born to Mr. and Mrs. Chance, of Wichita, Kan., a babe, who weighed 15 ounces when she was three weeks old. She was perfect in form.

In 1904, Mr. and Mrs. Beatty, of Steadman, Mo., were the parents of a one-pound male child. A finger ring passed over the hand and up to the elbow.

My mother weighed one and a half pounds when born. She was one of a pair of twins—the other died. I came within one of not having any mamma. I am glad that they saved what there was of my mamma.

---

"We had to remove the main source (D. D. Palmer) of all discontent; this required 'nerve' (and imprisonment of the Founder of Chiropractic), and with no little feeling in the matter we had a housecleaning among the faculty of The P. S. C." That which is included in parenthesis has been added for explanation.

For the next year and a half after that "housecleaning" each arrival was told that I was on a vacation and that I might return any day. Many letters are in my possession to that effect.

## THE PATH THE CALF MADE.

One day through the primeval wood,
A calf walked home as good calves should,
But made a trail all bent askew,
A crooked trail, as all calves do.

Since then two hundred years have fled,
And, I infer, the calf is dead;
But still, he left behind his trail,
And thereby hangs my moral tale.

The trail was taken up next day
By a lone dog that passed that way;
And then a wise bell-wether sheep
Pursued the trail o'er vale and steep.

And drew his flocks behind him, too,
As good bell-wethers always do.
And from that day, o'er hill and glade,
Through those old woods a path was made.

And many men wound in and out,
And dodged and turned and bent about,
But still they followed—do not laugh—
The first migrations of that calf;

And through the winding wood way stalked,
Because he wobbled when he walked.
This forest path became a lane
That bent and turned and turned again;

This crooked lane became a road
Where many a poor horse with his load
Toiled on beneath the burning sun
And traveled some three miles in one.

And thus a century and a half,
They trod the footsteps of that calf.
The years passed on in swiftness fleet,
The road became a village street.

And this, before men were aware,
A city's crowded thoroughfare;
And soon the central street was this
Of a renowned metropolis.

And men two centuries and a half
Trod in the footsteps of that calf.
Each day a hundred thousand rout
Followed the zigzag calf about;

And o'er its crooked journey went
The traffic of a continent.
A hundred thousand men were led
By one calf near three centuries dead.

They followed still his crooked way.
And lost one hundred years a day.
For thus such reverence is lent
To well-established precedent.

A moral lesson this might teach
Were I ordained and called to preach,
For men are prone to go it blind
Along the calf paths of the mind;

They follow in the beaten track,
And out and in and forth and back,
And work away from sun to sun
To do what other men have done.

They go two miles instead of one,
To follow a path that was begun
By one lone calf; and to this day
They follow this old crooked way.

If each and every wise M. D.
The wisdom of these lines could see,
They would look back along their path,
And see the folly of the calf.

Years and years, o'er tortuous way,
They've given physic—made it pay,
And our straight Chiropractic plan
They laugh at, to a single man.

Their noxious drugs, no more we'll drink,
But think we are the ones to wink,
When viewing this devious path,
Made by some medicinal calf.

We hail with most sincere delight,
The dawn of scientific light,
That leads us from the old, old way
To this, our Chiropractic day.

## SUBLUXATION OR APPROXIMATION OF VERTEBRAE THE CAUSE OF IMPINGEMENT.

"A man of eighty years is from two to three inches shorter than he was at the age of twenty-five years. This shortening of the spinal column that comes with age is mostly or entirely at the expense of the intervertebral cartilages."

"When from two to three inches is deducted from the combined thickness of all the segments of the intervertebral discs or cartilages, which is originally about four to five inches, there must be a loss of nearly one-half of the thickness of the intervertebral cartilages."

The difference in the height of a man at twenty-five and eighty, barring abnormal curvatures and luxations, considering the natural shortening or approximation of the vertebrae, does not exceed one inch, usually less than half an inch. This shrinkage must be divided between the twenty-nine articulations from occiput to ankle. A slight bending of the neck of the femur should be considered. Dividing this contraction between all the articulations, it would average one-thirtieth of an inch. It should also be remembered that the spinal nerves become slightly firmer and narrowed in diameter as age advances, and, we might also say, slightly contracted in length.

When we consider that the spinal cord is freely movable within the spinal canal and that the spinal nerves are afforded ample space for their emergence from the intervertebral foramina, we will see that normal movement do not compress either the spinal cord or spinal nerves. The very slight difference in the size of the spinal foramina between the age of twenty-five years and eighty, would not be worth considering. How much of a squeeze would be made on the first pair of cervical nerves? Take into consideration the play, the amount of space between the occipital and the posterior arch of the atlas and the size of the nerves which pass out over the grooves, and that, between the atlas and the occiput there is no intervertebral cartilage, only a very thin hyaline, articular cartilage, which, if half of its thickness was shrunken, or if it was all absorbed, would make no appreciable difference in the gap between the atlas and occiput, sufficient to compress or pinch a nerve—even if such were the case, would not the bending of the head forward ever so little relieve the compression?

Take your spinal column in hand. Do you not see that there is no intervertebral cartilage between the atlas and axis? Do you not see that the long, wide gap between the atlas and axis affords no possible chance for nerve compression—no more than there is between the atlas and occiput? If you think that the first or second spinal nerves can be pinched, compressed or squeezed by the approximation of the atlas and the axis or the drawing together of the occiput and the atlas, just try to explain such a condition to your next prospective patient. The same kind of pressure that causes corns and bunions, and the many diseases which arise from the impingement of the first and second pairs of cervical nerves, must also cause diseases elsewhere.

The spinal column of an adult measures about two feet two inches. The intervertebral discs occupy about one-fourth of this space, or about six inches all told. The average thickness of all the intervertebral cartilages is about one-fourth of an inch. They increase in thickness from an eighth of an inch, in the cervical, to half an inch in the lumbar region.

The fact that the intervertebral cartilage is very thin in the cervical region and that there is none either between the atlas and occiput or the atlas and axis, renders the following statement erroneous.

"Narrowing of the foramen. Since the intervertebral foramina are between the pedicles of the vertebrae, and being formed by notches in the pedicles, this thinning of the intervertebral cartilages, while permitting the bodies of the vertebrae to come nearer together, will cause an approximation of pedicles above and below, and thus narrow the foramina. This effect is general in all sections of the spine and causes a general narrowing of all the sections of the spine and causes a general narrowing of all the intervertebral foramina.

"This general contraction of the lumen of the foramina, by interfering with spinal nourishment, will cause a general atonic condition of all the organs, or the transmission of nerve impulse may be mechanically interfered with because of a slight impingement."

"Lumen of the foramina."

Foramina have no lumen, tubular vessels have.

"A slight impingement."

The narrowing of foramina by the thinning of the intervertebral discs, or the approximation of vertebrae, might pinch, compress or squeeze a nerve, but never impinge on or strike against it.

"The vertebral column is that vertical line shaft of man or beast expressing mechanical actions."

The vertebral column is viewed as vertical in man, but not in beast. It is no wise a line-shaft used to support pulleys, flywheels and a transmitter of power or motion. It does not express mechanical action; does not pertain to machinery. **All action of the vertebral column is of the will—not mechanical.**

"Pressure: That condition where nerves or nerve fibrillae (soft tissue) are entirely surrounded by osseous (hard structure), intervertebral foramina, the lumen of which decreases in size and shape according to the constriction thereof, producing a squeezing or crushing upon the contents passing through."

Intervertebral foramina, composed of two bones, **cannot constrict, draw together, contract, or make the intervening tissue smaller by constriction.** Two bones may squeeze or crush, but **never constrict.** Foramina composed of two bones, may be made smaller, but it does not constrict. A foramen may be **decreased** in size, but not **in shape.**

---

"Practically all impingement of nerves is produced by subluxation or approximation of adjacent vertebrae, causing an alteration and narrowing of intervertebral foramina. The nerves at this point pass between the pedicles of adjacent vertebrae, and are surrounded by movable bone.

"The spinal column (a cut) showing the intervertebral foramina which may become narrowed by undue approximation of vertebrae, due to contraction of ligaments.

"A person who has not studied the subject of subluxations or the approximation of vertebrae interfering with the intervertebral foramina would suppose a possibility of a subluxation to be at least of very rare occurrence. **Sprains,** injuries and reflex action **cause ligaments to become contracted and shortened.**

"The subluxation of a vertebra is a slight deviation from its normal relation to adjacent vertebrae.

"**The atlas,** the first cervical vertebra, the one that articulates with the occipital bone, **is very often subluxated. The atlas may be forcibly slipped to one side**—to either the right or left—**which lesion constitutes a lateral subluxation.**"

The above five paragraphs are quoted from "Spinal Adjustment." All impingements upon nerves are produced by subluxations or approximation of vertebrae—which?

Narrowing of intervertebral foramina might squeeze, pinch or compress the outgoing nerves, but impinge upon them, never. The author should have said movable bones, not bone.

A sprain is the result of an injury or strain.

If the forcibly slipping of the atlas to the right or left side constitutes a subluxation, why may not a similar abnormal position of other vertebrae, also, form a subluxation? If a sliding of the atlas to either side causes an impingement upon or against a nerve, why not the same rule hold good with other vertebrae?

"We are not opposed to agencies which neutralize the poisons and remove the accumulated waste material and thus give nature an opportunity to assert itself, and aid the entire system to harmonize itself in every part and organ in the body."

Poisons introduced in the body by injection or ingestion, impair the functions of one or more organs by its action on the nervous system. Poisons relax or contract the nervous tissue. McFarlan says, "It is a knowledge of these specific actions of poisonous substances that forms the foundation of therapeutics, and it is only a thorough knowledge of pharmacology that gives medicine a firm scientific station." Dunglison substantiates McFarlan's statement by saying, "The most energetic poisons are used therapeutically, and often with considerable advantage. They have, of course, to be administered in extremely small doses to avoid the production of true poisoning."

The medical profession look upon disease as a change in the structure of tissue and its functions; these conditions are concomitant, they always accompany each other. It is impossible to have abnormal functions without abnormal tissue, and on the other hand, normal tissue and normal functions are coexistent. The medical profession consider the disturbing element to be poison. Therefore, poisons are used as medicines, remedies, counter-poisons, which, by their counteraction, are capable of antagonizing or combatting the effects of a poison.

A poison is pathological, disease producing, when administered to a person in health; physiological, when it exerts an effect upon the system contrary to that of the pathological poison, for which an antidote is desired.

A poison taken accidentally or purposely by one who is not a toxicologist, is disease producing, but if administered by one who is versed in poisons, it is physiological—health producing. The distinction makes the difference.

Displacements of the osseous frame-work of the body are directly caused by injuries and accidents. Indirectly, thru poisons which contract the fibers of the nervous system, which in turn act on muscles, thereby drawing bones out of alignment.

The medical man uses remedies to "neutralize the poison," which disturb the ordinary action of vital organs. Poisons, thru the nervous and muscular system, draw vertebrae out of alignment. Antidotal poisons, by their action on nerves and muscles, realign vertebrae.

The Chiropractor places vertebrae in line by hand, thereby removing impingements and returning the nerves to their normal tonicity. Normal tension produces normal functions, harmony and health.

## THE SPLEEN.

Baker City, Ore., December 21, 1909.

Dr. D. D. Palmer:—

I note your description of the spleen—in your last Adjuster—and cannot understand where you find a description like the one you give in that number. Your multiple spleens and the thickness are exceptional, so far as my knowledge goes.

Fraternally, A. P. DAVIS.

Dr. Davis refers to my description of the spleen found on page 45 of number seven Adjuster. As his "knowledge goes," where he "understands," therefore, this adjusting.

Because the amount of vibration which transmits an impulse and gives it force may be either too much or not enough, causing functions to be performed excessively or insufficiently, the spleen, like other organs, is subject to many diseased conditions. Stengel says on page 400, when referring to hyperplasia (excessive formation of tissue) of the spleen: "The spleen is **large** in size and **firm.** The capsule may be greatly **thickened.** The **thickening** is either diffused or circumscribed. Patches of cartilaginous **hardness** may occur." Dr. Davis can find more information about the question by referring to Prudden's Anatomy, pages 457 and 458, McFarland, pagè 596, and Hare, page 311.

The Doctor does not know where I got my information regarding accessory and multiple spleens, so I will tell him; it may be news to others.

Lippincott says: "Occasionally there is one or more accessory spleens in the greater omentum or in the pancreas."

Dorland states: "Accessory spleen, a detached and outlying portion, or exclave, of the spleen."

Gould says: "Accessory spleen, a loose portion of splenic tissue in the neighborhood of the spleen."

Prudden says on page 452: "Small, accessory spleens, from the size of a hazelnut to that of a walnut, are not infrequent. They usually lie close to the spleen, but may be at a considerable distance from it; thus they have been found imbedded in the head of the pancreas. Two spleens of about equal size have been observed."

McFadden tells us on page 595: "Frequently accessory or supernumerary spleens are observed. These are usually the size of a pea, or may be as large as a cherry. They may be single or multiple. They are readily recognized by their color and consistence. Marsh observed two quite well-formed spleens in the same person."

Stengel, on page 397, speaks of accessory spleens the size of a pea or a marble being very often found.

McMurrich corroborates other writers when he says: "Supplementary spleens are found near the hilus in the gastrosplenic ligament, or less often in the great omentum. From one to twenty of these small bodies may be met with. They are red and round, of the same structure as the spleen and vary in size from a pea to a walnut."

Gray's knowledge goes. He says on page 1355: "Accessory spleens vary in size from that of a pea to that of a plum; these are known as supernumerary or accessory spleens."

Cunningham is not in the dark. He says on page 1212: "Small globular masses of splenic tissue are not infrequently found in the neighborhood of the spleen. These are termed accessory spleens."

Even Gerrish knows of these supernumerary spleens. On page 795 he says: "Frequently accessory spleens are found. They are globular and small, but otherwise look like the principal spleen, near which they are situated."

Cabrolius and Morgagni found two spleens in one subject. Cheselden and Fallopius reports three. Fatoni found four in one person. Guy and Patin saw five.

A case was shown at the Vienna Medical Society with a large number of spleens in the mesogastrium, peritoneum, on the messentery and transverse mesocolon and Douglas pouch. Every one of these spleens had a capsule, was covered by peritoneum and exhibited the histologic appearance of splenic tissue.

Bro. Davis:—You better get busy. There is much you may learn regarding spleens and Chiropractic.

---

"Chiropractic is a natural, **scientific method** of removing the cause of disease by **adjusting the anatomy.**"

Chiropractic is a science, it is not a method, the method is the art. Scientific is that which relates to and based on science, having a knowledge of the science, a systematic knowledge, as a scientific chemist, a scientific reasoner, a scientific argument. The science and the method are entirely and distinctly two different things, the method may be based on scientific principles.

Anatomy is the dissection of organized bodies, whether human, brute-animal, or vegetative. Human anatomy is the dissection of man. The science of anatomy has for its aim a knowledge of the structure of organized bodies, not their adjusting. There are many branches of anatomy, they all refer to the study and knowledge of structure, not adjusting, adjusting is an art, is not dissection.

## MALARIAL FEVERS.

Medical men divide malarial fevers into four kinds, intermittent, pernicious intermittent, remitting and yellow fever.

Intermittent fever is, also, known as dumb ague. In this form the febrile exacerbations occur at regular periods with a continuance of a lesser degree of fever between them. It is rarely attended with danger but it is very discouraging to the patient. A typical malarial paroxysm consists of a cold, a hot and a sweating stage.

Pernicious intermittent fever is distinguished from the above by the violence of its onset; it may prove fatal within a few hours. Pernicious means highly destructive; of intense severity; deadly; fatal. When the clinical thermometer indicates 104 degrees Fahrenheit or over, the fever is said to be "high."

Remittent fever is designated as bilious fever or bilious intermittent.

Yellow fever occurs only in certain months and in limited districts. In the United States it is confined to the border of the Gulf of Mexico and the south part of the Atlantic Sea Board.

These diseases are due to inhaling miasmata, noxious effluvia, which contaminate the atmosphere. The first three mentioned forms are predominant in prairie sections where there is much decomposition of upturned sod; it is prevalent near marshy regions where vegetation is decaying.

Yellow fever occurs on sea coasts at or near places where large streams empty their polluted waters. A continuation of high temperature of about eighty degrees for one or two months, in connection with excessive moisture in the atmosphere and the decomposition of animal and vegetable matter, make conditions favorable for yellow fever. The prevailing currents of the atmosphere direct and transport the miasmata to certain localities.

Malaria of any form is certainly an air-borne disease, altho great diversity of opinions has prevailed regarding its cause and mode of action.

The conditions favorable and necessary for the development of malaria, are, marshy soil, atmospherical humidity and high temperature. The medical fraternity have positively (?) demonstrated that, when certain mosquitoes are allowed to feed upon malarial patients and later upon those who are free from malaria, the latter acquire the disease. What is now troubling the mosquito men is, where did the first quadrimaculata culex get his proboscis filled with microgametocytes.

Chiropractors will find that malarial fevers, like all other general fevers, can be relieved by adjusting the fourth dorsal vertebra, so as to replace the osseous tissue which has been drawn out of alignment by the action of poison on the nervous system, relieving the impingement of the fifth pair of nerves.

---

Some of our readers may think The Adjuster is a rough Adjuster. They should read the July Ophthalmologist. It publishes monthly 6,000 copies. When it has anything to say, it just spits it right out. It does not replace names with dashes either.

We give credit to the Ophthalmologist for the following five items:

John Alexander Dowie, fanatic, did something no other mortal ever did in the history of the world. He built a city of 10,000 people in two years and it contained no saloons, no drug stores, no cigar stores, no gambling houses, no sporting houses, no doctors, less sickness than any other city of its size in history, and fewer deaths; eight propositions which put all other municipalities to shame.

Representative Gorman, of Peoria, Ill., offered a Medical Trust Compulsory Vaccination bill in the Illinois House of Representatives. It was killed May 26, by a vote of 67 to 22.

Osteopaths seeking the privilege of performing minor surgery, and using drugs in certain cases, are confessing to the Legislature and the public the weakness of their "system."

Homeopaths who graduate as such, with a materia-medica absolutely different from Allopaths, secure licenses as physicians and then proceed to practice Allopathy for which they are no more qualified than is the Osteopath.

Cattle Plague—Smallpox Virus: the Late Foot and Mouth Epidemic Traced to Vaccination Serum.

The recent outbreak of foot and mouth disease among cattle in New York, Pennsylvania, Michigan and Maryland, has been investigated by the Agricultural Department at Washington, and its cause has been traced to calves that had been used for vaccine purposes by Parke, Davis & Co., of Detroit, and by the H. K. Mulford Co., of Glenden, Pa.

This is the kind of stuff that the great State of Pennsylvania has declared by specific legislation shall be injected into the children of that State before they can enter school.

Will the people of Pennsylvania submit to such outrages, or will they meet the Medical Trust Doctors (who attempt to enforce the law for the dollars there is in it), with armed resistance?

## NEUROPATHY—SPINAL TREATMENT.

"If the manipulations (xv.) explained in Neuropathy be understood and properly applied, there will be but little use of the osteopathic manipulations in very many conditions. There is such a far reaching effect of the **spinal treatment,** as performed by adept Neuropaths, that but a few movements as shown in osteopathy, are necessary to accomplish the purpose intended through manipulations."

The whole proposition turns on that first word "if." Remember, Neuropathy is Chiropractic with the "Fad" of "Two Forces" added. Chiropractic has supplanted manipulations with adjustment. Dr. Davis uses these two terms as synonyms. The adjustments, or manipulations, are not intended to adjust, replace displaced osseous tissue, but to unite the two forces, which are supposed to have their union about the 4th dorsal vertebra. Concerning this he says on page 37, "That the force or power which controls this body of ours should be somewhere is self-evident; but what that is, we are as ignorant of as if such a thing did not exist." And yet the author of Neuropathy has built a philosophy on this ignorance of the force or forces which control this body. He imagines that the human body is under the control of not only one force but two, the positive and the negative, which he attempts to explain on page 76. "There is no power in a dynamo, but it generates power. This power is created by friction; the power is electricity and this is conducted through wire." After making a lengthy comparison of man to a dynamo, he says on page 367: "From the foregoing it would seem unfitting to call the human system a machine. That term originated in ignorance, has been perpetuated in ignorance, and used inappropriately in reference to the human body without regard to its components. There is no semblance or resemblance to an inert machine, that has neither sense nor motion—simply moved by mechanical force."

The following will be found on page 39 and is given as Neuropathic treatment of the spinal nervous system. It will be observed that he treats some diseases by manipulating down the spine and others by manipulating upward.

"It is well to use gentle pressure above and along the vertebra until the tender spot is located and treat all tenderspots found at each seance. The prominences are made by the irritation of the nervous system ending in the muscles attached to the process, or sides of the process, whence we find the prominence—most generally. Thus we discover that it is altogether a nervous condition we have to treat, and not bone.

"The reverse course of treatment should be made in cases of diarrhea, or to stop discharges from the uterus. The way to do it is to begin the treatment down at, and just above, the sacrum, and let a strong treatment be made there, then one a bone or two higher up, then the next one higher, and so on until the second lumbar has been reached."

The above is spinal treatment by adept Neuropaths.

Page 699. "The uniting of the two forces is the most valuable discovery for the relief of human ills of this century, or any preceding it, to the world, in the art of healing, and the philosophy of healing through the science of Neuropathy will go down to the ages, when understood, as the best means possible for the purpose intended." Yes, "when understood."

---

## "THE HUMAN SYSTEM."

"Mr. Palmer explained that the practice of the science differed from the practice of medicine in that Chiropractors look for the primary cause and not effects and that the cause of all disease was in the spine and center or the nerve centers."

To practice Chiropractic or medicine, is to exercise their professional duties. To look for the cause of disease comes under diagnosis, not the practice. Practice and diagnosis are two quite different terms, one relates to the official duties of the profession and the other to the discrimination of disease. The cause of all diseases are not in the spine, more especially when defined by the word "primary." Quite a large per cent have their origin from concussion and pressure on the brain, because of blows on the skull, or an indirect force transmitted to the base thru the occipito-atloid articulation from a blow on the head or a fall on the feet or buttocks with sufficient force by transmission, expends its force at this point. This is known as indirect force. An illustration is afforded by the case of President Lincoln, in which the bullet, after having pierced the left side of the occiput, went to the cranial base below the anterior lobe. The autopsy revealed a fracture in the roof of the right orbit, which had not been touched by the bullet. Corns and bunions are from displaced toe-joints. A nerve-center is any nerve ganglion from the brain itself down to the smallest which are not visible to the naked eye. They serve individually as centers of nervous influence for certain organs or localities. There are many ganglia of nervous influence for certain organs or localities. There are many ganglia or nerve centers in the brain and spinal cord, but no one is or can be "the center of the nerve centers."

## DEVIATION.

Elsewhere, we have noticed the deviations of the osseous, nervous and muscular systems. To know of these deviations and their liability to occur in any normal tissue as a result of morbidity, is of interest to a Chiropractor, inasmuch as there can be no set rules for diseased conditions, normal variations, nor for the adjusting thereof. Modifications are also dependent upon developmental processes. The division of arteries into branches are not always the same. The localities traversed and regions furnished vary. Variations may be rare or so common as to make it difficult to determine the normal; certain arteries, veins and capillaries are fairly constant, while others are extremely variable. Cunningham takes ten pages to describe the variation of the lymphatics and the vascular system.

Dr. G. Harlan Wells, of Hahnemann Hospital, at a meeting of the Philadelphia Academy of Medicine, on May 28, 1910, exhibited a man who enjoys perfect health despite the fact that his vital organs are situated on the side of the body opposite to that in which they are usually found. The subject is a Philadelphian, 45 years of age, and a machinist by trade. His heart is on the right side, the stomach on the left, the spleen on the right, the liver on the left and his intestines also are reversely arranged.

A review of medical literature shows that there have been 300 similar cases noticed since 1643. This is the first case reported in Philadelphia in a decade. Individuals with situs viscerum inversus, an anomaly in which the viscera of the body are changed from the normal to the opposite side, live as long and as well as those with normally placed organs.

Herrick refers to a case of a young man of twenty-five in whom the viscera were transposed. Barbieux mentions a case of transposition of viscera. The liver was on the left side, the spleen and heart on the right. Young reports a woman of eighty-five who died at Hammersmith, London. A post mortem examination exposed a complete transposition of the viscera. The heart lay with its base toward the left, its apex toward the right, reaching the lower border of the 4th rib, under the right mamma. The vena cava was on the left side and passed into the pulmonary cavity of the heart, which was also on the left side, the aorta and systemic ventricle being on the right. The left splenic vein was lying on the superior vena cava, the liver under the left ribs, and the spleen on the right side underneath the heart. The esophagus was on the right of the aorta, and the location of the two ends of the stomach was reversed; the sigmoid flexure being on the right side. The names of eighteen more who report instances of transposition and inversion of the viscera might be given.

In cases like the above, the nerves which supply the heart, stomach, liver, spleen and intestines will be found to emerge from foramina directly opposite those from which they usually find exit, from the opposite side to that of the ordinary, a fact that should be remembered by the Chiropractor.

The above cases are anomalous, abnormal, they deviate from the ordinary; they do not conform to the general rule.

---

The physician believes in his prescriptions: the pharmacist in the hidden power of drugs—superstitious therapeutics.

---

The December weekly budget of The Palmer School contains this statement:

"The fecal matter in the bowels may be a poison; Innate immediately converts it into a liquid state and is thus more quickly passed from the body." Better to have said, the feces may contain poison taken in the food or administered by the physician as a physic. Innate gathers water from the surrounding tissue for the purpose of assisting in its expulsion.

"It is a positive fact that fibers lead from the eye to the 4th cervical." It is a fact demonstrated on the cadaver by anatomists, that the optic nerve springs from the brain, passes through the optic foramen and, slightly above that opening, enters the eyeball at the posterior portion, passes through the eye to the front, gradually enlarging until it forms the expansion nåmed the retina. The optic nerve, including the retina, in all its relations and makeup, seems a part of the brain. The nerves traced by Chiropractors are from the 4th cervical.

"It is true there is an optic nerve leading from the eyeball to the brain—of that there can be no question, but there is also another set of nerves which were not known to have existed, at least, have not been mentioned by medicine, which lead from the eyeball to the 4th cervical." There are motor, sensory and sympathetic nerves which enter the orbit through the superior orbital fissure. The sympathetic branch is traced to the carotid plexus, from thence to the superior cervical ganglion, and back through the mixed, short, spinal nerve trunk, through the foramen to the spinal cord and to the brain. In tracing, we follow the sympathetic branch. The spinal trunk is so short and in front of the transverse processes, that it cannot be palpated. All anatomists mention these nerves. The teacher who does not know of them is a back number.

## THE HUMAN MIND.

The capacity of the human mind to absorb and retain knowledge varies greatly. Some minds are easily satisfied, while others are always hungry for science and philosophy; again there are those who care more for bread, meat and potatoes. Some are mentally limited in their ability to accumulate an education, while others seem unlimited. As soon as any person thinks he knows it all, he ceases to learn, or at least, until he has fully digested what has been acquired; while there are others who realize that they know but little in comparison to what there is to be known. There are those who are capable of accumulating knowledge in one direction or line and not in another; others are capable of comprehending any branch of education.

In my fifteen years of teaching the science—principles and art of Chiropractic, I have found but few who are capable of learning it as a science. I cannot, at present, remember a Chiropractor whom I have seen analyze a case, correctly locate the displaced vertebra and adjust it for the ailment from which the patient desired to be free. All invariably adjust from two to two dozen vertebrae. There are very few who comprehend Chiropractic as a science, making it specific, adjusting definitely for a certain ailment.

Some persons are able to compose and write lengthy articles, while others are pleased to copy sufficient of the coveted information to make an article or a booklet.

The following is from an article which was wholly copied, except the portion below. It contained nothing original, not a thot or expression but was copied, except the portion mentioned, yet the author was proud of his attainment, as also of his ability to copy cuts, at which he is an expert. He was so appreciative of his article that he read it to me three times and to Mrs. Palmer twice (I had previously read it to her). After reading about half of his article, the author (?) swelled with pride as he looked over his copy and said:

"Dad Palmer has given to the world impinged nerves as the cause of disease—the greatest blessing ever received. And yet Dad, or his son B. J., with all their hard study, failed to solve the problem. I do not mention this to censure, but to show that one or two minds have been unable to elucidate all the principles involved in Chiropractic. Remember, the mind which gave us the science and art, did not give us the various uses of electricity or wireless telegraphy. It takes a peculiar character of mind to develop peculiar ideas. Those advanced were the best those minds were able to produce. Their incorrectness prevented the science from being generally accepted. It therefore remained for some one to come forth who has studied human anatomy, one who comprehends the anatomical structure of the vertebral column, to explain the how and why of impinged nerves. That is the object of this article."

What has electricity, telegraphy, machines, steam pipes, telephones and dynamos to do with Chiropractic or animate, organic functions? Was not the giving to the world the science and art of Chiropractic enough, without expecting the same mind to discover and develop electricity and wireless telegraphy?

I do not know what problem the author refers to which "Dad" and his son failed to solve. The mention of their failures was not made to censure, but for the purpose of showing that at last "one man had come forth who had studied human anatomy, one who comprehends the anatomical structure of the vertebral column, one who can explain the how and why of impinged nerves, "one from whom the world generally will accept Chiropractic. "The incorrect ideas of the Palmers (which have but little or any resemblance) prevented their general acceptance. But now, since this self-wise man has come forth, the world will be enlightened, for he will, no doubt, publish a book of copied cuts and literature.

As soon as the world knows that this man, who learned to adjust while sitting behind a curtain, has come forth, being one who has studied human anatomy, one who comprehends the anatomical structure of the vertebral column, the problem will be solved, then the science of Chiropractic will be generally accepted.

---

"What is the difference, if any, between a functional and an organic disease?"

A functional disease consists of a derangement of normal action, functional disturbance, abnormal functionating of an organ without structural derangement.

An organic disease is one in which the actual substance of an organ is affected, the tissue itself being altered from its normal consistency.

Abnormal structure cannot do otherwise than produce abnormal functions.

An organ may functionate abnormally and yet remain normal in structure. For example, diabetes of the kidneys from derangement of the pancreas and functional disturbances of the stomach because of the entrance of bile or the absence of splenic fluid.

## NEUROPATHY.

"Recognizing the fact (page 22) that two forces are to be considered in all movements to adjust the spine when treating the patient for any ailment, we should aim to unite them so that harmony of action at once begins, and this is done by the hands along the spine, so placed as to bear down suddenly at given places along the spinal column.

"The operator should be elevated at the side of patient high enough so that he can throw his weight downward on his own hands, which he places on the body of the patient—on or at sides of the spinous processes; one hand resting flat on the palm on back of patient, as seen in cut, and the other hand on the back of it."

"The operator (page 53) to place his hand or hands in such a position on the body, near the spinal processes and at about the lower edge of the bones called scapulae, holding them against the body, one hand on either side of the spinal processes, with the balls of the thumbs near together, and in this position he presses gently, but suddenly, against the body without any other motion, holding his hands in this position."

The cut referred to is on page 100. Underneath the cut are the words, "This cut shows the manner of placing the hands when giving Chiropractic adjustment."

What I specially object to, is that Dr. A. P. Davis tells us, what he calls Neuropathy is Chiropractic, when the facts are, he does not know what Chiropractic is; is not acquainted with its principles, nor its art of adjusting. All observing Chiropractors, who are scientific adjusters, will recognize from the above description and the cut, that the discoverer of Neuropathy is ignorant of Chiropractic as a science and an art.

I do not think that Dr. Davis means to misrepresent Chiropractic, but it is a "notorious fact" that what Dr. Davis don't know, he does not know. I have shown the cut referred to to many Chiropractors. They never fail to express pity for the ignorance of the author.

One of the very first principles enunciated by me was that of using the spinous and transverse processes as levers to rack vertebrae into their former, natural position.

Dr. Davis lays his flat hands upon the patient on the outside of all clothing. His consideration is not the replacing of displaced vertebrae, but that of pressure which by some means, unknown, unites the two antagonistic forces causing them to be harmonious, thereby neutralizing their antagonism.

As a direct illustration of the difference between relieving an impingement by adjusting a vertebra and that of uniting the two forces by pressure, we will refer to the cataract—a complete opacity of the crystaline lens—in the right eye of Dr. Davis. He took five adjustments. I used the spinous processes of a certain vertebra, throwing it in a special direction. He was perceptibly benefited. He thot that he could show his good wife how to unite the two forces. It was useless for me to try to convince him that he could not do so, so I informed him that he would improve for a few more days, which he did. His wife's downward pressure did not adjust the vertebra, continue to return it to its former and normal position. This difference he cannot see.

There is only one way to adjust—return a vertebra to its normal position—and several moves which would not do so.

---

"Suppose 100 per cent of impulses are passing through a wire; to section that wire would be to cut off 100 per cent, and Dr. Morat says there is a loss of motion when we cut off 100 per cent, or if by pressure we impede 50 per cent of transmission, then 50 per cent of loss of action must result, and the latter idea is purely that of Chiropractic."

It is not that of Chiropractic by a long ways. Disease is either too much energy or not enough, an excess of nutrition or a lack of it. According to the illustration there never could be too much action, 100 per cent being normal. The large proportion of diseases are because nerves are irritated, excited; they carry impulse in an exaggerated amount, away above normal.

"Suppose we were to cut an efferent fiber carrying 100 per cent of vibration to the mind, we have interfered with feeling because the vibration does not reach the periphery. Supposing we produce pressure upon that nerve, cutting off 50 per cent of afferent impressions. Now what occurs? We have just one-half the interpretation that should take place—one-half is absent. We have abnormal sensation, consequently pain following—again proving the Chiropractic basic principle."

This proposition has the same basis as the above. The basic principle of Chiropractic is that disease is either too much or not enough functionating; energy supplied in a degree either greater or less than normal. In these illustrations, there are no provisions made for excessive transmission, only for those that are normal or less than normal.

## LESION.

What constitutes a lesion, is not generally understood. Taking Gould's Dictionary of Medicine as a standard, we quote:

Any injury, hurt or wound in any part of the body is a lesion.

In pathology, any morbid change in the tissue is a lesion.

There are many kinds of lesions, among which are the following given by Gould:

A central lesion is one **affecting** the central nervous system.

A diffused lesion is one **involving** (implicating) all the tissues of an organ.

A focal lesion is a circumscribed (inclosed within certain limits) lesion **giving rise** to distinctive and localizing symptoms.

The **initial** lesion of syphilis is the chancre, i. e., the chancre is the beginning, the commencement of many structural and cutaneous lesions. From the chancre it extends to the skin-mucosa and to nearly all the tissues of the body, even to the bones. A chancre is the primary lesion of syphilis. From the point of inoculation a focus of inflammation develops—**the initial sclerosis, is the lesion from which the chancre is developed.**

An irritative lesion is one in the nervous system which **excites** the functions of the part wherein it is situated.

A lesion of nutrition, is any pathological alteration in the capillary system, consisting of an increase or decrease in the amount of nutritious blood required for assimilation and absorption.

An organic lesion is one in which is manifested a morbid structural change in the tissues of an organ. There must of necessity be abnormal functions to produce structural change.

Secondary lesions comprises those of syphilis, erosions, ulcers, rhagades, squamae, cicatrices, scars, crusts and pigmentation; they are due to irritation and development of the primary lesion.

Toxic lesions are due to poisons.

Traumatic lesions are owing to injuries.

Any injury, hurt or wound is a lesion.

A pathologic lesion is one which disturbs functions, or changes the structure of tissue.

---

Chiropractic seldom fails, and never does harm when properly handled.

"You state in your letter that you will be pleased to know that our school is teaching specific Chiropractic. This is, indeed, the very essential; we are using every possible precaution and tact to stick to strictly pure, unadulterated Chiropractic; no mixing goes here, nor do we teach religion or politics, or anything else but Chiropractic."

Very few realize what is meant by being specific, scientific in either teaching the science or practicing the art of Chiropractic. The above writer, no doubt, thot it meant unadulterated, not "mixing."

I believe that every Chiropractor thinks that he is specific in his or her adjusting. There are those who adjust every vertebrae for any and every disease; others who adjust every other one on the first day and the alternate ones on the next, thus, in the two days, they surely do not miss any; and still others who adjust any vertebrae which seems to be out of line. They all think they are specific.

To be specific, scientific, to make a scienec of Chiropractic, is to know **which vertebra** to adjust for curvature of the spine, **which one** for smallpox, **which one** for diphtheria, **which one** for hemiplegia, **which one** for paraplegia, **which one** for typhoid, **which one** for ptomain poison, and so on, for any disease.

To be specific, is to exhibit a knowledge of the principles and art of adjusting; a comprehension of facts so systematized that they are available for the relief of disease.

The writer of the above letter, no doubt, thot "strictly pure, unadulterated Chiropractic" was specific in the art of adjusting.

Specific adjusting requires a knowledge of pathology, diagnosis and where and how to adjust the one vertebra which, by its displacement, is causing the one or more symptoms or ailments from which the patient desires relief.

---

The following is a copy of a postscript to a personal letter which was not for publication, therefore it is without date or address.

"Not for **my sake,** nor for the **other fellow's sake,** but **for God's sake, Dad, write a book on Chiro** and **everything pertaining to it,** from **'A' to date, for everybody's sake,** so we all will know who is the **'Real genuine Discoverer, Founder and Developer** of this **grand science,** and **proclaim it from the Fountain-Head** and **settle this question once and for all,** so prospective **students** and **practitioners** in the field **will know where they are at** and **where to go;** so that **parties** and **readers** will **know where to locate** the **genuine Fountain-Head.**"

## NEUROPATHY.

For several reasons I have become interested in reading Neuropathy.

"**We wish** (page 64) **it distinctly understood that the term Neuropathy embraces and includes all means which aid in relieving the nervous system.**"

I find that Neuropathy embraces and includes Osteopathy, Chiropractic, Ophthalmology, Magnetic, Phrenology and Medicine.

"So far (page 663) as any medicine system is concerned, we think Dr. W. H. Burgess system the most plausible."

"The medicines are put up in convenient form and not costly, and they get right to the work of neutralizing the toxins, removing the retained poisons and toning up the nervous system." That reads like the ordinary medical ad. It is quite Allopathic in its tone.

"It would be (page 104) disregarding a large field of our nature to neglect to say something about tissue elements, when these are what constitute the physical make-up of our bodies. These elements are sometimes deficient in the food we live on. No case will be in a normal condition unless the elements are supplied, either by the use of the food containing them, or supplied by direct means—that of furnishing them to the patient.

"They are best supplied in the form of two-grain tablets obtainable at any homeopathic pharmacy, or of almost any homeopathic physician.

"To object to this would only exhibit a narrow-minded prejudice, unworthy the thought of any intelligent person. Nature demands a substance to manifest itself in, on or through. The Shussler Tissue Elements are the best in general use and are nicely put up in bottles in potencies. The third to the sixth potency are the most commonly used.

"So far (page 257) as medicines are concerned, the homeopathic approaches nearer to science than any other medical system and supplies the molecular with the elements needed in a way that changes conditions and harmonizes the entire body with itself."

If metabolism is not performed in a normal manner and the body is not supplied with the right proportion of the different elements which constitute tissue, why not find the cause of the abnormality and adjust the lesion?

Would it not be better and more in harmony with science to have the usual kind and amount of tissue elements furnished by metabolism?

To furnish such elements, thru food or medicine, as we may find lacking because of abnormal metabolism—to use the Shussler Tissue Elements, might be in accord with Neuropathy, but is not with Chiropractic.

"Is it not time (page 27) to call a halt on medicine and to look upon its administrators with 'sharpened, sly inspection.' "?

I was surprised to find in the Medical Department and elsewhere in Neuropathy, over 100 medical prescriptions associated with sciences which claim to heal without drugs.

"We need not stop (page 202) to argue this question, for we have been through all the pathies of this country to qualify for the effectual treatment of diseases and claim to be skilled in the science of healing, having eliminated all superfluous measures, medicines and foreign substances not needed in the treatment of any disease known to humanity."

I fully realize that Dr. Davis has been thru all the pathies in order to qualify himself to treat human ailments, so much so, that he now hardly knows where he is at. His many years of study and observation should have informed him that pathy treatments have been a dismal failure. Eliminate all medicines and medical substances for they are not needed to correct the cause of disease.

"There are no medicines (page 288) necessary, neither does this book recommend drugs.

"To object to homeopathic remedies only exhibits a narrow-minded prejudice."

I hear what you say, but your recommendations belie your statement. It is the lawbreaker who is constantly crying "thief, thief."

"Our system (page 114) is—a drugless system of healing."

Neuropathy—a drugless system—is like seedless fruit with the seed left in.

"We have (page 202) a method, **or methods,** by which we stop the waste, the leakage, and remove the strain, **and that, too, without drugs,** and all sorts of functional disturbances, recognized as diseases, get well."

The Neuropathic method "embraces and includes all means which aid in relieving the nervous system ("and that, too, without drugs") such as we find prescribed on pages 664 and 665, viz., sulphate of soda, bitartrate of potassium, tincture of camphor, coal oil, turpentine, olive oil, tannin, alum, chloroform, tobacco, mustard, vinegar and black pepper. These substances are known as drugs and are used by A. P. Davis and others as medicine. Dr. Davis prescribes these remedies, on these two pages, for thirteen diseases. "There are no medicines necessary, neither does this book prescribe them."

## THE VAGUS NERVE.

The pneumogastric or vagus nerve is the tenth cranial. It is called the pneumo-gastric, because it supplies the lungs and stomach with vital force. The term vagus is applied to it because it takes a long and wandering course. This nerve originates in the cranium. It is the longest and the most extensively distributed of any of the cranial nerves. It sends an auricular branch to the external ear, a pharingeal to the pharynx, a superior and inferior laryngeal to the larynx, a cardiac to the heart, a pulmonary to the lungs, an esophageal to the esophagus, a gastric to the stomach, an hepatic to the liver and a recurrent meningeal to the meninges of the brain. The terminal filaments are the gastric branches. The right pneumogastric sends branches to the sympathetic nerve-plexus, the splenic plexus and the renal plexus of the kidneys.

The sympathetic and the vagus are the only nerves which reach and enervate the viscera of the abdominal cavity; the former from the spinal cord and the latter from the medulla oblongata. The vagus has a small ganglion in the jugular foramen from which it sends communicants to the glosso-pharyngeal and the sympathetic nerves.

The jugular foramina are irregular openings varying from a quarter to a half-inch in diameter. They are to be found outward of the occipital condyles, the open space formed by the jugular notches of the temporal and occipital bones, the enclosed petro-occipital suture. This passage serves for the transmission, outward, of the glosso-pharyngeal, spinal accessory, a meningeal branch and the vagus. There is often a considerable difference in the size of the right and left jugular foramina: they may be divided by spicules of bone similar to the vertebraterial foramina.

The vagus nerves (a pair, one on each side) descend close to and on the outside of the sympathetic ganglionic chains.

The pneumogastric nerve originates in the oblongata by a junction of eight to fifteen filaments. Here, as well as elsewhere, we find the rule is to vary in their makeup. The pathways of the right and left vagus nerves differ very much. They lie against the sides of the vertebral column and therefore are liable to the same interruption, by an impingement upon them of the displaced vertebrae and the heads of the ribs upon which they rest, as are the sympathetic ganglionic chains.

The vagus nerve is composed of motor and sensory filaments. It supplies the organs of voice and respiration with motor and sensory fibers; the pharynx, esophagus, stomach and heart with motor fibers.

The pneumogastric receives filaments from the spinal accessory, the glosso-pharyngeal, hypoglossal, the facial nerve, the loop of a large sympathetic nerve between the first two cervical nerves, and an ascending filament from the superior cervical ganglion. McMurrich says, "The cervical portion is characterized by forming numerous connections with almost all the neighboring nerves."

The pneumogastric passes thru the jugular foramen, down the neck, thru the chest and diaphragm and into the abdomen.

The eleventh cerebral nerve, the spinal accessory, arises from the medulla and the cervical portion of the spinal cord. It is accessory to the pneumogastric, supplying one or two branches to the jugular ganglion of the vagus. From thence it goes to the pharynx and larynx. It also sends some branches to the cervical nerves. It has a **double origin**: the **accessory** portion, **within**, by four or five filaments from the side of the medulla below the vagus roots, and the **spinal** portion **outside**, the cranial cavity. The spinal portion arises from the spinal cord as low as the sixth cervical nerve, and, sometimes, it associates with the dorsal roots of the upper two spinal nerves. **Ascending** into the subdural space between the ligamentum denticulus and the posterior roots of the spinal nerves, **it enters the cranium thru the foramen magnum** to unite with the cranial portion, and **passes out of the cranial cavity, thru the jugular foramen**, in the same sheath as the pneumogastric nerve.

The cranial nerves make their exit thru openings in the base and front of the skull, and all, except the spinal portion of the spinal accessory, arise from the encephalon.

We have given the ramifications of the sympathetic nervous system elsewhere. Therefore we will only briefly refer to it here. The sympathetic nervous system consists of a series of ganglia connected by a gangliated cord which extends from the base of the skull to the coccyx. Its ganglionated chains are **distributing agents of motor impulses.** Remember that there are two **gangliated cords,** one on either side of the vertebral column. Each of **these extends into the cranial cavity,** passing thru the carotid canal, representing the direct continuation of the sympathetic trunk into the cranial cavity where it forms the internal carotid and the cavernous plexuses. These furnish branches to several of the cranial nerves.

We, as Chiropractors, are concerned in knowing where the filaments of the vagus nerves may be impinged upon. It will be seen that much of its makeup is from the spinal cord where they are liable to be impinged upon by vertebral and rib displacement. The first cervical vertebra, because of its close proximity, may by its subluxation, cause tension of some of its filaments, more especially by impinging upon the gangliated chains which pass thru its vertebraterial foramina.

"Direct mental impulse" would cut out the wandering vagus nerve, the same as was done with the sympathetic nervous system. But, as long as we find this complex arrangement existing in man, we will have to study it as it is.

---

The word Innate and its use, as one of the principles added to Chiropractic literature, was originated by me, as were all the principles of Chiropractic. The only principle added by B. J. Palmer was that of greed and graft, aspiring to be the discoverer, developer, founder and the fountain head of a science brought forth by his father while he was a lad in his teens.

Oh what a tangled web we weave,
When first we practice to deceive.
—Scott.

---

Is it possible for a man to "master every branch of study which would qualify him" for a Chiropractor in two years? I have known those who thot they had become master of the whole science and art in two or three months, but had they? The originator of every principle of the science and art does not know it all; there remains much for him to learn. But the man who knows it all has no room in his "think-box" for another idea.

---

Before me lies a Chiropractic leaflet. It is not straight Chiropractic, therefore, I desire to correct the luxations.

"Chiropractic was discovered by Dr. D. D. Palmer in September, 1895, and developed into a science and philosophy by his son." If a lack of knowledge of laws, anatomy, reason, philosophy, science and the phenomena of Chiropractic constitute development then truly the above is correct.

"The cause of all diseases is in subluxations." How about corns and bunions? There are no intervertebral foramina wherein the first and second pair of sub-occipital nerves may be pinched, squeezed or compressed.

"Spinal foramina at **various regions.**" A region is a space of indefinite extent. Spinal foramina occupy **definite** localities; **they do not vary.**

This "D. O. Oph., D. C." tells us that mental impulses shut off from the brain, by constricted nerves, are the cause of disease. Mental impulses are never shut off from the brain. All impulses, nerve energy, go out from the brain, **not to it.** Much the larger share of diseases are caused by too much impulse, an excess of energy, a surplus of life, an overplus of action.

He "locates the **point** of **obstruction.**" A point has no length, breadth or thickness. A point is only an imaginary, supposed indefinite, space. The cause or place might be located, but not a point. Osteopaths talk much of the obstruction of the circulation of the blood. Chiropractors do not understand that nerves are obstructed. Nerves may be impinged upon, causing either a repressed or an excited condition, a lack of, or too much, carrying capacity of energy.

He tells us that the Chiropractor uses his art to adjust. Chiropractors do not use a "basis" or an "art" to adjust. Adjusting is an art. Chiropractors use their hands to adjust.

"This condition is called health, 'fevers,' or as we term it, excessive heat, is a slight pressure upon a calorific nerve resulting in 'fever,' or excessive heat at periphery or nerve ending, and by adjusting the vertebrae concerned, the 'fever' is speedily abated." It is said that pupils imitate their teachers in thought, actions and language. I have seen similar "jargonities" in your instructor's writings. A slight pressure on nerves causes **local inflammation. General heat,** named fever, is the result. When the pressure is removed the inflammation and fever decrease. It is a question whether the heat of the body is regulated by certain nerves named calorific and frigorific, or whether Innate controls the temperature through the sympathetic nerves, each nerve carrying its own temperature. I see no reason why the same nerve of communication cannot be used for various impulses or different functions.

"Since the beginning of time, there has never been a magazine that dared to hit within their own ranks for justice; defend specific, pure, unadulterated, philosophical Chiropractic, as the Chiropractor does. It strikes the 'spot' and we want you to know it and profit thereby."

The above was written before The Adjuster appeared. If The Chiropractor had known that The Adjuster was then undergoing the period of gestation and would be duly born of the same parent who gave The Chiropractor birth it would not have given utterance to the above, nor to "**Chiropractic was taught you** (O. G. Smith) **ten years ago** (1899) **by D. D. Palmer as original principles, the product of a masterful mind that dared to conceive, teach and prove** the efficacy of that which you are trying to give others."

**The Adjuster dares to hit within its own ranks for justice. "It strikes the 'spot,'" it hits the bull's-eye every time. "We want you to know it and profit thereby."**

## NEUROPATHY.

"For corns (page 673). Take off the pressure and keep it off. If on the toes, wrap a soft twine around the toe loosely between corn and foot, avoiding pressure on the corn, and wear it for several days, anointing the corn every night with castor oil."

The pressure referred to is that of the shoe or boot—the time-honored excuse for the presence of corns. How the shoes cause corns on the plantar surface of the foot, or soft corns between the toes is not explained.

Corns are the result of slightly displaced joints, usually the one near the corn.

Chiropractors should know that the cuticle of the neck becomes thickened because of inflammation, the result of a displaced cervical vertebra; also that a displaced tarsal or metatarsal bone impinges upon and inflames nerves which end in the cuticle. We do not say take the pressure from the corn; but rather remove the pressure from the nerve by replacing the displaced bone. Many corns are relieved by one adjustment. Others may take weeks or months, because of osseous ankyloses.

Hello! Is that you, Dr. Davis? Say Doctor, **why not correct the luxated joint, take off the nerve pressure, unite the positive and negative forces** (?), thereby cure corns?

"For warts. Apply tincture of iodine on end of warts every day until they disappear. Another remedy is to apply a solution of acetic acid to wart once or twice a day. This will cure in about ten days. The warts go when not expecting them; seemingly suddenly. Bathe them in Epsom Salts, one ounce to a pint of water, several times a day. Some can charm them off, so they say."

Page 2. "Medicines are not needed." Page 33. "That medicines are indicated in any case is hypothetical." Page 160. "Medicine is not a necessary desideratum in what we term the healing art." Page 202. "The hardest thing we have to do is to convince the afflicted that they do not need medicine." Page 203. "When we get the attention of the afflicted we convince them that medicine is not needed." Page 209. "It does seem as if suffering humanity would learn to doubt the curative effects of medicine." Page 288. "There are no medicines necessary, neither does this book recommend drugs." Page 414. "Our system is * * * a drugless system of healing."

Warts also are the result of impingement. Warts on the hands may have their cause in luxated joints of the carpal, or metacarpal bones of the dorsal vertebrae.

"Bunions are painful and caused by a dislocated toe joint. Set the joint by pulling it in place and then securing it there with a pledget of cotton between the toes."

Hello! Is that you, Dr. Davis? Have you not discovered that it is easier to **set joints of the toes, the joints of the vertebral column** and other joints of the body, by having them **as lax as possible?** Do you not find that when you go to **pulling**, that the muscles contract, that **counter-resistant force** is exerted against you? When setting joints, do not pull them. **Always use the long bones and the processes of vertebrae as levers, and what you do, do quickly.**

Why not try castor oil on bunions? If that don't do, try tincture of iodine, or a solution of acetic acid, or bathe them in Epsom salts. As you state on page 666, "In medicine we have certain kinds for given conditions and these constitute the curriculum of specifics, as it were, and the routinist having tried his specific for a given condition and failed to obtain relief, his limit is reached and he improvises other means."

Say, Doctor! Instead of "**pulling it in place,**" **why not get the knack of adjusting** other joints as readily as you do those of the vertebral column?

"For ingrowing toe nails. Cut the nails square across and thin the top of nail by paring it down on the center, on top, as may be borne and cut a notch in center of toe nail, at the end, V-shaped, and wear cotton pledgets under corners of nail so as to turn them up and away from the fleshy part. If corners are sore, apply compound tincture of benzoine once or twice a day.

"Cases which have gone so far as that the nail has grown down into the flesh may have to be operated upon to cure."

Hello! Oh! You are there yet. Say, Doctor, **did you ever try adjusting the lumbar vertebrae for ingrowing toe nails? I** know you have not. **If you knew how easily and quickly such cases are relieved**—often by one adjustment—**you would never prescribe the above painful operation.**

"What is that you say? Oh! You don't see how replacing the lumbar vertebrae and the joints of the feet and hands will often, instantaneously, relieve ingrowing toe nails, corns, warts and bunions. Yes, I understand, **you don't see where the two forces—the positive and negative—come in. Yes, I see; you would have no use for the theorem. Say, Doctor; call that a theory instead of a theorem.**"

---

"Chiropractic is a system of manual therapeutics."

Chiropractic is manual—done by the hand, but is not therapeutical, does not use remedies.

## THE HUMAN AURA.

Psychologists and metaphysicians have given this subject much attention.

All observers realize that we are surrounded with an aura; that we pass from our bodies a subtle, invisible substance known as magnetism; that this emanation may be either repellant or attractive. On the one hand it is known as an affinity, an attraction; on the other hand it may be repulsive, causing a discordant sensation.

Heat, magnetism, odor and no doubt other unseen forces emanate from our bodies in all directions. It is said that each nationality has its peculiar odor, which, although not recognized by themselves, is readily perceived by others. Some persons give off an effluvium that is nauseating, sickening to those who inhale it. Effluvia may be pathologic or physiologic. By this odor, aroma, essence or scent which emanates or exhales from persons, dogs know their masters, hounds distinguish one person from another or trail their prey for miles.

There is an emanation from us, not magical or miraculous, but a subtle, invisible substance, capable of perception, which consciously or unconsciously magnetizes, influences, more or less, every person and object with which we come in contact. The rooms we occupy, the furniture used, the food and water handled, is more or less permeated with, and becomes a part of, it.

Have you not noticed your ease in the presence of certain persons, and of discomfort in the company of others? Also, have you not experienced a feeling of uneasiness and depression that pervades some rooms and houses, and the sense of calmness and pleasure that is present in others. Have you not observed that certain store-rooms seem to be hoodooed; no one succeeds in them, altho their neighbors thrive? You like to trade at certain stores, not because you are treated any better there than elsewhere, but because a feeling of ease and welcome is felt. On the contrary, there are other business houses in which you are uncomfortable; you feel anxious to leave and become at ease as soon as the door is closed behind you.

In selecting rooms for a residence or for an office, not only the location should be studied, but the impression made upon you by the rooms should be considered. Remember that your callers will be affected by the same conditions, the same emanations, the same sensations from the walls and furnishings as you are. The previous occupants have magnetized each room and every pieec of furniture with their effluvia; have impregnated everything with their successes and failures, good fortunes and reverses, triumphs and blunders, victories and defeats, omissions and commissions, encouragement and discouragement, contentment and dissatisfaction, a desire to remain or to get out. If the impressions are not agreeable, it will take much time to remagnetize them to your approval. This work will require an undoing as well as doing, and time is money.

Some persons seem to be surcharged with magnetism, are highly magnetic. They are always giving off their life-force, they affect not only persons, but animals and plants as well; while others seem to be shut up like clams and some are even absorbents—living upon those with whom they are associated. House plants thrive under the care of some persons, and wither and die by the handling of others whose very presence seems to be poisonous. Persons of a highly sensitive organization are affected pleasantly or otherwise by those whom they meet. Those who are delicate in health may be made to feel stronger or weaker by a call from a neighbor. Some persons seem to tire, while others enliven; one person exhausts the invalid while another refreshes.

These facts have been recognized for many centuries; they have survived all sorts of opposition, ridicule and argument.

---

A Chiropractor's newspaper add reads, "Chiropractor and Optometrist.

"Heals as Nature heals, in accordance with the Nature's laws. Compelling the body to do its own healing with its own forces.

"Yours for health's sake."

Nature's method of healing is a process of repair. If the lips of a clean incised wound are drawn together by sutures or plasters and kept closely apposed, rapid healing occurs, this is called healing by immediate union.

If the lips of a wound become red, swollen and slightly glazed, it is known as healing by first intention.

Healing by scab, when the healing is performed under a scab.

If the healing is more slow and granulations appear, it is called healing by second intention, or by granulations.

Where wounds gap, the healing takes place by direct union of the filled-in granulated surfaces, this is named healing by third intention.

This Chiropractor of the "Drugless Health Institute compels the body to do its own healing with its own forces."

He has a new method, healing instead of adjusting. It is certainly painless.

## THE NERVOUS SYSTEM.

The encephalon includes all of the brain matter situated in the cranium. The term brain is not definite as it may include all of the encephalon or only a portion of it. Thru the foramen magnum, at the base of the cranium, all of the nerve matter, except the cranial nerves, is continued down the back in a bony canal (the spinal canal), forming the spinal cord or spinal marrow. This spinal cord, medulla spinalis, contains all the nerves which go to and make up the spinal nerves and filaments from those of the sympathetic nervous system. A spinal nerve contains somatic, sympathetic and cranial fibers.

The encephalon (cerebrum and cerebellum) and the spinal cord form the cerebro-spinal center or axis, from which proceed all the cranial and spinal nerves and those of the sympathetic, for they are included in the spinal nerves. The cranial nerves are those which leave the cranium thru openings other than the foramen magnum. The spinal nerves leave the spinal canal by way of the intervertebral foramina. They contain fibers which become accessory to the cranial nerves.

The cranial and spinal nerves are voluntary (under the control of the human will). They are the nerves of animal life; whereas, the sympathetic nerves (a portion of the spinal nerves) are nerves of organic life; they supply innervation for the vegetative functions. These latter are called the involuntary nerves, because they are not under the control of the human will. Yet, as far as Innate (spirit) is concerned, they are voluntary. These two kinds of divisions of nerves, the voluntary and involuntary, the nerves of animal and organic life, are separate in their functions. The vegetative functions depend upon vital energy for their ability to perform growth of tissue. To the living, conscious being belong the intellectual functions by whose action, when expressed, external labor is performed. Vital functions proceed from Innate when active vegetative functionating is the result.

All of the visceral branches of the spinal nerves on each side of the vertebral column collect to form the sympathetic ganglionic chains. These two gangliated cords extend, on either side of the spine, from the coccyx to the base of the skull. From the upper portion of the superior cervical ganglion they enter the cranium by a plexus of nerves.

These two vertebral nerve-trunks consist of ganglia connected by nerves. The two cords are connected by commissural cords of nerve filaments—cross nerves, which pass in front of the vertebrae from one vertebral cord to another. These two gangliated nerve cords are permanently connected with the spinal system by one of the four branches of each spinal nerve. From these, nerve-fibers pass to the various viscera of the head, chest, abdomen and pelvis, where they again form ganglionic plexuses from which fibers endowed with varied functions pass to the different organs.

---

## BUNIONS AND CORNS.

The amount of agony and torment suffered on account of corns, bunions and ingrowing toe-nails is beyond estimation, as the parties who suffer from their presence are not sick and often suffer without complaining. Our business, as Chiropractors should be to relieve human suffering, no matter whether it comes from a corn or cancer. It is a general opinion among the laity that Chiropractors know nothing about corns, bunions or ingrowing toe-nails, in that they are right.

I have never felt it beneath my dignity to do anything to relieve human suffering. The relief given bunions and corns by adjusting is proof positive that subluxated joints do cause disease.

These toe ailments often inflict enough torment to ofset all the comforts of life, upset one's disposition, making a chronic grumbler of its possessor.

Lippincott describes a bunion as an "Inflamation and distention of the bursa mucosa at the ball of the great toe, induration of the adjacent parts, enlargement of the joint."

Sayre says, "A bunion is an enlargement and inflammation of the bursa situated upon the side of the great toe, at the metatarso—phalangeal junction. Inflammation of this bursa is frequently so severe that the reflex contractions which follow produce a subluxation at this joint. In consequence of the subluxation, the phalanx is made to press against the nerve that supplies this portion of the great-toe to such an extent as to produce the most exquisite and torturing pain.

"Occasionally these bunions produce periostitis, or end in caries of the joint or ankylosed.

"A corn is simply a localized hypertrophy of the skin, caused by abnormal pressure. The irritation produced by pressure upon these formations may give rise to reflex muscular contractions, which will draw the toes up, and it is not at all uncommon to see a row of corns over the second phalangeal articulations, caused by the elevations of these joints against the shoe from this reflex muscular contraction."

## THE VERTEBRATERIAL FORAMINA.

These foramina are also known as the transverse foramina, the costo-transverse foramina and the transversarium foramina.

Each transverse process is formed by two roots. The anterior root is known as the costal process, the homologue of the costa or rib of the dorsal region of the spine. The posterior root springs from the junction of the pedicle with the lamina and corresponds with the real transverse process in the dorsal region. In the coalescing of these two roots, an inter-space is left for the passage of the vertebral vessels.

The seven cervical vertebrae are specially recognized by the foramina in the transverse processes. The transversariums are usually of large size, more especially those of the seventh, which may more than equal the extreme diameter of the atlas. One of the transverse processes of the seventh may be formed from two ossifying centers and create a seventh cervical rib.

The foramina of the cervical vertebrae are known as transverse foramina, because they are in the transverse processes. As they occupy a space between the rib and the homologue transverse portion, they are sometimes called costo-transverse foramina. They are also named vertebraterial—a combination of vertebra and artery — the vertebra-arterial foramina and transversarium foramina, transversarium meaning a crossbeam. A cross-piece on a cross-staff was an instrument, formerly used at sea, consisting of a graduated pole with one or more sliding cross-pieces called transversariums.

The transverse processes of the seventh cervical vary greatly in size and shape, depending upon whether they resemble the cervical or the dorsal in their transition. Their foramina, one of which is occasionally lacking, partake of similar changes in form.

The foramina of the cervical transverse processes are for the transmission of the vertebral artery and vein, and a plexus of the sympathetic nerves, the arteries and veins being well supplied with both medullated and non-medullated nerve-fibers. The fibers form dense plexuses on the outer surface of the vessels from which filaments pass to the middle coat to be distributed almost entirely to its muscular fibers.

The foramina of the seventh cervical occasionally allows the vertebral artery to use it on the left side; frequently the vertebral vein traverses it on both sides, but it is usual for both artery and vein to pass in front of the transverse process and not thru the foramina. This canal is continued in the dorsal region by a space between the neck of the rib and the front of the transverse process which serves for the passage of the post-costal anastomotic artery.

The transverse processes of the cervical vertebrae consist of two parts, the portion behind the foramen which springs from the neural arch which is the true transverse process ending in the posterior tubercle, and the portion in front of the foramen, the vestigial rib of the thoracic vertebrae, which ends in the anterior tubercle. Each process is deeply grooved on the superior surface, especially noticeable at the distal end between the tubercles. The spinal nerve passes outward thru this groove.

The sympathetic trunks form two gangliated cords, a double axis of the sympathetic system extending vertically, one on each side of the ventral aspect of the vertebral column, parallel with each other from the base of the skull to the first segment of the coccyx. In the cervical region, the sympathetic trunks lie in front of the transverse processes; in the thoracic region they lie at the sides of the vertebral bodies and on the heads of the ribs.

On account of the relation of these two series of ganglia to the vertebral column, the great sympathetic system has been called the "vertebral nerve," the "nervous system of the automatic functions" and the "trisplanchnic nerve," as it gives origin to the three splanchnic (visceral or intestinal) nerves.

The two ganglionated chains of the sympathetic nervous system consist of twenty-four pairs of ganglia (three cervical, twelve dorsal, four lumbar and five sacral), connected by communicating branches with each other. According to some authors, the two ganglionic chains are also connected with the ganglion of Ribes, a nervous ganglion, the alleged upper termination of the sympathetic nerve chains, upon the anterior communicating artery of the brain at the point of junction of the right and left trunks of the sympathetic. Upon the posterior (sensory) roots of the spinal nerves are thirty pairs of ganglia, which are more or less intimately connected with the sympathetic system. If we include these with the ganglia found in connection with the cranial nerves, we will have one hundred and thirty ganglia. There are also twelve great ganglia, parts of the brain, the center of the cerebro-spinal system. Counting the small ganglia in the substance of the heart and the two large gangliform masses in connection with the solar plexus, will make all told one hundred and forty-four sympathetic ganglionic centers.

These gangliated cords are connected superiorly with the upper cranial nerves by branches which enter the cranium with the internal carotid artery. The internal carotid nerve, the ascending branch from the superior cervical sympathetic ganglionated chain, may be regarded as an upward prolongation of the primitive sympathetic trunk. It arises from the upper end of the superior cervical ganglion and passes thru the carotid canal, a large circular aperture to the front and on either side of the occipital condyles, into the cranial cavity where it divides into two branches, the internal carotid plexus and the cavernous plexus. Filaments from the carotid plexus occasionally form a small gangliform swelling on the under surface of the artery, called the carotid ganglion. The internal carotid plexus communicates with the Gasserian ganglion, with the sixth nerve and the spheno-palatine ganglion and distributes filaments to the wall of the carotid artery and to the dura mater; while in the carotid canal it communicates with Jacobson's nerve, which is the tympanic branch of the glossopharyngeal. The cavernous plexus communicates with the third, fourth, fifth and sixth cranial nerves and the ophthalmic ganglion. The sympathetic root of the ciliary ganglion and filaments to the pituitary body are also derived from this plexus. The hypophysis cerebri, the pituitary body or gland, was so called from the erroneous notion formerly entertained, that it secreted the mucus (pituita) which is discharged from the nose. This small ellipsoid organ occupying a depression in the sphenoid bone, is attached to the brain by a pedicle. This body is believed to be a ductless gland which furnishes two substances, a "pressor" and a "depressor," which are supposed to increase and lower the blood-pressure. The pituitary body has attracted much attention on account of its pathological changes in its structure in certain obscure (that in pathology is not definite) diseases, such as acromegalia and myxedemia. In Marie's disease it enlarges in proportion to the hypertrophy of the hands, feet, face, etc.

The sympathetic nervous system serves to rearrange fibers derived from the cerebro-spinal system and distribute them to the viscera and vessels of the splanchnic area. It transmits to the cerebro-spinal system afferent fibers from the viscera and fibers to the vessels, involuntary muscles and glands in the course of the somatic divisions of the spinal nerves. To a certain extent it is a separate system. It presents a distinct contrast to the canal and spinal nerves, in that it includes and furnishes for the most part the nerves to the viscera and blood vessels. Its functions are separate and distinctly different from the somatic, perivisiceral cavity. It is connected to the central nervous system by rami-communicantes. In contrast to the cerebro-spinal system, its functions are said to be involuntary—performed independently of the will, a term applied to certain motions and functions of the various organs of the body that are not controlled by, or are not dependent on the will.

The trunks connecting the ganglia of the vertebral chains

contain three varieties of fibers. Fibers which have entered from the spinal nerves of higher or lower areas, desiring to terminate in other ganglia, either above or below, or in ganglia not belonging to the ganglionic chains; fibers originating in sympathetic ganglia, above or below, passing upward or downward to terminate in other ganglia of the trunk, or to go from the trunk to more peripheral ganglia, or to ganglia of the opposite vertebral ganglionic chain and splanchnic afferent fibers, and sensory fibers arising in the spinal ganglia, or sensory sympathetic fibers arising in sympathetic ganglia and passing in the trunk to go to spinal ganglia above or below.

The spinal nerves emerge from the intervertebral foramina and immediately divide each into two primary divisions, named the posterior and anterior primary divisions. Just before their division, each nerve gives off a slender recurrent branch which re-enters the vertebral canal, after affecting a junction with a branch of the sympathetic cord, and is distributed to the spinal cord and its membranes.

The posterior and anterior primary divisions of the spinal nerves are responsible for the innervation of the skeletal muscles and the skin covering the trunk and limbs. They are thus, properly speaking, the somatic (the walls of the body-cavity as distinguished from its contents) branches of the spinal nerve. The anterior primary division supplies, unaided, the intercostal muscles of the segment in which it lies. The nerve supply of the spinal column is from the spinal nerves of that contiguous region. The articulations of the ribs with the vertebral bodies receive their arterial supply from the intercostal arteries; the costo-transverse articulations from the posterior branches of the intercostal arteries. The nerve supply of the former comes from the anterior primary branches of the inter-costal nerves and the latter from the posterior branches of the intercostal.

To designate the different portions of nerves, anatomists have seen fit to use the same terms that we apply to trees, namely, rootlets, roots, trunks, branches and twigs. Let us repeat. We find the rootlets springing from the spinal cord; they form the posterior (sensory) root and the anterior (motor) root. These together form the trunk. The divisions of the trunk nerves are named branches and the ends of branches, twigs.

The spinal nerves give off a small recurrent or meningeal branch which is joined by a branch of the sympathetic. These united, form one nerve and pass inward. It is a question whether each filament of the sympathetic does or does not go to and reach the encephalon, or only to its appropriate ganglionic brain from which each motor nerve has its function directed by a sensory nerve.

Inasmuch as the heart continues to beat after removal or detruncation, "the snake will live until the sun goes down," it is evident that the stimulus does not originate in the brain, the central nerve ganglion. Hence, may we not rightfully conclude that the impulse which directs the heart and those which run other functions, are neurogenous, each having its own specific ganglion and nerves; that functions are rythmically and automatically conducted by ganglia, each organic function by its special ganglionic brain.

There is in all organic beings a vital principle called nerve force, nerve energy, vital force or nerve impulse.

The vibrations of an artery is known as pulse, a pulse wave, which varies with the rigidity of the vascular tube; the more rigid, the more rapid the wave pulse. If the vascular tubes become flaccid, soft and weak, the pulse will be feeble. The pulse may be large and heavy (pulses magnum), or small and weak (pulsus parvus), or rapid (pulsus celer), or it may be a prolonged beat (pulsus tardus). Modification of temperature causes the variation in the tensity of the blood vessels, likewise, an alteration in the pulse waves.

When a nerve is stimulated, the change produced is known as a nervous impulse. An impulse travels along the nerve in waves, known as vibration, similar to the vascular pulse wave, only much more rapid. A nervous impulse is not that of electricity. Nerve impulses are conducted in only one direction; in efferent (motor) nerves from, and afferent (sensory) nerves to, the ganglionic centers.

We will now return to the spinal or vertebral canal, foramen vertebrale, composed of twenty-five vertebral foramina. It affords an abundance of room for the spinal cord. It is larger in those regions in which the spine has the greatest freedom of movement, as in the neck and loins, where it is wide and triangular. It is comparatively narrow and rounded in the dorsal region, where motion is more limited.

The pedicles consist of bars of bone which join the body of the vertebra to the articular processes. Their vertical breadth is half that of the height of the vertebral body and the intervening cartilage. It will be observed that their breadth corresponds to the vertical thickness of the vertebra to which they are attached. The intervertebral foramina, all told, occupies a full half of the length of the spinal column.

The intervertebral foramina are each bounded in front by the body of the vertebra and the intervertebral disc, on the back by the articular process, above and below by the pedicles. The surfaces of the intervertebral foramina which bound it are smooth, even the superior and inferior borders of the pedicles are rounded. These openings form communicating channels for the passage of nerves and blood vessels to and from the neural canal, similar to that afforded by the vertebral foramina for the spinal cord. The very slight movements between vertebrae are in no wise likely to compress the spinal cord or spinal nerves, as neither occupy but a small portion of the vertebral or intervertebral space. These foramina are formed by the intervertebral grooves, often misnamed notches of the pedicles. They are in no wise notches, for a notch is a V-shaped indentation; whereas a groove is a shallow channel or gutter.

The first and second pairs of nerves pass out from the neural canal, thru long gaps where it is impossible for them to be pinched, squeezed or be impinged upon.

The size of the intervertebral foramina and spinal nerves, which find an exit thereat, vary. The spinal cord is larger in the cervical and lumbar regions because of the innervation required for the upper and lower limbs, so the nerves of these regions are larger than elsewhere.

The spinal cord does not nearly fill the space of the vertebral canal. The spinal arachnoid cavity is filled with a loose spongy, web-like reticulum which has no special nerves or blood vessels. The dura mater and pia mater of the spinal cord cover the spinal nerve in a manner similar to that by which the bark of the tree covers its branches.

Tone is that state of tension or firmness in nerves and organs necessary for normal transmission of impulses and the proper performance of functions. It is the effect of tonicity, the vital energy that determines the general tone of nerves and muscles. Excessive tonicity (tension) causes erethism, irritation, augmentation of the vital phenomena in any organ or tissue in which it is concerned. Deficient tonicity creates atony or weakness. It is a well known fact that the nearer the point of stimulation (whatever excites), irritation, is to the central nervous system the greater is the contraction.

The cerebro-spinal nerves arise directly from the brain or spinal cord. Those which pass out of the cranium thru foramina in the skull are called cranial nerves. Those which spring from the spinal cord and emerge thru the intervertebral foramina are spinal nerves—except the first spinal nerve which arises from the medulla oblongata and emerges from the neural canal between the occipital bone and the atlas, and the last spinal or coccygeal nerve which passes out thru the lower end of the neural canal.

The spinal nerves after emerging from the intervertebral foramina, divide each into primary and posterior divisions, the branches of which are distributed to the body-wall and limbs, the posterior division passing backward between the transverse processes, the anterior division going forward between the ribs, yet remaining in the anterior body-wall. These two divisions innervate the skeletal muscles and the skin of the trunk and limbs. Just before the division mentioned, a small recurrent nerve forms a junction with a branch from the sympathetic cord and is distributed to the spinal cord and its membranes. The anterior primary division supplies the communicating branch to the sympathetic ganglionic chain. The trunks of the spinal nerves are very short, from a half inch to three-fourths of an inch long. The divisions mentioned are embraced in a small area. These nerves must have normal tension—tone—to forward motor or sensory impulses with normal force. If they are lax there is atony, if contracted by poisons, or by being impinged upon by a hard substance or an intense, continued thot, there is undue tension.

Before me is a spinal column, which reveals some information on the cause of pathological conditions. The first and second lumbar vertebrae have been destroyed by Pott's disease, caries. There is absent all of the body of the first lumbar vertebrae, the two pedicles and the left transverse and left superior articular processes. Of the second lumbar, the upper two-thirds of the body is absent. A portion of the body has oozed, forming a lip on the anterior-inferior margin. The inferior articular processes of the first and the superior articular processes of the second lumbar are ankylosed. See cuts on the following pages.

In describing the position of a displaced vertebra it is customary to consider the lower vertebra as normal in position and the upper as the one subluxated. As ankylosed, the spinous process is upward and to the right of the usual position; the right transverse process is forward five-eighths of an inch from its normal position; the right inferior articular process is forward and the left backward of the normal; consequently the body of the vertebra must have been wrenched to the left and torn loose by fracturing the intervening cartilage.

This displacement must have of necessity caused extreme tension of the spinal trunk nerve, or one or more of its divisions described above. Tension, vibration and excessive heat are concomitant. This excessive heat caused the destruction, disintegration, named Pott's disease, or caries.

If this condition had been the result of "pinched nerves," then surely the destruction of both bodies by caries, ulceration,

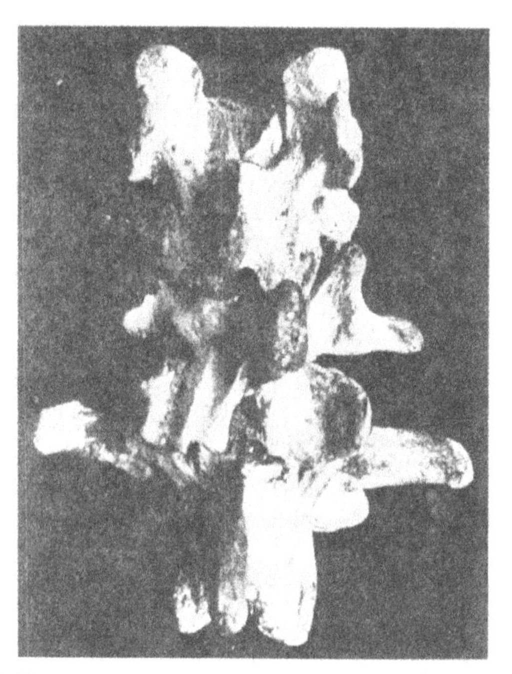

Last dorsal, first, second and third lumbar vertebrae. See description on page 329.

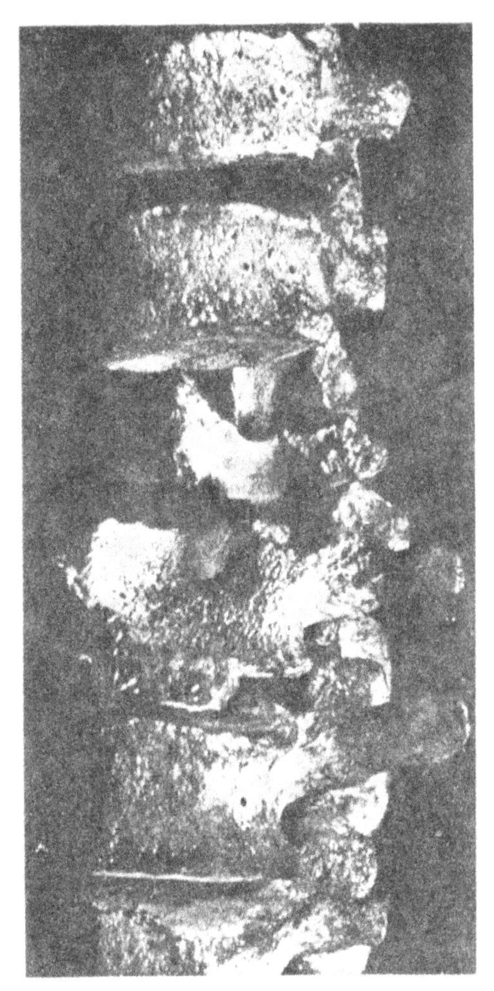

Last two dorsal and first three lumbar vertebrae. See page 329 for description.

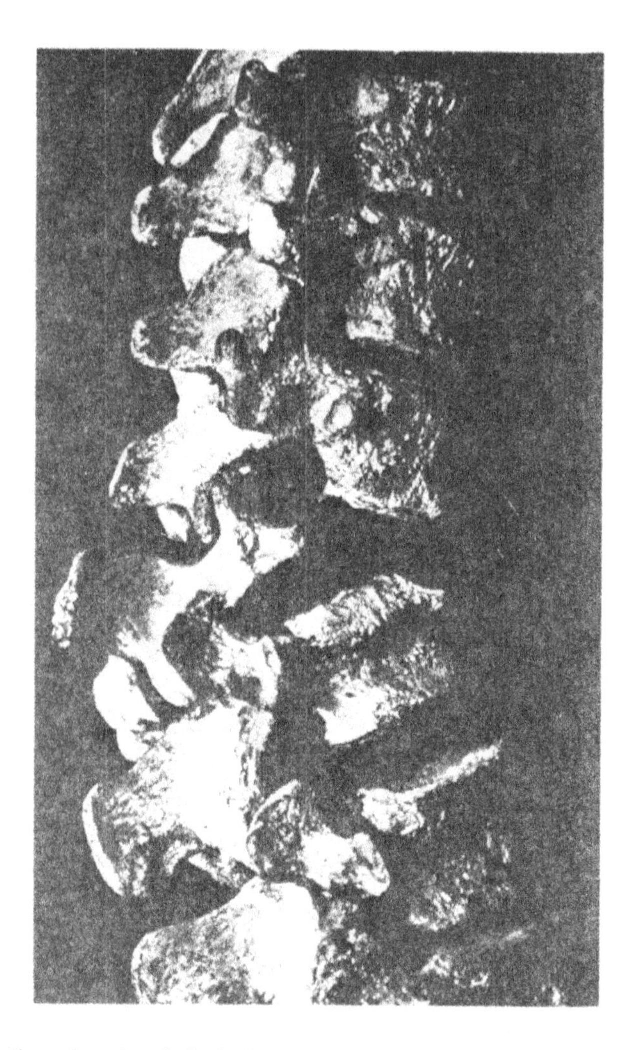

Last three dorsal and first three lumbar vertebrae. For description see page 329.

ought to have relieved the "squeezed" condition of the "pinched nerves."

A Chiropractor would have replaced the displaced lumbar vertebrae, thereby relieving tension, the tightened condition of nerves and saved life and much suffering.

The most wonderful part of this controversial question is that where a state of atony or tension exists, that tonicity, the normal condition of tone or tension, may be restored by replacing the bony structure, more particularly the vertebrae.

These facts are so potent and easy of demonstration that those who have no knowledge of pathology, neurology, myology or are ignorant of biology or anatomy, are able to place the physician in an awkward position. The physician with his superior knowledge may remedy his trouble by learning how and why the success of those who are inferior in medical education, altho superior in qualification and results. The physician should be able by his higher education and the skill, which he may acquire, to do even better than those who are illiterate.

In "The Science of Chiropractic," 1906, page 410, published by B. J. Palmer, I find: "It has taken Dr. D. D. Palmer many years of hard study to localize the cause of different diseases, and many more of laborious application of unusual genius to develop this unique method of adjustment." In volume two of "The Science of Chiropractic," date 1907, page 61, written by the same author, I find: "I knew a peculiar sort of a crank. As odd as he was and is considered to be, he has succeeded in keeping people a guessing as to what he would do next. His actions and thots are sharp, alert and ahead of the times. He holds today an enviable honored position because others are being taught to reach his intellectual level. His every thought was, **Why?** Originality combined with strict discipline and stick-to-itiveness joined with principle and honor has made him many enemies, the majority of which are, knowing him better, turning from enmity to respect and reverence. Many students have been placed on the royal road to wealth, and a very few have, for mercenary, avaricious, greedy, hoggish, reasons that, childlike, to undermine his honor, and they are still the cowards that are failing at every turn of the road.

"He would study two bones, and by comparison, would find one normal and its opposite very much abnormal. **Why?** would be the first question."

Here I am that same "peculiar sort of a crank" studying bones by comparison, always with the question "Why?" I am well aware that the man who is "ahead of the times" and possesses that which the other man wants is often considered a mono-maniac, but there is much satisfaction in knowing that I have been able to give Chiropractic to the world. Avaricious, hoggish greed has caused my imprisonment and created a few cowards, who try to undermine my honor, because I am ahead of the times and possess by hard study that which the other fellow desires to rob me of. In a few years I will have passed to the beyond, then I will receive the honor and respect due the man who **gave Chiropractic to the world.**

---

Lodi, Cal., Feb. 23, 1909

D. D. Palmer:

I have just received a copy of The Chiropractor Adjuster.

"Thorough efficiency and up to date" is my slogan. I have been in Chiro. long enough to know that a smattering of it is N. G. **Proficiency** spells **success**; that I have had.

Chiro is a healthy boy; he is developing mentally and physically. He is in every way progressive and up to date.

Chiropractors must "brush up" and step lively to keep up with that kid. The embryo must have been perfect, as the child is good to look upon.

I want to keep abreast of the youngster and continue with him to manhood.

I do not want a "correspondence course," for I know how fruitless they are.

Truly yours,

C. E. EDDY, D. C.

Brother Eddy:—Chiro. is again looking quite well. When I recaptured him his face was awry—looked as though he had been hung on a nail by his mouth. I soon learned that he had been badly mistreated by his captors. They sought to make such changes that his father would not recognize him. They had deprived him of the cranial nerves, which made him look like a fool; they had taken out the sympathetic nervous system —truly, he did need sympathy—his vital functions were below par, he looked pinched and grim. His clothes hung on him like a mother hubbard on a bean pole.

The Adjuster has returned his cranial and sympathetic nerves. He is once more a thinker, has a good appetite, all vital and intellectual functions are performed normally. I think before the Summer is through that he will not know what hurt him.

Our subscribers will have to keep in hand an anatomy, dictionary and a vertebral column, so they may keep in touch with this youngster.

"Practice of the Science." The knowledge of principles or facts, can not be practiced; however, the art of Chiropractic may be practiced by one who has a knowledge of the principles which form the science. There are two classes of Chiropractors, those who desire to know all they can of physiology, pathology, neurology and anatomy, and those who have an aversion for intelligence, do not want to take effect into consideration, depending only upon an examination of the spinous processes.

"Mr. Palmer claims that the human system is simply an electric dynamo, and that it was such a long time before electricity was discovered; that the spinal column is the main wire distributing the light throughout the system, over the smaller wires, which are the nerves, and to prove this, the skeleton was lighted with electric wires, running from the spine, with bulbs for heart, lungs, liver, kidneys, etc."

"Mr. Palmer" is the only author or lecturer who refers to the human body as a "human system." In biology a system is composed of those organs collectively which specially contribute toward one of the more important and complex vital functions, as the aliamentary, vascular, or nervous system. A dynamo is a machine. The human body is not a machine. A dynamo is used for converting mechanical force into electrical power. Mechanical, electric, chemical and vital are entirely different forces. Vital force is not mechanical, chemical or electric. "To prove this, the skeleton was lighted with electric wires." The skeleton was not lighted with wires, it was electric. Lighting the skeleton with "electric wires" did not prove anything in biology, it certainly was not biological, did not pertain to biology. Did it prove anything in the line of electricity. "That the spinal column is the main wire." The spinal column consists of a number of bones and intervertebral discs; it has no resemblance whatever to a wire in material, appearance or function. I presume he meant to have said spinal cord instead of spinal column; if so, there is no similarity between the spinal cord which is composed largely of nerve-fibres arranged in bundles which are the conducting elements of the nervous system. The ignorance displayed in these write-ups should not be blamed upon the reporters, for "Mr. Palmer" is voluminous and willingly pays for all "frills or furbelows" at so much per. The above are some of the "masterful developments" of "Dr. B. J. Palmer, Ph. C., D. C."

---

Chiropractic includes the art of adjusting vertebrae and the reason for doing so.

## UNJUST MEDICAL LEGISLATION.

The Journal of Osteopathy has well said, under the heading of "The Effects of Unjust Medical Legislation:"

It is ignorance clad in authority.

It is contrary to progress and liberty.

It is aimed not at failure, but at success.

It is against common justice and equal rights.

It limits personal liberty in the interest of drug dealers.

It cannot stand the light of day, or a searching investigation.

It restricts the citizen from employing the physician of thon's choice.

It is against the opinion of judges and jurys of this fair land of liberty.

It is taxation without representation—restrictive, oppressive and unjust.

It protects certain schools to the exclusion of others equally meritorious.

It curtails rather than expands the means applied to alleviate human ills.

It is a violation of individual liberty and an insult to the intelligence of a free people.

It can but shackle and obstruct, hinder and smother, more sane and rational modes of treatment.

It protects those who administer poison against competition with superior, natural, drugless methods.

It furnishes the means whereby medical trust methods are made effectual in regulating demand and supply by absolute control.

It permits no doctor, however learned, reputable and zealous, to practice his profession without enlisting in one of the four medical schools.

It is class legislation of the worst type, building a fence around medical doctors and giving them exclusive license to practice unmolested.

It cuts off the entire public from the freedom to choose their doctor, except that he gives medicine and wears the collar and brand of the State Medical Board.

It creates a medical monopoly and excludes from practice some of the most skillful, progressive, painstaking, conscientious proctitioners our country has produced.

It is a fraud upon society; clothes four schools with legalized monopoly; its influence is so restrictive and oppressive, its effects upon civilization so debasing, that liberty-loving citizens cannot help but evince the most loathsome contempt for its promoters and beneficiaries.

## INFLAMMATION.

Inflammation considered as a prominent symptom, or as a disease, is present in the larger number of cases. The word inflame is from the Greek and means, a flame: I burn as a flame. Inflammation is a condition of inflaming or being inflamed. As Webster says: "A morbid condition consisting in congestion of the blood vessels and exudation of serum and blood corpuscles with resulting hyperplasia. It is manifested outwardly by redness and swelling, attended with heat and pain."

Morbid is used as a technical or scientific term in contradistinction to the term healthy—simply meaning disease.

By congestion is meant an excessive accumulation of the contents of any of the blood-vessels or ducts. An engorgement of blood; an accumulation of blood in an organ. Congestion, as understood by the pathologist, is an important symptom in all febrile diseases. It is supposed to be the result of an extraordinary flow of blood by the arteries or from a difficulty in the return of blood to the heart by the veins. Therefore occur the terms venous congestion, stasis, stagnation, lack of drainage, detained blood, stoppage of blood, obstructed blood, strangulated blood vessels, detention of blood, pressure on blood vessels, bad blood, impure blood, poisoned blood, lack of blood, diseased blood, nourishing blood, perverted circulation, shortage of blood and blood fermentation.

Exudation is the oozing of a liquid thru the pores of a membrane. The material which has oozed thru is known as an exudate. Inflammatory effusions are spoken of as exudates; dropsical effusions as transudates. They present the same general appearance, being clear fluids of a yellowish green color. It is difficult to tell a dropsical from an inflammatory fluid by chemical or a personal examination; the liquids appear very similar.

Serum is the clear portion of any animal liquid separated from its more solid elements; especially the clear liquid which separates in the clotting of blood from the clot and the corpuscles.

Blood corpuscles are the body or solid material of the blood, minute, concave, flat discs, circular in man, elliptic in the camel and oval in birds and reptiles.

Hyperplasia is an abnormal or unusual increase in the elements composing a part; hypertrophy is an increase in bulk of pre-existing normal elements.

**Inflammation is the most common source of structural lesions**; it is itself a developing lesion. It advances from a simple form to one more complex in structure and function, becoming more and more manifest as heat increases. Inflammation is a name given to a condition of vital action which causes a change of functions and tissue structure. It may be seated in any organ or tissue of the body, excepting the cuticle, hair and nails, yet, some organs or parts are more frequently affected than others. The phenomena characterizing inflammation, the changes in the circulating and secreted fluids; the effects produced by them locally and constitutionally; the remarkable variations these present in the same and different systems, at different ages; their exciting causes, and the liability of any organ or tissue to be affected, combine to cause the utmost interest in regard to the nature, cause and proper treatment of this most common, but imperfectly understood, deviation from a healthy condition.

Very many opinions have been entertained respecting the proximate cause of inflammation. Nearly all have been built upon the supposition of there being some kind of an obstruction to the circulation of the blood in the inflamed part.

The earliest conception of inflammation was that of a **specific entity,** and the treatment that of exorcism.

Before the discovery of blood-circulation, the **humor theory** was generally accepted. The physicians believed in four humors: blood, phlegm, choler or yellow bile, and melancholy or black bile. These were conceived as entering into the constitution of the body and determining by their relative proportions a person's health and temperament. Physiologists, before Harvey's time, believed phlegm was cold and moist, and caused sluggishness. An excess of phlegmatic humor caused a person to have a phlegmatic constitution. In ancient physiology, the relative proportions of the elements, dry, moist, hot and cold, affected the body according to their relative quantities. Hence, in modern usage, the peculiar physical and mental character of an individual; as, the sanguine, phlegmatic, choleric, bilious or melancholic temperament, denoting types formerly believed to be due to the preponderance of one or other of these humors.

Gould says under the head of pathology: "Pathologic humoral, the old doctrine that all disease is due to abnormal conditions of the blood. It has been revived in recent times in a modified form, and is now based on the theory that both immunity and susceptibility to disease reside in the juices of the body."

Dorland: "Humoral pathology, the opinion that disease is due to abnormal conditions of the fluids of the body."

Solidism.—A doctrine of solidism, who referred all diseases to alterations, condensation and rarefaction because of contraction and expansion of the solid parts of the body. They maintained that the solids only were endowed with vital properties; that they alone could receive the impressions of morbific agents and be made the seat of pathologic phenomena. Viewing the effects of inflammation as causes, as the medical world has always done, they apparently had good reasons for their belief.

While the circulation of the blood was unknown and the nervous system hardly thot of, the hypothetical notions of the power of the liver, in preparing and sending forth this humorous fluid, continued to prevail. Physicians were so fully persuaded of the existence and influence of different humors, and **so little did they know of the regular and constant motion of the blood and the nervous transference of impulses**, that they believed in the possibility of depositions and congestions of the blood, the bile and lymph, acknowledging these as the cause of inflammation. Their anatomists taught them, and the professors of physic supported the opinion, that the liver was the center of the vascular system from which the blood went forth by day to the extremities and returned again by night. If any peccant humors irritated the liver, the blood was sent out more forcibly; if any part of the body was weakened, or disposed to receive a greater quantity of fluid than the rest, a swelling was produced by the flow of humors to that place. Fluxions, or flows of humor to a place might happen either from weakness of the part or organ which allowed the humors to enter more abundantly than usual, or from the place attracting the humors, in consequence of the application of heat, cold draughts or the drinking of cold water. The peculiar nature of the swelling was supposed to depend upon the kind of humor. Blood produced the true phlegmon; bile, erysipelas, etc. An idea was entertained that the blood and humors might slowly stagnate in a part from want of expulsive power. Such an affection was known as congestion, while the expression fluxion or defluxion was used to denote any swelling arising from the sudden flow of humors from a distant part.

After the discovery of blood circulation, fluxion and congestion were quite incompatible and physiologists turned their attention to obstructions of the circulation. The blood was too thin, too thick or viscid. In diseased conditions, of which, then as now, the larger share were of inflammatory origin, the blood was lentus, pliant, tough or sluggish, or the larger globules of the blood passed into the smaller vessels and thus plugged them up. The blood might become thickened, as manifested by diarrhea, profuse sweating or a too copious flow of urine; these conditions dissipated the thinner parts of the blood. A resistance in one part of the body to free circulation, caused an increase in another part, creating an excited, irritated condition behind the obstruction. This was considered the cause of heat and pain, and the accumulation of blood produced redness. These ideas are entertained by many today.

The theory of acrimony of the blood and lymph had its day. The humoralists attributed a pungent, acrid condition, irritating, as the cause of many diseases.

Date 1776: "Acute inflammatory maladies differ very much one from another, in refpect to the parts and emunctories towards which the matter of the fever inclines to be fettled. The nature of an epidemical diftemper (of that time) was generally inclined to depofite the febrile matter towards the inteftines, caufing fometimes dyfenteries, fometimes dry-gripes, and fometimes the most violent fits of the colic and iliac paffion. But this diftemper arofe with a fever; which, after raging a few hours, ended in the moft fevere pains of the bowels. They affirmed, that the iliac paffion can only be properly fo called when **acrid or malignant humours** are thrown by a tumultuous fever upon the ftomach and inteftines; for if the faid diftemper fhould arife from an hernia, indurated faeces, or the like, it ought rather to be called a falfe or baftard iliac paffion.

"The inteftines, but more efpecially the fmall ones, are, like the ftomach, very frequently **invaded with an acute inflammation** in their membranes, either from the common or general caufes of a phlegmon operating upon, or particularly tranfferred to, thefe parts; or from fomething **acrimonious taken into the body**, under the form of drink, foods, preferves, medicines, or poifons, which being conveyed into the inteftines are retained and arrefted betwixt their valve-like folds; or from fome morbific matter, acrimonious, putrid, fetid, purulent, ichorous, gengrenous, bilious, or atrabiliary, tranflated or coming from the oefophagus, ftomach, liver, fpleen, pancreas, or omentum, to thefe nervous parts of membranes, and there fettling fo as to corrode them; or laftly, from fome violent cramps or convulfive confrictions foregoing in the bowels, and either creating an inflammation of them, or fuppreffing the motion by which they drive on their contents, and by that means producing an inflammation."

The **salutary explanation of inflammation** was and is yet accepted by many. According to this theory inflammation is considered only as a disturbed state of parts which require a new, but salutary mode of action to restore them to a condition wherein a natural mode of action alone is necessary. From such a view of the subject, therefore, **inflammation, in itself, is not to be considered as a disease, but as a salutary (health-**

**ful) operation**, consequent upon some violence or some disease. The act of inflammation is considered as an increased action of the vessels, or of distension beyond their natural size. This increase depends upon a diminution of the muscular power of the vessels and at the same time the elastic power of the artery must be dilated in the same proportion. This was considered something more than a common relaxation: an action in the parts to produce an increase of size for particular purposes, was known as an act of dilatation. The whole was considered as a **necessary benign operation of nature.** Owing to the blood-vessels being stretched beyond their normal dimensions, there is a greater quantity of blood circulating in the part which, they thot, was according to the rules of animal economy; for, whenever a part has more to do than simply to support itself, the blood is sent to that portion in larger quantity. The swelling was supposed to be produced by an extravasation of coagulate lymph, with some serum. They reasoned that this lymph differed from common lymph in consequence of passing thru inflamed vessels. It was this lymph which became the uniting medium of inflamed parts, therefore, salutary, or healthful. This new tissue was supposed to have the power of becoming vascular, or of having vessels shoot into it. The pain came from spasm. The redness was produced by the arteries being more dilated than the veins or because the blood was not changed in the veins. As the vessels became larger, the part became more the color of blood. It was supposed that there was more blood in the part, and as the true inflammatory color is scarlet, or that color which the blood has when in the arteries, they concluded that the arteries were principally dilated, or at least, the veins were equally distended, and that the blood underwent no change in its passage from the arteries to the veins while passing thru the inflammatory portion. When a part was unable to be restored to health, after an injury, by inflammation alone, or by adhesion, then suppuration, as a preparatory step to the formation of granulations, and the consequent restoration of the part, took place. The blood-vessels were supposed to be nearly in the same state as in inflammation but more quiescent, having acquired a new mode of action. This theory is advocated by some of the medical profession today, as will be seen from future quotations.

A writer of 1822 said: "The remote causes of inflammation are infinite in number, but divisible into two classes. **The first includes all such agents as operate by stimulation, including mineral, vegetable and animal poisons. The second class of causes are those which act mechanically, such as bruises,**

**wounds, pressure and friction.**" This same writer states: "Fevers often seem to become causes of local inflammation." Strange it is, that in attributing inflammatory causes to the two classes, that he had not observed that fever was diffused heat from a local inflammation, and that inflammation always precedes fever.

The inequality of blood distribution has had and still has its advocates. This inequality of blood distribution was supposed to throw an unusual quantity into certain vessels, and, in order to relieve the congestion, the vis medicatrix naturae, which, as in all febrile diseases, it relieves by forming a spasm on their extremities. "**A spasm** of the extreme arteries supporting an increased action in the course of them, **may**, therefore, **be considered as the proximate cause of inflammation**; at least, in all cases not arising from direct stimuli applied; and even in those, the stimuli may be supposed to produce a spasm of the extreme vessels."

**The increased action of the blood-vessels have been held as a proximate cause of inflammation.** The irritating nature of the blood when applied to any living, or sensible parts occasion such increased action of the vessels. "That the proximate cause of inflammation consists in an increased vital action of some particular artery, or arteries, by which the blood is propelled with greater force than usual, into the communicating lymphatic and colourless vessels.

"The advocates for each hypothesis agree in admitting, 1st, that inflammation has its seat in the capillary vessels; and 2dly, that the redness in inflammation is owing to an unusual quantity of blood in the vessels of the inflamed part, and consequently that the capillary arteries are much dilated during the state of inflammation. The contraction of these vessels, indeed, it has been said, are increased also in a ratio proportional to the dilations; but, this is an assertion, which has not yet been proved, either in the way of experiments, or of observation."

Dr. Hastings says: "It is proved that the healthy circulation of the blood essentially depends upon a due degree of action in the vessels throughout the system; that **the application of stimuli, whilst it increases the action of the vessels, produces none of the symptoms of inflammation.** When, however, the excessive action of these stimuli has impaired the excitability of the small vessels, the phenomena of inflammation are fully manifested; and when their excitability is restored, the inflammation subsides. It may be logically inferred, therefore, that inflammation consists in a weakened action of the capillaries, by which the equilibrium between the larger and smaller vessels is destroyed, and the latter become distended."

Many physicians have supposed that the redness of inflammation is occasioned by the generation of new blood-vessels.

Copland defines inflammation as an "**Alteration of the vital actions of a part** manifested by morbid sensibility or pain, by redness, increased temperature, and swelling, generally with more or less febrile commotion of the system."

Pain is a distressing or an agonizing sensation. It is usually due to irritation of a sensory nerve. Pain is a conscious representation of a change produced in a nerve-center by a certain mode of excitation. Pain is generally symptomatic. It is called acute when sharp and violent; when short and sudden, a twinge; and when more violent, a pang; pungent when it resembles that which would be produced by a sharp instrument run into the part; heavy, when attended with a sensation of weight; tensive, when the part seems distended; boring, terebrant, or terebrating, when resembling that which might be caused by boring with a gimlet; lancinating, when occurring in shoots; fulgerant or lightning, when intense, but momentary; lacerating or tearing, when the part seems to be tearing; burning, when resembling that produced by a burn; throbbing, when beating regularly like the pulse. Why such a variety of sensations?

Inflammation, hyperthermia, excessive heat, modified function, pain and diffused heat, is concomitant with contraction longitudinally and expansion diametrically of nerve tissue.

Febrile, pertaining to or having the symptoms of fever—diffused inflammation.

Gould defines inflammation as "**A condition of** nutritive **disturbance** characterized by hyperemia, with proliferation of the cells of a tissue or organ, and attended by one or more of the symptoms of pain, heat and swelling, discoloration, and disordered function."

Hyperemia is an excess of blood in any part of the body, due to increased influx, or obstruction of the outflow.

Proliferation.—Reproduction of similar forms, both normal and morbid.

Normal temperature insures normal functions. An excess of heat means an excess of action, of nutrition, circulation, cell growth—disordered functions.

Dorland says that inflammation is "**A morbid condition** characterized by pain, heat, redness and swelling, and histologically by hyperemia, stasis, changes in the blood and walls of the small vessels, and by various exudations."

Stasis.—Stoppage of the flow of any of the fluids of the body, more especially of the blood.

An excess of heat produces the conditions named by Dorland. Stasis would result from a thickening of the transudating membrane and the walls of the blood-vessels.

Dunglison states.—"**The process of inflammation** comprises changes in the blood vessels and circulation, exudation of fluid and of blood corpuscles from the vessels, and changes in the inflamed tissues. All these changes go on together."

A process is a procedure, a method of performing an operation.

An excessive action of the heat functions causes the walls of the blood vessels, by muscular contraction, to become more tense and rigid up to a certain degree of temperature. Under the influence of a temperature higher than this the walls of the blood vessels become softened, and there is an exudation of the fluid and blood corpuscles thru their softened tubular walls, for as Dunglison says, "these changes accompany each other."

Landois tells us: "When a vascular part is subjected to severe irritation, hyperemic reddening and swelling of the part are at once observed. It has been shown by microscopic examination of transparent parts that both the capillaries and the smaller vessels become dilated with blood-cells; sometimes dilation is preceded by a temporary contraction of brief duration. At the same time, a change in the velocity of the blood-stream is observed in the vessels. Donders points out the greater number of leukocytes in stagnating blood and believes correctly that this **accumulation of leukocytes is a greater obstacle** to their progress, as compared with the erythrocytes. While these processes are going on, the migration of the leukocytes and rarely also of the red cells takes place."

Landois concurs in the statement that **irritation, contraction, dilatation, engorgement, hyperemia and the velocity of the blood stream all keep apace.**

McFarland says: "**Inflammation is** the sum of the phenomena manifested by an injured tissue. The phenomena are, for the most part, **reactionary and reparative; some are destructive and disintegrative.**

"The clinical manifestations by which inflammation was originally recognized were pain, heat, redness and swelling.

"An organ or tissue in which active hyperemia is in proggress; in which the resulting swelling becomes painful, in which nutritional changes are in progress and into which an inflammatory exudate takes place, is one in which the performance of function must be interrupted.

"A careful analysis of the phenomena of inflammation leads us to the broad generalization that they are **conservative in**

**tendency benign in disposition, and evidently the result of a carefully adjusted protective mechanism.''**

McFarland, evidently, sees two sides to these inflammatory phenomena; that of destructive and reparatory, disintegrative and reactionary, wasteful and conservative, merciless and benign, pathological and physiological, death-dealing and health-giving. In all inflammatory processes there is evidently a fight on hand, the bad against the good, our friends against our foes. The doctor calls daily with his arsenal, his whole armamentarium of instruments, medicines, surgical appliances and note-book, in which the nurse's reports are recorded, showing the wave-lines and fluctuations of the battle. This book is a daily record of the battle of life against death.

Samuel Cooper says: ''By the term inflammation is generally understood the state of a part, in which it is painful, hotter, redder and somewhat more turgid than it naturally is; which topical symptoms, when present in any considerable degree, or when they affect very sensible parts, are attended with fever, or a general disturbance of the system.

''The susceptibility of the body for **inflammation is of two kinds**; the one original, constituting a part of the animal economy, and beyond the reach of human investigation; the other acquired from the influence of climate, habits of life, and state of the mind over the constitution. The first kind of susceptibility, being innate, cannot be diminished by art; the second may be lessened by the mere avoidance of the particular causes, upon which it depends.

''**Inflammation** may, with great propriety, be divided into **healthy and unhealthy.** Of the first there can be only one kind, though divisible into different stages; of the second, there must be an infinite number of species, according to the peculiarities of different constitutions, and the nature of diseases, which are numberless.''

Turgid.—Swollen, congested, plethoric.

Topical.—Local, pertaining to a particular part or situation of the body.

Cooper considers **two kinds of inflammation**, one innate, the elevation of temperature for a physiological purpose, the healing of wounds and fractured bones. This physiological elevation of temperature may be studied as readily as that which is pathological; it does not disturb the normal action of the system; there is no pain, congestion or fever attending its manifestation. The other relates to diseased conditions.

Lippincott says inflammation is ''the **local reaction to irritation,** usually bacterial in origin, but sometimes physical or chemical, which tends to counteract the injurious agent or repair its deleterious effects; the condition of hyperemia, exudation, and degenerative or proliferative tissue-changes manifested by the cardinal symptoms of celsus, rubor (redness), dolor (pain), calor (heat), and tumor (swelling), to which list the fifth symptom of functio laesa (impaired function) was added by later writers."

Reaction.—An increase of the vital functions succeeding their depression. An action induced by vital resistance to some other action; depression or exhaustion of vital force consequent on overexertion or overstimulation; heightened activity and overaction succeeding depression or shock. The response of an organ, tissue, or the system, to a stimulus, agent, or influence; the state of activity in vital processes which succeeds the depression caused by physical shock; reciprocal or return action or influence, as when one commits an injustice there is a reaction on himself.

According to the philosophy of Chiropractic there is no reaction which is bacterial or chemical.

DaCosta: "When the tissues are injured they react or respond, and this **reaction or response is known as inflammation.**"

Metabolism—anabolism and catabolism, constructive and destructive—is present in all tissue, whether somatic as a whole, or confined to germ cells. Injury to the nervous system, traumatic or toxic, causes excitation, irritation, overaction, local inflammation which when diffused is known as fever. The body thruout is subject to the same general law of waste and repair.

Wharton and Curtis: "**Inflammation** may be defined as **the reaction of the tissues against injurious influences.** This definition is satisfactory from the clinical standpoint, but not entirely so from a pathological point of view, for it is difficult, if not impossible, to draw a sharp line between the changes which take place in the injuries and the alterations which occur as a result of true inflammation, although it is important not to confuse the two.

"The cause of inflammation is an injury to the tissues by mechanical, thermic or chemical means, by the effect of electricity, or by the growth of bacteria."

Inflammation, by its superabundant heat, changes physiological to pathological processes. There is nothing reactionary in so doing. To produce greater heat than normal, it is absolutely necessary to create more tension of some portion of the nervous system. Normal tension is extended to the nervous system by its attachment and extension to the neuroskeleton. By the displacement of any portion of the bony frame, by fracture or luxation, a modification is made in the tension of the nervous system.

Delafield and Prudden state that "**inflammation is a modification of physiological processes.**

"The conception of inflammation was originally a clinical one in which the process was marked by special symptoms—redness, heat, swelling, pain and impaired function. This conception was gradually enlarged to embrace the new formation of tissue which might be associated with or follow these symptoms, or which might be independent of them.

"It is only within the past decade or two that the processes and lesions involved in inflammation have been seriously considered in the light of comparative pathology, and as biological problems divorced for purposes of research from the dominance of traditional clinial conceptions.

"The death of tissue from trauma, and degenerative alterations in the tissues in the presence of various forms of poisons are often important factors in the inflammatory processes.

"A comprehensive survey of the conditions under which inflammation most frequently takes place shows at once that it is almost always associated with some form of injury. This may be direct trauma, or excessive heat or cold. It may be poisons of various kinds—from the cruder inorganic poisons inducing immediate and gross tissue destruction to the subtle toxic substances which result from the metabolism of micro-organisms, or from the aberrant metabolism or degeneration of the body cells themselves. Dead cells or foreign substances or many kinds within the body are common of the inflammatory processes."

"Aberrant metabolism."

Metabolism is the process by which energy replaces the discarded worn-out tissue. This is a double process; destructive metabolism, katabolism, a change of worn-out tissue into excrementitious products; and constructive metabolism, anabolism, the changing of nutritious substances into body tissue.

Stengel asserts, "**Inflammation is a combination of pathologic processes** representing the reaction of the tissues to various forms of irritation; it is characterized by hyperemia, excessive emigration of leukocytes from the blood-vessels, exduation or more or less altered blood-plasma and secondarily and less essentially by reproductive cellular processes and by degenerative changes in the affected tissues.

"Emigration of leukocytes."

A leukocyte is a white blood corpuscle. Erythrocytes are the red corpuscles. In fever, as I have stated elsewhere, the percentage of the leukocytes are decreased and the erythrocytes increased.

"At the present day inflammation is generally regarded as

purely reactive in nature, the irritation causing sometimes one and sometimes another primary lesion.

"Local excess of heat produces various lesions. Moderate excess leads to relaxation of the walls of the blood-vessels; with increasing grades of temperature; there is in addition necrotic change in the cells of the part, and exudation of serum causes vesicle formation. Still **higher grades of temperature produce immediate destruction**, perhaps with charring, of large or small areas, while the surrounding tissues suffer from reactive inflammation and hyperemia."

The American Text-Book of Surgery affirms: "**Inflammation is a disturbance of the mechanism of nutrition** and affects the structures concerned in this function. It is the 'response of living tissue to injury.' This injury is caused by micro-organisms in the great majority of cases. **It is probable, however, that some injuries, such as simple fracture, produce many if not all the symptoms of inflammation without the concurrent action of bacteria.** The condition is then one of hyperemia with exudation, and should be distinguished from true inflammation. As the result of either form of disturbance, however, we have conditions favorable for the process of repair or for the neutralization or removal of the primary microbe cause. These changes give rise to the five cardinal symptoms of inflammation—pain, heat, redness, swelling, and impaired function.

"One of the most constant symptoms of inflammation is the swelling. This is rarely absent, and is seen even in non-vascular parts. **The increased amount of blood in the vessels in the part does not add materially to its size. We must seek for an explanation of this phenomena in the altered condition of the tissues.**

"The next symptom of inflammation is pain, which is due to the pressure or tension produced by the swelling upon the terminal branches of the nerves. It is the most severe in the early stages of the inflammation, before the tissues have had an opportunity to accommodate themselves to the pressure exerted by the exudation. It will vary greatly with the anatomical nature of the part. In bone, where the tissues yield less rapidly than elsewhere, it will be very severe, and even in the chronic forms of inflammation the pain will be of a boring character, which is proverbially hard to bear. The throbbing pain is due to the pulsation of the hyperemic vessels of the part, and the peculiar lancinating pain which pus causes in its efforts to escape is characteristic of an abscess which is about to discharge. **Pain may**, however, **be entirely wanting. This is the case in nerveless tissue,** and also in severe inflammations which rapidly destroy the vitality of the part.

"The fifth symptom of inflammation, disturbance of function, will show itself in various ways, according to the part affected: an inflamed muscle will become rigid and contracted; an inflamed gland will cease to give forth its natural secretion. The special senses may also be impaired, or even permanently affected, by the inflammatory process.

"The symptoms of inflammation are brought about by the disturbed functions of tissues which have been damaged.

"Cohnheim believed that all these agencies acted upon the walls of the blood-vessels and produced a **molecular change** in them by **means of which the phenomena of inflammation were produced.** Virchow advanced the **'abstration' theory,** in which the cells of the tissues played a prominent part. Landerer does not think we ought to separate the capillaries from the tissues in which they lie in considering the seat of inflammation. When the cause of inflammation acts upon the tissues they become relaxed, the equilibrium between blood and tissues is disturbed, and we have a leakage or exudation into the inflamed part.

"The principal method of treating inflammation a generation ago was the so-called **antiphlogistic treatment.** This was based on the theory that **inflammation was an inflammable condition** of the part, which, like a fire, **must be subdued** by appropriate measures. It did not take into account the causes of the process, which are now so much better understood. This method consisted in the use of emetics, venesection, cupping and leeching, and the administration of drugs, like mercury, which were supposed to have an antiphlogistic tendency. This method has given place to antiseptic treatment, which has the important advantage of dealing directly with the cause of disease. Some of the older measures are, however, still retained, and may occasionally be used to advantage in relieving some of the symptoms of inflammation. Counter-irritation was another of the weapons of the anti-phlogistic system, although much less used at the present time than formerly, has not been wholly discarded."

"The causes of the processes" are now no better understood by physicians than formerly. They do not "deal directly with the cause of disease."

The "**abstraction theory.**"

Venesection; blood-letting; the abstraction of blood.

The advocates of the **phlogiston doctrine** held to the hypothetical principle of **fire,** or inflammability, **regarded as a material substance.** According to this peculiar belief, every combustible (phlogisticated) substance is a compound of phlogiston, and the phenomena of combustion are due to the phlogiston, and sulphur as being very rich in it. This theory held sway for a century. The saphir was used as a phlogiston. From an old book, 1716. I copy in part: "It is either Oriental or Occidental, and of each there are Males and Females. The Oriental are found in Zeilan, Calecut, Bifnagar, Canaor, and Pegu, in which last place are the best. The Occidental are found in Silefia and Bohemia. It is a glorious, clear, tranfparent Blue, or Sky Colour'd Stone, thefe are the Males. The Females are white and unripe, fo they want Colour. The most tranfparent and deep Colour'd are eafily divefted of that Beauty by a little Heat of the Fire. It is cold and dry, aftringent, glutinative, ophthalmic, cordial, alexipharmic, and analeptic. It comforts and ftrengthens the Body, cures Difeafes of the Skin, caufes a good Colour, and refifts Melancholy and Witchcraft. Applied to the Pulfes it cures Agues. It cools inflammations, and dries up Rheums in the Eyes."

As I have said of the earliest conception of inflammation, so I could say of all phases of disease, that they were considered of an entity, a being of intelligence, one which was supposed to be "going to and fro in the earth." A good illustration is that of Job, 3543 years ago, whom satan "smote with sore boils from the sole of his foot unto his crown."

A. P. Davis in Osteopathy declares that "fever is only a symptom, and not a disease. Where is the trouble? What produces the fever? We regard fever as the result of chemical changes in the elements—friction of the molecules, due, in many instances to capillary disturbances, resulting in congestion, or hyperemia (which means too much blood in parts). Decomposition (tissue metamorphoses of a degenerative character) takes place, friction ensues, heat is the result.

"Whether obstructions occur as a result of changes in the weather, direct cold, or to continuous exposure of the body, or any part of it, to a lower temperature than normal, or to direct pressure, such as bandages, tight lacing, over-crowded vessels, impediment due to lack of fluidity of the blood, paralysis of nerves controlling the circulation in any or many parts of the body, any one or all of these causes may be and are the cause or causes of the pathological conditions that afflict mankind. **Our whole theory has its origin, support, conclusion, on this idea, this fundamental and unheard-of cause of disease, and perhaps unthought-of by other diagnosticians.** And while we would not desire to appear dogmatic in this regard, we firmly believe that **all pathologic conditions are traceable to obstructed circulation** somewhere in the system, and that removed, the patient has a better opportunity of recovery than from the possible influence of medication. It surely seems more rational to take off the pressure producing the pain of a morbid condition, than to impose more labor, to care for some other foreign substance that has no earthly relationship with the system, and can not possibly have, with the idea of the necessity involved in the premises. It is like goading an already over-burdened animal, or pressing the head of a drowning man under water to keep him from death! Oh, if we could induce the doctors to think!"

When Dr. Davis reads this article, he will see that his "theory" of "obstructed circulation" and "lack of fluidity of the blood," has been "thought-of" and "heard-of" by "diagnosticians" ever since Harvey discovered the circulation of the blood. "Oh, if we could induce the doctors to think!"

Dr. Davis further says: "In all fevers the friction is caused by decomposition of the elements.

"Fever.—The phenomena in the body characterized by a rise of temperature, increased circulation of the blood, marked tissue change to a greater or less degree, disturbance in the secretions, mental excitement or depression.

"The causes of fever are a mooted question. Many theories are advocated, but the most plausible seems to be that of central disturbance near the corpus striatum, due to blood pressure. The cause of the blood pressure is as much a mooted question as the cause of fever."

Potter says of fever: "The primary cause of the fever phenomena is still a mooted question, and is either a disorder of the sympathetic nervous system giving rise to disturbances of the vaso-motor filaments, or a derangement of the nerve-centers located adjacent to the corpus striatum, which have been found, by experiment, to govern the processes of heat-production, distribution, and dissipation."

Pathologists have considered effects as causes. A suppositious fluid, recognized as humor; chemical changes; capillary disturbances; congestion; occlusion; an unbalanced condition of the two forces, positive and negative, acid and alkaline; decomposition; friction and the Still combustion theory of gas; the acrimony of the fluids (sharp, acrid, corrosive quality, biting to the tongue); the condensation and rarefaction of solid tissue; the salutary explanation—inflammation, a physiological process, health restoring, reactionary and reparative, conservative in tendency and benigh in disposition; the arterial spasm theory; increased action of the blood vessels; obstructed circulation, accounted for by the accumulation of leukocytes, thickened or viscous quality of the blood, have been assigned as causes of inflammation and disease.

Is inflammation a symptom or a disease? Is fever a symptom or a disease?

A symptom is any perceptible change recognized by the senses in any organ or function connected with morbific influence.

Disease is a condition of the body marked by inharmonious action of one or more of the various organs, owing to abnormal condition or structural change.

I have examined many authors regarding the functions of the two brain ganglia, the corpus striata. A. P. Davis is the only one who designates their use, saying, "central disturbances **near** the corpus striatum." The why of the rise of temperature, chemical changes, capillary disturbance, heat and friction are wholly theoretical and a mooted question.

In Neuropathy, date 1909, A. P. Davis states: "Repeated suggestion will bring one under complete control of the suggester, is an undeniable fact; but how suggestion cures disease or in any way changes pathological conditions is not easily defined, described or understood. The fixed thought on any assertion, if believed, brings corresponding results. If all men who have disease had strong enough faith in their inherent recuperative powers to persist in the thought, and do the things necessary to carry out the thought, all functional ills would get out of the body and leave it 'swept and garnished.' Diseases seem to resolve themselves into a mental ideality, which may be eliminated by intense thought in the direction indicating such a desideratum. Many diseases have been permanently dispelled by this means. There is a power in this science which surpasses human comprehension, and can be positively used for good or harm."

Tone is a term used to denote a normal degree of vigor, tension, activity, strength and excitability of nerves and muscles, as observed in a state of health—the effect of tonicity. Tonicity determines the tone. Excessive tonicity causes an augmentation of vital phenomena; a deficiency of tonicity a want of tone, a loss or diminution of muscular or vital strength. The quality of irritability gives tone. Tone or tonicity is that normal tension which belongs to the involuntary nerves and muscles, the insensible irritation and contractility of the nervous and muscular systems manifested in the vital operations of circulation, transudation, secretion, nutrition and absorption.

Inordinate excitement of the moral and malevolent emotions unduly irritates the nervous system, both the voluntary and involuntary.

By nerve and muscle tone, I mean a continuous shortening or contraction, which under normal conditions is slight, varying from time to time. This condition is dependent upon the connection of the muscles with the nerve centers, which are continually sending nerve impulses into the muscles, the result is, the muscles have a continuous contraction known as tone. This normal tension plays an important part in controlling and furnishing the heat of the body. **By a disturbance of this**

**tone**—normal tension—**we have a condition known as inflammation.** The intensity of tone depends upon the amount of vibrations of the transmitting medium—nerves. It is well known that a gradually weaker and weaker sounding string exhibits a corresponding smaller amount of vibration. The intensity of a sound, or tone, corresponds to the degree of illumination of brightness to our vision.

Gregory defines inflammation: "An inflammation is a derangement of the trophic, thermic, and secretory action of an organ, which is due to pressure or irritation of the nerves.

"Four characteristic symptoms mark all inflammatory processes—viz., heat, pain, redness and swelling. Inflammation is the result of irritation and consequent excitation and derangement of the nerve supply."

Dr. Gregory should have said, and probably intended to state: "Derangement of the trophic, thermic, and secretory action of an organ is caused by inflammation." It is the excessive heat which causes deranged metabolic action.

Carver defines inflammation as a swelling accompanied by an elevated temperature, caused primarily by an occlusion. An occlusion is the state of being occluded, shut up, closed as the transient approximation of the edges of a natural opening, as of the eyelids. He says an occlusion may be the result of a displacement of a vertebra or vertebrae by direct injury, or the result of a motor reaction from some irritation producing a vertebral constriction and consequent occlusion of nerves, or it may be the result of an occlusion produced by a constriction resulting from a motor reaction from irritation of sensory nerves.

I presume the "vertebral constriction and consequent occlusion of nerves," referred to, is the closing of the intervertebral foramina. If so, they do not constrict, do not close an orifice or passage **by binding in a circular direction. Neither do they occlude or shut up.**

In 1905—five years ago—Friend Carver was a suggester (a woman is a suggestress). He believed in and practiced suggestive therapeutics. He wrote me: "There are a large number of ills which affect the human body that have nothing whatever to do, per se, with the bony structure."

Under date of March 2, 1910, Dr. Carver wrote Dr. Davis, "If you are anything, of course, you are a therapeutist. If so I am a scientist. You could not expect the two to agree, since there is not a single basic truth in the whole of therapy and I will give you a thousand dollars to disprove that statement." If the reader will turn to "Suggestive Therapeutics, "thon will see a radical change is Dr. Carver's views on therapeutics, but, like some others I might mention, he has gone off on another tangent which has no more to do with Chiropractic than had suggestive Therapeutics. I am glad to see the change and to know that he has outgrown therapeutics, replacing it with adjusting. Now, if Friend Carver will learn the fundamental principle of Chiropractic, then, build thereon, the science and philosophy, then learn specific adjusting, there will be no need of adding vagaries as adjuncts.

A. T. Still says: "Phosphorous with oxygen air, assisted by nerve and blood motion, aided by electricity produces a union between the oxygen and phosphorous and the addition of nitrogen which occupies much cellular space in the body, produces the combustion known as fever heat.

"As we line up to learn something of the causes of fever, we are met by heat, a living fact. Does that put the machinery of your mind in motion? If not, what will arouse your mental energy? You see that heat is not like cold. It is not a horse with eyes, head, neck, body, limbs and tail, but it is as much of a being as a horse. It is a being of heat. If cause made the horse and cause made the heat, why not devote energy in seeking the cause of both? Who says **heat is** not a **union** of the **human gases with oxygen and other substances** . . . how fast must the heart or life-current run to **ignite the gases of the body and set a person on fire to fever heat?** We know man is . . . a motor which would be incomplete if it could not burn its own gases.

"So far I think we are safe to say that all evidence is favorable to the fact that bones, teeth, muscles, tendons, nerves, blood-vessels, hair, and organs of the body have had their origin from gas, and are only condensed gas. **Now, we as chemists of good health, to succeed in curing our patients, must keep the gas-making machinery in good mechanical condition to do laboratory work, or we surely will fail to cure or even relieve our patients.**

"Is it not just as reasonable to suppose those high temperatures of the body are Nature's furnaces, making fires to burn out . . . these substances . . . in a gaseous form? What better effort could Nature offer than through its gas-generating furnace? I know of none that my reason can grasp.

"Fever is electric heat only."

While it is a fact, that thots are things, are entities, that we influence each other and ourselves for good or bad by our thinking, it is also a fact that it is a mental condition, in and of ourselves. It is one of the three methods I recognize of creating normal and abnormal nerve and muscle tension.

In auto-suggestion, as manifested in hysteria simulating almost every disease, we have results of pathological nerve tension. In auto-suggestion of so-called spiritual mediums, we get impromptu speeches and poetry.

The faculty of receiving mental impressions thru sensory or sense organs of the body, those of sight, hearing, smell, taste, touch, perception, apprehension, recognition, understanding, discernment and appreciation of our physical surroundings; the occult and spiritual of intuition and immediate perception of truth and immaterial insight; the internal of imagination and memory; the discriminating qualities of intensification, extension and temporal; the effective feeling of tone attaches to each sensation, determined by the amount of tension, is conscious intelligence. Physiological tension is the usual or normal; an over or under amount of strain is pathological. **The amount of nerve tension depends upon the position of individual bones of the osseous frame (the keyboard) to which the nerves are attached.**

---

"Spinal Adjustments the Wonder of the Age." P. W. Johnson.

---

If the readers of The Chiropractor's Adjuster will give to these articles containing new advanced thoughts on the science of Chiropractic, one tenth of the hard study that I did in digging them out, they can surely comprehend and make them their own. How contemptible, mean, and sordid to say that I steal these ideas from some unknown source as fast as I advance them. Can't my accusers find the source from which I draw these ideas? If so, they can assist instead of hindering me, and cease being jealous of honor justly due one who is not only willing but dares to study.

---

The Adjuster finds a portion of an eight-page booklet by a D. C. is Chiropractic and some is not.

In part he says: "Chiropractic is the discovery of D. D. Palmer in the year 1895. He discovered and perfected the art of Chiropractic adjusting. Chiropractic is a science of spinal adjusting. Ninety-five per cent of deranged functions are made so by displacements of joints in the spinal column, causing pressure on nerves."

Those who are going to put out literature may profit by the study of our criticisms. Do not copy; you should be able to compose a few pages, even if it takes you days to do it.

"Chiropractors use the **spinal** processes and **handles** to adjust these displacements."

The process which extends posteriorly from the laminae of the vertebra in which it is rooted, is never called "a **spinal** process." This process is so named because it has the form of a thorn or spine. Spinal is an adjective and always pertains to the spine or backbone. Hence, we say spinal column, spinal canal, spinal cord, spinal nerves, spinal artery, spinal veins, but never **spinal** process. Chiropractors never use the processes as handles, but as levers and the axial centers as fulcra.

"The Chiropractor is a master mechanic, curing disease by mechanical adjustment."

By adjusting he removes the cause of disease, thereby relieving the patient of his illness.

"Disease **is always** due to some form of vertebral sub-luxation."

About 95 per cent of diseases are due to vertebrae being racked out of alignment; the remainder is caused by sub-luxations of other joints. An example of the latter cause is the case of a sprained knee which a student has just relieved by one adjustment. Replacing the projecting portion of the knee which was impinging upon a nerve gave immediate relief.

"**Chiropractic** has been **used in the treatment** of diseases."

Diseases are treated by a great many remedies; but I have never known Chiropractic to be used for such a purpose. You can treat a disease or its symptoms, but a disease or symptom cannot be adjusted.

"This **new** science deals mostly with cases that **all other schools of healing** had failed to **cure.**"

Chiropractic is not a "**new**" science. The principles of which it is composed are as old as the vertebrata. "All other schools of healing." Chiropractors do not "heal," they are not "healers": salves heal. They do not "cure," charms cure. Medicines cure by virtue of the hidden magic contained therein.

"Dr. Palmer says: 'All aches, pains and miseries are the impressions of the nerves.' "

He should have quoted "There is not an ache or pain which is not the sensation of nerves." Nerves never impress or make an effect on the senses of the intellect. Sensations are the consciousness of impressions.

"All acts or movements of any part of the body are done by **brain impulses.**"

He should have copied correctly, if at all. "All acts of any part of the body are functions performed by nerves." According to Chiropractic the **apparent origin** of impulses is in the brain, but Innate is the originator and distributor of them.

## PATHOLOGICAL PHYSIOLOGY.

Pathological processes are but variations of physiological actions, modifications of physiological functions. General physiology refers to the normal laws of life; special physiology to the nature and functions of certain specified organs. Physiology is also qualified as normal or hygiene physiology in contradistinction to morbid or pathological physiology.

Pathology is subdivided into etiology, the cause of disease, and morbid or pathological anatomy, which considers structural changes other than normal. Morbid or pathologic physiology refers to the disturbance of functions, their variation from normal. Pathology is divided into general and special pathology. The former treats of the cause of disease, or pathologic conditions irrespective of any individual part; the latter specializes it as referring to a certain organ or portion. Thus, fever is a diseased state or condition found present in many diseases—general pathology. Typhoid fever is a febrile condition with definite symptomatology—special pathology. General pathology deals with certain diseased processes of tissue or functions common to the whole organism, as degeneration, gangrene, etc., and special pathology to diseases of certain specialized organs. To comprehend pathology, we should have a clear and accurate knowledge of normal physiology and normal anatomy. Physiology is that subdivision of biology which considers life in its normal relations, while pathology studies it in its variations from the normal.

Health exists when the normally constructed body properly performs its functions. Disease is a condition in which the organs or organism is abnormally related to internal or external influences which relates to our welfare, physically, mentally or spiritually. Disease is, therefore, a general term signifying any variation from the normal either in functions or tissue or both. An alteration of function cannot occur without a corresponding change in the structure of tissue. It is possible, however, that the structural change in the functionary organ may be so slight as to remain undetected by the most precise method of differential diagnosis known by pathological investigators.

Nevertheless, Chiropractors, when confronted by a condition of this kind, should be able to locate the bone lesion and the sensitive, enlarged, contracted, tense, rigid, nerve that is impinged upon.

When we specialize disease by giving it a name, we recognize a certain type of abnormality which is characterized by the occurrence of definite phenomena.

Morbid or pathological anatomy refers to gross anatomy as studied by direct observation without the aid of a microscope. Morbid histology contemplates the minute structure as revealed by the microscope. Normal histology is the study of the structure of healthy tissue.

All functional acts necessary for the production of vital phenomena result from the releasing of stored energy. The storing and liberating of energy in health is under certain fixed and definite conditions. The amount of stored energy depends upon the capacity of the organ and its absorbing quality; the quantity liberated makes possible all expressions of life in any degree ever known.

Superstitious ideas concerning health, disease, life and death have been perpetuated by unthinking persons. The superstitious belief that disease is an entity, something foreign to the body which may enter it from without; that diseases is goetic, magical; that wizards, witches, sorcerers and sorceresses, possess a supernatural or magical power and have a compact with devils, demons and evil spirits to use this power to injure destroy mankind and animals, and thru their devilish black art and magic, stir up storms, damage crops, bring sickness and death, confound and change the laws of nature; and all this by an express agreement with the evil ones; that disease is a creature of intelligence with which the body must struggle, fight and conquer, or succumb to its ravages, is no longer tenable.

Students of Chiropractic should constantly remember that disease is not a thing, but a condition. It is an abnormal performance of certain morphological alterations of the body. Agencies and conditions which the body cannot adapt itself to, sway the capacities of energy above or below normal, inducing the functional aberrations and structural alterations known as disease.

The symptoms of disease are the expressions of abnormal functional activity—pathological physiology. Functional abnormalities, structural changes, make up the signs, symptoms and lesions of disease. A symptom serves to point out the nature, character and seat of disease; it is a subjective manifestation in contradistinction to a physical sign which is objective. The signs of disease may be objective or physical, apparent to the examiner of the patient; or subjective, perceptive only to the one affected. We study disease by the symptoms exhibited. A lesion is an injury, hurt or wound in any part of the body, or a morbid change in the exercise of functions or the texture of organs. Lesions do not involve any expression of function which the normal body does not already possess; they are simply diminished or increased, perverted or abolished. The body in disease, manifests no new functions, develops no new forms of energy. It has acquired only an abnormal capacity. The body as an organism is incapable of creating any new forces. It is able to accumulate and store energy direct from without, in its organs or organism, and release it under established and restricted conditions.

There is a subtle transmission of physiological impulses, which by augmentation or diminution may become pathological. This modification, from health to disease, has been a tenuous, complex problem for pathologists. The interrelationship of innervation, circulation and transudation, which the organs share in common, have very important bearings upon morphology, functions expressed physiologically and pathologically.

When studying the etiology of disease, we should remember, that underlying the manifestations of health and disease, are, the ceaseless, complex vital transformations which supply energy in varying amounts, which maintain life as expressed in health and disease.

Impingements, poisons and intense thinking, auto-suggestion, unrelieved change of thot, insufficient rest and sleep, increase or decrease the momentum of impulses. In the study of pathology we should look to the etiological factors which, by their exciting or debilitating effects, retard or liberate stored up energy, resulting in abnormal functionating and morbid structure.

Functional disturbance is known as pathological physiology, a condition recognized by the symptoms presented. Pathological morphology deals with the abnormal forms, relations, metamorphoses and phylogenetic development of organs—the organs apart from their functions. Pathological morphology includes morbid anatomy, pathological histology and embryonic malformations.

The determining cause of disease are traumatism, poison and auto-suggestion.

Trauma, singular (traumata, plural), a wound or injury or lesion. A lesion, however, also, means a pathological alteration of tissue. Traumatic means pertaining to, or caused by, a wound or injury. A traumatic medicine is used for the cure of wounds. A traumatic cataract is one due to injury. Traumatic fever is caused by a wound—not by poison. Traumatic inflammation is due to an injury, usually to fractures of the long bones. The displaced fragments cause pressure, impingement upon nerves, tension being the result. Fever is diffused inflammation. Lesions caused by physical agencies are said to be traumatic. Traumatic suggestion is a peculiar condition occurring after a railroad accident attributed to auto-suggestion; so says the railroad attorney. A dislocation is traumatic when it is the result of violence; pathological when the bones have become displaced by destructive changes in the joint. A traumatic back is a condition marked by tenderness, pain on movement, and spasm of the rector spinae muscle, due to a blow or wrench. Traumatism is a morbid condition of the system due to trauma, the condition of one suffering from injury.

Chiropractors are especially concerned in traumatism, because of the fact that all displaced osseous tissue is attended with modification of temperature, either above or below normal. All diseases are the result of altered temperature; temperature variation depends upon the amount of nerve tension and abnormal nerve tension upon traumatism.

Poison is any animal, vegetable or mineral substance which, when applied externally or taken into the body by ingestion or injection, causes such a change in the animal economy as to produce abnormal functionating, disease or death.

Irritant or acid poisoning, produces tension, a stretched, or strained condition of stiffness of nervous tissue, nerve irritation or inflammation. Narcotic poisons produce stupor or delirium due to loss of sensibility, a suspended or diminished activity of the sensory nerves. A sedative poison is one which directly reduces the vital powers, lowers functional activity.

In auto-suggestion, which is also known as psychological suggestion and traumatic suggestion, the will and judgment are more or less suppressed and auto-traumatic action is directed to any organ or portion of the body, thereby modifying bodily functions, exciting or relieving morbid conditions by mental processes independently of external influence. This condition is due to an underlying psychical impressionability exhibited in paralysis, contracture of muscles, impairment of vision, sensory and functional disturbance, more or less of the nervous system.

All acts or functions are performed by muscles under the control of the nervous system. Tonicity is the normal condition or tone or tension which gives to each organ or tissue its proper firmness.

The neuro-skeleton, the endo-skeleton, or the true skeleton, serves to protect the whole of the nervous system, more especially the central nervous system. The endo-skeleton and the exo-skeleton in animals are frame-supports for the soft tissue. In man the neuro-skeleton affords special protection to the cerebral and spinal portions and by extension it affords tone to the whole nervous system and firmness to the viscera of the four cavities. If any portion of this neuro-(nerve)skeleton is displaced it modifies the tension or tone of that portion of the nervous system which it normally supports. This being the case, Chiropractors should have a knowledge of muscles, nerves and bones.

---

When a person is suffering with boils on the neck for weeks or months it is because the cutaneous nerves of the neck, which spring from the spinal cord and remain as spinal nerves, are impinged upon by a cervical vertebra which has been wrenched from its normal position. We find the vertebra which causes the impingement and give relief by replacing it.

In neuralgia of the face, tic douloureux, an affection of the facial division of the 7th cranial nerve, we trace the cause back through the posterior auricular nerve and from thence to the 2d and 3d cervical.

If we find the lining membrane of the nose, the tonsils, the soft or hard palate affected, we know that such conditions are because the palatine branch distributes too much or not enough function. We trace the palatine branch back through Meckel's ganglion, the Vidian nerve, through the spheno-palatine ganglion. This has motor, sensory and sympathetic communicants. We still pursue this disturbed filament to the spheno-palatine branch, from thence to the superior maxillary branch, then to the Gasserian (semilunar) ganglion, through the carotid plexus and the superior cervical ganglion, through the intervertebral foramen between the 3d and 4th cervical vertebrae. If you prefer, you can trace this nerve anatomically from the cervical to the palatine branch. To be sure, the digital examination, the tracing by palpation answers all practical purposes; but it is quite satisfactory to know the ramification of an affected nerve.

---

Baker City, Ore., February 18, 1909.

Dr. D. D. Palmer: Dear Sir and Doctor—I shall be glad to know what "**Innate**" has to do with **governing the body**, and **controlling the functions.** Do you mean by "**Innate,**" **mind?**

If there is an **inborn** something that **controls the body, mind being a product, and it controls,** does it not follow that **more than one thing controls? How is this?**

I would be glad to know what particular move is calculated to **do harm—when adjustments are made?** If adjustments **free** the impingements what are the results but freedom of the **nerve-filaments**, so **they can carry the intelligence to their endings**—where function is performed?

I think the idea of "**harm,**" **as a result** of "adjustment," is an unsafe idea to present to the world—or to be taught to a class.

My eye is seemingly getting better—film thinner. I can see **more of what I see** plainer—a little more distinctly.

Kind regards to your good wife, self and the class.

Sincerely yours, A. P. DAVIS.

A. P. Davis, N. D., Oph. D.: I am pleased to answer your questions. There may be many of our readers who have these self-same questions in mind.

Innate has all to do with the control of the vital functions, and thru them, indirectly, the control of the intellectual functions. Innate is not the mind. Innate is the intelligence back of and controller of the mind as well as of every thought.

There is an inborn intelligence in every living being, and in every plant that grows. Mind is a product of Innate, and is sane or insane in proportion as the nervous mass, the encephalon, and its radiating branches, the nerves, possesses normal or abnormal carrying capacity.

Harm can be done; the diseased condition can be augmented, as well as decreased; or other diseased conditions may be created. The nerves which contain filaments that find their way to the eyeball, emerge from the right side of the dorsal vertebrae, where they are liable to be impinged upon after they have left the intervertebral foramen and have entered the sympathetic ganglion. If the vertebra is racked by the adjuster so as to increase the impingement, "harm is done."

You should have noticed that I always stood on your right and used the spinous process as a lever, throwing it toward the left shoulder. To have reversed this movement would have increased the tension. Adjustments free impingements if the movement is such as will take the pressure from the nerve, otherwise the impingement is made greater.

It is unsafe and unwise to teach adjusting, unless it is taught intelligently. Much harm, as well as good, has been done by those who know nothing of it as a **specific science.**

Innate "uses the sympathetic nervous system" as channels through which to transmit its orders, the actions resulting from these directions, whether normal or abnormal, are what we are pleased to name functions. Actions are not executed thru the nervous system by mental control—the mind.

## TONE AND FUNCTIONS.

What is the basic principle of Chiropractic, the elementary proposition from which all other principles of Chiropractic have sprung? It is tone.

What is tone. Normal tension.

What is tension? It is the renitency, the elasticity of tissue in a healthy state.

What is renitent? It is the normal resisting pressure acting against an impulse by elastic force, known as tonicity.

What is tonicity? It is the state of healthy tension or partial, normal, contraction of muscles, ligaments and nerves.

What is contraction? It is the shortening of living fibers with consequent thickening by the application of a stimulus; it may be traumatic, toxic, auto or nervous.

What is a stimulus? It is anything which rouses or excites the vital energies of an organ or part of the body to increased functional activity.

What is energy? It is the power to produce action, the ability to overcome resistance.

What is functional activity? It is the action of an organ, whether physiological or pathological.

From whence does this power originate. It is inherent and dependent upon the tension of the organ whose function is being performed.

What is physiological action? The normal functionating of the body or organs.

What is pathological action? It is vital action expressed in too great a degree, or of less than normal, resulting abnormal functionating and morbid tissue.

What is morbid tissue? The tissue of an organ in disease. Morbid is used as a technical or scientific term in contradistinction to the term healthy.

What is disease? A condition consisting of a change in position, or structure of a part or an organ, also, a change in one or more of its functions. Abnormal functions and morbid tissue are co-existent.

What view does the medical man take of disease? "An abnormal condition, general or local, marked by more or less characteristic changes of structure and function, generally having a definite cause, and running a more or less typical course, so, it may be considered as a distinct entity; a vigorous effort of nature to throw off morbific matter, and thus to recover the patient."

What are the most prominent symptoms of disease? Increased or decreased respiration, temperature and pulse. The vital tripod, the tripod of life, consists of the heart, lungs and brain;

so named because their united action is necessary to the maintenance of life.

Why are abnormal functions and morbid tissue contemporaneous? Because normal and abnormal tissue can only perform functions becoming their condition; their structure and function depending upon their tension.

Why are not the functions of respiration, pulsation and temperature equally affected in disease? Because the impingement, poison or auto-suggestion may not make a like change in the tension of the innervating nerves of all.

---

"Function is any specific power of action which belongs to an agent. The operator is behind the energy which is the cause of action. This definition covers the two functions of energy—vital and intellectual. The vegetative and cumulative functions are not those of energy; they consist in the performance of the two functions of force. The energy which innervates these functions is the vital. Pressure on nerves breaks the continuity of its molecules and renders it unable to transmit vibrations or impulses."

Before offering any criticisms on the above, I shall define some special terms.

**Thots** are entities; they exist, are created by imagination, reflection, meditation, judgment and reason; they are elaborated.

The power or force of thot depends upon its momentum, and the momentum upon the impetus received from nerve vibration during transmission. Vibration receives its force from the amount of heat contained in nerves. The quantity of heat depends upon the tension and tension upon excitation. Normal stimulus is furnished by Innate, the spirit, a segment of Universal Intelligence. Too much or too little excitation, stimulation, is the result of pressure and nerve toxication.

An **impulse** is a spontaneous incitement arising from the feelings of the mind or spirit in the form of an **abrupt and vivid suggestion prompting some premeditated action. An impulse suddenly starts or drives a thot forward to action.** Morbid impulses are qualified as animal, destructive, homicidal, suicidal, uncontrollable and especially those of an insane character. Impulse denotes action, not an entity.

**Function** is the special and normal action of any organ or part of a living animal. This includes the natural action of any mental faculty. Pathological functions are those performed in a greater or lesser degree than normal.

**Force** is that power which produces or arrests motion, that which may be converted into motion, the rate of transforming energy.

**Vitality** is the vigorous active principle upon which individual life depends.

**Vital force** is that principle of life which imparts energy. It is inherent in each organ of an organism.

**Energy** is the internal, inherent power, the product of activity, that which is aroused by one's feelings.

**Nerve-vibration** carries thots, the commands, the orders—**not impulses. Impulses liberate thots, start them into action.**

An impulse refers to the thot which is carried, or to the vibratory wave-movement of the nerve by which it is transferred.

**Thots gather force, an impetus,** while being transmitted; the amount depending upon the quantity of nerve-vibration.

**Momentum** is the force of motion acquired by the movement of thots, the impetus received from nerve-vibration.

Tone is the normal activity, strength and excitability of the various organs and functions as observed in health. A response of tonicity.

Tonicity is the normal elasticity of the filamentary or thread-like structures of the body.

To **innervate** is to supply with nerve-force. To **enervate** is to deprive of nerve-force.

The above quoted paragraph refers to physiology, that branch of biology dealing with the processes, activities and phenomena incidental to, and characteristic of life, or of living organisms; as such we shall criticise it.

In the first sentence the author should have used the word organ instead of agent, as he referred to physiology—not to law. When writing upon any subject, we ought to be technical, otherwise our language lacks proper expression and force.

In the second sentence, we are told that energy is the cause of action. On the contrary, energy is the product of activity. The principle, Innate or spirit, the creator, the originator, is behind thot. **Impulse is the prime mover of thot. The force of thot rouses energy to action.** Energy is the capacity for performing function.

My criticism of the third sentence is that energy has no individualized functions to perform. The words vital and intellectual should be used as adjectives; they tell what kind of energy.

The fourth sentence is misleading. The vegetative function is one of physical growth. The cumulative is of the mental, corresponding to the vegetative; it is mental growth. These two functions are dependent upon the organism as a whole, not upon one quality.

The fifth sentence teaches an error. ' Energy does not innervate functions. Functions are aroused, stimulated into activity by the force of thots.

The sixth and last sentence is incorrect, inasmuch, as **nerve-vibration and impulses are not transmitted.** Nerve-vibration, like the vibrations of the strings of an instrument, may be increased or decreased, but not transferred; it may become pathological—disease producing. As we have said, **impulses are not transmitted**; it is the function of an impulse to start, suddenly impel or drive thots forward, causing immediate motion. **Impulses act on thots and have to do with the motor nerves only.**

The ganglia may be considered as small brains, or nerve centers, and like the great ganglionic nerve-center—the brain, are centers of nervous action, relay stations, depots for the exchange of sensation from sensory nerves to that of motion on the motor nerves, impulse being the same in function in the smaller brains as in the greater. Sensation, or impressions —**not impulses**—are transferred from the peripheral nerve-endings to their appropriate ganglia, which are found on the posterior, sensory roots of each spinal nerve and on the posterior sensory root of the fifth cranial nerve. The motor roots have no transferring stations.

"Students of Chiropractic have no occasion to know materia medica, theory and practice of medicine, medical chemistry, surgery or obstetrics, therefore, we do not take up these branches."

Chemistry is the science which treats of the elements and atomic relations of matter, and of the various compounds of the elements. Analytic chemistry deals with the analysis of substances. Synthetical chemistry has to do with the building-up of substances from their constituents. This includes all there is of chemistry. Some add inorganic chemistry, that branch which deals with non-organized bodies. This is included in the above two forms of chemistry. Mineral chemistry is also included under the first two. Organic chemistry deals with organic substances, not the vital principle of organs. To these some physiologists add that of physiological chemistry, the chemistry of nutrition, the changes wrought upon nutrition by chemotaxis, positive and negative chemotaxis. It is an impossibility to analyze or compound chemically any part of a living body. That which is referred to—"chemistry of nutrition"—is metalobism. Metabolism is vital and chemistry non-vital, they are in no way related, they have no similarity; one is physiological and the other chemical.

"Subjects taught: Anatomy, histology, osteology, physiology, hygiene, bacteriology, Chiropractic principles, orthopedia, diagnosis, nerve tracing, clinic, symptomatology."

Histology is the minute or microscopic study of anatomy—useless to a Chiropractor. As to hygiene: the Innate Intelligence which runs all the digestive functions knows far more in regard to them than we will ever know; so, let Innate run them. Students of Chiropractic have no occasion to know "bacteriology." Orthopedia as known in books is not Chiropractic; Chiropractic orthopedy is quite another thing. A "clinic" is not a subject to be studied; it includes instruction at the bedside, or in the class-room, on the condition of a patient who is present.

"The brain covers itself by a number of bones."

The brain is incased; but it did not do that work of itself.

"The spinal cord incases itself within hollow bones, twenty five in number."

The occipital bone has a foramen magnum and each of the twenty-four vertebrae has a spinal foramen. The vertebrae are not hollow; they have no empty space within, or a cavity; they are not excavated on the interior, as is a hollow tree. The spinal cord does not pass thru the foramen magnum, but that foramen surrounds the medulla oblongata. The spinal cord does not extend below the lower border of the first lumbar vertebra, nor above the upper surface of the atlas, hence twenty vertebrae incase the spinal cord instead of twenty-five.

"Emanating from these openings are the great trunk nerves that ramify and absolutely control every organ of the viscera and every portion of the tissue."

If the thirty-one pairs of the great spinal trunk nerves control every organ within the four great cavities, the cranium, thorax, abdominal cavity, pelvis and the somatic portion, what is there left for the cranial and the sympathetic nerves to do? What about the organs of the eye, nose and ear? Are they controlled by these spinal trunk nerves?

"Each one of these trunk nerves has a specific function to perform."

There are sixty-two of these trunk-nerves—sixty-two functions to perform—pray tell me what performs the balance of the multitudinous functions?

"Each cerebro-spinal nerve-trunk controls a certain organ or portion of the body."

There are thirty-two teeth, each one is an organ with a certain function to perform; this leaves only thirty nerve-trunks for other organs and portions—there is not near enough to go around.

"The science of adjusting."

Adjusting is an art, not a science. The science is the know-how and the art is the doing.

"The free flow of nerve stimuli is cut off, the nerves are shriveled, and disease of the organs to which these nerves lead is the inevitable result."

Stimuli does not flow, it is not a fluid. Functional energy is inherent in the organ or organism. It does not flow, is not obstructed, occluded or cut off. Nerves do not shrivel, do not shrink or wrinkle; they do not become corrugated. Leaves shrivel in the hot sun; the skin shrivels with age. Nerves may become lax or tense, but shrivel—never.

"These handles I use in adjusting **mis**placed vertebrae."

The spinous and transverse processes have not the appearance, use or function of handles; however, we may use them as levers by which to rack displaced vertebrae into their normal position.

Vertebrae are not **mis**placed; they may be **dis**placed, moved out of the place where they properly belong. We misplace an article when we put it where it should not be; we misplace our confidence; what we have misplaced we do not know where to find. Vertebrae moved out of place are displaced.

"Shutting off the life current."

A current runs, moves and flows; life does neither. Chiropractors have no use for a person who has the life shut off. Chiropractors should think twice before they write books or attempt to teach Chiropractic.

"Vertebrae become slightly out of normal apposition, partially closing one or more of the spinal windows, and impinging certain trunk nerves, which restricts the flow of the life-giving power from the brain to the organ which those nerves ramify."

Parts are said to be in apposition or contact, as the edges of a wound or the fragments of a bone. Apposition is a wrong term to use to express the displacement of a vertebra. The spine has no windows, no openings for the admission of light and air. "Life-giving power" does not "flow from the brain to the organ." Thots and impressions are the only entities which are transmitted over nerves. Impressions are transmitted inward and thots outward by vibration.

"Release the impinged nerves and allow the unoccluded life impulse to be conveyed to all parts of the body."

Instead of releasing the impinged nerve, "why not remove the impinging bone? Webster's latest dictionary does not know such a word as "unoccluded." To occlude is to close or shut up. "Unoccluded life impulse" would mean not to have the impulses of life shut up. That must be some of that "strictly pure unadulterated Chiropractic."

## SPASM.

Spasms, cramps and convulsions are terms used interchangeably. A spasm is a sudden, violent, involuntary, rigid, muscular contraction. When persistent, continuous, tension or rigidity and immobility of the muscles exist, it is called partonia or tonic spasm. Clonic spasms, which consist of alternate contracture and relaxation of the affected muscle or muscles, are of various degrees of severity. The mildest variety of clonic muscular contraction is termed tremor. If very widespread they are spoken of as convulsions, as seen typically in epilepsy. A sudden but transitory contraction of a passage, canal or orifice is known as a spasm. Some kinds are attended by pain, derangement of function, involuntary movements and distortion.

There are many forms of spasm, the most prominent of which are the following: Spasm of the ciliary (eyelid) muscles, producing excess of visual **accommodation** of near-by objects—Adjust third cervical. **Athetoid** spasm, in which there is a continuous movement of the fingers and toes, usually found in children. **Bell's** convulsive facial tic, a spasmodic movement or twitching of the face. See tic douloureux, a spasmodic, facial neuralgia. In **blepharofacial** spasm there are paroxysmal spastic contractions of the obicularis palpebrarum and other facial muscles. This spasm often tightly closes the lids. Generally in children there is also photophobia with the spasm of the eyelids, which is often tonic in character and generally bilateral. **This condition has associated with it spots near the supra-orbital foramen or over the vertebrae, which, when pressed on, cause sudden relaxation of the spasm.** These should always be sought for, as they aid in locating the lesion and giving relief to the patient. **Bronchial** spasm, known as asthma, which see. Spasm of the stomach, **cardialgia,** which see. **Canine** or cynic spasm, a tetanic grin or involuntary smile; adjust third cervical. **Carpopedal** spasm of the wrist or foot, thumb or large toes; adjust fourth dorsal. **Cholera morbus, colic convulsive;** griping pain in the bowels, accompanied by vomiting, purging and colic, occurring in the hot months; a manifestation of food poisoning; adjust some one of the vertebra from the sixth dorsal to second lumbar. **Chorea,** St. Vitus dance, is characterized by spasmodic and convulsive contraction, jerking and non-rythmic actions of the muscles of the face and limbs; see chorea. **Croup spasms,** spasmodic affection of the chest and larynx, accompanied by suffocating convulsions, usually occurring between the third and ninth month, characterized by great difficulty in breathing and a loud, croupy noise on inspiration; adjust fifth dorsal. **Enterospasm,** spasmodic constipation; enteralgia may be present; the stools may assume the form of a ribbon, or of rounded masses and may be covered with mucus. These conditions are pathognomonic. The Chiropractor would look to the second lumbar for an impingement on the nerves which go to those parts, creating these conditions. **Epilepsy** is a chronic functional disease characterized by spasms or fits, in which there is loss of consciousness and the power of coordination of motion, with a succession of tonic or clonic convulsions. Mental and physical traumatism are the causes. **Ergotism** or ergotismus is a chronic poisoning from excessive use of ergot as a medicine or from the eating of bread made from spurred rye, ergotized grain; it is marked by cerebro-spinal symptoms, spasms and cramps: ergot is a dark purple club-shaped body which is found in the place of rye grain; ergot is used as a medicine on account of its contractile effects; ergotism is manifested by severe cramps in the muscles of the legs, ending in tonic contraction—spasms. Facial or mimic spasms, a clonic contraction and relaxation of the muscles supplied by the facial nerve. It may involve the entire side of the face, or only around the eye; see facial paralysis. **Habit** spasm, consists of grimaces, winking, twitching of certain muscles of the face, a quick toss of the head and sometimes a peculiar sniff; adjust third cervical. **Hydrophobia,** a specific infectious disease, peculiar to carnivora, which may be communicated to the herbivora and man. It is characterized by slight fever, spasm of the larynx and pharynx, delirium, paralysis, coma and death. **Hysteric** tonic spasm. One of the many and varied symptoms of hysteria, consciously or unconsciously; a functional disorder not dependable upon any discoverable lesion. A disease mainly of impressionable young women, known as feigned disease, caused by auto-suggestion. Hysteria presents every variety of motor, sensory and psychic symptoms. It is distinguished by morbid self-consciousness, an exaggeration of the effects of sensory impressions and simulation of various disorders. The patient using hysterical auto-suggestional effects to induce sympathy or concessions. A cure is effected by complying with her request, or by adjusting a bucket of cold water to her person to arouse her to self-consciousness and a normal condition. There is no danger of the patient having an attack when alone. Future attacks may be warded off by reminding her of the water treatment. Anders says of this feigned, wilful simulation of disease, thru malice, or for the purpose of attaining a desired end: "A condition of the general nervous system partaking of the natures of both a neurosis and a psychosis, and characterized by a vast multiplicity of clinical manifestations, all indicative of a loss of voluntary control over the inhibitory will-powers. Hysteria is to be regarded as essentially a morbid entity, without, however, any tangible pathologic features. The most careful postmortem examinations of subjects who have while in life manifested pronounced hysteric symptoms have failed to reveal any organic nervous alterations, however slight. The occurrence of the affliction in men as well as in women excludes the former theory of a uterine pathology, which, though an idle fancy, held sway for many centuries and gave origin to the name by which the condition is generally recognized. A curious phenomena that is worthy of mention is the apparent contagiousness of hysteria; moreover, the baleful influence one neurotic individual exerts over the unfortunates of this temperament, explains the so-called 'hysteric epidemics' that have swept over communities, and even over vast tracts of land or entire countries, at different periods of the world's history. Similar, though limited, outbreaks may still be seen in the nervous wards of hospitals or in religious and political conventions, and these depend largely upon the general prevalence of the neurotic disposition untempered by a virile will-power. The hysteric temperament may be, and often is fostered by improper and pernicious modes of life, especially by luxurious and sensuous living and by the habit of gratifying every desire of the will during early life. It is manifested at this early stage of the individual's existence by hyper-sensitiveness, brilliancy, undue enthusiasm, and a more or less erratic turn of mind. A very influential factor in the production of the disease is the lack of proper mental development. It stands to reason that those who are sensitive, yet illiterate, and who have not been taught the lessons of self-denial and self-control, and who are subject to the various and multiplex superstitions that are ever prevalent among the masses, will respond more quickly and more generally to the causes that tend to destroy mental equilibrium. Hence, hysteria or insanity shows its rankest development among those whose education and culture are defective. This is, however, by no means an inevitable law, for over-stimulation of the faculties may be just as deleterious as under-stimulation, and some of the brightest lights of the world have manifested at various periods of their lives decided hysteric symptoms. True hysteric patients never die of the disease, nor does the hysteric spasm ever result fatally. As to an ultimate cure, however, the prognosis is very doubtful.'' I will say that the cold water treatment is effectual. On one occasion I used a hose that was handy, to the surprise and immediate relief of the patient. She complained of her clothing being wet, but was assured that the cold water was an unfailing remedy; that her clothes would not be considered. That was her last spell of hysteria. **Lock** spasm, a form of writer's cramp in which the fingers become rigidly contracted upon the pen; adjust third or fourth dorsal. **Masticatory** spasm may be tonic or clonic. In tonic spasm, trismus or lockjaw, the jaw is firmly set, the muscles hard, rigid and sometimes painful. When clonic, it is more or less continuous or intermittent. The tongue or cheeks may be bitten during the attack. In acute cerebral meningitis, which may be due to traumatism or toxins, there may be ptosis, squint, optic neuritis, facial paralysis, or spasm of the muscles at the back of the neck; adjust third cervical. **Nictitation,** winking spasm, an involuntary winking or twitching of the fibers of the obicularis (eyelid) muscle. To the transient flickering of a few muscle fibers, the term myokymia is applied. It is most often seen in the obicularies palpebrarum; it is an indication of fatigue or debility; adjust third cervical. **Nodding spasm,** a clonic spasm of the sternomastoid muscles; see nodding spasm. The spasms in **pallagra** are due to poisoning by eating contaminated corn meal bread. **Paramyoclonus multiplex,** a convulsive tremor characterized by clonic spasms in a number of symmetrical muscles. The spasms cease during sleep and do not interfere with voluntary movements. It is hysterical, choreic or due to a central vertebral lesion. Perineal spasm, vaginodynia, muscular contraction of the whole vaginal canal. In vaginismus the contraction is merely at the introitus; adjust second or third lumbar. **Phonetic** spasm of the glottis, spastic aphonia, an interference with respiration; adjust third cervical. **Saalam,** salatory spasm of the leg, causing a jumping or springing movement; adjust fourth or fifth lumbar. **Sewing** spasm, an affection of tailors, seamstresses and shoemakers, in which tonic or clonic spasms affect the forearm and hand when attempting to use them; adjust third or fourth cervical. **Smith's** spasm, hepistic-hemiplegia, occurs in those engaged in the manufacturing of cutlery. It consists of spasmodic movements of the arm, final paralysis of the affected member; adjust fourth or fifth dorsal. **Synclonic** or synclonus spasm, paralysis agitans, a tremulous, simultaneous, chronic agitation of various muscles; see paralysis agitans. **Tetanus,** emprosthotonos, a form of tetanus which brings the head and feet forward and the whole body tense; pleuro-thotonos, a tetanic bending of the body to one side; opisthotonos, a form of tetanic spasm in which the head and heels are bent backward and the body bowed forward. From the fact that the affection is of the extremities, as well as the whole body, I would look to "center place" the sixth dorsal. **Tetany,** painful tonic spasm of the muscles of the extremities. It occurs after typhoid fever and excision of the thyroid gland and in rickets. The fingers, hands and wrists are the parts usually affected. Tetanic spasm is observed in its completest form in strychnine poisoning, hydrophobia and some forms of hysterical fits; adjust sixth dorsal. **General tic** is a spasmodic affectation which is considered wholly psychic in nature and character. It consists of apparently purposeful coordinated spasmodic movements, explosive sounds or words and imperative ideas without intellectual disturbance. The patient may repeat many times some apparently purposeful and coordinated movement as tho brushing flies away. They may make sounds as tho imitating some animal, as the barking of a dog or crowing of a cock, or the repetition of some word. Thon may imitate sounds just heard or movements observed. The **tongue** is subject to spasms. They may be bilateral or unilateral; it is usually associated with other affections. **Torticollis,** spasmodic wry-neck; see wry-neck. **Toxic** spasms, those caused by the action of poisons. Poison may enter a wound; if so, the lesion is toxic; adjust according to the kind of poison, the place of entrance and the part affected. For egested poisons, those taken into the stomach, adjust the sixth dorsal, standing on the left side and throw to the right shoulder. **Traumatic** tetanus or spasm is one following a wound. **Writers'** palsy or cramp, known as pen-palsy, a clonic contraction of the muscles of the fingers, professional neurosis, a kind of stammering, a functional spasm of the fingers, in which they are unable to hold the pen, in which one or more muscles of the fingers are irregularly and unresistibly contracted; adjust third or fourth dorsal.

Spasms may be due to traumatism, toxins or auto-suggestion. A general increase in the normal activity, strength and excitability of the various organs and functions, as observed in a state of health, is spoken of as hypertonia; a general diminution as hypotonia; while a sudden, violent, involuntary, rigid contraction of muscles is called a spasm. Tetanus consists of a more or less continuous contraction of one or more muscles, measured by the intervals of time between the stimuli, irritation, and the contraction. It is complete or incomplete owing to the number of stimuli which vibrate in the muscle in a second of time. If the rate of stimulation is increased up to the number when the interval between each vibration is less than the duration of the entire contraction process, then the muscle does not have time to completely relax before the arrival of the next stimulus.

Traumatic suggestion is a term applied to the peculiar mental state often occurring after accidents, in which the will and judgment are partially obscured; suggestions are easily received and stick; so. the slightest injury to a part induces a hysteric paralysis, contracture, dysesthesia, arthralgia and neurasthenic affections.

Spasm is one of the most troublesome complications of simple fracture which the surgeon has to deal with. It arises from the fragments irritating and stretching the nerves which supply the muscles contracted—irritation causes tension. It is sometimes so severe and uncontrollable as to tax any means used for relief. The tension causes great pain because of the displaced fragments impinging upon sensitive nerves. As a rule there is more or less spasm until the fracture is reduced; after the broken ends are replaced, the spasm and pain cease immediately.

Alkaloids are animal, ptomain or leukomain; or cadaveric, putrefactive ptomain; or artificial alkaloids that are made by chemical processes. These are considered of great value by the medical profession on account of their active poisoning principles and disease provoking. They poison, irritate, cause contraction of a portion or all of the nervous system, when egested or injected. It is these destructive qualities which give to drugs their great value (?).

In this city a few months ago, two men on the same day had each a tooth extracted; their gums were anesthetized. One of these was J. E. Lavalley, D. C. I was called and found him in persistent tonic spasm. I relieved him. In less than an hour I left him free of the effects of poison and out of danger. The other case was taken to the hospital and died the same day.

Spasm, muscular contraction, nerve tension, is because of auto-suggestion, poison or impingement. I was the first to promulgate that the above mentioned caused vertebrae to be drawn out of alignment, and that by their replacement, tension was relieved. I now state that auto and hypnotic suggestion so modifies the action of the nervous system as to cause all the phenomena presented in hypnosis and auto-suggestion, including hysteria.

It is, or should be the business of the Chiropractor to restore to normal position any displaced portion of the bony framework, whether such a displacement be traumatic or toxic, so that nerves may have normal tension—normal tension means normal functionating—health.

Pathologists advise change of diet and climate, exercise and rest, diaphoretics and spasmodics, sedatives and tonics, nerve stretching and tenotomy, ending up with some one of the following discouraging but honest statements. The pathology of the disease is unknown. The prognosis is hopeless. No definite lesion can be ascribed. The exciting cause is usually some emotional disturbance. We have no specific. The disease is very obstinate and ordinarily continuous throughout life. The treatment is entirely symptomatic. Its etiology is obscure, idiopathic, self-originated, neither sympathetic nor traumatic, arising spontaneously without an obvious cause. No satisfactory treatment has been suggested. Some psychic disturbance. Neuropathic heredity. Nothing definite is known. A disease of unknown cause. No definite etiologic factor is known. The prognosis is unfavorable for cure. The medical management of the disease is absolutely without avail. No drug has been found to exercise the slightest influence. In those cases in which no cause can be discovered bromids are the only resource. As to an ultimate cure, the prognosis is very doubtful. Neuropathic heredity plays an important part. Nerve-stretching and tenotomy of the affected muscles is of very little value. Practically nothing can be done. **If the condition is due to pressure**, in some cases **relief may be obtained.** The cause of the functional forms we do not understand. The treatment is wholly mental and moral, with the occasional use of drugs to produce quiet and sleep.

In all that long list of discouraging statements, there is one and only one which sheds a ray of light upon the dismal gloom of these wretched unfortunates and reveals a scintillation of encouragement. It is: "If the condition is due to pressure, relief may be obtained." I have removed that "if," so the sentence may read: "Spasms are due to contractions of muscles, muscle contracture to nerve tension and nerve tension in some cases to pressure. In others it is due to poisons and in a small per cent of cases to violent emotions, mental excitement, an agitation of the passions or sensibilities in which the emotional and reflex excitability is exaggerated, is not under the constraint of the will, the patient losing mental control and becoming the victim of imaginary sensations, often falling into spasms or fits. The main symptoms are convulsions, tossing movements of the limbs and head, uncontrollable crying and laughing, vasomotor derangements, motor paralysis, anesthesia, hyperthesia or other sensory disturbances. Hysteria presents the most varied symptoms, often simulating those of the gravest diseases. As I have said, an application of a bucketful of cold water, with a promise of the same treatment in future attacks, will effect a permanent, safe and inexpensive cure.

Those muscular contractions due to traumatism or toxication are easily relieved by adjusting by hand such displacements of the osseous framework as are displaced by accidents or toxins, thereby relieving pressure and undue tension.

"Osteopathic Physicians." A physician is one who practices medicine. An Osteopathic Physician would be a medicine doctor who is osteopathic. An incongruity.

In the May number, Journal of Osteopathy, page 344: "Dr. Andrew Still, the fountain head of Osteopathy." This statement is correct, as much so, as "Dr. D. D. Palmer, the fountain head of Chiropractic." Would it not look strange and ridiculous to see the **Kirkville School** advertised as **the fountain head of Osteopathy?**

Fig. 4 is a profile showing the ramification of the cerebrospinal system, after leaving the canal.

If the reader will refer to these cuts as he peruses The Chiropractor Adjuster, he will the better comprehend the principles upon which the science of Chiropractic is founded. He will acquire a knowledge which thousands of physicians have sought a life time for and failed to attain, because they overlooked what a man of common education discovered.

Information upon this interesting and valuable method of adjusting the cause of disease will be presented in the Chiropractor Adjuster by the Discoverer, Developer and Founder of this simple, yet wonderful science.

"Mature" refers to successive stages through which anything has passed. Persons have mature judgment and give mature consideration when they arrive at mature age. Cartilage is changed into bone by ossification—the process by which phosphate of lime is deposited in cartilage. Bones are not fully ossified until the age of 25 or 30. Bones do not ripen or mature.

"The union of the soul with the body." The soul is intelligent life. It is the link which unites the immaterial with the material, the spirit with the body. What shall it profit a man, if he shall gain the whole world, and lose his own soul? Union implies contact without anything intervening. Bodies are connected by that which unites. The soul, the life, is the bond of union.

"If there be foreign bodies, such as a gall-stone, it may be difficult for Innate to remove the obstruction. Occlusion may be due to the presence of foreign bodies such as gall-stones."

Gall-stones are not foreign bodies. Dunglison says, "Foreign body. Extraneous body present in canals, or viscera, in which it may cause irritation or inflammation."

Gall-stones are solidified bile, made so by excessive heat. Bile, whether liquid or solid, is a natural product, is not foreign or extraneous by any means. It is no more foreign than pancreatic juice, spleenic fluid, or any other secretion. By adjusting, we remove impingements from nerves, restore them to their natural tonicity, vibrations become normal in quantity, excessive heat is removed, the liver is of ordinary temperature, gallstones (solidified bile) are liquefied, ordinary functions are performed.

"We have in various times heard a great deal about the value of the cranial nerves; that they were, or were not cranial nerves. Anatomy says there are, and **I say there are not**; that is generally considered as cranial nerves. I am not denying but what **these nerves are where they are found** to be under dissection; these nerves do have their point of exit in the skull and they go to the places where they have been traced, but in addition of all that, they are **not** performing the physical functions which they have been supposed to do. For instance, we have the location of many nerves which are supposed to be carrying out prominent functions, but under nerve tracing on the living individuals, that are suffering from a lack of specific function, we find and trace out altogether different nerves having a different point of origin or different paths and a different place of insertion and that former results prove all things. Anatomists or physicians by working on dissected so-called cranial nerves do not get results with the effects of these functions but the Chiropractor, following his tracing of those cases; finding their place of insertion in the spinal cord, in and between the vertebrae, releasing pressure upon nerves and thus restoring functions, consequently the results disprove that he does something to those nerves which he has traced out and by adjusting, has restored function and which had not been getting through those nerves, thus disproving that the nerves perform the function ascribed to them by dissection, and that in reality that function is performed by another nerve, as proved by results on a living body."

"The Student, Author and Teacher on any Phase of Chiropractic Philosophy, Science or Art, Anywhere at any Time" makes two statements in the above which are self-contradictory. He says, there are no cranial nerves; he also states that they are found just as anatomists state. The "Developer of the Philosophy, Science and Art of Chiropractic" means to say, that anatomists are correct in their description and location of the 12 pairs of cranial nerves, but, they do not perform the functions ascribed to them. He means we do not smell with the olfactory nerve; the optic nerve is not sensory—we do not see with it; we do not hear with the auditory nerve; the 3d, 4th, 6th, 11th and 12th are not motor in their functions; the 5th, 7th, 9th and 10th are not motor and sensory in their capacity, as stated by anatomists. If these nerves do not perform the functions ascribed to them, perhaps the "Developer of the Philosophy, Science and Art of Chiropractic" can enlighten us in regard to the character of the cranial nerves.

"The Student, Author and Teacher on any Phase of Chiropractic Philosophy, Science or Art, Anywhere at any Time," states that there are no cranial nerves, then admits that they do exist, but do not perform the functions they are supposed to execute. If not, what are their functions, of what use are they? Perhaps the "Developer of the Philosophy, Science and Art of Chiropractic" can tell us. Possibly "The Student, Author and Teacher on any Phase of Chiropractic Philosophy, Science or Art, Anywhere at any Time" can add an important item to physiology by discovering the real functions of the cranial nerves which have no existence, although they are found just where anatomists declare them to be.

If he would become acquainted with the cranial accessory nerves, those which establish communication between the cranial and certain spinal and sympathetic nerves, he would then understand how and why we can and do trace sensitive nerves from the spine to the cranium, and relieve impingements upon those nerves by adjusting vertebrae.

Remember, a nerve is an elongated, cord-like structure, made up of an aggregation of nerve-fibers. A nerve is composed of a sheath or covering, filled with a number of filaments. A fiber is not a nerve, it is one of the many thread-like structures which compose the interior of a nerve. These fibers may occupy a portion of a nerve, escape and become a part of another nerve or ganglion. Whatever nerve a fiber occupies, it is a part of that nerve and is so considered by all anatomists. The cranial nerves are composed partly of accesory nerves, nerves which have been added to and are therefore a part of the trunk. It is enclosed in some one of the branches, nerve of which they become a part. Thus a nerve filament originating in the nervous mass of the brain becomes a part of the spinal cord, one of the rootlets which form the roots, a part of the trunk, it is enclosed in some one of the branches, but always retains its individuality as expressed in its function. It is always a part of the nerve with which it is associated. The accessory nerves are auxiliary to the cranial nerves. They are the fibers which we trace from the spine to the cranium. The fibers which become a part of the cranial nerves. They may be impinged upon and we may release them and realize that they become associated with and are a part of the cranial nerves.

---

The following quotations are from a Chiropractor's card:

"A science which is able to locate the physical cause of disease."

It is the Chiropractor who locates the cause, not the science. There is as much difference between a science and the one who practices it as there is between a musician and his music. Physical is of, or pertaining to, the body. As may be seen in the article on spasm, disease may be caused by injuries, or poisons or from the mind.

"Chiropractic prevents disease."

Chiropractic is a science. A science in and of itself cannot prevent disease. The Chiropractor may make use of the art of adjusting; he may remove or relieve diseased condition. He should not make them, although many do.

"Allowing a free movement of the vital forces from the brain, along the nerves to the various organs of the body."

Vital force is that form of energy which is manifested in the phenomena of life (vital functions), especially when regarding it as distinct from other forces of nature, such as mechanical, chemical, etc. The vital forces are nerve force, neurism; thot force, phrenism, and bathmism, which includes all that is necessary to mature individual life, as constructed by the activity of a special form of energy known as growth-energy. These three vital forces are under the direction and control of the vital principle, Innate, Individual Spirit.

**Vital force is inherent in the organ or organism. Vital energy is the expression of the vital force** which is inherent in each organ. Function is energy expressed by or thru vital force; therefore, **vital force does not move "from the brain along the nerves to the organ."**

"The interrupted currents are set in motion again."

Currents is here used as a synonym for vital forces. Vital force does not possess a current, does not flow as a liquid, is not the swiftest part of a stream. Vital force is expressed in vital acts, functions. Functions do not flow as does a current of a stream or those of the ocean or atmosphere or electricity.

"Set in motion again."

**Could a person live if the "currents were interrupted and not in motion"?**

"Nature takes up the work of restoring the affected tissues."

Whatever is, is nature, natural, whether considered as a creative force or as the physical universe. Intelligent, vital force and matter or material is all there is. All action or forces are of nature. Nothing can be unnatural. The laws of the universe are those of nature; outside of nature there are no laws. The process of being warmed by the radiating heat of the stove and that of being burned by placing the hand on it, are alike in that one is as much a law of nature as is the other. Normal nerve tension insures normal temperature, normal vibration, normal transmission of thot; this is nature, natural, in accordance with the laws of nature. If a bone is luxated, presses against, impinges upon a nerve, the result is an undue amount of tension, excessive vibration, an excess of heat, all of which is nature, in accordance with the inevitable law of nature. If the temperature becomes sufficiently great, there is softening of tissue, necrosis, that is nature, according to nature, one of the laws of nature. It is a law of nature that heat, at a certain temperature, will liquidize not only the soft tissue but bone also. All diseases are the result of nature's laws. **Whatever is, is nature.** The impairment and restoration are both the work of nature.

The last line of the card reads, "The Chiropractor removes the obstacles to nature's healing processes."

The first four lines tell us that the science of Chiropractic locates the cause of disease, provides means of removal and prevents disease, **why not furnish the science to the patients; it will locate, remove and prevent disease (?)?** The last line states that the Chiropractor removes the obstacles. **Who or what is running the business, the science or the Chiropractor?**

Thot force (impulse) impels, drives onward with a sudden force. Force, so communicated as to provide motion suddenly, is an impulse. Innate or Spirit thinks, produces thots. Thots are entities, things. Vital force and currents are not entities or things. **Thots are started, driven onward. Neurism, nerve force, vibration, transmits thots to their destination. Thots receive their impetus, phrenism, or thot force, the momentum, from the rate of transit.**

"Expert Chiropractic adjustments."

Expert is a technical term; it applies to the person who does, not to what is done. Hence, we can say, Dr. Blank was an expert witness, or that he is an expert surgeon, or an expert adjuster, meaning that he possesses superior knowledge or skill, that he is a specialist in the line mentioned. One is an expert whose knowledge and experience make him an authoritative specialist, as, he is an expert in handwriting, or in surgery, or in adjusting. The writing or surgery or adjusting is not an expert. Adjustments can not be expert.

---

"Is there a prospect of eliminating disease?"

Not while our surroundings are unsanitary; not while we are being inoculated with the poison of infectious diseases, vaccine lymph taken from the pustles of an animal; not while we are subject to traumatic accidents which displace some portion of the osseous framework.

## DR. DAVIS, A MEMBER OF THE ADJUSTER CLASS.

As I am the discoverer, developer and founder of Chiropractic, and also a teacher of this science both in the school-room and through the columns of The Adjuster, I have earned the right to be the chief instructor.

The readers of The Adjuster are students desiring information concerning this new science. The students of The Adjuster are like those in the class-room; some desire information in one line, and some in another. The teacher should be the judge of what is most necessary and how much of it should be given in one lesson. It is but fair to presume, in fact, I do not need presume, that students in The Adjuster class are as varied in their previous education, their likes and dislikes, as those immediately under my personal instruction. Pupils in either class have the right and privilege "to talk back." There are those in either class who may feel hurt for the time being when they are criticised. But, remember, that your teacher means to conduct the recitation in the manner he thinks will be for the edification of all concerned. Therefore, we give space to the following letter.

I am personally acquainted with Dr. Davis. I know him to be a scholar and one who has given the nervous system much study. He has paid his fee as a student and is also a subscriber to The Adjuster. The teacher often picks up valuable information from his students; they, too, may observe mistakes.

To be brief and comprehensive, I shall quote his letter by paragraphs, answering each in turn.

Baker City, Ore., May 6, 1909.

Dr. D. D. Palmer.

My Dear Sir and Doctor: I have your number 4 Adjuster and your recent letter. I am surprised at your stating that the optic nerve ends in the lens.

(I was also surprised when I noticed the mistake. It should have read retina, for in it the fibers of the optic nerve expand and terminate. The sensitive portion of the retina is known as the ora serrata (serrated edge). The "recent letter" contained an offer by me to give him further free adjustments for cataract. After I had made marked improvement by four adjustments, diminishing the opacity of the lens, by removing a part of the deposit in the capsule, he did not see why his good wife could not do that adjusting as well as I could myself. Chiropractors know why.)

I agree with you that nerves are "**Innate**"—inborn, for they could not be placed there after birth. They are not innate as to education. They are the conveyancers of thought. Thought is a result of **impressions.** The impressions are conveyed to the brain through one or all of the five senses—and no thought ever enters into the brain except through these avenues—and when received into the brain they are formulated into words.

(Did I say anything about nerves being Innate? Nerves are not Innate, any more than they are spirit. Spirit, as generally understood, is what I designate as Innate. Nerves and Innate are not synonyms, they do not mean one and the same thing. Did any one else get the idea that nerves were Innate? If Dr. Davis had been as close a student as he was eleven years ago, he would have known better.)

Through words or signs, we express ideas—these properly arranged, we denominate intelligence—and intelligence only applies to the mind, however it may be expressed. The word "Innate" is wrongly applied when you say it is the director of the mind. God is the author of mind, and the media through which mind is conveyed. The mind is expressed through the Nervous System to each and every part of the body.

(Innate **is** the director of the mind—the manager of all functions—vital, vegetative and intellectual. God is the author of all intelligence. Innate is a personified portion of The All Wise —the sum total of which is God.)

The prime cause of all aberrations of the muscular system is traceable to nerve irritation, and the irritation causes muscular contraction; and the contraction squeezes the nerves which pass through the muscular tissue, and mitigates, lessens **or destroys nerve function where the nerves end.**

(I have never known of such a condition as an "aberration of the muscular system." Aberration may refer to "a disordered state of the intellect," a "derangement of the intellectual faculties," or "mental derangement." Nerves may be irritated by pressure. They can only be acted upon by poison or by a substance harder than themselves. Bones are the hardest tissue of the body. They may press against nerves and cause impingement. Either poison or bones may irritate nerves and cause atomic agitation. A nerve, over-excited, becomes enlarged, rigid, tense, sensitive to the patient when palpated. Its rigidity causes an excessive vibration. Molecular action produces heat. Tensity of nerves and too much heat produce aberration of the intellect, because of increased nerve vibration. Functions mitigated, a lessening of nerve function, produces anemia or paralysis in the parts which have less than normal function. To destroy nerve function would produce gangrene, death of the portion which lacked function. Excessive heat intensifies, increases function. An undue amount of heat softens tissue, produces necrosis. When functions are performed normally, health becomes reinstated.)

The Thermal-nerve theory of yours is without reason, without proof.

(Reason depends upon education. Much of life which was unreasonable to you and me twenty-five years ago is reasonable today. Dorland says, heat is a form of kinetic energy. Landois says, under "Animal Heat": The heat of the body is a form of kinetic energy, appearing without interruption, and must be conceived as depending upon vibrations of the atoms of the body. If a leaden weight be thrown from the summit of a tower to the earth and there encounter an unyielding surface, its movements in mass will come to rest, but the kinetic energy, which to the eye appears dissipated, is transformed into an **actively vibratory movement of the atoms.** On striking the ground heat is generated, the amount of which is proportionate to the kinetic energy that is transformed by the impact. At the moment of contact on the part of the falling weight **the atoms are set into vibration by the concussion. They impinge upon one another** and then rebound in consequence of the potential energy that tends to prevent their immediate apposition; they separate to a maximum degree in so far as the power of attraction of the ponderable **atoms permit** and they **oscillate to and fro** in this manner. **All atoms oscillate** like a pendulum until the heat of the heated mass is radiated. **Heat is a vibratory movement of the atoms.** As the amount of heat generated is proportionate to the kinetic energy that is transformed by the impact, it must be possible to find an adequate measure for both forms of force.

"The transformation of the kinetic mechanical energy of the viscera furnishes heat as the work done cannot be conveyed to the outside. Thus all of the kinetic energy of the heart is transformed into heat through the resistance opposed to the blood-stream. The same may be said of the kinetic energy of certain muscular viscera. Thus the torsion of the costal cartilages and the friction of the current of air in the respiratory organs of the contents of the digestive tract yield a certain amount of heat."

Gould states that **heat is** a mode or **rate of vibration** of etheral **atomic,** or **molecular,** or **wave-motion.** Webster affirms that **heat** in its nature **is a mode of motion,** being in general a form of **molecular disturbance or vibration.** The Twentieth Century Dictionary sets forth that **heat** is a phenomena believed to **consist** in a **certain motion or vibration of the ultimate molecules** of which bodies are composed.

Lippincott says that "Heat is a form of energy which when

applied to matter causes its expansion, elevates its temperature, converts it from the solid into the fluid state and from the fluid into the gaseous."

Landois says on page 390: "Like all bodies, the human body undergoes expansion at elevated temperatures. A man * * * will expand * * * with an increase of his bodily temperature. Of the different tissues, connective tissue (tendon, nerves, muscles) is expanded by heat, while elastic tissue and skin are contracted like rubber.)

(Nerves are contracted longitudinally and expanded transversely by overheat. The more rigid and tense, the greater the vibrations and molecular action. The temperature may increase until the nerves become softened; as they do so they relax, and the fever subsides. Nerves may become so soft by an undue amount of heat that their carrying capacity is nil; if so, Innate can no longer send impulses over the lines; communication ceases, no function is performed and death is the result.

The dynamic theory of heat, ascribes it to the moving of ultimate particles of matter—not to a kind of fluid. Caloric was the name given to the agent to which all phenomena of heat was formerly assigned. Caloric is not now used in scientific nomenclature, but occasionally as a general term for heat. I trust that the authorities quoted will justify my using the kinetic "Thermal—nerve theory," and hope that Dr. Davis will not think it is "without reason, without proof.")

"Nerve tracing," as you call it, is absolutely misleading, and should not be considered at all.

(Nerve tracing is one of the fine arts of Chiropractic which I had not developed when Dr. A. P. Davis was my student, nearly eleven years ago. Following a sensitive, swollen nerve from the place of impingement to its peripheral ending, or vice versa, by a discriminating touch; tracing it before adjustment by its rigidity and tenseness; then finding that it has become lax and not sensitive immediately after adjustment, is important in diagnosing many morbid conditions and proof positive that the lesion has been located and removed. Surely knowledge thus obtained which shows the relation of, and enables us to distinguish between, cause and effect, is not "absolutely misleading." Every Chiropractor will smile audibly when he reads "Nerve tracing * * * is absolutely misleading and should not be considered." It is direct pathological diagnosis; knowledge versus theory and ignorance; it is Innate's assistance in making a diagnosis.)

Your answer to my questions regarding the eye for cataract is unreasonable, it has no possible relationship with the nervous system, and cannot be reached through the nervous system.

Cataract is a degenerative phenomena, and is only affected by stimulation or irritation through ciliary muscle action, and this action is absolutely mechanical—due to irritaton of the ciliary nerve terminals.

(Cataract is a deposit in the membrane inclosing the lens of the eye, caused by a lack of vital functionating, a deficiency of innervation in a functional communicative fiber which has its origin at S. P. on the right. The vegetative functions of secretion and excretion are not fully performed; when they are, the opacity of the crystalline lens will be relieved by the deposit being absorbed and excreted. A Chiropractor should know just where those fibers are impinged and how to relieve them. The fact that quite a portion of the white deposit was removed by five adjustments is proof positive that the Allopaths, Homeopaths, Osteopaths and Ophthalmologists, from each of whose schools you are a graduate, are mistaken in their etiology, diagnosis, prognosis and the proper treatment as given by you in your last quoted paragraph. To say that your "good wife is an excellent adjuster, and gets responses every time the adjustment is made," lacks confirmation. I presume that she has had no education along this line except from one who cannot see how harm can be done by moving the vertebra in a wrong direction; one who does not believe the adjuster moves a vertebra; who does not believe a nerve can be impinged upon; who does not believe a vertebra can be luxated, would be a poor teacher to give his wife lessons on adjusting when he is the subject.

You say, "Cataract has no possible relationship with the nervous system," that it "is a degenerative phenomena." All organic phenomena, physiological or degenerative are due to impulses either in normal force, or too much or not enough impulse momentum.

(Doctor, come down and stay with me two weeks; I wish to use your case for the clinic. I will do the adjusting of the displaced vertebra, remove the impingement from the sympathetic nerve fiber which is a part of the spinal trunk that emerges from the spinal canal. That accessory fiber should communicate certain functions to the retina which, owing to impingement, fails to functionate properly. Come; I will finish removing the deposit. That will be a pleasant and positive answer to your questions, a proof that will be appreciated, one which ought to cause you to change your mode of reasoning.)

My system does affect the entire nervous system—your strictures to the contrary notwithstanding.

(In consideration, as you told me, that Ophthalmologists do not treat cataractous conditions, and that your system reaches and affects the entire nervous system, shall we understand that the ora serrata, the wavy zizzag sensitive portion of the retina, or the capsule, or the crystalline lens—the optic portion of the eye—is not a part of the nervous system? Or is it a "degenerative phenomena" which Neurology cannot reach?)

Ninety-five per cent of disease is not caused by vertebrae being out of alignment, or from "luxations" of the spine, as you claim. The clicking is no evidence of luxation. Crack one of your fingers, and tell me if it was luxated.

(The replacing of luxated joints, their forcible separation, or the rubbing of rheumatic articulations, whose surfaces are void of cartilage, are attended with audible sounds. The normal movements of joints do not emit any noise. We have the audible crack of the atlas when it is driven by the hand from one side to the other; the striking of the tubercle against the odontoid process. The forcible separation or the replacing of the vertebral joints, whether by accident or the hand of the Chiropractor, is usually accompanied by a distinct sound, varying from a click to that of a crash, which, with the sensation is distinctly felt by the patient and by the hand of the adjuster.)

Contraction of muscular fiber draws the facets tightly together and the sudden spring against the muscle, stretching it, produces the sound as the relaxation takes place—the air is introduced between the joints.

(Do you wish to be understood as saying that the sound heard and the sensation felt when joints are moved, is because of the sudden expulsion or introduction of air from or into the joint? This is Osteopathy. A. T. Still states, on page 130 and 131 in his book on Osteopothy, that the cause of rheumatism, neuralgia, sciatica, consumption, dropsy, tumors, fits, gray hair, baldness "and so on to a surprising number of diseases," "not accounted for to date by our philosophers," are because "gas or wind has left the joints," "thus electricity burns because of bone friction." Why not crack some air into the joints?)

I would that you would eliminate all your theories from your literature, and teach facts, and let criticism of other sciences alone.

(Doctor, if you and I were to eliminate from our literature all of which the other fellow calls theories we would have only blank covers left. When you wrote your book—Neurology—you did not fail to criticise Chiropractic. In your forthcoming book I presume that Chiropractic will receive its share of criticism. That is human nature, and I think, all right, whether it tickles or hurts the one criticised.)

You will find what I teach, by reading my book Neurology, about your "Heat Nerves" and luxations.

(I have your books, Osteopathy and Neurology. Your last is plentifully supplied with criticisms on the science of Chiropractic.)

I have said in kindness what I think, and mean it thus. Fraternally with best wishes for all. A. P. DAVIS.

P. S.—Starting with you early in the Chiropractic science, and getting from you all you knew about spinal adjustment—as you claimed, and possessing perhaps as much ability as yourself, why should I not have had the same opportunity to grow in the knowledge as yourself?

(Yes, Doctor, I taught you in two weeks, eleven years ago, all I then knew of Chiropractic, but I fail to see where you have made any advancement along Chiropractic lines. You had the ability to advance, in fact, were far more qualified to discover and develop the science of Chiropractic than myself; but for some reason you have retrograded instead of advancing. Why did you physically grow to the height of six feet and I only to five-feet four? Because you were A. P. Davis and I D. D. Palmer. Thus have we mentally grown different. You may have had the same opportunities, but you were not "Old Chiro." Thousands may have had the same opening, but their surrounding environments were not the same; they were not the men for the occasion; they failed to find the cause of disease. They started wrong and investigated in the wrong direction. Therefore, they did not discover the principles the combining of which made the science which I had the pleasure of naming Chiropractic.)

(You have not grown in Chiropractic knowledge. You have not learned that vertebrae may be luxated. You know nothing about specific adjusting. You do not recognize the tracing of enlarged, sensitive, tense, rigid, inflamed nerves. You do not comprehend what Chiropractors understand by Innate—the Spiritual Intelligence which is back of and controls the mind. Chiropractically, you do not know the cause of disease. You do not comprehend any one of the principles of Chiropractic. You should at least be able to embrace the simplest and basic principles of Chiropractic—that sub-luxated joints cause pressure on nerves; that displaced bones impinge upon nerves, more especially those of the vertebral column; that nerves become excited, because of pressure; that atomic agitation creates heat; that caloric causes nerves to become swollen and rigid; that vibration depends upon nerve tension, and that the greater the tension the greater the number of vibrations in a given length of time; that the amount of functionating depends upon the laxity or rigidity of nerves; that the ability of nerves to carry impulses depends upon their firmness; that compactness is determined by the amount of heat; that inco-ordination is because of too much or too little functionating; that any vital vegetative or intellectual function performed in either an excessive or insufficient degree is disease.)

Friend Davis, what do you know about Chiropractic as a science?

The class will excuse me for using seven pages. That boy talking back gave me a chance to say something; some of which is new to every member of The Adjuster class.

---

The following is copied from page 527 of the **Practice of Physic,** date Nov. 1, 1908:

"Issues and blisters, skillfully managed, are important remedies in the treatment of consumption, whether the object be prevention or cure. To be really useful, their action should be **long continued,** for a **chronic remedy** is always necessary in a chronic disease.

"On the treatment of pulmonary consumption generally, we have but little to say—at furthest, very little that is worthy of attention. Like that of other physicians, our practice, in the complaint, has been exceedingly discouraging. We hold it useless, therefore, to trouble our readers with a tedious account of what has been attempted, on the subject, to so little purpose. Although we would not hastily fall into the ranks of those who pronounce the disease definitely **incurable**; we must, notwithstanding, acknowledge it to be true, that physicians are, **at present,** unable to cure it. We flatter ourselves, however, that this is to be attributed, not to the **necessary fatality** of the complaint, but to the defective state of the healing art; and that some powerful panacea, or efficacious mode of treatment, is yet in reserve, for the many interesting subjects that fall by this disease.

"In Great Britain and the United States, where pulmonary consumption has been more thoroughly studied, and is better understood, than in any other country, the remedies and expedients, by which its cure has been attempted, are numerous and powerful. Notwithstanding this, the disease, when completely formed, has almost uniformly proceeded, with more or less rapidity in different cases, to a fatal termination. **Radical cures** have, indeed, ofttimes appeared, in **medical reports**; but we doubt their appearance in **medical practice.**

"In the treatment of this disease, our only rational hope is placed in preventive measures."

## OSTEOPATHY VS. CHIROPRACTIC.

It will be observed that in 1906 and 1907, the Kirksville School of Osteopathy did not teach Chiropractic; did not know anything about it. A year later they learned that Palmer took a few treatments at their infirmary, and, now, it claims Chiropractic to be the same as Osteopathy.

The Osteopathic College at Franklin, Ky., and the one at San Francisco, affirm that Chiropractic is not taught in any Osteopath school.

The College of Osteopathy at Boston, Mass., says there is a wide difference between Osteopathy and Chiropractic, and so says A. P. Davis, D. O., D. C.

The Osteopathic College at Des Moines, Iowa, says Chiropractic is Massage, although Chiropractors try to make it appear that Osteopathy and Chiropractors are one and the same.

The Osteopathic College at Los Angeles, Cal., **thinks** "Chiropractic is a mechanical manipulator, while an Osteopath is an all round physician." A physician is one skilled in physic, a doctor of medicine. As Osteopaths do not use medicine to physic their patients, they are certainly not physic-ians.

One college states there is a wide difference between Osteopathy and Chiropractic; while two colleges state that Chiropractors try to make it appear that the two sciences are the same. One says, Chiropractic is only Massage; another, that it is a mechanical manipulation. Dr. Fiske swore on the stand at La Crosse, Wis., that Chiropractic is nothing but Osteopathy. It took the jury but twenty minutes to decide, as did Dr. A. P. Davis, after taking a course under the founder of each system, that they are entirely two distinct systems. Where the testimony of witnesses is so conflicting as the following from Osteopath schools, any jury would decide that none of them know what constitutes Chiropractic.

At Hutchinson, Kans., on Aug. 10, 1910, during the trial of P. W. Johnson, D. C., for practicing Osteopathy, the jury wanted to be shown the difference between Osteopathic treatments and Chiropractic Adjustments. The prosecution, the state, the Osteopaths objected to displaying the difference between Osteopathy and Chiropractic, but as the jury insisted upon being shown, B. J. Palmer was made the recipient of an Osteopathic treatment and a Chiropractic adjustment. It took the jury 28 minutes to decide that P. W. Johnson, while practicing Chiropractic was not practicing Osteopathy.

See The P. S. C. Announcements, No. 4, page 139, for the following opinions secured by B. J. Palmer:

From the American School of Osteopathy:

Kirksville, Mo., Dec. 29, 1906.

Mrs. S. J. Rice, Davenport, Iowa.

Dear Madam: We do not teach the so-called system of Chiropractic, nor can we tell you anything about it.

(Signed) WARREN HAMILTON, Sec.

American School of Osteopathy,

Kirksville, Mo., Jan. 5, '07.

N. L. Brownell, White Bear, Minn.,

Dear Sir: We do not teach Chiropractic, nor do we know anything about it. Yours truly,

(Signed) WARREN HAMILTON, Sec. and Treas.

Southern College of Osteopathy,

Franklin, Ky., Jan. 8, 1907.

Mr. N. L. Brownell, White Bear, Minn.

Dear Sir: We will state that we do not teach Chiropractic in our college, nor is it taught in any reputable osteopathic school. We are not able to tell you just what it is, as we do not know very much about it—in fact, it is not known over the South at all. Yours very truly,

(Signed) W. J. GOOCH, Bus. Manager.

Southern College of Osteopathy,

Franklin, Ky., Jan. 8, '07.

Mrs. J. S. Rice, Davenport, Iowa.

Dear Madam: Replying to your inquiry of recent date, we beg to advise you that we do not teach Chiropractic in our college nor is it taught in any reputable osteopathic school. Yours very truly,

(Signed) W. J. GOOCH, Bus. Manager.

Osteopathic Association of the State of California,

San Francisco, Cal., Jan. 7, 1907.

Mrs. J. Rice, Davenport, Iowa.

Dear Madam: Your letter making inquiries concerning Chiropractic has just been received. In reply, will state that we do not teach it in our college. It is not taught in any of the Osteopathic Colleges. Sincerely yours,

(Signed) EFFIE E. YORK.

Dean of the California College.

Osteopathic Association of the State of California,

San Francisco, Cal., Jan. 9, '07.

Mr. N. L. Brownell, White Bear, Minn.

Dear Sir: In our college we teach only Osteopathy, and have nothing to do with Chiropractic. Some one has misinformed you. Yours very truly,

(Signed) EFFIE E. YORK,

Dean of the California College of Osteopathy.

Office of Busar, Mass., College of Osteopathy,
Boston, Mass., Jan. 7, 1909.

Mr. N. L. Brownell, White Bear, Minn.

Dear Sir: Yours of Jan. 2d received, and in reply would state there is a wide difference between Osteopathy and Chiropractic. We do not teach Chiropractic. We do not teach Chiropractic at this school. Yours very truly,

(Signed) HOWARD F. CRAWFORD.

Still College of Osteopathy,
Des Moines, Iowa, Jan. 5, 1907.

Mr. N. L. Brownell, White Bear, Minn.

Dear Sir: Chiropractic is nothing more than massage. Chiropractors try to make it appear that it is the same, but this is not correct. If it is the same, they would come and take it in a recognized college. We don't teach Chiropractic.

Very sincerely yours,

(Signed) W. E. RUMMEL,
Sec. and Manager.

The Pacific College of Osteopathy,
Los Angeles, Cal., Jan. 9, '07.

Mr. N. L. Brownell, White Bear, Minn.

My Dear Sir: You ask for the difference between Chiropractic and Osteopathy. Briefly state, I think the difference is that the Chiropractic is a mechanical manipulator, while the Osteopath is an all round physician. Very respectfully yours,

(Signed) C. A. WHITING,
Chairman of Faculty.

American School of Osteopathy, Kirksville, Mo., 2-4-'08.

J. F. Petritsch, Logan, Utah.

Dear Sir: You ask what Chiropractic is. I can tell you in very few words of the difference in Chiropractic and Osteopathy. Some few years ago a man by the name of Palmer, from Iowa, came here for Osteopathic treatment and remained only a short time. After his return home he conceived the idea that he could establish a school which he called Chiropractic and has undertaken to teach a system of treatment claiming it to be the same as Osteopathy. It is absolutely a farce on his part.

I would be glad to have you investigate further if you have any doubt as to the correctness of my statements. Very respectfully, J. A. QUINTAL, Sec. and Treas.

The Chiropractic Adjuster No. 2, January, page 19, contained the above and the following. There has been no answer—they have swallowed the false statements.

In answer to the above, I will say that D. D. "Palmer from

Iowa" was never in Kirksville, Mo., therefore never was in "The American School of Osteopathy," That I, D. D. Palmer, never took Osteopathic treatment of, in or at "The American School of Osteopathy," or elsewhere. That I, D. D. Palmer, will be pleased to give space to J. A. Quintal, or anyone else, who will inform the public of the date on which D. D. Palmer took treatment in "The American School of Osteopathy." I will pay for a photograph of my signature with the date, copied from the register of patients in "The American School of Osteopathy." I will make a cut of the same and publish it in 1,000 copies of The Chiropractor Adjuster. This monthly is for the purpose of adjusting just such misrepresentations as the above.

I will give J. A. Quintal $10 for each copy of the Adjuster wherein I claim Chiropractic to be the same as Osteopathy. Here is a chance for him to adjust himself; if he don't we will.

I will be pleased to have him or the school he represents give me $10 for a copy each time I have stated in the Chiropractor and elsewhere that there is little or no resemblance between Chiropractic and Osteopathy.

The above statement made by J. A. Quintal is false. He purposely or ignorantly states what is not true. It is up to him to either prove himself a man of truth and veracity, for which purpose space will be given him freely in this journal, or apologize to me for slander and misrepresentation.

In order that J. A. Quintal may realize and know that there is but little or no resemblance between Chiropractic and Osteopathy, so that he will not again wilfully or ignorantly misrepresent Chiropractic, and not repeat that D. D. Palmer claims Chiropractic to be the same as Osteopathy, I am going to send him a marked copy of this Adjuster.

The following sworn statement of Dr. A. P. Davis is self-explanatory:

State of Illinois,
Rock Island County, ss.

I, A. P. Davis, M. D., of the city of Rock Island, in said county, a medical practitioner of forty years' standing, being duly sworn, on oath state that I am familiar with the science of Osteopathy as originally taught by Dr. A. T. Still, of Kirksville, Missouri, having been with it from its very beginning; having been a teacher in the first Osteopath school, in which said science was taught, having learned it from personal contact and by "word of mouth" from Dr. Still himself and having written and had published the only book explaining Osteopathy, entitled "Osteopathy Illustrated"; that I am also acquainted with the science of "Chiropractic" as taught by Dr. D. D.

Palmer, of Davenport, Iowa, having taken the Chiropractic course of instruction of Dr. Palmer, and being perfectly familiar therewith, I would state that the said two sciences above named are as distinct from each other as regards application, as day is from night, that either can be practiced without the other or the knowledge of its existence, and therefore they are entirely different sciences, applied differently, are in no way related to each other, and are independently and absolutely different.

(Signed) A. P. DAVIS, M. D.

Subscribed and sworn to by said Dr. A. P. Davis before me this 15th day of December, A. D. 1903.

(Signed) MARION E. SWEENEY,
Notary Public.

---

True friendship is always the richest in days of greatest need.

---

THON.—That one; he, she or it. A pronoun of the third person, common gender, a solidified and contracted form of **that one**. It is proposed as a substitute in any case where the use of a restrictive pronoun involves either inaccuracy or obscurity, or the non-employment necessitates an awkward repetition.—**The Standard Dictionary.**

This is a word that deserves universal recognition, for the reason that it obviates the use of the awkward form "he, she or they," "his, her or their," etc. It is said to be in common use in some parts of Great Britain with the meaning given above. **Thon** is used in the singular or plural, as a nominative or objective, the possessive form being **thon's.—Proofreaders' Style Book.**

Webster's International Dictionary, date 1910, says, "Thon (Contraction of that one.) A proposed genderless pronoun of the third person."

---

"We are taught, as fundamental in Chiropractic, that there must be pressure or constriction of nerves to interfere with transmission of currents, and if we were to believe that the twelve crainal nerves, as taught today, have an exit external to the spinal cord, they would not be subject to pressure, and we would be open to a great deal of ridicule as to how we get results, unless those fibers do enter those places and are impinged."

"How many times have we traced nerve fibers from S. P. on the right around to that throat, and adjustment at S. P. alone restored the sense of taste. How many times have we traced the fibers from fourth cervical to the eyes, finding the nerve directly at its exit from the inter-vertebral foramen, tracing directly to the eye, and adjustments there have restored sight. How many times have we traced fibers from the ears to the atlas, and adjusted them there, restoring hearing; how many adjustments following tracing from nose to fourth cervical have restored smell!"

Instead of there being "pressure or constriction of nerves interfering with the transmission of currents," their carrying capacity was too great or too weak, due to an impingement which either excites or allays their transmitting qualities.

The cranial nerves, like the spinal nerves, are developed from cells of the **primitive tube,** of which we have spoken freely elsewhere, beginning with the fifth pair downwards; all the sensory nerves are developed from the cells of the neutral crest like the sensory components or dorsal roots of the spinal nerves. The area where the nerve-fibers leave or enter the brain substance is the superficial attachment—**the apparent origin.** The group of cells deep in the brain material from which the fibers spring **is their real origin.**

The cranial nerves never leave the cranium. They, however, leave the interior thru the foramina other than the foramen magnum. If this were all "we would be open to a great deal of ridicule as to how we get results." As shown elsewhere, there are nerves which branch off from the spinal cord and pass to the cranial nerves inside of the spinal canal; others pass by way of the spinal cord, spinal trunk nerves, to the ganglia of the sympathetic; from thence to the cranial nerves by way of the carotid canal, keeping company with the carotid artery. These nervi communicantes—nerves communicating sensation and motion—are filaments from the spinal cord by way of the spinal nerves; they are liable to impingement as they emerge from the inter-vertebral foramina.

The nerve fibers traced from S. P. to the throat; from the fourth cervical to the eyes; from the atlas to the ears; from the fourth cervical to the nose, were accessory nerves, communicating either sensation or motion to the nerves affected. These were the nerves impinged upon. When freed from pressure their normal activity and sensation were restored.

Now, my boy, make another step—recognize the cranial nerves, as you have the sympathetic. Then learn how nerves communicate with each other. "Wide awake. Right you are."

## METABOLISM.

Metabolism is a physiological process by which food is converted into tissue; that act of vital energy by which suitable substances are changed from inanimate to animate material.

Stengel says: "Concerning metabolism, there is little systematic knowledge."

Landois states that "little is at present known concerning metabolism in nerves."

McFarland says: "The metabolic processes, while believed to be chemical are, as yet, inexplicable."

Kirke states: "There is little doubt that metabolism—the chemical changes which occur during nutrition—has to deal with the trophic influence of nerves."

Landois, referring to this complex process, says: "The explanation of the vital phenomena in the organism by the simple principles of physics and chemistry is rendered extremely difficult and in many respects appears impossible."

The Ioatrochemical School looks upon metabolism as a fermentative process in which the substances introduced are decomposed in conjunction with the bodily juices. They refer all physiological and pathological processes to chemical action. Their theory is that disease and its treatment are explicable on a chemical basis; that chemistry is the basis of all therapeutics.

Delafield thinks the chemical changes in metabolism are induced by micro-organisms, that the processes of fermentation are extremely complex and little understood; that the prevalent views as to the importance of disturbed metabolism in the body which may lead to the excretion of abnormal, harmful products, favor the conjecture that in many cases, at least, both the degenerative and the productive processes may be the marks of a persistent auto-intoxication.

While thousands of defenseless animals have been subjected, for examination and investigation, to cruel torture, pathologists do not comprehend the process by which living cells or organisms incorporate the material obtained from food, into, and as a part of, their own structure.

In order to accomplish metabolism, there are two quite opposite results to be attained; that of constructing living cells out of dead material, named anabolism, and the conversion of living matter into lifeless material—waste products—named catabolism. The process of transforming food into nutritive material so that it may become a part of the human economy, is known as assimilation or constructive metabolism. The converting of living cells into waste products is dissimilation, physiologic tissue disintegration. These two processes are constantly going on. In health they balance each other.

In order that food may serve the purposes of nutrition, it must be digested, absorbed and assimilated. The body does not remain in this stable condition while it is being supplied with nutrition. There are changes constantly going on; constructive and destructive processes proceeding at the same time. While food is being taken in and converted into living tissue, destructive metabolism is excreting the waste product by expired air, urine, sweat and feces. If these two processes equal each other, there is health; if not, we should find wherein the mechanism is at fault and correct it, not by adding some chemical ingredient which we think is lacking, but by mechanical adjustment.

Metabolic equilibrium exists when an equal amount of the material that is taken from the food and assimilated for the maintenance and growth of the body, is discharged from it, by the excretory organs, in the form of waste materials or end-products of retrogressive, tissue metamorphosis. Proteid metabolism is the essential characteristic of vitality.

The force of gravitation acts upon particles of matter without reference to their character. There is another kind of attraction, of quite a different nature, which is confined to all living organisms; a force known as chemical affinity, the attraction of certain organs for special substances.

The glands secrete bile, saliva, splenic, enteric, pancreatic and gastric juices; products for use in the body economy. Each of these has its special function in metabolism; bile being the only one secreted during fetal life.

Each of these fluids or semi-fluids has its chemical affinity. If the temperature of the body remains normal the chemical relationship is not disturbed; each is produced in normal amount and transferred as required.

Any of these glands may become inflamed. The osseous framework may be displaced by accident or drawn out of alignment by irritating poisons, causing direct or indirect pressure on nerves thru which all impulses are transmitted for functional expression. An over-excited condition of nerves produces a surplus of innervation.

Structural and functional alterations of the various organs lead to complex departures from the normal. An occlusion of the gall ducts may lead to digestive disturbances and icterus, a deposition of pigment. Pigmentation is a deposit of pigment which discolors the tissue. Functional disturbances and structural lesions always accompany each other. Pathological physiology cannot exist without either abnormal structure or displacement.

McFarland says of pigmentation (melanin), that its chemistry is somewhat obscure. He certainly would be in the dark regarding Melanosis (abnormal pigmentary deposits).

Pigment may be yellow, brown, black or reddish, depending upon its origin.

Many diseases are accompanied by pigmentation; it is one of the subjective signs of disease. Normal alterations in color may occur from exposure to sun and weather; but it is the abnormal colorations which interest us from a diagnostic standpoint. The most common disease due to pigmentation is jaundice in which there is found a catarrhal **inflammation** of the bile ducts. The color of the deposited matter varies from a slight yellowish tinge to a dark, citron or olive-green hue. This pigment is transferred and distributed thru the body by seepage. Jaundice may be accompanied by gall stones—hardened bile—because of inflammation.

Chronic silver poisoning causes the skin to become a bluish-slate color which is more pronounced in the face. Owing to the disuse of silver preparations by physicians, this discoloration is now quite rare.

A yellow tinge of the cuticle exists in carcinoma patients.

Kidney affections may cause a darkened discoloration of the skin.

Patches of brown pigmentation may result from fly blisters, or mustard platsers which were used as counter irritants.

Pigmentations denote secretions, in excess, which transude, exosmose and are deposited in other tissue.

Normal heat means natural metabolism. Too much or not enough heat disturbs the equilibrium of secretion and excretion. Local inflammation or general fever excites or interrupts functional activity.

---

The June number of the Journal of Osteopathy is at hand.

Advertisements of Malted Milk, Antiphlogistine, Listerine and Bovinine seem to be out of place in a journal opposed to drug medication.

Dr. A. T. Still states, before his class, that the human body is a laboratory which prepares chemicals and pharmaceutical drugs for the use of the body. It is difficult for a physician to get away from his medical training.

The doctor states that all diseases, except those which are infectious or contagious, can be managed by mechanics. Chiropractors take pleasure in **accepting** those which Osteopaths **except.**

He says that tuberculosis is caused by paralysis of the pneumogastric, which allows the blood to stagnate, ferment and deposit a cheesy matter in the cells of the lungs.

The above pathology is not that of Chiropractic.

Under Field Notes, we find No. 3 had a bad case of hives. To stop the itching he bathed the parts with 1 dram of cyanide of potassium. Is that Osteopathy?

Mrs. Gunn, a neighbor, came to me one day last May with intolerable itching, because of hives. I gave her permanent relief by one Chiropractic adjustment; that was Chiropractic. Very much unlike Osteopathy.

Osteopathic treatment of effects and Chiropractic adjustments of the cause of hives are certainly dissimilar.

No. 5 reports a case of phagocytosis (ingestion of bacteria) following smallpox five years previously. The left limb is greatly enlarged and has a continued lymph exudate discharge. He says there is no spinal lesion.

The Chiropractor finds a lesion at 5th cervical for smallpox. and one in the lumbar for the discharging ulcer. There is no lesional relation between the two.

Between the two systems there is a vast difference in pathology. The Osteopath finds no lesion—the Chiropractor does. Their treatment and adjusting are also very unlike.

One reports a case diagnosed as abdominal tumor, floating kidneys and enlarged spleen. He says: "It will require a surgical operation to determine just what it is and where located."

It seems to me, that Osteopathy, of late, is sliding back into medicine and surgery. Better advance by accepting Chiropractic.

I would be ashamed to know that I had graduated one who could not diagnose between the above three pathological conditions without turning the patient over to the surgeon.

One Osteopath has a Turkish bath outfit and two electric light bath cabinets. These may be appropriate, they may look well, may even be necessary in an Osteopath's operating room, but they would be out of place in a Chiropractor's adjusting room.

No. 5 "gives as a reason for not prosecuting the Chiros that the American people are too much in sympathy with the man who seems to be persecuted and it will only react in his favor and against the prosecutor." No. 5, "Your head is level. You do not forget the early days of Osteopathy, nor the two legal meetings of Osteopathy and Chiropractic in Wisconsin.

## CHIROPRACTIC DEFINED.

**The Philosophy of Chiropractic** is founded upon the knowledge of the manner in which vital functions are performed by Innate in health and disease. When this controlling intelligence is able to transmit mental impulses to all parts of the body, free and unobstructed, we have normal action which is health.

Innate directs its vital energy thru the nervous system to specialize the co-ordination of sensation and volition thru the cumulative and vegetative functions.

Displacement of any part of the skeletal frame may press against nerves, which are the channels of communication, intensifying or decreasing their carrying capacity, creating either too much or not enough functionating, an aberration known as disease. The nature of the affection depends upon the shape of the bone, the amount of pressure, age of patient, character of nerves impinged upon and the individual make-up.

**Chiropractors** adjust, by hand, all displacements of the 200 bones, more especially those of the vertebral column, for the purpose of removing nerve impingements which are the cause of deranged functions. The long bones and the vertebral processes are used as levers by which to adjust displacements of osseous tissue of the body. By so doing, normal transmission of nerve-force is restored.

Vital functions are individualized, physical expressions

Knowing that our physical health and the intellectual progress of Innate (the personified portion of Universal Intelligence) depend upon the proper alignment of the skeletal frame, we feel it our bounden duty to replace any displaced bones so that physical and spiritual health, happiness and the full fruition of earthly life may be fully enjoyed.

Chiropractic resembles Osteopathy more so than any other method; yet they are as different as day is from night. In practice, Osteopaths are absorbing Chiropractic. Osteopaths state that Chiropractic is a part of Osteopathy; yet their schools affirm that they do not teach it.

That the investigator may see the difference between the two methods, I append a definition of Osteopathy given by Dr. William H. Cobble, an Osteopath:

"Osteopathy is a science of drugless healing, based upon the principle that the body has been endowed by Nature with all the fluids and forces necessary for the preservation of health and recovery from disease, providing the mechanism which produces and distributes these fluids and forces is in perfect mechanical adjustment."

Dr. A. P. Davis, a student of the first class in Osteopathy under A. T. Still, the founder, states in his masterly work of 851 pages:

"Diseases are recognized as only the result of the interruption of the onward flow of the fluids of the body, in their various rounds to build up and tear down the various tissues in itself, and that when these tissues are normally built up and the waste material properly eliminated, health is the inevitable result."

Osteopathy is thus defined by A. T. Still, the founder:

"Natural flow of blood in health and disease is the effect of local or general disturbance of blood—that to excite the nerves causes muscles to contract and compress venous flow of blood to the heart; and the bones could be used as levers to relieve pressure on nerves, veins and arteries."

"Historical: Osteopathy was discovered by A. T. Still, of Baldwin, Kan., 1874."

---

"Chiropractic Physician." A Chiropractor is one who is versed in the science of Chiropractic and the art of adjusting displaced vertebrae. A physician is one who has received the degree of M. D., Doctor of Medicine, and is licensed to practice medicine. It is barely possible that the author of this card is a Chiropractor and a physician. But the expression, a Chiropractic physician, or a physician Chiropractor, is the joining of two words of opposite meaning. "Disease is a result of deranged functions." Disease is a disturbance of function or an abnormal condition of any part of the body. "Disease is imperfect co-ordination of mind and body." In many diseases the mind and body co-ordinate. The reasoning of an insane mind is co-ordinated by muscular movements of the body. A diseased condition may exist, a condition in which Innate is not able to transmit an impulse as given, and yet the mind and body may have the same degree; may be in harmony with each other and yet not be in accord with Innate. "Chiropractic adjustments eliminate the cause and effects." Effects cannot be adjusted; causes can be. "Abnormal conditions in the spine are **at the bottom** of every ailment." What is at the top? "Innate intelligence" is, or should be personified, used as a proper noun, therefore, should commence with capitals. "After other healing systems have failed." Chiropractic is not a healing system. It has nothing in common with any other system and is not therapeutical, does not use remedies, does not treat, cure or heal.

## "SEROUS CIRCULATION."

The human body contains about 60 per cent of its weight in water. It is said "All organisms must have running water." The human structure has moving water transuding through all tissues. Water in the human economy performs important functions. When these are accomplished in a normal manner the result is health. When the circulation is too rapid or too slow it unbalances that equilibrium. By water the solid foods are dissolved so they may be digested, absorbed and assimilated. The waste products leave the body in the urine as an aqueous solution, through the skin as insensible perspiration and by the way of the intestines as a semi-solid stool.

The water in the human body must transudate in order to perform its functions. Its stagnation means a lack of function, the result being one of the many forms of dropsy, which are named according to the portions of the body in which the infiltrated fluid finds lodgement.

The transuded fluid is known as lymph. When functions are properly performed, when the tissue drainage is normal, when no more fluid is exuded into the capillary tubes than is needed, the proper amount escaping from the tissues by exudation into the compound tubular glands of the kidneys, the physiologic balance is maintained and there is health.

When it is considered that water is constantly being thrown off in the urine and feces, also by the skin and lungs, the importance of a constant supply and continued renewal of it will be apparent.

All foods contain more or less water; it is therefore, a constituent part of food. But in and of itself it is not a food, although thought to be so by some writers. No greater mistake could be made, than to state: "**Water is a liquid food** which is digested and assimilated." Food is that which is eaten by animals, digested and assimilated as nourishment. Water is not separated into the nutritive and non-nutritive elements, as is food, in its passage through the alimentary canal. Water is not converted into fluid or solid nutriment by the process of digestion and absorption. Water does not contain fats, proteids or carbohydrates, nutritive materials for the animal economy. Physiologists divide all foods into nitrogenous and non-nitrogenous. Water does not contain albumens or fats, therefore it is not a food, it is only a distributor. Water does not contain proteids, extractives or salts until it becomes a transudating fluid in the body.

Ott refers to the infiltration and transudation of water through the capillaries; also to the capillary circulation of fluids in animals and plants. He says that "water has an im-portant function to perform. When proteids are inefficient water accumulates in the tissues."

The American Text Book of Physiology states that the re-moval of from 5 to 6 per cent of water from the body, in cholera, causes the blood to flow slowly; that no urine is secreted and the nerves become especially irritable.

Stewart refers to the circulation in the capillaries and the **existence of channels** between arteries and veins.

Landois speaks of this "serous circulation" as "a regulated, chemical transformation of the tissues."

Kirkes' Physiology refers to "the circulation through the capillaries" as "the **capillary flow.**"

Dutton's Anatomy states: "The lymphatics **carry** lymph, a **clear fluid** or chyle. The lymphatic vessels constitute a sys-tem of minute, delicate, transparent vessels, which have their origin in the lymph **spaces,** or capillary plexuses, **of almost every organ in the body;** and, after passing through one or more lymph-nodes, or glands, finally **empty** into the veins and **general circulation.** These **vessels resemble the veins, but are smaller and more numerous.** They are often called **absorbents.**"

Gerrish thus describes this "Serous Circulation." "The lym-phatic system begins in the microscopic crevices between the cells and fibers of almost all tissues. **These diminutive spaces are called 'juice channels' or 'juice canals,'** because they are the **receptacles of the fluids which exude** from the adjacent blood-vessels and tissues."

Gray is acquainted with this "Serous Circulation." He says: "The lymph **canalicular system is the system of spaces in areolar tissue.** . . . they form connections with each other by **anastomotic channels** and constitute **a system of spaces and channels.**"

Cunningham did not forget to mention the passage of lymph through intervening tissues by transudation. He says: "Lymphatic **vessels anastomose freely** together, and the major-ity form **communicating channels.**"

Sobotta describes this "Serous Circulation" as an appendage to the vascular system. He says: "They (the lymphatic ves-sels) pursue a relatively straight and extended course, with but little inclination to anastomose."

McFarland, when referring to this "Serous Circulation," uses such terms as, imperfect circulation, serous infiltration, transuded fluid, circulatory disturbances, serous exudate and system of tissue drainage.

Much more might be cited on "Serous Circulation." Then why should any one make such remarks as "No physiology or anatomy gives these new thoughts. Serous circulation is an original theme. This dogma is mine."

Morris gives the dates of the first knowledge of the lymphatic system, which includes its transudation as well as its functions. "Lymphatic vessels were discovered in 1622 by Asellio, and the receptaculum chyli and thoracic duct by Pecquet in 1647. From that time onward the system was diligently studied, and, in 1797, Mascagni published a comprehensive account of it."

"The dogma" of the "Serous Circulation" was discovered nearly 300 years ago.

"I am aware this is a broad jump, and one in which ridicule will be heaped upon me by all professions, but it is because I, at least, and those keen students who imbue it thoroughly that agree with me, that encourages me to speak what I think. At first reading it will appear the height of ridiculousness, but **studying** (not reading) will open a cloud now and then, for these paragraphs are full of meat if the shell be broken."

The author of "Serous Circulation" did not have to "jump" to get his thoughts, for they are found in every book on anatomy, physiology and pathology. A jump may be long or short, but never "broad." Educational professors have an opportunity to ridicule the article referred to. It is not the province of a profession, but of the professors to criticise. A student may have a keen understanding—but a "keen student" —never. "Imbue" is a transitive verb—requires an object to complete a sentence. We could say, students who **imbibe** it have their minds imbued or tinctured by those sentiments. I can see how prejudice will cloud men's minds and impair their honesty, but I fail to see how "studying will open a cloud."

I have cracked some of the paragraph shells and find that what is new is of no value and what is of worth is given in every book on anatomy, physiology and pathology. It is ridiculous for any one to state that "Serous Circulation has never been conceived before." It certainly never has been.

---

From a Chiropractic's booklet I copy, "The spine is the line shaft of the body."

A line-shaft is the main bar of steel syndrical, solid or hollow, used to support rotating pulleys, flywheels, transmitting power by rotation in a shop or factory.

The human body is not a shop or factory, it does not manufacture goods, wares, or utensils. There is no resemblance whatever between a line shaft and the spine or backbone. In appearance they are as unlike as any two objects on earth; they are not similar in shape, material, structure and very unlike in their use. Why not talk Chiropractic instead of childish nonsense?

"A stiff, irregular spine is a **sure** indication of mental or physical disturbance."

There are many, very many, exceptions to the above, in fact, the exception is the rule. Hunchbacks are as free of disease, or more so and as frequently live to a ripe old age as the ordinary.

"These (the above) are axioms upon which the science of Chiropractic is founded."

An axiom is a self-evident truth; a proposition or quality of being true which is so evident that no reason or demonstration can make it plainer. I see nothing in the above two copied lines, except absurd stultiloquy. I hope no one will think for a moment that I built the science of Chiropractic on such nonsensical absurdities.

Chiropractic as a science is founded on tone. Its philosophy deals with the knowledge of biological phenomena, that state of a body, or any of its organs or parts, in which the animal and organic functions are performed with normal vigor. Biological philosophy deals with the origin, development, structure, functions and occurring phenomena accompanying in life, growth and reproduction. The one who reduces these principles to practice, gives philosophical reasons for their cause, energy and the laws governing vital action and those of the intellectual of the human economy, is a philosopher. The science of Chiropractic is not founded on chemistry, shops, factories, line-shafts or machinery.

"Most of diseases have their origin in a combination of pressure."

I am frank to say, I am not onto the combination. I prefer being specific, definite and precise in locating causes and just as explicit and exact in adjusting.

"In typhoid fever there is always pressure at second lumbar, fifth and tenth dorsal, first and fifth cervical."

I have given relief to many typhoid cases by adjusting the sixth dorsal and no where else. Why adjust five places? This "combination system" does not seem to harmonize with "the direct brain system?"

"Acute diseases yield rapidly to adjustments."

To be rapid is to advance with haste or speed. To yield is to give up, to surrender, relinquish. My boy you have used the wrong words; words of nearly opposite meaning; words which do not express what you desire to say.

"The intervertebral discs should be normally a fourth of an inch in length."

You certainly intended referring to their thickness; discs have no length. A flat, round circular plate of iron, paper or cartilage has no length; it has circumference, diameter and thickness.

"From subluxations come the pressure which holds back from the organs and tissues the vitalizing currents."

Hello! You have vital energy and electric fluid mixed. Their mixing looks bad on paper and causes death in the human body. Vital energy cannot be mixed with mechanical, electric, thermal or chemical. I have not known of anyone trying to mix vital force of the human body with the magneto-electric dynamic. The mixing of them in our literature kills the principles of Chiropractic.

"Consultation on this matter is invited."

A consultation is the meeting of two or more physicians to consult or deliberate on a particular phase of disease, usually in the presence of the patient. A prospective patient may consult the physician in regard to his case or for advice, but that is not a consultation.

"In all cases of tuberculosis there is pressure found upon the nerves supplying vitality to the lungs, stomach, liver and kidneys."

In tuberculosis the lungs, are most frequently affected and hence the term is often used in the sense of pulmonary tuberculosis. In children the lymphatic glands, bones and joints are more often tuberculated. The brain, spleen, intestines, kidneys, liver, skin, mucos membranes and the peritoneum are subject to such an affection. The stomach is exempt.

Nerves do not supply vitality to the organs. Vital energy is a permanent attribute, it is not an adjunct to any organ, it is a part of its being, it belongs to it. An organ and its energy, vital force, are inseparable, they are coexistant, as much so as human economy and life.

"One of the foundation principles of Chiropractic may be thus stated—"Chiropractic simplifies the problem of the restoration of health by recognizing the fact that a few abnormal conditions may, by combination, have many manifestations or symptoms. But the cause of all diseases is found in the conditions, not in the symptoms. Its work is to remove the conditions. Then the disease by whatever name it is called, ceases to exist."

The foundation principle of Chiropractic is contained in four letters, it does not take 300 to express it, and, even then, in all the above there is not a fundamental principle. I see it is quoted. The author of that paragraph is always talking and writing about the foundation of Chiropractic and its basic principles, but, no one ever heard him state the principle upon which this science is founded. That quoted paragraph is not the philosophy of Chiropractic.

"The problem of the restoration of health."

A problem is a question to be solved; it requires a mental solution. To solve this problem is a question of philosophy—not a principle. Chiropractors do not "remove conditions," they change them. Disease is a condition or relaxation, abnormal function and structural change. Disease is not any thing added which must be removed; conditions need changing.

"Legally the Chiropractor stands with the physical culturist and the masseur."

The Chiropractor has no legal standing. No state or country has recognized thon or the science.

"Allowing a free movement of the vital forces from the brain, along the nerves to the various organs of the body."

The physical strength or vigor or a living being, the energy which characterizes a living being from inanimate objects, known as vital force, a power dependent upon life, is not manufactured in the brain or elsewhere, to be transported, in, thru, on, or along the nerves.

Vital force is that form of energy which is manifested in the phenomena of life, being distinct from other forces of nature such as mechanical, electrical, and chemical.

Tone manifests itself by its renitency, its elastic resistance to impressions, whether from the center or the peripheral. The momentum of an impulse, a thot passing over the nerves, is measured by the renitency of the nerves over which it is carried.

"Chiropractic's work is to remove the conditions."

Is not that the work of the Chiropractor instead of the science?

A Ph. C. (the title in this instance was conferred by the class—you tickle me and I will tickle you,) says "Chiropractic is the name of a drugless theory."

Chiropractic is not a theory, it never was with the founder; each case demonstrated it to be built on facts. Theory is opposed to practice, the actual performance or application of knowledge, a plan or scheme theoretically constructed, not demonstrated.

"It is founded upon the philosophical and physiological laws."

A law is simply a rule or an ascertained order of succession of phenomena, whereby one becomes the premonitory sign of another. Philosophy is a general systematic conception, the knowledge of laws. A law, under certain conditions, is invariable in its phenomena, whether its philosophy is understood or not.

"It is unfailing in its results, when applied by a competent hand."

This "competent hand" uses massage for costiveness instead of adjusting the 12th dorsal.

"At the time the theory of Chiropractic was discovered."

I did not discover the theory. That which I named Chiropractic was a theory but twenty minutes previous to adjusting Harvey Lillard. As soon as I demonstrated it to be a fact, it was no longer a theory. I discovered facts, not theories. Any one can theorize; a philosopher demonstrates his reasons to be based on facts.

"He (Harvey Lillard) told that while working under a building, he forgot himself, and suddenly straightening up struck his head against the floor."

Harvey Lillard never told me or any one else the above story; why not state facts?

"As he did so he heard something crack in his neck."

He felt something give way in his back; that is what he told me. I adjusted the 4th dorsal, not a cervical, relieving him by one adjustment, however, he returned the third day for examination.

"By a crude attempt of the adjustment of the lesion."

That "crude adjustment" has never been equalled by the teacher of the "Imperial College."

"The theory of Chiropractic is based upon the philosophical possibilities of displaced bones."

The principles of Chiropractic never was a theory with me; the first adjustment demonstrated it to be a fact. Chiropractic is demonstrable and always was. It is not based on "philosophical possibilities." Theorists theorize on "possibilities," philosophers reduce their reasoning to practice by demonstration.

"Chiropracticly; disease is a change in function, either above or below normal, which is nicely illustrated in Bright's disease, and diabetes; in the former there is a lack of action, in the latter there is too much."

"Chiropracticly" is not known by Webster's dictionary.

Bright's disease and diabetes are not suitable to illustrate a change, the two extremes of functionating, as Bright's disease is an inflammatory condition of the kidneys, while diabetes is the result of an inflammation of the pancreas.

"The fact remains that nerves are the means through which the functionary energy is carried to the different organs.

Energy which produces function is not carried or transported from one part or portion to another. The energy of each organ depends upon its vigor or tonicity.

"The vertebra are very likely to subluxation."

The above "Ph. C." (philosophical Chiropractor) should have said, "The vertebrae are liable to be subluxated."

A comprehension of the philosophy of Chiropractic makes a distinction between it and all other methods. An understanding of the principles lays the foundation for the superstructure of Chiropractic. The know how, skill and practice makes one proficient in the art. This self-labled philosophical Chiropractor knows but little about the philosophy of Chiropractic.

---

I can consistently and justly claim to be **The Fountain Head** of Chiropractic, the primary source from which issued the original first principle of the science which I had the pleasure of naming. See Rev. Weed's letters on pages 102, 103 and 104.

I am the Founder by virtue of the fact, that by years of teaching, by word of mouth and public writings, I have disseminated its principles, and by my original method of hand-adjusting of vertebrae which peculiarly belongs therewith. As the **author** of these principles, and of the hand-adjusting, I laid the foundation, and **built thereon, the science of Chiropractic.**

The first Chiropractic Adjustment was given Harvey Lillard in September, 1895. The principles upon which Chiropractic is based lie in that first vertebral adjustment given by me. For years I had questioned physicians and others, asking what difference there was, in two persons who were similarly situated, that caused one to have a certain ailment while the other remained free from it. That important question was answered by the discovery that displaced (sub-luxated) vertebrae impinged upon nerves, which are but tubular cords of the same substance as that which composes the brain and spinal cord and whose functions are to convey impulses and sensations to and from the nerve centers. This pressure caused by projections, modifies the force of Innate's desire; therefore, disease is but aberrated impulse, increased or decreased from that which is normal. If it was so in this case of deafness, why is it not so in other diseases? Disease is nothing more nor less than functions performed in either a too great or too little degree. If they are performed in a normal or a natural amount, as desired by Innate, we have health. Pressure on nerves causes irritation and tension with deranged functions as a result. Why not release the pressure? Why not adjust causes instead of treating effects. Why not?

## TUBERCULOSIS.

Definition: This disease is often called consumption or phthisis. Tuberculosis refers to the growth and development of tubercles, small tumors or nodules in the substance of organs. It must be remembered, however, that tuberculosis may occur without a single definite tubercle. Inflammation is always present. It may affect any organ or tissue in the body. It is not always a disease of the lungs. The intestines and the brain are especially liable to be the seat of this disease, especially in those who are under the age of puberty. The disease is one and the same, in process, wherever it may occur, altho the details may vary. In this disease, as in others, age makes a difference; it attacks the lungs in the adult and the intestines in children. The bones and joints are frequently affected by it in the form of caries or necrosis.

Etiology:—Tuberculosis is the result of mechanical lesions in the spine, the region depending upon the portion or organ affected. McFarland's pathology says of this disease, "the origin and source of infection is unknown."

Pathological Anatomy:—Tuberculosis is characterized by an inflammatory, necrotic process and an eruption of small nodules, known as milliary tubercles, which vary from the size of a pinhead to that of a small pea. They are attended by inflammatory lesions which coalesce and cause the affected tissue to assume a cheesy appearance — caseous degeneration. These centers of caseous necrosis may become liquified, causing cavities which are filled with purulent liquid and degenerated matter. On a free surface, it forms ulcers. They may involve not only the soft tissue, but the bones also. Tubercles tend to coalesce and form large tubercular masses and sometimes distinct tuberculous tumors. These lesions are due to inflammation. It should be remembered that similar nodules are found in other diseases.

Pathological Physiology:—The patient is weak, anemic and emaciated and has a hectic fever and night sweats. The skin becomes pale and white, the fingers enlarge at the tips and the nails curve over their ends.

Locality:—The most frequent seats of tuberculosis are the lungs, intestinal tract, lymphatic glands, serous membranes, bones, skin, testes, brain, fallopian tubes, uterus and spleen.

Consumption of the bowels is usually a secondary lesion following consumption of the lungs. The extension of the disease to the intestines is indicated by a persistent and watery diarrhea. The stools are thin often yellow, and contain pus and small fragments of the lining membrane. Occasionally a small amount of blood is seen. This is because of necrosis of the intestine due to an excessive amount of heat. At a later stage, the abdomen becomes full and tender, the patient is feverish, rapidly loses flesh and becomes exceedingly feeble. In children, tumors the size of the fist can occasionally be felt in the abdomen.

---

The following is from The Journal of Osteopathy. "There are foramina between the vertebrae through which all spinal nerves pass out before reaching soft tissue and a very slight deviation of vertebrae will compress these nerves; and may cause all kinds of trouble depending on the severity of pressure and distribution of these certain nerves, their various functions and distribution.

"The trouble with the Osteopaths and M. D.'s is we do not wish to admit that there is any better way than ours.

"**All** spinal and vaso-motor **nerves pass out through the foramina between the vertebrae, a slight deviation of which will compress these out-going nerves and cause all kinds of trouble.**"

This kind of talk in the year 1910 sounds like Chiropractic of ten years ago, seems good to hear it. It does not coincide with Osteopathy of 1902, when Dr. A. T. Still said, dried ear wax was the cause of croup, sore throat, tonsillitis, pneumonia and all diseases of the lungs, nose and head; and a rational cure therefor, which any mother could appreciate, perfectly safe, putting glycerin in a child's ear. See A. T. Still's book on Osteopathy, date 1902, pages 295, 299 and 300. With my book in hand they can now make further progress.

The Science Circle of Osteopathy says: It seems to me that **if we discard vaccination and the newer serum and vaccine theories that we are tearing down the very framework on which our science is based and admitting that osteopathy with its theory of impeded flow of pure blood with all its germicidal powers is faulty. We are not using drugs but simply assisting nature in as true a sense as when we reduce a bony lesion.**"

The science of Osteopathy is based upon the same theory, flow of pure blood, as that of medication.

**A drug is any medicine used to cure disease. Vaccine virus and toxic serum are not used to cure disease, but to create them; therefore, they are not drugs, they are poisons.**

"Assisting nature" is the slogan of the medical and Osteopathic professions, and I am sorry to know that term is used by many Chiropractors. Assisting nature by making disease is Allopathic and now I learn that it is Osteopathic, also.

Nature is a term loosely used to cover indiscriminately both biologic and non-living phenomena, the energy by which the innumerable phenomena we see daily occurring are produced. Everything is nature, natural, could not be otherwise. The processes of health and disease are of nature—the inevitable law of nature. We, aş Chiropractors, simply **adjust the tensor-frame in order to return nerves and thru them muscles and organs to tone, normal tension.** Nature is producing phenomena just as much under the condition of too much or not enough tension, a condition known as disease, as tone, normal tension.

A writer in The Journal of Osteopathy says: "On examination I found the **second cervical vertebra up and twisted to the right.**

"In making my examination I found that **all the vertebrae from the second cervical down to the fifth dorsal, were out of place,** the second, third and fourth dorsals being decidedly anterior."

A vertebra is one of the bones which by their union form the vertebral column. A vertebra is composed of a body, spinous process, two transverse processes, the four oblique articulating processes, two pedicles, and an arch or laminae. It takes all these parts combined to constitute a vertebra. He did not find the vertebra **up, higher in the vertebral column than it should be**; neither did he find the vertebra twisted. He found, at least, he thot he had, the spinous process to the right of the median line. As to the second cervical vertebra being tilted, tipped, so that the spinous process was upward, crowding against the spinous process of the second, is a question difficult to determine because of its being so much smaller and shorter than the adjoining processes. As to the spinous process being "twisted to the right," is not only using a wrong term, but a condition which is very doubtful. We refer to the spinal column being twisted, a condition of torsion, but not of the spinous process or vertebra when making an examination of the distal ends of the spinous processes on the living body; as to the determination of the spinous process of the second cervical being to the right of the median line, is difficult to determine. We must remember that the spinous process of the second cervical vertebra consists of two prongs that are frequently unequal in length, or perhaps one or both are absent owing to fracture or morphological defects, which would make an apparent difference when palpating.

In the second statement, "Found all the vertebrae from the second cervical down to the fifth dorsal out of place." A vertebrae displaced is not in juxtaposition with its adjoining neighbors, and not a half dozen above or below.

"The second, third and fourth dorsal being decidedly anterior." An examination of the oblique articulating processes show that the condition of one or some vertebrae being anterior of their neighbors is an impossibility without a fracture having occurred of one or more of the articulating processes.

Osteopaths have from time to time changed their definition of Osteopathy. To do so is perfectly right, but they should remember that they are progressing, or at least a portion of them are, in practice as well as in definition. The following is found in the June number of The Osteopath Journal: it aims to cover the whole field, or at least all that is contained in an Osteopathic view. Should Dr. Heath chance to peruse this volume, he will see a need of revising his proposed legal definition.

"Osteopathy as a therapeutic art, includes an educated and skillful use of the hands in manipulating the structures and tissues of the body so as to restore normal conditions, and includes all forms of hand manipulations and movements under whatever name; such as putting all joints and structures through their normal motions to ascertain their condition, stretching and relaxing muscles and ligaments by lateral tension, springing and rotating the spine by lateral pressure to overcome any rigidity or misplacements or curvatures, stimulating or inhibiting the circulation or nerve supply by pressure over the vaso-motor centers, circular and vibratory movements with the hand over groups of muscles to stimulate their activity, and working congested organs in the direction of their drainage by a massage movement and giving a chopping movement over inactive organs to stimulate their activity, to which is added such suggestions as the condition of the mind seems to indicate and the habit."

The Chiropractor has no use for any of the principles, philosophy or movements mentioned by Dr. Heath.

The one move of the Chiropractor falls far short of being a manipulation. The Chiropractor does not spring or rotate the spine by lateral pressure to overcome rigidity, misplacements or curvatures.

The Osteopaths will have to get busy, be in a hurry, if they catch up with the science, art and philosophy of Chiropractic as developed by the founder.

---

"Mr. Brown," said the doctor, "you have a very sick wife. She is at death's door, but I think I can pull her through."

Mrs. Brown died. Now, Mr. Brown is wondering which door the doctor meant.

## NEUROLOGY—CHEMISTRY.

"As all heat (page 505) is due to molecular change or friction, or chemical changes, it is very reasonable to attribute the cause of fever to bi-chemical changes, causing increased molecular action."

While it is true that **heat is generated by** both **molecular and chemical change**, there is a vast difference between these two forces, which are in no way related to, or responsible for, each other.

**Molecular action creates heat,** the amount being determined by the quantity of **atomic friction. Chemical heat is induced by a combination** of substances of varying qualities.

Molecular change creates heat by and thru the **force of gravitation** acting upon particles of matter without reference to their character. There is another form of force found in the realm of atoms, which is effective **between** the atoms of **chemically different bodies,** that of **chemical affinity.**

**Both mechanical action and chemical combination create heat,** but by quite different processes.

**Gravitation and affinity** are very different forces.

Molecular change of atoms is caused by the **interaction of forces,** while chemical change, known as **chemism, is dependent upon elective attraction, affinity,** the tendency or ability of one substance to unite with another.

The force which unites the particles of any single body is known as **gravitation**; that which **combines,** fuses, **two or more** bodies of different natures into one, is called chemical affinity.

Molecular or anatomic friction creates heat by **vibration** of its particles. In a chemical process, when affinities are satisfied, heat is set free—generated by the **force of unition,** the intermingling, while forming a compound, of the molecules of unlike substances, because of their affinity.

**These two forces, gravitation and affinity,** are present in both the human body and the chemical laboratory. The former is operated by an **intelligent vital force** which I saw fit to name Innate—born with. The latter is directed by the **educated mind of man.** One is governed by an **unerring intelligence,** the other is **laboratory experimentation.** These two branches of knowledge are known as **metabolism and chemism.** The laws of **gravitation and affinity** are present in both. **Innate Intelligence runs the former** and a **chemist,** one given to chemical investigation, one versed in chemistry, **the latter.**

**Adhesion** (molecular gravitation) and **chemism,** the force exerted between the atoms of elementary substances, whereby they unite to form chemical compounds, and chemical affinity are quite different attractions.

A laboratory is the workroom of a chemist, a place devoted to experiments in any branch of natural science.

I think it will be readily seen, that **all changes in the body are molecular** and **those in the laboratory are chemical. Molecular action, therefore, is not caused by chemical or bi-chemical changes. Molecular and chemical changes are in no way related to or dependent upon each other.**

**It is not reasonable, logical or within the realm of facts, to state that, chemical or bi-chemical changes cause increased molecular action, inflammation or fever.**

"Neuropathy" tells us, on page 77: "Nature is continually demonstrating the fact that **affinity is a product** of certain chemical constituents."

Biological affinity is the physiologic relationship between organs. In chemistry it is the attraction occurring between heterogenous substances, resulting in compounds.

In metabolism, food comes in contact with saliva, gastric juice, succus entericus, pancreatic juice and bile. This active, attractive transference is physiologic affinity. Chemical affinity is the attractive force between the atoms of different materials, which induce them to unite and form a new substance—a compound. Instead of affinity being a product, it is attraction—physiologic or chemical.

If an undue amount of heat is confined in one locality of the body, it is known as inflammation. If this elevation of temperature is generally diffused thruout the body it is termed fever.

In health, heat production and heat dissipation are evenly balanced. In fever, the body is in a large measure incapacitated for normal activity; anabolism is decreased and katabolism is increased. The pores of the protecting covering of the body are closed, preventing the escape of the superabundant heat. In health, if heat production is increased, so also is heat dissipation. Under normal conditions there can be no elevation of temperature or an accumulation of heat.

Fever is an overproduction of heat and its retention in the body by the closing of the pores of the cuticle.

To determine the composition of the human body, a dead body is subjected to chemical analysis.

Functional activity is not chemical analysis.

Chemical analysis of any or all portions of a dead body does not give a correct understanding of the intimate nature of physiological processes. The chemical analysis of a dead body is easily made, but it does not give us knowledge of the successive stages through which food passed before it was changed into living tissue. The methods used for chemical analysis destroy the composition and vitality of the substance. The products obtained from a living body are peculiar to a living body—not to a dead one.

Chemical analysis can only be performed on a dead body. There can not be such a process as chemic physiology, or physiologic chemistry.

By chemical analysis the body can be reduced to a number of liquid and solid compounds which belong to the organic and inorganic realms of matter. These are proximate principles of the living body. They cannot be analyzed in the living body.

---

The nervous system is anatomically and functionally highly developed.

The nervous and vascular systems are the first to appear. As such they are vitally important, for they furnish the energy and material for the development of the ovum, the forming of the embryo and the growth of the fetus.

The spermatozoa give life, furnish vital function to the nucleus of the ovum. The yolk supplies food, the spermatozoon vital force, the vegetative function growth. The spermatozoon, yolk, heat and moisture create a parasite.

The villi of the chorin are nervous vascular projections on the surface of the impregnated ovum, which adapt it for living on the body of its host. With its tufts of hair-like appendages, it penetrates deeply into the uterine mucosa, even into the ducts of its glands, using its villi like roots in a loose soil, thereby becoming a parasite. These villi receive the energy to perform the vegetative function of growth from the spermatozoon.

After the ovum has lodged itself in the wall of the uterus, the villi perform the function of absorbing nutriment for the building of the embryo. Thus the host is compelled to furnish nutrition for its guest.

In time the embryo builds the placenta and receives its nutrition through endosmosis. The nervous system supplies the energy, the vital functionating necessary to run the vegetative function of growth. Thus the co-ordination of these two systems (nervous and vascular) furnishes the nutriment and creates the embryo.

We have good reasons to believe that the vascular and nervous systems are co-related, one furnishing the material, the other the energy, until the fetus becomes an infant and breathes the breath of life.

"Chiropractic is the science of locating and removing pressure from nerves. Every organ in the body is controlled by impulses from the brain, which it transmits through the nerves: Pressure interferes with its transmission. Disease is the expression of an impulse so interfered with. Normal impulse expresses health.

"Chiropractors adjust those displaced bones of the spine which are pressing on the nerves as they branch from the spinal cord."

Chiropractic **as a science** defines the laws of life and embodies them into a system for the preservation of health. Chiropractic, also, includes the art of adjusting, by hand, any or all subluxations of the 300 articulations of the human body, more particularly those of the vertebral column, so that Innate may have perfect control of the vital functions.

The second sentence tells us that impulses start from the brain; that the brain transmits them through the nerves; that the brain is the intelligence which controls every organ in the body. The true Chiropractic idea is that Innate controls the communicating force known as impulse, through an elongated structure, which is cord-like, and contains filaments for the conductors of nervous impulses from and to the brain. It also affords a central path for reflex actions. The third sentence is indefinite. It would be better to have said that an impingement modifies the force of an impulse. The thought contained in the fourth sentence is more correctly stated as follows: A deranged communicated force causes diseased conditions.

"Normal impulse." An impulse is the desire of Innate for the performance of a certain act. This impulse, or desire, cannot be otherwise than normal. Innate wants every act performed just right, otherwise it would be unnatural. There cannot be an abnormal impulse, a wrong desire. A nerve, the channel through which Innate sends its messages, may be impinged upon, pressed against, bent, stretched or irritated so that the communicative force, or impulse, is transmitted too slowly or too rapidly.

"Pressing on the nerves as they branch from the spinal cord." The spinal nerves are rooted in the spinal cord; they spring from it. The anterior and posterior roots form a nerve called the trunk, which does not branch until after it leaves the spinal canal. This mixed trunk, named spinal nerve, contains afferent and efferent nerves. Upon its exit, it divides into four branches, one of which connects with the sympathetic nervous system and furnishes it with innervating force, and through its channels Innate forwards its impulses to and from the vital organs and the vascular system.

## HEMORRHAGE IN DISEASE.

Hemorrhage in disease is confined to an exudation of blood thru capillaries or its forcible flow thru ruptured blood-vessels.

McFarland states that about half of the cadávers examined show seepage of blood into the stomach. The eroded surface of cancers and ulcers oozes blood into that organ. Hemorrhage escaping from the mouth is, usually, termed "coffee-ground vomit," as the blood is modified by gastric juice and arterialization.

Pulmonary hemorrhage is of common occurrence. There are several diseases of the lungs, as tuberculosis pulmonalis, hyperemia, ulceration and gangrene, in which hemorrhage is one of the symptoms. If capillaries are eroded, the hemorrhage is slight, the sputum being merely stained with blood. If large vessels are ruptured, the hemorrhage may be extensive, perhaps fatal.

McFarland states: "Hemorrhage from the lungs—hemoptysis—may occur from the oozing of blood from the eroded capillaries, usually situated in the walls of the cavities. It may occur from the direct erosion of a blood-vessel of considerable size, but is usually preceded by aneurysmal dilation resulting from weakening of the walls of the vessel. The hemorrhages are of all degrees of severity—sometimes only sufficient to tinge the expectoration slightly red, sometimes large enough to cause the death of the patient from loss of blood. When large hemorrhages are not fatal they are usually distinctly detrimental, in that the blood which escapes by way of the air-vessels is sucked back into the bronchioles and air-cells with each inspiratory effort, thus lessening the already diminished breathing space, increasing the amount of effete matter contained within the lungs. Hemorrhages are sometimes followed by gangrene of the lung."

Hemorrhages of the brain and spinal cord may be minute or massive. The escaped blood is partly infiltrated into the brain substance and perivascular spaces. This is accompanied with softening of the brain or cord. These characteristic changes are necrotic and belong to the class of colliquation necrosis.

McFarland says: Hemorrhage between bone and periosteum may cause superficial necrosis. He should have said necrosis of the periosteum may cause hemorrhage.

Arthritis or inflammation of joints may create a slight hemorrhage and an accumulation of blood in the joint. As the inflammation subsides the blood is absorbed.

Hemorrhage from the bowels, in small quantities, imparts a chocolate color to the stool. Excessive hemorrhages depend upon the denudation of large vessels—the detachment of masses of exfoliating tissue. If bright blood appears with the stool, it is from the rectum.

For vicarious menstruation, see Anomalies and Curiosities of Medicine by Gould and Pyle, a book of nearly 1,000 pages, containing the most information for the price of any book I ever read.

Mechanical injuries—bones displaced by accidents or poisons—impinge upon nerves and create an excess of heat which softens the walls of blood-vessels, thereby causing hemorrhage.

---

Dr. D. D. Palmer:

I wish to ask a few questions which I think will be of interest to Chiropractors. (These have been answered in these columns; but the Adjuster class is like the one under my personal supervision, they need to be told and retold.)

1st. How can a laterally-bent spinous process be differentiated from a lateral sub-luxation, where one cannot be guided by nerve-tracing on account of paralysis of sensation?

While a large share of diseases are febrile, known by the nerve being inflamed, enlarged and sensitive, there are cases in which the nerves have lost part of their firmness, tonicity and vibration. Consequently, there is a lack of impulse, conduction and sensation. Nerves which are impinged upon become hypersensitive until they arrive at a temperature which will soften their tissue.

When we refer to a luxated vertebra, we consider the **position of the body,** because its displacement to the left or right, may impinge upon, press against, the vertical, sympathetic chain, **upon one or both sides.** If to the left it may impinge upon the vertical nerve trunk on that side, upon the opposite side, or upon both sides. The projecting vertebra on the left, or the two adjoining bodies, may press against the sensitive sympathetic trunks. By the displacement of a vertebra to either side, it of a necessity draws with it (because of its attachments), the vertical chain of ganglia. In doing so, the sympathetic trunk is pressed against by the bodies of the vertebrae above and below.

As inferred from the question, there may be no sensation. If so, we cannot determine by palpation whether the nerve is impinged upon or not. Can we determine by an examination of the spinous process, judging by its position, whether the vertebra is displaced? As only a small per cent of vertebral columns have spinous processes projecting in a vertical line, the larger share being bent to the right or left, more especially those of the center six dorsal, and those not in regular order, their normal position would be misleading to one who thought they were in line. The same can be said of the spaces between the distal ends of the processes. I most emphatically state that an examination of the spines will not determine the position of the vertebra.

To say that a vertebra is displaced, does not express its relative position. I prefer to consider it as being racked, tipped from its normal position. Take your vertebral column (every Chiropractor should have one), tip a vertebra, throw the spine upward, keeping the anterior of the body in line, and you will see that the spinous process (more especially those which are oblique) projects backward. Thus it will be seen that the vertebra is racked, rather than displaced posteriorly. Thus, we cannot determine its position by the lateral curves, although posterior alignment is usually reliable. Spines are frequently lengthened by the spinous ligament being ossified and attached to the distal end. There is no rule without exceptions.

There are so many exceptions, that it is almost impossible to give them in a journal; each should be noted in the clinic as they are presented by individual cases.

3d. As the axes of the lumbar vertebrae differ in position from those of the cervical and dorsal, the former being posterior to the bodies and the latter anterior, does it not require a different kind of move to give a proper adjustment in the different localities? Should not the cervicals and dorsals be adjusted more quickly, while the lumbars require a slower and heavier move, as there is more weight (the entire body of the vertebra) to be moved in the lumbar?

As to the force and quickness required in adjusting, the movements should be as light and as quick as possible.

An example will explain more than a description. Dr. N. J. B.'s wife took six weeks adjusting from two of my graduates. They gave her such forcible adjusting that she had to be helped off the table, and for a few minutes was unable to walk. Dr. B. spoke of taking her to the "Old Doctor," but was partly discouraged by being told that the old man adjusted much more severely. Mrs. B. however, came, took an adjustment and remarked that I did not give adjustments as heavy as my son. They are now taking a course of instruction under the "Old Doctor," where they may learn specific adjusting.

4th. In case of excessive heat or any function in excess, caused by a slight impingement, should the vertebra be moved by a light adjustment and where there is paralysis, give a heavy adjustment?

Thanking you in advance for the information desired, with my best wishes, I am one of the Chiros.

"Natural Science."

The above is the title of a book now on the way by a Chiropractor. Did you ever hear of an unnatural science? A science could not be otherwise than natural. A system would not be a science if it was not natural. To refer to a science as being "natural" implies that the writer knows of one or more sciences which are not natural.

"Our anatomists tell us that one branch arises from the outer cord and another from the inner cord." Neurology, page 422.

There are no anatomists who tell us that nerve-branches arise from the cord. The nerve-trunk is composed of two roots; the posterior is composed of root-filaments which are of the peripheral origin of spinal cord. The anterior root is composed of root filaments which emerge from the cord. These two roots form the nerve-trunk. **The trunk divides into branches,** ultimately, into terminal filaments. Just think of a tree—do not get the branches on the root end.

---

In The Chiropractor of May, 1908, we find the following: "All other schools are branches or graduates of The Palmer School." How about The D. D. Palmer School at Portland, Ore.?

I am the originator, the developer of Chiropractic. Back of me every Chiropractor traces his Chiropractic lineage. From this Chiropractic tree originated every Chiropractic scion. The teachers of the above school and all others are branches from the one taught by me, or cuts from those branches. I am the one from whom all trace their knowledge of Chiropractic. The original Chiropractor has been transported from his primary soil to Portland, Ore., where he will again send off branches from the original stock. The students under me are receiving a Chiropractic education first handed. **No others are.** Is not "The Palmer School" in a similar position as "The Palmer-Gregory School" and "The Gorby and Hinkley School," over all of which I once presided? Each school was fortunate in having The Founder as its acknowledged head for a time. The D. D. Palmer Chiropractic College of Portland is now the Fountain Head of Chiropractic and no others are.

I am not a graduate of "The Palmer School." I am the man to whom all Chiropractors are indebted for the basic principles of a science and art which I have discovered and developed and which are taught with more or less fidelity by all schools, of whatever name, from which students receive their degree of D. C.

## MUMPS.

"A lecturer of great ability, who is beyond a doubt the ablest instructor in the Chiropractic world; one who has been vitally connected with the science for the past ten years, who stands at the head of the science of Chiropractic." Thus he speaks of himself; if he don't know, who does? I can vouch for the statement that he has been vitally connected with the science for the last ten years, for he was relieved of consumption about that long ago by the writer. This result created in him such an interest in the science that he took a three months' course two and a half years ago, under Dr. Parker, of Ottumwa, Iowa, the latter having just finished a nine months' course under me.

This lecturer of great ability stated in one of his discourses: "We understand that the salivary glands and the testes and the ovaries are the same kind of organs—they are ramified heavily or richly from the kidney nerves." "You can see that in case of great inflammation of the parotid gland there would be a severe irritation on the periphery of sensory nerves and would produce a motor reaction and a contraction of the muscles at kidney place, which might impinge the filaments that extended down the ureters and ramify the testes or ovaries, and of course, we understand there are filaments from kidney place that ramify the mammary gland, especially the lymphoid tissue surrounding the mammary gland."

"You can see that it may produce such constriction at kidney place as to leave the person with pressure upon the nerves at kidney place that will eventually produce kidney disease; it may leave inflammation constant, chronic, of the testes or ovaries and might result in such severe pressure of the nerves ramifying the mammary glands, especially the lymphoid tissue near the gland as to cause it eventually to thicken with the heavy deposit, and this might also be true of the parotid gland so as to produce, finally, a cancer or tumor or some of those various conditions of destruction of tissue under that head. So that, even in a case of mumps it is a pretty good idea, before you let it alone, to find that you are in thorough adjustment."

He follows this up by saying that the early condition of blood stasis is followed by inflammation.

Doctor, your explanation does not explain the situation, does not elucidate the metastatic parotiditis, the change of the disease from the parotid gland to the mammae, testes or ovaries.

I do not understand that the above glands "are ramified heavily or richly from the kidney nerves." In fact I do not see where the nerves of the kidneys have anything to do with mumps or their metastasis in any one of the six glands which are frequently connected, or that blood stasis is the cause of inflammation. It is in the province of this Adjuster to adjust any misstatements made under the head of Chiropractic.

Inflammation is but excessive heat, caused by an impingement upon calorific nerves. This impingement excites the functions of these fibers, thereby increasing heat function.

The student of anatomy will understand that the parotid glands, mammae, testes and ovaries are glands connected by the lymphatic thoracic duct which extends from the neck to the lumbar region.

The parotid gland is connected with the spinal nerves through the carotid plexus, which is a branch of the superior cervical ganglon of the great sympathetic. Thus Chiropractors analyze the condition, trace the line of communication back to the cause and from cause to effect.

Poisons act on sensory nerves; they in turn draw vertebrae out of alignment, impinging upon nerves and creating an excess of heat—named inflammation. There is a rise in the bodily temperature in consequence of this local excess of heat which we name fever. An overstimulation of nerves by pressure causes enlargement of those filaments, more especially at their peripheral endings; thus we have parotitis. This inflammatory condition may pass to the mammae and down the thoracic duct to the testes or ovaries.

---

"If you watch anatomy closely you will find many places, especially in connection with the brain and nerves, where that word **apparent** comes in. It expresses a **questioning** thought in the mind of the man who wrote it."

Dunglison says: "**Apparent origin, superficial origin.** Deep origin, nucleus of cells in brain or cord to which the fibers of a nerve penetrate. Ectal origin, superficial. Ental origin, deep origin. **Superficial origin, point on the surface of the brain or cord where a nerve emerges.**"

Gould states: "Origin deep, of a nerve, its beginning in the cells of the nerve center. Origin superficial, of a nerve; the point at which it emerges from the brain or cord."

Dorland makes this question plain by stating: "**Origin. Apparent origin.** Ectal origin. **Superficial origin, the point at which a cranial nerve emerges from the surface of the brain.** Deep origin, Ental origin, the true beginning of the brain-fibers of a nerve within the substance of the brain."

Gray says on page 826: "**The point where the nerve-root or roots emerge from the nervous center is named the superficial or apparent origin,** but the fibers of which the nerve consists can be traced for a certain distance into the nervous center to some portion of the gray substance, which constitutes the **deep or real origin of the nerve.**"

## CHIROPRACTORS.

During vacation I had the pleasure of meeting a dozen Chiropractors in Seattle.

While passing an office, I noticed on a window, Chiropractic among several methods of treating the sick. I called: the doctor was not in. A lady answered my call and many questions. She informed me that they had several different methods; that they picked the best of each; that Osteopaths used the fingers and the Chiropractors the thumbs when treating. She showed me an Osteopathic chart, which contained cuts of four spines. From it, and her explanations, I learned that disease was caused by the vertebrae compressing the cartilage, making it thinner and the holes which pinched the nerves smaller. When satisfied that I had learned enough for one lesson, I introduced myself by giving her my card and hand, and informed her that she knew nothing about Chiropractic.

I called at the office of another Chiropractor. The doctor was not in. A patient answered several questions. She told me that it took Dr. Blank an hour to give a treatment; that he sometimes used his thumbs, fingers and fists. She had also taken Osteopathic treatments. She thought one was about as good as the other, if not better. The main difference was that the Chiropractor used a vibrator and the Osteopath did not. Dr. Blank had paid $500 to learn Chiropractic. She had lumbago. The doctor used the vibrator to strengthen her back. She said he was a nice man; he was studying everything he could find on Chiropractic.

I called upon another Chiropractor. I could not play green with him for he had seen my picture. That was not the first time that my picture prevented me from learning something. He treated me nicely; took me in his adjusting room. A vibrator told me that it was also a treating-room. Patient had hemiplegia. I saw him make an examination. I watched him several minutes, how many more he would have needed to complete it I do not know. Tiring of seeing him pinch the cuticle over and around the spine, I gave one stroke with my hand and showed him the vertebra displaced. He had not made a single palpating move. He then began stretching the spine with his hands so that he might adjust the vertebra. He was pleased to receive instructions. He was not above learning as are some practitioners who hold me off at arm's length and receive nothing. The Chiropractor Adjuster is certainly needed to teach the principles of the science and adjust pseudo Chiropractic.

A physician in Seattle told me that a dressmaker took a six-weeks' course and hung out her shingle as a Chiropractor. I know of a more extraordinary incident than this. One Goldsmith listened to an hour's lecture, ,attended a clinic, immediately secured an office in East Portland and placed on his windows in four-inch gold letters, "Dr. Goldsmith, Chiropractic Spinologist." His disappearance was almost as sudden as his appearance. As Chiropractors increase, the incompetents will be weeded out. Therefore, it stands each practitioner in hand to make himself competent. If he is not, he will be as a weed in the way of advancement.

---

"Why would it be a pretty good guess to say asthma is caused from 4th cervical?" Ans.—That would be a pretty good guess, but Chiropractors are not doing guesswork.

From thirteen years' experience as a Chiropractor, I would say that it is not a "good guess to say asthma is caused from 4th cervical." Of the many cases of asthma of which I have given relief—one in this Hotel Scott—I have invariably found that asthma comes from a luxated dorsal.

The vagus and sympathetic contribute to form the pulmonary plexuses in front and behind the root of the lung from which branches go to accompany bronchial arteries; a smaller number accompany the air-tubes.

The vagus is also known as the 10th cranial and the pneumogastric nerve. It receives the last name because it supplies the lung and stomach with innervation. It is connected with the ninth, eleventh and twelfth cranial nerves and also the sympathetic.

"I know of no other portion of the body, aside from the spinal column, where the nerves (soft substances) are surrounded, entirely, by hard substances. I know that frequently they lie up against a hard substance and may be surrounded by same on three sides, but there is always a remaining avenue of escape on the other side, and it is only when they are entirely surrounded that they can be constricted, not otherwise."

True, the spinal nerves, as they emerge from the spinal canal, are entirely surrounded by bones. Nerves cannot be **constricted** by bones even if they are surrounded on three or more sides.

Compression and constriction are not synonyms; they have quite different meanings. Nerves may be compressed, squeezed or pinched by pressure between two or more bones. But in order to constrict, to **make smaller,** to contract a portion in size, it is necessary that the nerve, artery or other tubular canal, must be surrounded by a substance which is pliable, as a thread, string, cord or rubber which may be used as a ligature. Unyielding bones would make poor bands; no one would think of ligating with bones.

"The highest compliment any one can pay me is to quote my views on the Sympathetic Nervous System, because they are entirely contradictory to any authority dealing with the nervous system today. The development of the Educated Nervous System has been more or less understood to be a system directly in communication with the brain. The fibers are supposed to pass directly from the spinal cord to the tissue where they receive their power."

I do not desire any such compliment. Allow me to go on record as being with "all authority dealing with the nervous system." Every anatomical examination of the nervous system shows three systems of nerves, viz., spinal, sympathetic and cranial. It is strange that all anatomists find these nerves if they do not exist. It is more strange that a youth of 26 years, who has had but little or no experience in dissecting should array himself against every anatomist.

What's that? The fibers are supposed to receive their power from the tissue?

"Chiropractors have at all times denied the existence of the 12 cranial nerves as found in anatomies today." The writer should not be so sweeping in his denunciations. He is the only Chiropractor I know (or have heard of) who insists that all dissectors are either dishonest or have mistaken muscles or ligaments for nerves. It is simply too bad that he could not spare one day with scalpel in hand, and a dozen of our most eminent anatomists at his side, to make just one demonstration that would open their eyes! He follows up his incorrect statements by referring to nerve tracings. In these statements he is correct with one important exception. The nerves which he and his students trace under the impression that they are cranial nerves, are the nervi communicantes, accessory nerves to the cranial from the spinal and sympathetic nerves. He knows nothing of the accessory nerves as communicants. If he did, he would appreciate the nervous system as a grand masterpiece of **workmanship.**

"We are taught as a fundamental in Chiropractic that there must be pressure or constriction of nerves to interfere with transmission of currents and if we were to believe that the 12 cranial nerves, as taught today, have an exit external to the spinal cord, they would not be subject to pressure, and we would be open to a great deal of ridicule as to how we get results unless those fibers do enter those places and are impinged." The superficial attachments of the twelve pair of cranial nerves are in the encephalon inside of the cranium. These nerves ramify the interior and exterior of the cranium, but never proceed down the spinal canal. Instead, they are supplied with branches from the spinal and sympathetic systems. These communicating nerves are the filaments which are mistaken for cranial nerves.

"I want to go on record as saying that the so-called Optic Nerve is a part of the spinal cord. The Optic Nerve has nine divisions. The big optic nerve (of medicine, if you will) may contain all functions but visual one, for all I know, but I do know that this passes down through the Foramen Magnum and emits from the Spinal Cord at 4th Cervical."

Dr. B. J. Palmer is the first man to go on record who says that there are no spinal or sympathetic nerves; that all nerves are rooted in the brain, pass down and in the spinal cord, through the intervertebral foramina, and from thence to the various parts to which they are assigned Even the optic nerve, which is a very few inches in length, becomes a part of the spinal cord, emerges from the spinal canal through the cervical intervertebral foramen, then back to the eye and from thence to the brain. I am at a loss to know what those nine divisions of the optic nerve are. I am also ignorant of such a nerve as the "big optic nerve of medicine." It must be a "big" fellow to "contain all functions but visual." It must have got mixed up with ophthalmology.

"When I saw there was no use for a Sympathetic Nervous System, I threw it out, and then just had to put something better in its place, so I discovered Direct Mental Impulse."

I think I have fully shown that there is a system of nerves known as the sympathetic nervous system; that Innate, through this system, controls all the vital functions; that all thinking persons have use for those nerves; that even fools are depending upon them for their vital actions, and would not think otherwise, if it were not for their kleptomaniac proclivities. I am truly ashamed to have such ignorance passed off for Chiropractic. Therefore I will continue to adjust all dislocations found in Chiropractic literature. Such clothing does not belong to Chiropractic, does not fit the boy Chiro. It makes a laughing stock both of him and those who accept such teachings.

---

"Lack of current is the cause of disease."

The current referred to is mental impulse. Much of the larger share of diseases are because of too much impulse. Functions are then performed with a degree of rigidity above the normal rate instead of below it.

Gould says of impulse.—Any communicated force. Dunglison.—Force directly employed. Webster.—Impulsion. Force so communicated as to produce motion suddenly or immediately.

## FEVER.

The function called heat is conducted by means of the nerves; they are the source of all heat production. The processes of heat production and heat dissipation are regulated in an orderly manner under the influence of the nervous system.

Fever may be defined as a disturbance of this uniformity of temperature. It is distinguished by a quickened pulse, rapid respiration, increased tissue-waste and disordered secretions. Fever differs from inflammation in that in the former there is a rise of temperature thruout the body, whereas in the latter augmented temperature is confined to a locality.

Delafield says: "Exactly **how these** various substances (toxins, endotoxins and autotoxins) **act** in the incitement of fever **is unknown.** Stengel states: "Special centers for the production, dissipation and regulation of heat have been described by physiologists, though **their location and method of operation still remain in doubt.** Whatever the exact mechanism may be found to be, **it is quite certain that in some way the nervous system exercises a control over production and discharge of heat.**" Dunglison says: "In the treatment of fevers it is important to bear in mind their tendency, particularly the exanthemata (any eruptive disease), **to run a definite course** and terminate in restoration to health." I discovered that heat either above or below normal depends upon the molecular activity of nerves, and that pressure on nerves irritates them, excites them to greater activity, causing an excess of heat designated as fever.

High temperature—fever—is the cause of many, perhaps all disorders. An undue amount of heat is the cause of all pathological consequences. **It is in no sense conservative or useful.** Fever always denotes a diseased state of the system and a general derangement of the functions. It is the prominent symptom of many diseases.

McFarland says that "Fever may be traumatic or infectious. **Traumatic fever remains unexplained,** but seems to be not infrequent after fractures." There is a Chiropractic beam of light in that sentence. Many accidents cause not only fractures but displacements of the osseous frame-work. These displaced bones press on sensitive nerves, exciting their activity and causing an increase of temperature. All of the tissues, as well as all the functions, of the body become morbid when subjected to **high** bodily temperature—fever. All organs are found, after death from fear, to be in a state of cloudy swelling The heart and voluntary muscles show degenerative changes. During fever the respiration is accelerated in the ratio of the increased frequency of the pulse. The glandular secretions are profoundly altered and universally diminished. The skin is hot and dry, and the secretion of sweat suppressed. The urine is scanty, dark colored and of high specific gravity. The mammary secretion is diminished in quantity and altered in quality. The nervous system suffers from the very beginning of fever. The metabolic processes are greatly modified. There are many kinds of fever, each designated according to modifying conditions.

---

There are only two classes in the world—doctors and patients.

---

The terms, anterior, posterior, superior, inferior, lateral, ventral, dorsal, distal and proximal, are used by the author for the same positions and directions as they are by all anatomists and lexicographers, who regard man in an upright position. Whether reclining on the side, front or back, or in an erect position, anterior and ventral is toward the front and away from the median line. Lateral is toward the side. Superior is the more elevated position and inferior the lower situation. Distal is the farthest from the center of the trunk and proximal the nearer portion toward the center of the body.

---

## PARALYSIS.

Abolition or great diminution of voluntary or involuntary movements or of sensation in one or more parts of the body is named paralysis. When the right or the left half of the body is included, it is named hemiplegia; when it concerns the lower half, paraplegia.

Pathologists name from 50 to 100 kinds of paralysis, depending upon the portion of the body affected, how long standing and the lesion.

Chiropractors find pressure on some portion of the nervous system to be the cause of any kind of paralysis.

In hemiplegia the lesion will be found at center place. In paraplegia, in the lower portion of the spine, depending upon how much of the lower half is affected.

Paralysis agitans, shaking palsy, is a disease of later life. It is attended with profuse sweating, sensations of heat and cold. The lesion will be found at k. p.

---

A pupil in a school near Chatham Square, New York City, thus defined the word "spine":

"A spine is a long limber bone. Your head sets on one end and you set on the other."—Lippincott's Magazine.

## ADJUSTING.

Willard Carver, D. C., says: "Adustment is the art of securing by hand the proper relation of the elements of a joint." This would have been well said, if he had used the words, articular surfaces, instead of elements. An element is one of the simple substances or principles of which the physical universe is composed. In chemistry, an element is one of a limited number of distinct varieties of matter which, singly or in combination, compose every material substance. An element is a substance which cannot be separated into particles different from itself; at least, by ordinary chemical processes. We have alkaline elements and acid compounds, but a joint is not composed of elements or compounds. The number of known elements is about eighty.

A principle is a fundamental substance or energy; a law or doctrine from which others are derived or founded.

Dr. Gregory in **Spinal Adjustment** says: "In making an adjustment, observe the rule to always tighten the hand against the part to be adjusted, because if you slacken, or if you are not against the process before adjusting, you will usually fail to get the adjustment. After the quick application of force, get your hand away immediately, so as to permit a rebound movement."

He directs the reader to an illustrated cut, wherein the adjuster has his underhand flat on the cervical region, covering the first six cervicals. It should be so situated that the edge will be snugly and firmly held against the process to be used as a lever.

Many Chiropractors allow themselves to get into habits. One of which is to adjust standing on one side only; another is to raise the hands up several times, so that the adjuster might give the patient a good hard thrust. In doing this they lose the precise location necessary to use a certain spinous process as a lever, and they use force instead of knack.

Vol. III. by Dr. B. J. Palmer says: "Make every move tell by that quick, energetic, light, metallic touch that makes the Chiropractor's adjustment different from anything which has preceded him."

This sentence is all right, except that of "metallic touch." Can you fancy a touch whose characteristic qualities or nature is that of metal?

"To again restore Innate Intelligence to her dwelling place." This phrase is more poetical than truthful, and not much of either.

"Chiropractors make an external agitation, but Innate creates the recoil and then the simultaneous action corrects the cause. We, by using our hands against vertebral processes, in a quick, energetic manner, create a demand for resistance which is met by an internal intellectual response; it is this answer to our call that exactly shifts or transfers the vertebra into normal position."

Chiropractors should not create an external or internal agitation, an excited condition. "Innate creates a recoil!" Innate gets thon's back up when thon is going to get his back set; that is natural when thon is going to be jumped upon. If the adjuster will prepare the patient before giving the adjustment by making a few appropriate remarks and have the patient to lay thon's arms alongside of the body or the hands upon the buttocks, the adjuster will find the patient has but little or no desire to buck against the adjuster.

"It is this internal, intellectual response to our call that exactly shifts the vertebrae into normal position." This is more prosacial than truthful and but very little of either. What is that? "An intellectual response from the internal; an answer to our call, shifts or transfers the vertebra into normal position?"

That is the limit. The adjuster calls, cries out with a loud voice to Innate, giving thon directions what to do. Innate responds from the internal, by shifting the vertebra from one position to another, or transferring it from one place to another, until thon gets the vertebrae into position. Adjusting is the result of intellectual and mechanical force on the part of Educated—not of Innate.

"**Immediately after** the adjustment the vertebra is heard by the adjuster and felt by the patient to return to its normal position."

Those adjusters and their patients are slower in their hearing and sensation than any I ever met.

---

The vital and mental functions in our domestic animals are similar to those in mankind. Those of insects must be very different. Their eyes are immovable and compound. Investigators are led to believe that fish, ants, bees, wasps and insects in general do not possess the sense of hearing. Taste, smell and sight seem to be highly developed in insects. Lobsters, crabs and insects are provided with touch-hairs and feelers from which they derive much information of each other and their surroundings.

## RHEUMATISM.

Rheumatism sets in with, and is attended by, fever. The joints become swollen and painful. The skin around and over the affected part is red and tender. The movements cause severe pain. The weight of the bedclothes may become unbearable. The inflammation may be confined to one or more joints or shift from one to another. In severe cases every joint may become affected. Usually the corresponding joints on the two sides of the body are simultaneously affected.

Acute rheumatism is associated with fever; therefore it is often called rheumatic fever. The appetite is impaired, there is great thirst, the tongue is thickly coated, the bowels constipated. There is profuse sweating, more especially at night.

Chronic rheumatism is a disease of more or less permanency. The fever decreases, the joints become enlarged and stiff.

Gout is a form of rheumatism. The attack begins in one of the joints, usually in the great toe. It may be confined to one joint, or it may affect the corresponding one in the other foot, or the instep. Gout may be accompanied with indigestion, pain in the stomach and derangement of the bowels. Sooner or later, the feet become enlarged with a deposit resembling chalk. In time, the joints become deformed, stiffened and ankylosed. Fistulae discharges matter from around these affected joints. Other portions of the body are liable to be implicated in this disease. When the kidneys are affected the patient passes a large amount of urine.

Rheumatoid arthritis is known by alterations in the joints, such as softening, ulceration and erosion. The articular surfaces are denuded of cartilage and creak when moved, because of the friction caused by the articular bone surfaces rubbing against each other. Excessive heat is the prime factor in this cartilage destruction. Cartilage being a good conductor of heat is easily softened and distintegrated. Joints are frequently deformed, enlarged and luxated. Severe cases end in fibrous or bony adhesions, named ankylosis; the former inhibits the use of, while the latter obliterates, the joint.

Dunglison says: "Rheumatism is a word commonly used to denote a variety of clinical states, the underlying cause of which is supposed to be essentially the same. The disease may attack joints, muscles or fibrous, or serous structures; hence the terms muscular, articular, synovial, cardiac, cerebral, etc. It may be acute, sub-acute or chronic in its course and duration. It is characterized subjectively by pain, which may be severe, lancinating, shifting or dull and boring, according to the variety of the disease and to the structure involved. Objectively there may be fever, local redness, and swelling, when acute, or no perceptible change in the affected part or in certain cases great deformity may result from inflammatory changes with secondary contraction and disability. **The morbid anatomy and etiology of rheumatism remain doubtful.**"

Delafield says: "The excitant of acute rheumatism is unknown."

Do not forget for one moment that heat in a normal amount is health. Too much or not enough causes conditions named disease.

Heat in amount more than normal causes muscles and nerves to contract in length and expand in thickness. All stimuli, whether from traumatism or poison, produce destructive disorder in the exercise and harmony of functions. Vegetable, mineral or animal poison, when introduced into the human economy, act in a noxious manner on the vital properties or the texture of nerves and muscles, thereby drawing vertebrae out of alignment. Functions cannot be modified without a corresponding change in the texture of the lines of communication. Nerves and muscles, when irritated by pressure or poisons, are shortened and enlarged in diameter. When the length and thickness of a nerve is changed, all the fibers are included. The conductibility of nerves is in proportion to their rigidity. Poisons and impingements agitate the molecular groups of atoms of which muscles and nerves are composed. Greater activity causes an increased amount of heat.

In all rheumatics will be found certain vertebrae that have been displaced by accidents or drawn out of alignment by the contraction of nerves and muscles due to poison. These displaced vertebrae and the consequent nerve impingement, will be found to correspond to the parts of the body affected. Acute cases should be relieved by one or two adjustments. Chronic cases will take weeks or months because of the abnormal shape of the vertebrae and their ankylosed condition. Daily adjusting of the ankylosed vertebrae will loosen and return them to their normal shape and position.

No set rules can be given to determine the exact location of the displaced vertebra causing the impingement, because of their variation in rheumatism. They have to be located by an education acquired by experience.

---

The vaccination question is being aired in Tacoma, Wash. The Medical Board received a letter from Louis E. Miller, a high school pupil, who said that he would graduate next spring, that his parents were opposed to his being vaccinated, because two of his brothers died as a result of such treatment.

## "KIDNEY TROUBLE."

I find under the head of "Kidney Trouble" the following: "This affliction is so common, yet so difficult for any of the therapeutical methods to successfully handle, that it should be of great concern to the American people. In rheumatism, gout, Bright's disease, dropsy, cancers, ulcers, boils, and all skin eruptions, there is an abnormal condition of the kidneys. And the cause of this abnormal condition is that the nerve stimula to the kidneys is obstructed. The nerve force and vitality is shut off therefore it is impossible for the kidneys to function normally."

The writer of the above, although "a lecturer of great ability," was not well versed in Chiropractic. Chiropractic is readily recognized by its nomenclature.

We, as Chiropractors, do not believe that evil comes upon us, that we are **afflicted** with diseases by seen or unseen beings. We find the producing cause within the sufferer, not outside of him. If, by a vertebral luxation a nerve is impinged upon, inflammation created, extending to the twig ends of the nerves, creating boils, ulcers or cancers, we would not look after the afflictor, but, adjust the cause of these conditions.

While dropsy, diabetes and Bright's disease are the results of abnormal kidneys, rheumatism, gout, cancers, ulcers, boils and skin diseases are not.

The functions of the kidneys are secretion and excretion; the elaboration of urine and its expulsion. The kidneys are the terminals of the serous circulation. They drain from the body the fluid which is no longer needed in the animal economy.

If the action of the kidneys is performed normally, we have a natural flow of urine; if not, we have too much or not enough; (conditions known as Bright's disease and diabetes.) A slight impingement of the nerves which supply nerve force to the kidneys, creates too much heat—inflammation; a heavy impingement has the opposite effect. The one irritates and excities, the other prevents, the transmission of nerve-force. Gall-stones are formed in the liver and gall-bladder because of too much heat which dries the bile into hard concretions. In a similar way gravel is produced in the kidneys. Dropsy is owing to the serous fluid not being secreted by the kidneys, but left in the body; therefore not carried off. Abnormal functions are not because "the nerve force and vitality is shut off," as stated above.

"Rheumatism, gout, cancers, ulcers, boils and skin diseases" are not from "abnormal condition of the kidneys" as stated by this teacher who "stands at the head of Chiropractic." They each have different vertebral impingements, which should be relieved by adjusting their respective displaced vertebrae, thereby returning the articular processes to their normal position. Rheumatism, cancers, ulcers and boils may each have their special displacement, owing to the portion of the body affected. "The ablest instructor in the world" states that these diseases are always caused by lesion of the kidneys, therefore, he would adjust one vertebra for all, no matter what portion was affected. Whereas, the developer of the science finds it necessary to replace some one of all the vertebrae, depending upon the portion affected. This "teacher" and his students are not to blame for not knowing what they have not learned, namely, the principles of Chiropractic. They are only to be reproved when they assert that they know it all.

---

Drugs are delusive; they do not adjust anything.

---

"There is today only one person who says, and has continued to say for more than nine years, that he is the discoverer and originator of the Chiropractic principles and movements that are now used by all Chiropractors. That person is Dr. D. D. Palmer, who developed all there is of Chiropractic, except the bifid table, and Dr. Henry's "anti-bucker." Why should he not claim to be its originator? Why is he not the primary source from which all Chiropractors learned their lessons?"

This language can be repeated with the same force and truthfulness now, fifteen years later, in 1910, as when first uttered six years ago.

---

"If a subluxated vertebra is the cause of pneumonia, typhoid, etc., why do patients recover without having the displaced vertebra replaced?"

Some die during the fever stage. Quite a per cent have sequela following for months or years. These are corrected by returning the subluxated vertebra to its normal position and releasing the impinged nerves which cause functions to be either excessively or insufficiently performed. There is a portion, however, whose spines have not received due attention, but who nevertheless, recover from the primary illness without showing any secondary or chronic affections whose spine has not received any attention. How is this?

Excessive heat, named fever or local inflammation, has produced liquifaction of soft or hard tissue or both, a condition known as necrosis, by which the impingement has been removed. Innate has adjusted itself to the condition imposed upon it.

## NEUROPATHY.

"It is a notorious fact (page 427) that somehow, through nerve influence, there are maintained in the system two antagonizing elements—the Positive and the Negative—and that these are generated in certain parts of the system for special and distinct purposes, and that when the union of these poles takes place, the current established, neutrality occurs, and the excess of the acid or the alkali so changed as to reinstate normal action in the parts disturbed or exercised thereby. Whether the scientific world has observed such a condition in the system or not, we have not seen an account of it, but that it is so our observations in numerous instances have abundantly demonstrated. We have an example in point in the pathological condition called colic. The excessive acid in the stomach contracts the muscular fibers so as to compress the sensitive nerves in the stomach walls, hence pain. This excessive activity is due to inco-ordination of the pneumogastric nervous system and the splanchnic nervous system, one generating acid and the other alkaline secretions. Proper pressure—stimulation of the sympathetic filaments on the sides of the spinous processes over the splanchnics—corrects the acidity. Colic is instantaneously relieved by the proper manipulation in the splanchnic region."

"It is a notorious that **somehow" or other,** Dr. Davis cannot take in the simple fact that bones may become displaced, subluxated, nerves and muscles pressed against, thereby irritated, contracted and excited, creating an over-amount of functionating, which is known as disease. His early education sticks to him like a leech. He cannot get away from the medical idea that there are elements in man which are antagonistic, combative in their nature, fighting for supremacy.

The "somehow," or somewhere of the "two antagonizing elements maintained" or "generated" has not been "observed by the scientific world," and only conjectured by him.

Take his "colic" illustration. An excessive amount of acid in the stomach contracts muscles, which, in turn, "compresses" nerves. He says the "colic is instantaneously relieved by the proper manipulation in the splanchnic region."

Just think of Dr. Davis giving the "proper pressure" (adjustment); the patient receiving "instantaneous" relief. What is done with the excessive amount of acid which caused colic a moment before, he does not tell us. Is the acid dispersed, eliminated "instantaneously"? Has there been an equal amount of alkaline secretion formed and this acid neutralized "instantaneously''? Is not the statement, no matter how explained, an impossibility?

There are no organs or glands whose special duty is to secrete acid or alkali. The constituents of gastric juice are: Pepsin .41 to 1 17 per cent, and hydrochloric acid from .02 to .03 per cent, leaving about .825 per cent of water. Lactic acid may be present from indigestion, decaying food, fermentation.

In a normal condition, the walls of the stomach are covered with a protecting coat of mucus; otherwise they would be dissolved as food. In gastritis, inflammation of the stomach, the mucus becomes thickened and may peel off, in spots, from the size of a pea to that of a silver dollar, allowing the inner surface to be exposed to the dissolving effects of the gastric juice, thereby producing ulcers. These are known as gastric ulcers, and the condition as ulcerative gastritis.

Dr. Davis knows nothing of the positive and negative, attractive and repulsive poles, or of a current established between them, or of their antagonizing elements, or of their neutralizing each other.

If there are two secretions, positive and negative, having certain functions when united, and if, when they neutralize each other, their functions become inert, they destroy each other's qualities and influence, of what value are they in the human economy? How the proper pressure stimulates the sympathetic filaments, or corrects the acidity, the discoverer (borrower of Chiropractic) of Neuropathy has not the least idea.

Chiropractors do not give adjustments to produce the "proper pressure." They rack the vertebrae into their normal position and return them to normal shape by using the processes as levers. Adjustments require, as he states on page 57, a knack, a know how. "The ignorance of men (page 129) is sometimes apparent upon the very surface of their theories."

---

"If a woman were normal, there would be no menstruation." What is that you are giving us? If a woman was normal, she would not menstruate, would not have her terms, her monthly courses, no periodical discharge of ovum from the ovaries. That being the case, would an absence of menstruation be a natural condition, one denoting health? Is that one of the recent developments which has made a philosophy of the science of Chiropractic? Would that hypothesis hold good with other mammalia? If so, stockmen should be thankful for their female stock being abnormal. Is not that one of your "newly misplaced" developments?

## DIET.

"The occlusion causing catarrh of the stomach, on account of the errors in diet or habits of the individual with regard to eating, not infrequently becomes heavier instead of less grave, as is the general tendency.

"It must be understood that any catarrh is the incipient condition of a tumor.

"In ulcer of the stomach, a removal of the occlusion results in restored stimulus.

"Dilation of the stomach is not an inconsiderable symptom.

"Dyspepsia or chronic indigestion is usually the result of the grossest and most extravagant errors in eating and diet conceivable. However, it may be caused by occlusions produced by direct injury to the vertebral column.

"Inflammation of the stomach is very common and is most frequently produced by overeating, eating too frequently, eating without mastication, eating improperly combined foods, any of which conditions results in a fermentation, or in such chemical changes and combinations as to produce a poison or irritant.

"Digestion is reduced to the minimum, and absorption, of course, in any case, is greatly diminished, the substance absorbed being chemically abnormal and an auto-poison of dif-derent degrees of intensity.

"Abnormal chemical combinations, fermentations, and ptomain poisons. which, generally speaking, are but the results of eating too fast, too often, improper combinations, improper foods, and in excessive quantities."

Mucous membranes are covered with a semi-fluid secretion named mucus. When these membranes are subjected to excessive heat known as inflammation, the mucus becomes thickened and is secreted in greater quantity. This abnormal secretion is known as catarrh.

What has "errors of diet" to do with nasal catarrh? What has eating habits to do with the exudation of pharyngitis? How does the habits of an individual produce the uterine catarrh of metritis? What has the grossest errors in eating to do with the mucus discharge from the bladder, the result of cystitis? Wherein is it conceivable that extravagant errors in diet are connected with bronchial catarrh? How is it possible for overeating to produce the catarrh of hay fever? How does a certain combination of food produce the intestinal catarrh of enteritis? What connection is there between eating without mastication and the vaginal catarrh of vaginitis? What has mastication to do with catarrhal nephritis? Does eating too frequently cause catarrh of the ear? What has food to do with gastritis, enteritis or the catarrhs resulting therefrom?

What is that you say! Catarrh is the beginning of a tumor? The mucus discharge from an inflamed membrane and a morbid enlargement of tissue, with or without inflammation, have no necessary connection whatever.

The mucus of the stomach may be thickened, become detached, exposing the surface to the action of the gastric juice, causing ulcers.

"Restored stimulus."

The writer of this two-worded sentence considers that stimulus, the nervous energy, has been shut off, obstructed, when the facts are, it has been increased. Inflammation increases the circulation, produces an excess of heat and stimulation. Releasing the impingement does not restore stimulus, as there is already an over-amount.

We find the civilized nations who exhibit "the grossest and most extravagant errors in eating and diet conceivable, "do not have dyspepsia or chronic indigestion." Individuals of civilized nations have "dyspepsia or chronic indigestion," who observe special rules. "Take thine ease, eat, drink and be merry."

As to chemical changes, see another article on that subject.

"Abnormal chemical combinations."

Chemical combinations always produce certain compounds. They cannot do otherwise; there cannot be anything abnormal about that. It is perfectly natural for certain elements, when combined, to produce a definite compound.

"Ptomain poisons."

Any substance which, when introduced into the animal economy, acts in a noxious manner on the vital properties, on the textures of an organ, or on the system at large, is a poison. That which is poison to one may be food to another.

When we speak of ptomain poison, we refer to a peculiar product which is eliminated from vegetable or animal substances during decomposition. This putrefactive alkaloid may not act as a poison to all those who partake of it. Mark you, the putrefaction which produces ptomain is produced outside of the body, not inside, as we are told by the analyzer. Poisons do not depend upon "eating too fast, too often, improper combinations, improper foods, or food in excessive quantities."

---

Chiropractors have no starvation period; there is always plenty of work waiting for one who is able to do it.

## ANIMAL HEAT.

Heat is manifestly a kinetic force. All life depends upon its invigorating influence. Animated creation is indebted to it for its origin, development and the functions by which it continues an intelligent existence. It is the essential agent of life. By it we are endowed with vitality.

Heat is displayed in the rays of the sun, in combustion, in chemical and mechanical action, in fire, fusion and evaporation. It is created by a dynamic movement of atoms—a molecular vibration. It is not a subtle, imponderable flüid furnished by special nerves named calorific, and decreased by frigorific nerves.

The nervous system is intimately associated with the production, distribution and regulation of animal heat. By this function the body in health is kept at nearly a uniform temperature.

Inflammation is a **local** morbid condition characterized by pain, redness, swelling and an excessive amount of heat. It is known, histologically, by exudations and changes in the texture of tissue; also by an increased vascular action and preternatural nerve vibration. External inflammation is recognized by redness, heat, enlargement and pain upon pressure. Internal inflammation by swelling, disturbance of functions and soreness under constricting force.

Fever is a **general** condition of the body, known by increased heat in all its parts, an acceleration of the pulse, an augmentation of nerve vibration, and an excess of nervous impulses transmitted.

The heat of the body may be increased by exercise, electricity, poisons and undue pressure on nerves. Mechanical action excites; electricity stimulates; poisons increase molecular motion; impingement increases rigidity, and intensifies vibrations. Extremes of bodily temperature is incompatible with life. In health Innate maintains a normal temperature of 98 to 100 degrees. Heat above normal is an excitant, a lower degree is sedative. Excessive cold induces sleep. There are on record instances in which persons have withstood for a time 400 degrees above, and in the Arctic region, 83 degrees below zero. In these extremes of heat and cold, the temperature of the body varied but little, if any, because normal nerve vibration, upon which it depended for its warmth, did not allow it to depart from the temperature designated as animal heat.

Injuries may produce a pathological condition, that is, excessive heat, by exciting nerve action. We may have a healthy inflammation, as shown when Innate desires to produce a fusion of hard or soft tissue, it increases the amount of heat in that region, in order to produce an exudation of plastic mucous matter. This is known as adhesive inflammation.

Heat in excess causes nerves to become enlarged, swollen, intense, rigid: hence, pain is more intense in hard tissue, because it is less yielding than in soft material. The amount of functionating depends upon the amount of heat. The more intense the heat, the greater is the rigidity and tension of nerves; and their capacity to carry impulses is increased accordingly—nervous force when executed is function. Tension and rigidity determine the rapidity of oscillation, also the amount of heat. Colliquation, whether known as necrosis, caries or fusion, is because of liquifaction of tissue; it is the breaking down of an organ or tissue. Inflammation (excessive heat) causes the parts to become softer than natural.

The hardening of ear-wax is because of inflammation—high temperature. Gallstones are solidified bile, made so by overmuch heat. An undue amount of heat, if local, is known as inflammation; if general, as fever. All hemorrhages are due to softening of arteries and veins of the vascular system, making rupture possible.

Abnormal growths, as corns, goitres, boils, polypi, tumors and cancers, are because of too much action, surplus nutrition excited to excess by an immoderate amount of heat.

Dropsy, anemia and paralysis are due to a lack of heat, not enough action. Debilitated conditions are owing to a want of nerve energy. The nerves are lax, flaccid and flabby; they lack tonicity, the proper rigidity, therefore cannot conduct impulses in a vigorous manner.

Neuralgia and rheumatism, in fact, every ache and pain, is due to too much heat, which expands the nerves to too great a degree, causing them to be too rigid and tense; vibrations become too great, molecular action excessive.

The developer of Chiropractic does not hesitate to state that heat variation, either above or below normal, causes too much or not enough functionating. The greater the tension, the more vibrations there will be in a given length of time.

---

We are informed that a number of Chiropractors met some time ago for the purpose of renaming the science of Chiropractic. That was not the first effort to rename it. The science still retains the name given it by its founder. I would say to them, like the boy who said to his father who was driving a last in a boot, when he saw it coming out at the toe: "Drive on, Pap, it is coming."

## RHEUMATISM.

The generally conceived opinion of rheumatism is, that it is caused by exposure to cold; that there is a predisposition to it; that it runs in certain families; that it has a constitutional tendency; that it is hereditary. The belief that it is hereditary is confirmed, many think, by the fact of its occurrence in childhood and its repetition in the same person during life. Chiropractors have, in a measure, dispelled this erroneous idea by relieving thousands of rheumatics, by removing nerve pressure and thereby allowing Innate full control of all the avenues for the distribution of its intellectual impulses. However, the present idea of the medical schools is a step in advance of that entertained by the Ancient School of Medicine. This latter school declared rheumatism to be an evil which had to be driven out of the body Therefore, the most revolting, obnoxious remedies were used to exercise this evil influence.

Then arose the belief that diseases were caused by one of the four humors: blood, phlegm, yellow and black bile. Hence bleeding had its day of 100 years. This was slow progress, yet it was a step forward.

As we pass along and emerge into the era of rapid advancement, we find A. T. Still, an M. D., the founder of Osteopathy, stating in his book, page 130, date 1892, that rheumatism is because all gas or wind has left the joints; that it appears because the separating gas has been exhausted, and there follows friction and electric heat. He thus accounts for neuralgia, consumption, dropsy, tumors, fits, gray hair, baldness and so on to the full list of aches and pains and a surprising number of diseases not accounted for to date by our philosophers.

A. T. Still was hunting the joints for the cause of diseases. Although he did not find what he sought, he should have the credit of trying to **find it in the joints.**

Dr. Still's immediate followers took another step onward in stating that the cause was a disturbance in the circulation caused by the precipitation of acid crystals of lactic acid, sceptic wounds, digestive and hepatic disturbance, exposure to changes of temperature. It was hard for them to break away from Allopathic ideas.

Some of them held that **displacement** of viscera **pressing** on the vascular system, caused by physical strains was the cause of many diseases. It may seem that these were advancing toward Chiropractic, but the displacing of viscera by strains, causing them to press on blood vessels, was not the same as pressure on nerves through which Innate sends its messages to run the vital functions.

## NEUROPATHY.

"That (page 33) the most astonishing results take place within the body as a consequence of adjustment through this method called Neuropathy, no one who ever witnessed its effects will contradict; and that it is applicable to the most serious and the most malignant conditions is a matter easily demonstrated. Confidence should be had in a system after a successful application of it for six years under an adept in the science of healing and one who has passed the curriculum of the best medical colleges in the country, who, with long years of experience, ought to be able to compare methods and ascertain their distinctive merits."

Dr. Davis is here speaking of "**A method** (page 1) of application **called Chiropractice, really what we call Neuropathy.**" So, this method of adjustment, generally known as Chiropractic, Dr. Davis sees fit to call Neuropathy. Of this system, the Doctor tells us that "astonishing results take place." These results are truly astonishing to those who do not comprehend that the Chiropractor removes the osseous pressure from nerves and muscles.

Confidence should be had in a system after a successful practice of over fourteen years by the founder.

A. P. Davis may be an adept in the science (?) of healing, but not in the science of Chiropractic. "Passing the curriculum of the best medical colleges does not assist one in comprehending the principles of Chiropractic, but, on the contrary, it has a tendency to retard his progress, as he has much to unlearn while taking in principles of biology which he had never dreamed of.

Making a team out of the seven methods, driving all of them at one and the same time, should give him an opportunity to ascertain their distinctive merits unless their antipodal principles should operate in opposite directions.

The fourteen pages of illustrative cuts of nerves and their description is well worth the price of the book to Chiropractors who study them. Neuropathy may be had of the Author, A. P. Davis, Baker City, Ore.

---

"How is Dr. Jones getting on?"

"Doing wonderfully well."

"Do you suppose he will succeed in carving out a fortune?"

"I guess so; he removed the appendix of our wealthiest citizen a couple of weeks ago."

"The appendix, eh? What did he get out of it?"

"An automobile."

## AN INTERESTING CASE.

On page 174 of the Journal of Osteopathy there is an "interesting case, a very remarkable case," as stated. It is interesting to us to see the remarkable failure made by "numerous physicians, as well as the best specialists in Ohio," all or a part of whom were osteopaths. We are told that the "patient is a sister of an Osteopath" and had been treated for five years; that the credit of relief was due to surgery. If The Chiropractors were to report a case, in which relief was given by surgery, our readers would have the laugh on us. The quoted writer says: "Most practitioners find cases like this that they cannot handle without surgical assistance * * * which goes to show more than ever that the osteopath treatment combined with rational surgery will be the only logical treatment in time to come." The treatment for ovaritis, as told by this case, was the result of a mistaken diagnosis; a failure to discriminate between nephritis and ovaritis. It is difficult for every competent Chiropractor to understand how the result of a case of ovaritis, which, for five years, was successfully treated as one of nephritis and finally relieved by a surgical operation could be considered an osteopathic success worthy of publication.

Case report. Discussed before the last Ohio Osteopathic Association.

Patient is a sister of an osteopath, and first came for examination on December 1st, 1906. She was 19 years of age, stout, tending toward obesity, weighed 160 pounds, had ruddy complexion and was the very picture of health. Had been sick more than five years, and had been unsuccessfully treated by numerous physicians as well as the best specialists in Ohio. More attention had been given the kidneys than any of the other organs, but all had agreed that chemical analyses of urine proved them to be normal. Constipation had been very bad.

At the menstrual period she would be prostrated, experiencing a suppression of urine, lasting sometimes for 48 hours and even longer. Headaches were very severe and of nearly every type. The digestion was very poor.

The entire spine was extremely sensitive, with severe pains in the sub-occipital, lumbar and sacral regions. There was also a great deal of pain in the region of the 7th cervical and 1st dorsal. Pronounced lesion at atlas, third, fourth and seventh cervical, first and second dorsal, and the third, fourth and fifth lumbar. Right innominate was posterior. There was tenderness over the entire abdomen but it was greatest in the right iliac fossa.

In March, 1907, during her menstrual period, she was in bed

for a couple of weeks, at which time a muscular tremor developed. At first the tremor extended to the entire body, but in a few days disappeared excepting in the arms and hands, where it continued for about eighteen months.

April 19th, a sister fell down the stairs at the high school building, injuring her spine. The shock and excitement incident to this caused our patient to become much worse, having that night two or three convulsions, which lasted from fifteen minutes to an hour.

From this time she gradually grew worse, having slight convulsions every day and sleeping but two or three hours in twenty-four.

On May 12th, she became unconscious, remaining so for forty-eight hours, part of the time lying perfectly inert, and then again having hard convulsions.

On June 10th, a cross paralysis developed, the right side of the face and left side of the body being affected. This paralysis progressed gradually to the tongue and throat producing both aphasia and aphonia. Sensation was lost in the parts paralyzed and in the entire back region.

On June 14, A. M., sensation returned, and about twelve hours later there was a return of motion also. On June 15th, she became unconscious, and remained in this condition for eight days.

For three summer months the patient was under the constant care of a senior student of the A. S. O. A wheel chair was secured which was used until she was operated upon fifteen months later. From August 1st to October 15th she improved. Every night about eight or nine o'clock she would become unconscious, and after convulsions lasting an hour or so, would become quiet for the rest of the night. Attacks of unconsciousness lasting from two minutes to an hour would come on during the day. During December, 1907, and January, 1908, her condition remained about the same, some weeks better and some weeks worse. The first two weeks of February, a sister had a severe attack of pneumonia and the excitement incident to this caused her to be worse. For five days she again lay in an unconscious state, and for the first time in her whole sickness, had a fever; her temperature ranging from 101 to 104.

From October, 1907, to April, 1908, her menstrual periods were much easier. In May, however, she had a very hard time, and from that time until November they became worse. The pain did not last as long as it did a year or two previously, but it was much more severe.

During the past summer and fall she was always treated

during these unconscious states, and great efforts were made to correct the bony lesions.

Any work on the innominates, however, would cause her so much pain the following day, in fact, make her so much worse in every way, that work on those lesions had to be discontinued, and, while she was awake, it was impossible to do more than the lightest work in relaxing the muscles along the spine.

On November 11th, she was operated upon by Dr. George Still, Dr. Joss of Newark, O., administering the anesthetic.

There was found a cystic degeneration of the right ovary and tube, both of which were removed. Several watery cysts on the left ovary were punctured and sewed up, and the uterus suspended. The third day following the operation her menses appeared, and she suffered very little, if any, pain. The same has been true of each menstrual period since.

She is now learning to walk, not having stood on her feet since April 1st, 1907. Her progress since the operation, considering everything, has been very rapid, as she now walks around the house by herself.

For a year previous to the operation she complained of a burning pain high up in the vagina. This could be relieved by local treatment. In fact, during the fifteen months preceding the operation, she was treated locally two or three times a week, with seemingly more benefit than by anything else.

The case, as a whole, has been one of peculiar interest. To diagnose it, and give it a name from any of the standard medical works would be easy—namely, hysteria, but to accept their cause and treatment for the condition would be irrational, in fact, impossible.

Osler says, "To treat hysteria as a physical disorder is radically wrong. It is essentially a mental and emotional anomaly, and the important element in the treatment is moral control."

The day has come when the conscientious physician dare not, and be true to his calling, relegate all diseases which he cannot explain, to the functional neuroses, meaning by that, diseases which have no physical disorder as a basis and that the important element in treating is moral control.

Lancaster, O. J. M. LONG, A. M., D. O.

The surprising feature of the above case to a Chiropractor is that a girl 19 years of age, weighing 160 pounds, the picture of health, should be treated for over five years by numerous physicians, among whom were the best specialists in Ohio, for disease of the kidneys which an operation proved to be ovaritis. To publish this case with the failures and final success, shows at least one redeeming feature—honesty.

We are told that there were pronounced lesions of the atlas, 3d, 4th, 5th and 7th cervicals, 1st and 2d dorsals, 3d, 4th and 5th lumbars and both innominate bones. If a Chiropractor were to present such a case to me after five years of adjusting, I would think that he had bunglingly displaced eleven of the twelve lesions mentioned, and that he was the real cause of eleven-twelfths of her ailments, and especially when he had told me, "we made great efforts to correct the bony lesions."

Why did not an Osteopath relieve her sister of pneumonia, instead of allowing her to have "a severe attack"?

They "made great efforts to correct the bony lesions," but there were eleven displaced bones which they failed to replace. Better take a few lessons of a Chiropractor.

The medical schools have for many centuries resorted to the knife for those diseases for which they cannot find a physical cause. And now the "conscientious osteopath" does the same thing. It is certainly tempting to use the knife, when for five long years of suffering, a ruddy-complexioned lass of 19, the very picture of health, treated by numerous physicians, is reduced from robust health to feebleness, from an able-bodied woman to that of being bedfast; from an intellectual being to one of unconsciousness; instead of being vivacious, is spiritless —what else can they do?

---

Allopathy. "Opposites cure opposites." A method of treatment in which remedial agents are employed, the action of which produces symptoms different from those observed in the sick person.

Homeopathy. "Like cures like." A system of medicine which maintains that disordered actions in the human body can be cured by remedies which would produce the same in a well person.

---

The New Theology enunciated by me more than ten years ago as the basis of Chiropractic, is the identification of God with Life-Force. The Intelligent Life-Force of Creation is God. It is individualized in each of us. It desires to express itself in the best manner possible.

In every phase of life, vitality and action, man's highest aspiration should be to advance himself to a higher level, to make himself better mentally and physically.

God—The Universal Intelligence—The Life-Force of Creation—has been struggling for countless ages to improve upon itself—to express itself intellectually and physically higher in the scale of evolution.

## OSMOSIS.

Our remarks will be confined to metabolism, the process whereby organic beings transform food-stuffs into tissue elements.

Osmosis is what is known at The P. S. C. as the "Serous Circulation," an "original theme," of which the author says, "This dogma is mine." He was the discoverer and developer (?) of a transudation with which every writer on physiology is well acquainted. He tells us that he put in many months of study discovering and developing this "original theme," which became a "dogma" of his. Any high school-boy could have given him the desired information or referred him to a dozen works on physiology in which he could have found it.

Filtration is the operation of straining a liquid thru a filter.

Diffusion, endosmesis, is the act of spreading out, physiologically speaking, it means the diffusion of water throughout the fluids of the body.

Water is the most important constituent of our bodies and is indispensable to life. It is said that we live in water, as our bodies are more than half liquid. By it all food-stuff is dissolved. A wonderful discovery (?) to learn that water taken in the mouth reaches all parts of the body and is finally excreted by the kidneys, skin and lungs. Some one had to make it!

Water forms a part of all the tissues and fluids. The saliva is 99 per cent water. (Yes, that is right, to speak of a per cent of saliva as it can be divided into 100 parts, but impulse and function are not divisible.) The blood is 80 per cent water, the muscles 75 per cent, and two per cent of the enamel is water. A person weighing 175 pounds carries 125 pounds of water. Much of this water exists in a free condition, forming the fluids, the characteristic quality of which is fluidity. It holds in solution inorganic as well as some organic compounds. It is diffusable, making possible an interchange of materials thruout the body. It aids in the absorption of new material (anabolism) and transfers waste products until eliminated along with the water in which they are dissolved. The combination of water with tissue gives them characteristic properties, such as consistency, elasticity and pliability. The total amount of water eliminated by the kidneys daily is about six and a half pounds.

Diffusion, osmosis and filtration perform an important part in the physiologic processes of metabolism.

By diffusion the molecules of two or more liquids, when brought in contact by an attraction known as affinity, are gradually and spontaneously mixed.

When a soluble substance, as food or organic secretions, are placed in water, the molecules will separate and become diffused thruout the water, until the solution becomes homogenous. Although the dissolved substances possess weight, their specific gravity being greater than that of water, yet the solution remains homogeneous; the force of gravity is overcome by that of diffusion. The length of time required for substances to become diffused in the fluids of the body varies considerably, depending upon the quality of the substance and the temperature of the digestive tract.

Dialysis is the separation from liquids, through porous membranes, of different substances which are held in solution, but which differ in their degree of diffusibility.

There is a pressure exerted by the molecules of the substance held in solution against the enclosing wall, or membrane. known as osmotic pressure.

Filtration is the passage of water and of such substances as are dissolved in it, thru membranes. The amount passed will depend upon the force of filtration—the difference between the pressures on opposite sides of the membrane.

There are delicate membranes in the animal body thru which the fluids, containing organic and inorganic solutions, are constantly passing. Prepared food passes through the intestinal wall, into blood and lymph vessels; thru the walls of capillary vessels and various glands, into muscle fiber and into the interior of all tissue cells.

The waste products, the result of katabolism, pass thru their limiting membranes, into tissue spaces, and onward towards expulsion.

These processes are accomplished by diffusion, osmosis and filtration.

Laboratory experiments have been made with diffusion, osmosis and filtration by the use of non-living membranes, but the results obtained are not exactly in accord with those observed in the living body, hence are not strictly applicable to the elucidation of physiological processes.

"Uric acid is manufactured."

Articles of merchandise, such as cloth, nails, glass, shoes, harness and even machinery is manufactured by hand or machine; but, uric acid. gastric juice, bile and pancreatic juice are elaborated, not manufactured.

---

"Compulsory vaccination is an outrage and a gross interference with the liberty of the people in a land of freedom."

## "MEDULLATED AND NON-MEDULLATED NERVES."

"Two brains control functions of the body. Each has its set of fibers. The set which expresses the Educated mind is covered by white tissue, fatty in consistency—the medullary sheath. This shield is an insulator in function.

"The Innate voluntary brain has no fibers sheathed. The discrimination is to avoid crossing wires or intermingling of impulses.

"The various functions, representing impulses of each mind, cannot short circuit within itself, yet either could or would intermingle with those of the opposite. Innate, during foetal development, sheaths the fibres of the smaller bundle, thus using discerning and economic principles.

"Although brief, the above is the first article which has offered logical reason why the Innate body builder provided one set with sheaths and the opposite not. To state (as the M. D.'s and D. O.'s do) that these are the result of "reflex action" or "sympathetic results" does not intelligently attain the level of the wisdom performed."

"The above is the first article which has offered logical reason why." This same author offered "logical reasons why" there were no cranial nerves, no sympathetic nerves, and no reflex action; therefore he "discovered Direct Mental Impulse." I am pleased to note that The Chiropractor has ceased to repeat the above absurdities. I, as the discoverer and developer of the grandest and greatest science, would much prefer that the P. S. C. should teach Chiropractic. The Adjuster will continue the good work, trusting that the future will be as successful in straightening curvatures in Chiropractic literature as in the past. With the two-fold purpose of adjusting subluxations and advancing the science, we will present what is meant by medullated and non-medullated **fibres.**

The medulla is a fatty substance known as marrow, which occupies the interspaces of the cancellous tissue of the shafts of the long bones and their epiphyses, the vertebrae, sternum, ribs, the diploe of the cranial bones, in fact all cancelous tissues are filled with this oily material. The same can be said of the interspaces of nerve-fibres which compose nerves. As age advances, the marrow changes its color from red to yellow. Anatomists differ as to the function of the marrow; some think it is concerned in the formation of the corpuscles of the blood, while others are as emphatic in their assertions to the contrary. Innate, The All Wise Universal Intelligence, knows all about its use. If the osseous tissue is in normal position, Innate will provide for this filling of cancellous tissue.

The medullary sheath (covering) is a fatty substance in a semi-fluid state. It is supposed to insulate and protect the central part of the nerve—the axis-cylinder (the fibre).

The axis-cylinder, the essential part of the nerve-fibre, is always present; the other parts, the medullary sheath and the neurilemma (the sheath of a nerve-fibre or the fibrous membrane surrounding the nerves), being occasionally absent, especially at the origin and termination of the nerve-fibre. The axis-cylinder undergoes no interruption from its origin in the nerve-center to its peripheral termination; it is regarded as a prolongation of a nerve-cell. These central cores constitute one-half or one-third of the nerve-tube.

Nerve-fibres are arranged in bundles of greater or less bulk. They form the nerves which pervade every part of the body. They constitute the greater part of the brain and spinal cord. These nerve fibres are the conducting elements of the nervous system; they serve to bring the nerve-cells, as well as the various tissues of the body, into relation with each other.

Medullated nerve-fibres, when examined, frequently present a beaded, or varicose appearance. This is due to manipulation and pressure, causing the oily matter to collect in drops, and in consequence of the extreme delicacy of the primitive sheath (outside covering), even slight pressure will cause the transudation of the fatty matter which collects as drops of oil outside of the membrane.

There are different varieties of nerve-fibres, but, in all, the leading and essential constituent is a delicate thread-like band, termed the axis-cylinder or axone, the center of all nerve-fibres; this is the essential component of all nerves. Its function is to convey impulses.

**The medullated fibres** form the white part of the **brain and spinal cord,** and also the **greater part of the cerebro-spinal nerves,** giving to these structures their opaque, white aspect. When examined by transmitted light, a double outline, or contour, is presented, consisting of two parts. The central portion is named the axis-cylinder. Around this is a covering of fatty material which gives to the fibre its double delineation. The whole is enclosed in a delicate membrane the **primitive sheath.**

**Most of the nerves of the sympathetic system,** and **some of the cerebro-spinal** are non-medullated fibres; they consist of a core or axis-cylinder enclosed in an nucleated sheath.

In general all fibres of long courses acquire medullary sheaths a short distance from their cells of origin and lose them again just before termination.

Every nerve fibre arises in a nerve-cell of the brain, extends to nearby or more distant portions from its origin, branching at its peripheral endings in some certain tissue by a number of ramifications.

Axones, in the first stages of the cerebro-spinal nervous system in the embryo, are non-medullated. They acquire their sheaths of myelin (the medullary soft, oily covering which encloses the axis-cylinders of nerves) later; commencing about the fifth month.

Nerves are composed of nerve-fibres. The axis-cylinder is the central portion of a fibre. These thread-like bands are covered by one or two coats of myelin (a fatty substance) or they may be nude. When the axis-cylinder is coated by a more or less thick sheath of this oily substance, it is said to be myelinated or medullated. When the covering is lacking the fibre is called **non-myelated** or non-medullated. A second, thin, delicate membranous sheath may be present externally—the primitive sheath. Thus there are four forms of nerve fibres; the difference being in their covering—the non-medullated (the naked) and those with primitive sheaths—the medullated, those with and others without the primitive sheath.

Most of the neurones (unit of structure of the nervous system) with non-medullated and partially medullated axones (the center core of nerve-fibres) belong to the sympathetic nervous system. Some sympathetic axones are completely medullated (covered with a fatty substance); but their myelin sheaths (the covering of the fibres) are always thinner and never so well developed as those of the cerebro-spinal nerves. Certain axones (center of nerve-fibres) of short course in the central nervous system are non-medullated (not covered with medulla).

Nerves are composed of numbers of nerve-fibres bound into bundles; these are sometimes covered with medulla or myelin. Inflammation of the spinal cord is therefore called myelitis—inflammation of the myelin. Inflammation of a nerve is called neuritis.

The cranial nerves are all medullated except the fibres of the olfactory nerve. The olfactory nerve-fibres are gray. This nerve arises in a separate lobe of the encephalon, the rhinencephalon or olfactory brain.

The spinal nerve trunks are connected with the nearest ganglion of the vertically running ganglionic cord of the sympathetic nervous system. Every spinal nerve has at least one of these fibres, most have two and some three. The nerves of the cervical region usually have but one, which is composed largely of sympathetic fibres. Where there are two, one usually contains medullated fibres. The medullated fibres of the rami, chiefly from the spinal nerves which enter and course to their distribution through the sympathetic nerves, have been termed the visceral divisions of the spinal nerves.

The majority of axones (the central core which forms the essential conducting part of a nerve-fibre) acquire a protective and isolating envelope or sheath which begins a short distance from its cell of origin and loses this covering near its twig end of termination. There are axones with sheaths of all degrees of medullation. Most of the neurones (a neurone is a nerve-cell as a starting point, with its axone and terminal fibrillae) with non-medullated and partially medullated axones belong to the sympathetic nervous system. Some sympathetic axones are completely medullated, but their myelin sheaths are always thinner and never so well developed as those of the cerebro-spinal nerves. Some short axones in the central nervous system are non-medullated.

"Medullated and non-medullated nerves."

Nerves are never medullated; the fibres of which they are composed are frequently medullated.

"Two brains control functions of the body."

The special action of any organ or part of the body is its function. If functions are dependent upon two brains, what has Innate to do with them?

"The set which exercises the Educated mind."

Better to have said, "The nerves which give expression to the mind of Educated."

"The Innate voluntary brain."

The fibres or nerves presided over specially by Innate are involuntary when compared with the voluntary of Educated.

"The Innate has no fibres sheathed."

We find by our investigations that there are no set rules as to certain divisions of fibres being medullated or non-medullated. The same may be said in regard to the primitive sheaths. We therefore see no "logical reason why some are sheathed and others not."

"The functions representing * * * each mind."

The intellect, the understanding, the power which conceives, judges, reasons, the rational faculty in man is the mind, or rather, these are qualities of the mind. The mind exists in proportion as these make up the intellect. A thought is an idea, a mental conception, an opinion, a judgment, a fancy, a purpose or an intention audibly expressed or otherwise. It is a result—a product—of the brain. Mind is composed of thoughts. A thought expressed in action is a function.

The new-born babe has an intellectual mind that of the Innate, which understands how to run the vital functions; it uses judgment and reason in regard to the functions of its corporeal material, including repairs. In time Educated becomes mindful of providing for its bodily welfare externally. This knowledge is added to that which already exists. As the sympathetic, the visceral division of the nervous system, is dependent upon and is a part of the cerebro-spinal system, so the intellect is subject to and is a part of Innate's mind. Innate stores all the information and knowledge gleaned during a life-time. When Educated ceases to act, Innate will reserve all in the one primal mind—riper by its individualized experience.

As there is but one nervous system, there is but one mind. Educated thoughts are as dependent upon Innate as is the sympathetic system upon the cerebro-spinal nervous system. As we divide the nervous system into two or three systems for explanation and comprehension, so we speak of two intellects, two distinct thinking individualities; yet they are one and the same—start as one and end as one.

---

"He (D. D. Palmer) would study two bones, by comparison, he would find one normal and the other abnormal. His first question was, why?" He did not deny their existence, just because he could not comprehend the why.

On the same page, I quote, and comment upon in parenthesis, in order to be brief. "When, in his earlier pickings of osteological specimens, a pig's femur overlapped three inches as a result of an unset, overriding fracture. (The pig's femur did not overlap anything; the fractured extremities overlapped about three inches. The fact of its being so, shows it was "unset," the broken bones were not in proper apposition) and upon which was much porous surrounding spiculae. (There was nothing porous surrounding the slivered fragments. The useless pieces of bone were being absorbed; but there was nothing of a porous nature; disintegration did not use or need pores for transpiration or absorption. Innate Intelligence was removing those useless portions) and this was, gradually, being torn down in proportion as the fractured surfaces became better knit. (Innate was not tearing down; it was reducing useless portions to small particles for the purpose of removal to other parts where needed as repair callous, or as waste material to be carried off. "The fractured surfaces" were not knit, for the overriding would not permit it. Herein was manifested the intelligence I saw fit to name Innate. Uniting the two bones, as they lie side by side, disintegrating the spiculae and the two projecting ends; using the callous, the osseous material for reparation, which medical men are not able to accomplish; closing the medullary cavities of the two exposed ends, exhibited an intelligence unknown to the intellectual man.) To maintain that such was done by reflex action, or duplicature of the original conditions, which was a fracture reflected, ending or turned back, did and would not answer." (I have never known a person to maintain that the reparation of the pig's fractured femur was done by reflex action, duplicature or reflection. If such an idea had been presented to me I should have expressed the same thought in regard to it as did a P. S. C. student, who said: "He pursues too many will-o'-the-wisp vagaries, he does not get down to the fundamentals.")

Would it not be better to try to attain the intellectual level of the Founder of Chiropractic, than to be always tearing down and trying to knock the props from under the writings of wiser and better heads, with the vain hope of presenting something new, regardless of truth or value?

The following will be a fit closing of this review of no cranial nerves, no sympathetic nerves and no reflex action. "Not only does the language (of the following) in which ideas are couched belong to the author, but the very thoughts themselves were his from their inception." "When these questions have been definitely answered, the mystery blown away, the mist evaporated, we will have reached some conclusion; head and tail to our entity."

---

It is the boast of the Medical Trust that everybody in Korea has had smallpox. It can't be a very bad "disease," because the whole country is only as large as the State of Kansas, yet contains 12,000,000 people.—The Ophthalmologist.

---

As editor of The Chiropractor's Adjuster I shall endeavor to edit it for the benefit of Chiropractic and our subscribers; behind all, there is one whose conscious approval must be stamped on each page. I do not anticipate that every item or article will please every reader. An item or an article may palpate too heavily on an impinged sensitive nerve, but when released and the patient returns to the knowledge and principles of Chiropractic, thon will feel better and the adjuster will have a conscious feeling of having done what is right. If we make friends by firmly advocating that which we feel is right, we shall be pleased; if enemies are made, we hope they will feel the penetration of our remarks.

## ITEMS FROM THE MARCH NUMBER, JOURNAL OF OSTEOPATHY: ADJUSTED.

The Osteopaths are struggling with the legislatures of 17 States for recognition.

To apply State laws to Osteopathy is persecution; to apply them against Chiropractors is prosecution.

"The determination of the State society is to either drive undesirables out of business or make them reform in their methods of practice." That is Allopathic.

"It should be made plain that no one's rights are interfered with, nothing unfair is asked for, does not hinder progress or discoveries, does not interfere with other schools. Emphasize the point that every person has a right to choose his own physician."

"Doctors of Osteopathy, being among the leaders in modern thought along the lines of healing, are naturally enthusiastic in their endorsement of the Sheldon Spinal Appliance."

"The Osteopath can find no other aid equal to the Sheldon Appliance in his treatment of spinal troubles."

How is this for Osteopathy? "It seems probable that the disease (amoebic dysentery) has been introduced from Eastern Asia and the Philippine Islands."

"Bovinine is an ideal Food and tonic to build up and sustain Brain, Body, Blood and Bone. It does not disturb digestion and is readily absorbed into the circulation." The manufacturer says, "Oppose disease with the very power that will prevent or **overcome** it—live blood. Bovinine is the live arterial blood of the sturdy bullock. It is antiseptically prepared by cold process, and sterilized. It makes new and enriched blood quicker and better than any other known agent. It is Nature's Greatest Auxiliary, and a most efficient aid to any form of medication. Use it in Anemia, Consumption, Dyspepsia and all debilitated and impoverished conditions. Use it topically on Shronic ulcers, lupus, fistula, burns and bed sores; use it in obstetrical practice, and note **magical and** healthy healing, and prompt abolishment of pus, stench and pain."

"A very large number of man's physical ailments can be traced directly to a poor circulation of the blood. And this is the result of unhealthful brain action through hindered or **pinched nerve** threads or **soft wires.**"

"Chiropractics."—This mode of spelling is used by those who are ignorant of the science of Chiropractic, never by those who are conversant therewith.

The following is largely borrowed from Langworthy and Smith. "In between each two vertebrae there is a thick, spongy cushion, resilient like rubber. There are twenty-four of these, which are so placed that they help to **absorb** the jolts and jars and keep apart the vertebrae, **thus keeping open the windows** between the vertebrae through which come the spinal nerves. These buffers, or cushions, do not get too thick, but from constant use or from abuse they become thin, lose their resiliency, allowing the spine to shorten and **the windows in the spine** to become clogged and closed * * * until there is some breakdown or some sick spell from which he does not recuperate.

"He is told how **the little spinal windows**, through which the body receives its communications from the brain have been **closed** and **how the spinal cord,** the grand highway of the body impulses, **has become scarred through lack of the nourishment** which was **shut off by the closing of the little windows.** * * * The vertebrae which you wish to move is the one which is **tight** * * * He will also examine articulations and ascertain if the facets are correctly placed, and if not he will adjust them."

"I shall try to explain our whole bodily machinery in such a way that it will be no more necessary for us to suppose that the soul produces such movements as are not voluntary than it is to think there is in a clock a soul which causes it to show the hours."

If the above was intended for Chiropractors, it is far-fetched. Just keep studying Chiropractic principles; in time you may be able to comprehend its philosophy. The soul is the life guided by Innate. The soul, the life principle, does not produce any movements. The involuntary movements are under the control of Innate in proportion as the lines of communication are free from impingement.

"Believing that a loving, intelligent Maker of man had deposited in this body some place or through the whole system, drugs in abundance to cure all infirmities. On every voyage of exploration, I (A. T. Still) have been able to bring a cargo of indisputable truths that all remedies necessary to health exist in the human body. They can be administered by adjusting the body in such condition that the remedies may naturally associate themselves together, hear the cries and relieve the afflicted. Thus I have prosecuted the voyage from sea to sea, until I have discovered that Nature is never without necessary remedies. I am better prepared today, after a twenty years' voyage and close observation, to say that God or Nature is the only doctor whom man should respect. Man should study and use the drugs of this drug-store only."

Does the above look as though "Chiropractic is fundamentally osteopathic in principle"? Compare the above with my definition of Chiropractic, found in this book. Do the expressions, "drugs in abundance to cure all infirmities, remedies, afflicted, combat Nature, drugs of this drugstore," look like the principles of Chiropractic? One would think that A. T. Still had been reading A. P. Davis on Neurology, wherein the latter states that "all diseases are due to too much acid or alkaline elements in the body." "Adjusting" to "relieve" is Chiropractic. It will take a few more years for Osteopathy to change its original clothing for those of Chiropractic. It will have to be rebuilt, using Innate for a foundation.

Osteopathy has attempted to make another step forward toward Chiropractic by giving another definition for Osteopathy. "A system of drugless healing, by which a practitioner by a thorough knowledge of Anatomy and Physiology and by appropriate manipulations, adjusts structure, so that nature can restore conditions of normal function to the body.—J. R. Davis." Compare this definition with one of Chiropractic and the three of Osteopathy.—See index.

---

The Chiropractor of February, 1910, states, "Eventually only one school—the school of quality and honest delivery.

"Where is that school? It isn't far from where I am. THINK IT OVER."

The above prophesy and foresight into the future was published in the February number of The Chiropractor, 1910. Before the close of the year we see the beginning of the end of its fulfillment.

That school of quality and honest delivery is not far, only three blocks distant on the same street, 528 instead of 828. From what I hear, it is "the school of quality and honest delivery" just as foretold. "THINK IT OVER."

G. H. Patchen, M. D., D. C., in answer to the question: "What is the basic principle of Chiropractic," wisely remarks. "Both physicians and laymen have realized for many years that health depends upon normal tone of the nerves, but they have not known what means to use to promote or restore it when lacking. Having been educated to depend in all cases upon the efficacy of drugs; they have pinned their faith (in most cases with ultimate disappointment) to tones (TONE-ICS) and in spite of almost uniform defeat they still continue, like blind men groping in the dark, to look for something outside of the body, which will tone up the nerves, when tone is lacking, with the firm conviction that it will eventually be found.

"The Chiropractic thrust is the safest, quickest and most permanent method of restoring normal tone."

**Symptomatology** is that branch of pathology which observes and interprets the prognosis of disease. To be able to foretell and watch its progress is important and interesting to a pathologist.

Normal nerve vibrations create a temperature of 96.6 degrees. If nerves are impinged upon, pressed against, vibrations and heat are increased accordingly. This excess is known to M. D.s as fever. If the kidneys pass the normal amount of urine, we have health; if too much or not enough, we have conditions named disease. Any deviation of functional performance is known as disease. Disorders are but increased or decreased functional activity.

Our students are not required to spend hours daily in a laboratory mounting specimens of tissue on slides for examination under a microscope, just to see how they would look if they were 800 times as large; or in other words, to know how a man would appear if instead of weighing 180 pounds, his size should be increased to 144,000 pounds. These seeming exaggerations are of no value to the investigator who is in search of the cause of disease and its removal. Why is the activity of functions decreased or increased; or why are they performed in a normal manner, are far more important questions.

Chiropractors take symptoms in consideration in order to locate the cause thereof. If there is doubt or a desire to demonstrate the location of the cause, then trace the hypersensitive nerves from the affected portion to the impingement or vice versa.

Restoration is inherent if the pressure on nerves is removed. Special attention is given to outward signs, which point with unmistakable certainty to the location of the primary cause.

---

A letterhead has the two following statements, which we admire: "Chiropractic Adjustments remove the cause of 95 per cent of all Acute and Chronic Diseases."

"Every genuine Chiropractor adjusts the Cause of Disease by hand, therefore, does not use Drugs, Medicine, Knife or any other mechanical appliances."

The author of the above will be pleased to learn that I have but two criticisms to make on the above. Drugs and medicine are one and the same: therefore, use only one of the two. Why say "**any other**" mechanical appliances, as you have not mentioned any?

With the cut of himself, and two vertebral columns, in three colors, it makes a very nice letter head.

## EXOSTOSES AND ENOSTOSES.

Any abnormal protuberance of or on a bone is an exostosis. Enostoses are unusual bony growths on or of the **interior** surface of bones. They are found **in** the long bones and those of the face and cranium.

Abnormal growths of bones may be physiological or pathological. If Innate builds an abutment or pier to prevent further displacement or deposits callus to mend a fracture, such acts are physiological and are deemed necessary to accomplish certain purposes. Physiological exostoses are built to strengthen weak places caused by malacia, caries or fracture. They consist of osseous matter, diffused or nodular, deposited for a purpose on the surface of bones.

Pathological exostoses consist of morbid, osseous matter deposited on the surface of a bone or of an enlargement of the bone itself. Their structure, as well as their locations, vary. Bones in their makeup resemble the soft parts of the body and are liable to similar diseases. One or more bones, sometimes the whole skeleton, may be increased or decreased in size or changed in its consistency. Hyperthermia increases their softness and growth, while subnormal temperature condenses and hardens their substance by depositing a greater number of white corpuscles than are normal.

Pathological osseous growths are classified as true or false, that is, they are truly bony in their entire makeup, or else are more or less a spongy expansion of bone, containing fleshy, fungous matter (unossified) internally. This difference is accounted for by continued temperature, above normal, producing a surplus of red corpuscles—material for soft tissue, or a subnormal temperature which creates an increase of white corpuscles, the material for hard, compact tissue.

The periosteum of bones may become hardened by periostitis, inflammation of the covering of bone. Periosteal exostosis consists of a deposit of osseous matter between the external surface of the bone and the internal surface of the periosteum, firmly adherent to both. The abnormal growth may be of the medullary, a similar deposit of osseous matter on the medullary membrane and in the cancellated structure; for, be it remembered, that red and white corpuscles are supplied to these parts as elsewhere, and, that abnormality in the amount of heat and corpuscles cause a corresponding change in their structure.

Osseous tumors may be constructed of cartilaginous material ossified by ossific deposit. They differ in size, the larger ones are usually those known as false. While some bones are more subject to exostoses than others, yet, any bone of the skeletal frame may become the seat of this disease.

The bones of the cranium may be exostosed on either the outer or inner table. Or either one or both as well as the diploe, may be increased in thickness. The increased portion of the tables and the pericranium are of hard, bony consistence and attended with but little pain, while that of the increased diploe is fungous, more vascular and painful. Pain is a distressing sensation of the nerves, depending upon irritation or pressure, either at their endings or along their pathway. It is most severe where the tissue is unyielding, as in felons which occur upon the fingers in the stiff fascia thru which the nerves of sensation pass. Inflamed nerves which occupy loose cellular tissue are usually accompanied with little or no pain. An undue amount of heat increases the thickness of the diploe, while it may become entirely absent by continued subnormal temperature. The difference is caused by the amount of red corpuscles deposited in the diploe and of white corpuscles on the surfaces of the outer and inner tables.

The femur or other long bones may become enormous in size, while the medullary canal continues unchanged. In other cases, the outer and inner surfaces and the thickness of the bones are deformed by an augmentation of bulk, and the medullary cavities are more or less reduced in their caliber or totally closed. Or the bones may acquire great solidity and be as hard and white as ivory, the color and quality depending upon the amount of red or white corpuscles, which vary according to the temperature. A high temperature increases the number of red corpuscles, while subnormal temperature augments the per cent of leukocytes.

Medical writers have not been able to discover the cause of exostoses or enostoses. They are inclined to think scrofula and venereal diseases have much to do with their origin, but how, they do not say. The cause or causes of abnormal bone growths are not understood. Some consider them constitutional, that is, inherent, depending upon an abnormal structure of the body which causes a morbid development of the cells of nutrition, while others regard them as being composed of inorganic lime. To account for them as constitutional, scrofulous or venereal origin, is to make an explanation that is unexplainable.

Stengel tells us that "An underlying predisposition undoubtedly exists, which explains the occurrence of **congenital** multiple bony tumors. **Irritation** and **traumatism** undoubtedly play a part in the etiology, even in neoplasms unattached to the bone and in the case of bony outgrowths injury is generally the immediate cause. Secondary degenerative changes (softening) may occur."

Irritation and traumatism play a very important part in the etiology of all osseous and soft tissue growths. Nerves excited, express too much function, too much growth in the portion to which they extend and functionate. The exciting cause may be a toxic irritant or traumatic pressure.

Delafield and Prudden allow that "Osteoma may be the result of a peculiar inflammatory process or chronic inflammation. New-formed bone has been found in the soft parts of the body; in the brain substance, dura mater, and pia mater; in the pleura, diaphragm and pericardium; in the skin, choroid, air passages, lungs and other places."

The above parties are correct in their surmises. I have in my possession a spinal column whose first owner parted with it after using it about fifty years. In early life he met with an accident, receiving fractures of the articular processes between the sixth and seventh cervicals, also of those between the 11th and 12th thoracic, with consequent ankylosis at each place. There is also a healed fracture of the 5th sacral segment. I said in "early life," determined by a diminutive 12th pair of ribs, which are only one and a quarter inches each in length. This man possessed a 7th cervical rib. The special feature to which I wish to call the attention of the reader, is, that in consequence of hyperthermia, the injured vertebrae were softened, so that much of their substance oozed out, a part adhering to the anterior of their bodies and a mass, an inch by one and a quarter, being free in the tissue. The above conditions, resultant from lesions, were pathological. The spinal canal of the lower half of the thoracic region has piers built to prevent further displacement of those vertebrae. These enostoses are physiological.

John E. Erichsen says of exostoses: "The causes that immediately give rise to this disease are usually obscure. There can be no doubt that, in some instances, it is predisposed to by syphilis, scrofula, or cancerous affections; and that in other cases again, it is hereditary; but, in general, it occurs without any distinct or appreciable exciting cause. There is no means of ridding the patient of the tumor, but by the removal of the whole growth."

To assume that abnormal bone growths are because of heredity, syphilis, scrofula, cancerous affections, savors too much of throwing the blame for our ailments on Old Mother Eve. Chiropractic in its philosophy makes suitable explanations and with its science and art proves that by adjusting displacements of the skeleton frame, osseous enlargements may be removed. The medical profession have no idea that the absorbent vessels are able to remove the abnormal growths by particles in the reverse order of that by which the secerning arteries deposited them. Some writers refer to retrogressive degenration of caries or necrosis, or mucous metamorphosis. I have seen two scapulae which had met with severe fractures. Innate had taken quite a portion of the center of the blade and transported it to a place where it was most needed. The excavated portion was in an elongated vertical foramina. This act was physiological, done for a purpose.

Samuel Cooper honestly states: "Our ignorance of the pathology of exostoses, particularly their causes, accounts for the imperfection of our treatment of them."

Bayer acknowledges: "That the progress of exostoses can scarcely ever be checked by any general methodical treatment, the resolution of such tumors is almost impossible."

Bayer should have known, that all sciences were destined to advance, that those which did not would be left behind and others more fit would step in and lead.

The American Text Book of Surgery considers syphilis the cause, and "the only effective treatment for oxostoses is, removal of the growth by operation."

McDonald coincides with the above by saying: "The only effective remedy is extirpation. In some cases nothing short of amputation will suffice."

Malignant, osteoid tumors, such as osteo-cancer (osteosarcoma), osteo-cephaloma (encephaloid sarcoma) and osteoma, are true bone cancers.

An osteoma is a tumor composed of osseous tissue. Such tumors usually occur in connection with some part of the skeleton, but are occasionally found in the pia mater, the brain and the lung. In structure they may resemble the spongy tissue of the epiphyses of the bones, or the dense, ivory-like structure of the petrous portion of the temporal bone, or any intermediate density. Osteomata are the result of excessive growths resulting from inflammation.

Compact osteoma, dental exostosis, hypercementosis, inordinate growth, is an increase of cementum of a tooth. Osteoma durum, osteoma eberneum is a tumor of very hard, bone-like tissue. Osteoma spongiosum, medullosum or cancellous osteoma is composed of cancellated tissue. A diffused, widespread hypertrophy of bone is known as hyperostosis. Enchondromata is a tumor resembling cartillage in texture.

The ivory exostosis differs in its appearance and structure from true bone. It is extremely compact and white, and has a granular section resembling that of ivory. It contains more of the phosphate and less of the carbonate of lime and the proportion of animal matter is less. An osteoma may be eburnated, compact or cancellous, according to the proportionate amount of red and white corpuscles.

Bone tumors may be accompanied by secondary alterations of the bone tissue, such as osteo-porosis, osteo-sclerosis, ossifying periostitis. New growths may undergo calcification and ossification.

Spina ventosa is, by some, classified as an osteoid-cancer. It does not belong in that division, altho it is a disease of the osseous system. It is a rarefying form of osteitis in which the bone is eroded (destroyed by caries, the result of hyperthermia) and the superiosteal tissue and osseous marrow contain numerous small cells with transuded **red blood-corpuscles.**

As may be inferred from what I have said, red corpuscles form soft tissue and the white corpuscles produce bone. An excess of the red tends to soften bone tissue, while an excess of the white or bone-forming corpuscles produce an ossifying effect upon the soft tissue. In some instances osseous growths have necrosed and sloughed off without treatment.

Samuel Cooper states: "The fever, which commences at an early period of the disorder (exostoses), assumes a slow type and is continuous, together with the ichorous discharge and irritation may bring on the patient's dissolution."

Osteomata are closely allied to cartilaginous tumors; under certain heat conditions they are interchangeable, frequent transformations occur.

Stengel refers to "The bony changes of congenital syphilis," and "syphilitic diseases of the bones."

Enlargement of the facial bones in leontiasis ossea, acromegally and hypertrophic pulmonary osteo-arthropathy and ossifications of the muscles in myositis ossificans, are inflammatory hyperostosis.

Bones are created from leukocytes. A low temperature produces a larger per cent of white corpuscles. Hyperthermia increases the number of red corpuscles and lessens the white. Cartilage and soft tissue are composed of red, while the hard tissue is composed of white corpuscles. A normal temperature maintains an equilibrium of the red and the white. Because of the larger amount of soft tissue and its continued change, there is a necessity for a larger per cent of the red corpuscles. Heat is the producer and the regulator of the corpuscles. Its elevation and depression determines the proportion of them. The superabundance of either is directed to the area where the nerves which are impinged upon terminate. In osteomalacia of the whole skeleton we find the nerves of the 6th dorsal impinged, because of traumatic or toxic irritation.

In answer to The P. S. C. student, will say, the dorsal, cervical and atlas should be adjusted from the affected side. The lumbar from the opposite. An exception to this is the 3d cervical, because of the axial center being posterior to the articulating processes.

Please take a vertebral column, displace the atlas laterally—the only way it can be displaced—notice how the projecting edge of its inferior articular process strikes against the sympathetic ganglionic nerve chain as it passes in front of the transverse process, as Gerrish states: "The first cervical nerve (ventral division), after leaving the vertebral canal in the groove on the dorsal arch of the atlas, winds round to the front on the inner side of the vertebral artery and bends downward over the transverse process to join the second nerve. The central division of the second nerve leaves the vertebral canal behind the articular process of the axis; those of the rest of the cervical nerves pass outward in the intervertebral foramina, behind the vertebral artery and between the rectus capitis anterior major and the scalenus medius." Adjust from you, and the impingement and tension is relieved.

---

**Physiology** is the science which treats of the functions of organic beings. Morbid physiology pertains to those modified by disease. These vary according to the consistency of their lines of communication. The texture of connective tissue controls the amount of vital and intellectual functions transferred by the amount of molecular vibrations. According to the amount of energy carried, is the total of work accomplished by the cumulative and vegetative functions. The student should be familiar with physiology as taught by medical and osteopathic schools but, especial prominence should be given to those of Chiropractic as promulgated by the founder of this science.

Physiological chemistry of molecular and atomic structure, through which functions are operated, is comprehended by Innate far better than by the intellectual man. The vital and vegetative functions are under the control of Innate; all the acts of the body are regulated through the nervous system.

Chiropractic comes to the aid of morbid physiology by its rational explanation of heat, impulses, innervation and the work accomplished by the vegetative and cumulative functions.

This science has located the cause of organic and functional diseases. This achievement has been accomplished by clinical methods peculiar to the originator.

## CHIROPRACTIC.

Chiropractic was not evolved from any other system. Osteopathy was developed from and includes massage and Swedish movements. Neurology was "evolved out of Osteopathy, Chiropractic and the science of Ophthalmology."

Osteopathy has been found wanting, inasmuch, as its adherents use orthopedical machines, drugs and surgery.

The author of Neurology uses a vibrator, drugs, magnetism, suggestive therapeutics, phrenology and palmistry. His acts demonstrate that his science (which is but parts of three other methods) is not sufficient for the needs of all ills, although he says, "This science embraces the entire nervous system." It has been found lacking in cataract of the eye.

The principles of Chiropractic are being developed by the same mind which gave it birth—the fundamental ones being thots—disease is the result of too much or not enough function—and that—bone pressure on nerves causes impringements. Its origin and the principles upon which it is based, were included in that first adjustment.

Chiropractic came in its own good time. The world had grown to it—there was a demand for it—it was needed. It did not come to antagonize other methods. It was demanded, each of the others having served its time and purpose. Chiropractic came as an educator. Those practicing other methods are absorbing its principles and movements as fast as they are mentally able. The people demand that Medicine and Therapeutics shall move forward or step aside.

Chiropractic is a demonstrated fact; it is a science. As we become acquainted with its principles, founded upon laws as old as the vertebrata, we will make less failures. The science can only develop along the lines laid down by its founder.

The principles of Chiropractic should be recognized in the formation of the embryo, the development of the fetus, the growth of the infant and continue as a safeguard throughout life.

The cumulative function determines the mental qualifications. Therefore, the condition of the physical decides as to the contents of the mental store-house. We can but take with us, when the soul—intelligent life—ceases to exist, the sane thoughts, or the vagaries of the mind—monstrous conceptions—that we have conceived.

The man who had the intellectual capacity to comprehend the displacement of vertebrae, the mental ability to grasp the cause and effect of nerve impingement; the power to conceive and discriminate between the normal and abnormal; the foresight and wisdom to discern the outcome; the genius for originality; the brain caliber capable of reasoning on this perplexing question—the cause of disease; the sense of touch required to discover a racked vertebra, and the skill and tact to replace it, was the one destined to discover and develop the science which he was pleased to name Chiropractic. This philosophy will advance mankind mentally, physically and spiritually.

---

A forty-page Chiropractic booklet lies before me. It is well gotten up. Some portions are copied, but so well connected that one not well versed in Chiropractic literature would ever notice it.

The writer refers to nerves being impinged upon and pinched. These two terms are not synonyms—they have different meanings. A nerve can only be pinched or squeezed between two hard bodies, such as bones. An impinged nerve has pressure on one side only. The author of Chiropractic states that nerves may be impinged upon by any displaced bone, but pinched only by fracture and extreme displacement.

It is difficult to rid ourselves of stereotyped phrases, even when we know they are not correct, such as "every ill to which the human race is heir." We do not inherit our ills. "Other systems of healing." Chiropractic is not a system of healing; it is one of adjusting for relief. "Afflict the human race" implies that some one, an intelligent being, the evil one or a witch did the afflicting; such is not Chiropractic.

Remedies cure; adjusting relieves.

Page 12. The hands are not instruments. The thrust is not a rock.

"Straighten a displaced vertebra." By replacing the displaced vertebra he would straighten the spine; he cannot straighten a vertebra.

The liver, spleen, pancreas and kidneys are secretive and excretive—vegetative functions.

Page 21. "Nerves are life." Nerves are the conveyors of functions. Function expressed is action—life.

"Goitres disappear when the nerve supply has been restored that had been cut off by a cervical displacement." Goitres are growths because of an over-supply of nutrition—excessive vegetative functionating. Instead of functionating being cut off, there is too much functional activity. Goitres are because of impinged dorsal—not cervical nerves.

This Chiropractor wrote me: "I am a Chiropractor and practice nothing but Chiropractic." His book states on page 20 that he uses Chiropractic **with traction.** Traction is drawing or stretching the body by a machine; this is orthopedic, or osteopathic; **it is not Chiropractic.**

"By twisting the vertebra from its normal position that the nerve trunks are pinched and irritated, which certainly must disturb their function, which is nothing more or less than disease." This sentence states, function is nothing more or less than disease. He should have said, and no doubt intended to say, that deranged functions or structure harder or softer than normal or displaced organs result in disease. Some one or more of the fibers of the nerve-trunk may be impinged upon and irritated.

On page 6 he says, the dorsal nerves "divide into three branches," and gives their functions. He should understand that the spinal nerves of the dorsal region divide into **four** branches immediately upon leaving the spinal column. The recurrent nerve, which furnishes innervation to the meninges of the brain and spinal cord, because of an impingement, furnishes too much or not enough functionating, a surplus or a lack of heat to the brain and spinal cord, producing degeneration or calcification; myelitis or atrophy; hydromyelia or syringomyelia; tuberculosis or syphilis; meningitis or ischemia; malacia or sclerosis; this recurrent nerve he did not mention. As the president of a Chiropractic school, he should recognize this nerve which returns back to the spinal canal functionating the meninges of the brain and spinal cord. He should know it may be impinged upon and also how to relieve that pressure.

"It remained for the Chiropractic school to discover the exact relation, and to solve the problem of rectifying the wrong." I solved that problem years before he or anyone else had a school; long before he taught it to anyone. Why not tell it as it is? Why prevaricate? How could a school discover the principles upon which Chiropractic was founded? Some one had to know the relation between subluxation and impingement before a school was formed. No school discovered the relation between sub-luxated joints and the impingement of nerves; that these conditions excite the atoms which compose the nerves, creating too much heat; by its over-tension, vibrations are too great; carrying capacity increased, resulting in too much functionating, which is disease. I taught these principles to the writer of this booklet. Why should he say they were discovered by the Chiropractic School? Although he does not state that his school made this discovery, the reader, if he was not on his guard for misrepresentations, would be led to believe that his was the one referred to.

On the next page he repeats this falsehood by saying: "Chiropractic is positively the first school to adjust displaced osseous tissue." That is a positive lie, whether written by a Salvation Army Captain or the President of a Chiropractic School. I adjusted displaced osseous tissue (vertebrae) long before there was a school; years before I taught it to any one.

---

A recent graduate of the P. S. C. says: "A Chiropractor is qualified to diagnose without asking a single question."

I would think this a mistake or a mis-print, were it not that others have made the same statement. If such a thing is possible, I will pay liberally to be shown how it is done.

The statement is false, fraudulent, calculated to deceive, and obtain money by deception. I do not believe that The P. S. C. teaches that a Chiropractor can diagnose each and every case without asking a single question. Unless it can be done, the editor ought not to allow mention of it to go into its pages. Chiropractic is good enough without lying about it.

"Chiropract**ic** finds the cause of disease, removes it."

The Chiropract**or** finds the cause of disease and removes it. The science does not.

---

The Annual Announcement states that the P. S. C. was "established 1885."

The P. S. C. Announcement of "1904" states, on page 4, "We realize, after testing this science for **nine years,** that we have a method of inestimable value to suffering humanity, it is so considered by every physician who has had the courage. We have many graduates who are successfully practicing this science, proving beyond a doubt that others can do just what D. D. Palmer, the discoverer, is doing. Realizing that in order to have the benefits far reaching, it must be taught in all its entirety; therefore, with this end in view, **our school was started seven years ago.**"

The above is copied almost verbatim from 1904 Annual Announcement, page 4, which was written by D. D. Palmer. B. J. has developed much of my writing by copying. The above will be found as developed in the P. S. C. Announcement No. 4.

In 1904 the school had been opened seven years. There was one student in 1898; three in 1899; two in 1900; five in 1901, and four in 1902, among the latter was B. J. Palmer. The school was opened in 1897, but was not in session, did not have a student until in 1898. Counting the first student as the founding of the school, the P. S. C. has been running 11 years instead of (1885) 24 years. Why not tell it just as it is?

## A SPINE-SET PERSONIFIED.

I was shaped for a purpose; my designer was a thinker; he fashioned my body to his liking; he had an aim in view in my creation.

While passing through several phases of existence, being useful in each, I have become a firm believer in predestination and transformation. My earliest recollection is of an acorn existence. How comfortably I was cradled in my hard involucre of woody, indurated whorl of bracteole; my closely appressed bracteiform cradle was swung to and fro by the cooling breeze.

My mother who gave me an individualized existence, was a sturdy oak. For many months I was exposed to sunshine and showers, until I had grown to a fully matured acorn. One night during a terrific storm of rain, thunder and lightning, I was wrenched from my home on high. Daylight found me lying close to a rotten log covered with the same leaves which had given me shelter in my embryonic period of ovulation. I passed the long dreary winter, in a state of torpidity, protected from the frost by a covering of leaves which had gathered over my helpless form during that well-remembered night when the elements spent their fury. Spring came with its showers and sunshine. My insensible, indehiscent, pericarpial, syncarpous, ovarian germ was warmed into life and activity. The hidden powers that lay within my morphologically megasporangium began to swell, bursting my hardened shell. Not until then did I realize that within me were all the possibilities of my becoming a great and mighty oak. I well remember an orator when rehearsing his piece to the trees of the forest saying: "Great oaks from little acorns grow." During the spring and summer, I took advantage of the warmth and moisture to get well rooted and get a start in life. In time I became one of the mighty trees of the forest. In my branches the birds of the air built their nests and raised their young. I furnished shade and shelter to the beasts of the earth. To the graminivorous I gave nutritious food. I was useful in life and, as you will see, my dismembered body was shaped to benefit mankind. My existence has not been in vain.

One day, in September, two stout, husky men came with axes and saw. I heard them say: "That tree will make five cuts three and a half feet long for broom handles and a whole lot of firewood." That was a sad day for me. With many ugly, vicious blows of those cruel axes and with hours of gnawing and tearing my body with the continuous biting of those saw teeth, I was laid low. They hacked my limbs from my body and threw them in a pile to dry. My decapitated and dismembered trunk was cut in lengths of three and a half feet, as I heard them say, for broom handles. The next day after I had been mutilated beyond recognition, these same two men came with a sled and two horses. I recognized the team as one which had, on many Sundays, enjoyed the cool shade of my spreading branches. They hauled us, now named cuts, to a saw mill. I say "us," as I had been segmented into many parts, each becoming individualized.

We were sawed into inch-square strips, then, one by one, we were pushed into a machine which made our heads swim. When I came to my senses, I found that, with the exception of two inches at one end, we were round instead of square. We were tied in bundles and piled in a large shed where we had a season of rest. Eventually we were shipped to a broom factory here I learned what the two cruel butchers meant by "broom handles." We were ranked in a shed near a lot of broom corn which I remembered seeing in a near-by field. They, like me, had been grown from seed, but they were planted by the hand of man while I was a child of nature. They grew in rows, their growth increased and hurried by cultivation. While they were only robbed of their indeterminate inflorescent pendent, I was slaughtered for all that was in me. The broom corn had a jointed stem resembling that of sorghum, and bore a stiff-branched panicle, called a tassel.

Men polished and painted our bodies and wired a bunched skeleton of the pyramidal, loosely branched flower-cluster on our squared ends, giving us a tassel of simple, indeterminate, centripetal, inflorescence whose elongated axis had borne pedicellate flowers in acropetal succession. Thus we were adorned with skeleton plumes. We were neatly bound in dozen lots and placed in a car filled so closely that we were awfully crowded. We knew not where we were going but, at last, the door to our prison was opened and we were taken to a wholesale house from which we were distributed to retail dealers in dozen lots. I observed that each time we changed hands our value increased. The groceryman who bought a dozen, of which I was one, hung us up where we could be seen and not be trampled upon; he had an eye for business. This was a novel experience to me. I learned much about the tricks of trade.

One day a farmer's wife brought in her weekly produce of butter and eggs. She looked at us and asked, "Have you a good broom?" I wondered what she took us for. She handled three of us by jabbing us on the floor, and, with a dexterous sweep as much as to say, "You see I know how," took me as her choice. I was raised in the country and, really, I was glad to be able to breathe fresh air again.

It was late when we arrived at the farmer's home. The next day was sweeping day. Ma, that was what the family called my mistress, had a regular day for each part of the house work. That Thursday was the first day of hard labor I had ever known. Our next-door neighbor called, handled me and said: "A new broom sweeps clean, but the old one knows how to find the corners." When the day's work was done, I stood in the corner, behind the bed-room door, my broom-corn tassel uppermost.

I learned to hustle the dirt out of the back door, which Pa and the hired man brought in three times a day. Mrs. Brown, that was Ma's neighbor, said Ma was either a dirty house-keeper or a clean sweeper, judging from the amount of dirt I gathered each day. I learned to like my new home.

One day, in the early winter, it rained in the afternoon and turned very cold during the night, as I knew by the frost on the window pane. Daylight found the porch, steps and side-walk covered with ice and snow. Ma was up bright and early. She took me with her to clean the snow from the porch and walks. While she and I were sweeping the snow from the steps, Ma slipped and fell square on me, breaking me in two. I did not say a word, but Ma screamed for Pa. The hired man and Pa carried Ma into the house. Susie, one of the girls, went out to finish the sweeping and found me with a broken back. She wound a stout cord around my middle but my back was weak ever afterward.

Pa sent for our family physician. Ma was a good talker; she told the doctor all about her case. I could have told all about it in a minute, but she talked until the doctor got tired of listening. The doctor just looked at me but examined Ma's hip and leg. When he moved her leg, Ma screamed. The doctor said there were no bones broken but Ma had received a bad shock He left her some quieting powders.

Ma had a good bed to lie on while I had to stand, when not at work, behind the bed-room door where I could see and hear all that was said and done. Day after day and night after night passed and Ma got no better fast. On the tenth day, the doctor put a glass tube in Ma's mouth, held his gold watch in one hand and her wrist with the other. After a minute or two he looked wise and said Ma had some fever, that a kind of micro-organism named pyogenic cocci had developed.

Pa told the doctor that Ma was taken "worser and getting no better fast," that he must do something for her. So the doctor took a long time to tell us all about that infractious nerve. It was Sunday, so Pa and the doctor had plenty of time; and as for Ma and me, we had to hear it. I listened attentively to all that was said, for I was getting interested in doctoring. The doctor commenced by saying that neuralgia of the sciatic nerve was hard to cure; that nothing short of an operation would give Ma relief. He told us that this troublesome nerve was known by the names of sciatic, ischiatic and the great femoro-popliteal; that it was the largest nerve in the body, being about half an inch wide and a quarter of an inch thick; it was composed of fibers from the dorsal branches of the fourth and fifth lumbar and first, second and third sacral nerves. It issued from the pelvis, between the pyramidalis and the superior gemellus and descended along the posterior part of the thigh; it gave branches to the gemini, quadratus, obturator externus, gluteus maximus, semimembranosus, semitendinosus, biceps and third abductor muscles, dividing about the inferior third of the thigh into two branches, the external and internal popliteal; that this particular nerve was affected with neuritis; that is, inflammation of a nerve; that the real cause was tension but the cause of tension was not as yet well understood; that neuralgia was a paroxysmal pain in the area of the nerve or along its course; that it was an inflammatory disturbance in the nerve-trunk; that traumatism and poisons were exciting causes, there was no doubt; that lesions of the central nervous system give rise to attacks of neuralgia. The different forms of neuralgia were named according to their anatomic situation relative to the spinal cord, as trigeninal, tic douloureux or prosopalgia, cervico-occipital, cervico-bracial, intercostal, sciatica or ischias, coccygodynia, visceral neuralgia and cerebralgia.

The doctor said it was easy to produce pain and fever by nerve-tension, but not so easy to break a fever or release pain. That all nerves had a normal stimulation, which produced a normal tone; that tension was too much longitudinal traction; that a hammer could be used for mechanical stimulation of a nerve; that, as an instrument, it was not excelled by electricity in exciting contraction of nerves and muscles; that this method of shocking a nerve by rapid vibration is known as tetanizing or tetanization; it threw the nerves and muscles into a condition known as tetanus, a permanent contraction; that tetanus of a muscle was the fusion of a number of simple spasms into an apparently smooth, continuous effort, a tetanic contraction.

He told us that nux vomica, strychnine and brucine act, primarily, on the spinal cord, and, when taken in large quantities, produce tetanic spasms or convulsions. In cases of poisoning, the spasmodic seizures affect first the nerves and muscles near the point of inoculation; in mild affections it may be confined to those nerves and muscles only. The toxin travels by nerve cells, reaching the spinal cord through the axis cylinders. Nerves, affected by poison, often present symptoms of traumatic lesions with redness and swelling of the neurilemma. Tetanic convulsions are of spinal origin. Pressure on a nerve-trunk will often produce tetanus, spasm, convulsions or cramps. To insure such pathologic results the pressure must be applied several minutes. The best place to make the pressure for spasm effects is on the bicipital sulcus, or the crural sulcus. Sometimes pressure on the brachial plexus or on the popliteal space will produce an attack. Tapping with the finger tip or a rubber hammer over the anterior part of the zygomatic arch, the subcutaneous portion of the facial nerve, will often result in a spasm of the upper eyelid.

The doctor explained tetanus to Pa. He said that it was a continuous, spasmodic contraction of muscles, causing rigidity of the parts to which they are attached. That a spasm, or tetanus, is an extreme contraction caused by an immoderate vibration. Placing a vibrating tuning-fork, or a sounding string made to vibrate with a bow, in contact with a nerve, causes a rythmic tension according to the vibrations imparted to it, similar to that exhibited by a 'phone wire when impinged against by a telepgraph wire. If an exposed nerve is stretched, the tension up to a certain degree acts as an irritant; stronger stretching causes, for a time, a diminution of irritability, even temporary paralysis. A still greater degree of stretching finally gives rise to permanent paralysis; thus it is with an unexposed nerve. If a nerve is in a state of excessive irritability, as in a case of neuralgiform contraction, nerve-stretching may be useful by diminishing the irritability of the nerve. The nerve that is tense and superficial may be traced as a thick cord, a continuous, uninterrupted swelling; its course is sometimes marked by a red line, as in phlebitis or angioleucitis. The marked hyperthesia is followed by atrophy if the neuritis persists; hyperthesia will gradually give place to neurasthenia and finally to anesthesia.

Our doctor said that sciatica is a form of neuralgia; that there is a marked difference between rheumatism and neuritis. In the latter the pain occurs in the track of a nerve, later, it is differentiated by the sensory, motor, or trophic changes which set in. In neuralgia the pain is sharp and shooting and more diffused over the affected area. There is little or no rise of general or local temperature and usually no muscular spasm, although these symptoms are occasionally found in the peripheral endings of the fifth nerve.

I carefully made a mental note of all that our doctor said, for, thought I, "May I not become a doctor some day?" I longed to quit this ignoble slavish toil, this disagreeable drudgery, wearisome labor of sweep, sweep, nothing but dirt-sweeping.

I gave the doctor credit for having a storehouse of knowledge for every day he had a new treatment. He had the girls apply hot and cold compresses; at one time he blistered, and at another he cauterized Ma's leg. One day he brot a box and used what he called a galvanic current on Ma's leg and hip. I examined the box and discovered that the current was generated by the chemical action of accidulated water upon metallic plates. He said that in some cases galvanic currents are a good thing. Nothing seemed to help Ma. The doctor said her case was stubborn and would not yield to any treatment.

One day the doctor brought a small squirt gun with which he injected morphine, then atrophine, cocaine and lastly chloroform. He said in some cases of sciatic neuritis these preparations had been found of great value.

As I watched the many treatments given Ma, I thought that, if I was a doctor I would leave out all the "valuable, excellent remedies" and do something that would be of some benefit.

The doctor gave Ma morphine until he feared she would become a morphinomaniac.

Ma's leg was losing its natural feeling. The doctor said anesthesia was setting in so he used the faradic current with an electric brush. I saw that it was only a current of electricity produced by an electric coil. Part of the time he gave Ma quinine, or arsenic, or strychnine, or gelsemium for a change.

One day our doctor brought another doctor. His name was Brubaker—Dr. Brubaker. I thot at first he was going to make an Egyptian triangular harp out of Ma's leg. He said: "If a stethoscope or a myophone with telephone connections be placed on a muscle while in a condition of volitional tetanus and at the same time **kept** in a certain degree of **tension, there will be developed** in the observer **a sensation of sound or tone** which is spoken of as a muscle sound or tone. **It is also readily heard in the masseter muscle when** the side of the face is placed on a receiving body such as a pillow, and **the masseter muscles made to contract** volitionally. **This tone is attributed to a vibration or an alternate contraction or relaxation of the muscle or to an intermittent rhythmic variation in tension**, the result of the rate of stimulation. **This tone corresponds to a vibration** frequency **of from 18 to 20 per second** and is accepted as one of the proofs that the physiologic volitional tetanus is not continuous in character. If a muscle is tetanized with induced currents, the **tone increases in pitch** for a limited time as the frequency of the current per second increases up to a certain maximum."

They tried stretching the sciatic nerve by circumduction, a bloodless method. All the muscles of the hip and upper portion of the thigh were manipulated deeply, from side to side, to open the saphenous vein, so that the engorged veins might be reduced. Extension, abduction, adduction and flexion were thoroughly used. It hurt Ma awfully, but she felt easy for a while afterward, and took a good sleep without morphine. Our doctor saw that stretching the nerve did some good, gave temporary relief, so he told Pa that surgery offered relief for sciatica. That there was an operation, thank fortune, called neurectasia, neurectasis or neurectasy, nerve stretching, that had been used in many cases with excellent results. He allowed that contraction of the nerve, lengthwise, was the cause of all pain; that nerves could be stretched one inch in twenty, but care should be taken to not rupture the nerve; that it took a force of 82 to 288 pounds to fracture the ischiatic nerve, and that the leg or pelvis could be lifted by traction on the sciatic nerve.

The next day following this erudite and elaborate discourse, our doctor brought a neighboring physician. They gave Ma an anesthetic, using ether. They made an incision about four inches long in the middle line of the leg, beginning just below the gluteo-femoral crease, loosened the great sciatic nerve and stretched it in several different directions. I saw them lift Ma's leg by that nerve. I heard our doctor tell the strange doctor that, if this operation was not a success, they would perform an operation known as laminectomy; that is, cut out the laminae of one or two vertebrae, get to the spinal cord where the real seat of the trouble is, and exsect the sensory roots of the great femoropopliteal nerve. There will then be no sensation, so she will not be able to feel the tension. In this way they would surely make a success of this job. That operation they called an intraspinal section of the posterior roots.

During these operations and private consultations, no one was allowed in the room; they never once thought of putting me out. It would take a long time for me to tell you about all the treatments which Ma had, but there were some things of special interest to me, inasmuch as I was thinking of studying for a doctor. They tried to locate the lesion before operating. They were sure it was within three spinal segments, but to determine the exact vertebra was an impossibility, as any given surface or area derives its sensation from three or more nerve-roots. Practically every muscle is innervated from at least two segments of the cord. Furthermore, the efferent and afferent tracts run up above the exit, a variable distance in the substance of the cord. The cause of this particular disease may be much higher than the point of entrance of the exit of the nerve-root involved. So that the lesion is not always accurately determined by the spinous processes. I was not only an attentive listener, but I did some thinking, knowing that those who think govern those who toil.

I could not bear the idea of Ma going through any more operations and especially that of laminectomy.

After the doctors left, Pa and I had a long talk. I told him what the doctors proposed doing next. I advised him to take me to the wood-shed where he had some tools and a work-bench. He was willing to do anything for Ma. He did as I directed; sawed off five and a half inches of my upper end. Pa was quite ingenious and handy. I never saw a saw saw as that saw sawed. The saw tickled my sides so much that I could not lie still; I just rolled all over the bench, but Pa finally made as he said, an excision. I called him "Old Saw Bones" and he retaliated by calling me a "Holy Roller." He and I went to town. At the drug store he bought me a rubber cap for my head. I saw the druggist take it from the foot of a crutch. At the five-cent store he bought a solid rubber ball for foot-wear and at the hardware store he secured a rubber mallet.

When we got home, Pa cut a notch near the lower end of my body; then made a hole, a half-inch deep in the rubber ball, in which he crowded my foot. The notch acted as a stricture, holding my boot securely. Pa then cut a notch in the bottom of my boot so that it would not slip on the spinous process. He then placed my boot against the corner of a board and struck me over the head with the mallet, saying, "I think that will do the work."

Pa worked out the idea I got from the doctors. I had put a whole lot of what I heard the doctors say in my think-box and studied all of one night what to do. I remembered what our doctor said about the finger-tapping on the face, how it would produce a spasmodic tetanus; the vibrating hammer exciting nerves; nerve-stretching; the movements of extension, flection and circumduction and the operation they were going to perform. From all of these, together with what I had learned of anatomy and what I knew of Ma's injury, I thought that I could, at the worst, make no greater failure than those of our family physician. I saw the doctors examine and locate the cause of Ma's trouble in the last three lumbar vertebrae. I observed that the fourth lumbar was not in line, so I told Pa that, if he would help me, we would try to fix that vertebrae which had been wrenched out of alignment. Pa was a little nervous, but I encouraged him. After dinner, we told Ma that we were going to be her doctors; so she turned her case over to us. Pa laid Ma on her front and examined the five lumbar vertebrae. He found a very tender place on the left side and near the fourth lumbar vertebra. He put my notched foot against the spinous process of the fourth lumbar and raised the mallet to strike me on the head. He hesitated—I felt his hand shake—he was nervous. I encouraged him, telling him to strike quickly and drive the process upward which he did. I felt something move under my foot; Pa said he heard it; poor Ma screamed and thot we had broken her back. Ma took a good breath and said that she was like the boy who had a tooth pulled. He said: "Just as it was killing me it came out." Ma was easy for the first time since she was hurt. The next night Ma slept well without her morphine. In the morning she arose at her usual hour and superintended the morning's work.

After breakfast the two doctors arrived with their grips and surgical instruments. Susie had helped Ma to dress, so, when the doctors arrived, Ma was ready to receive callers. The doctors looked as surprised as Ma did pleased. The facial expressions of each were a study; pleasure, disappointment and astonishment were alternately manifested. Our old doctor said, "Well! Yesterday's operation was a success. I knew it would be." Ma made an explanation and offered the doctors chairs, but they were in a hurry for once.

The doctors left, believing, no doubt, that they had made the cure and ought to have the credit and that Pa was putting up a job on them.

Ma remained well and the Spine-Set cure was reported all over the country, much to the chagrin and mortification of the doctors who, in order to save their reputation, had Pa arrested for practicing medicine and surgery. The judge asked Ma to tell her story. It was a long pitiful one. Everybody just looked at Ma. When she sat down, the doctors were not in sight—they had some urgent cases that needed their attention.

A cut of two Spine Sets and their Drivers may be seen on the next page.

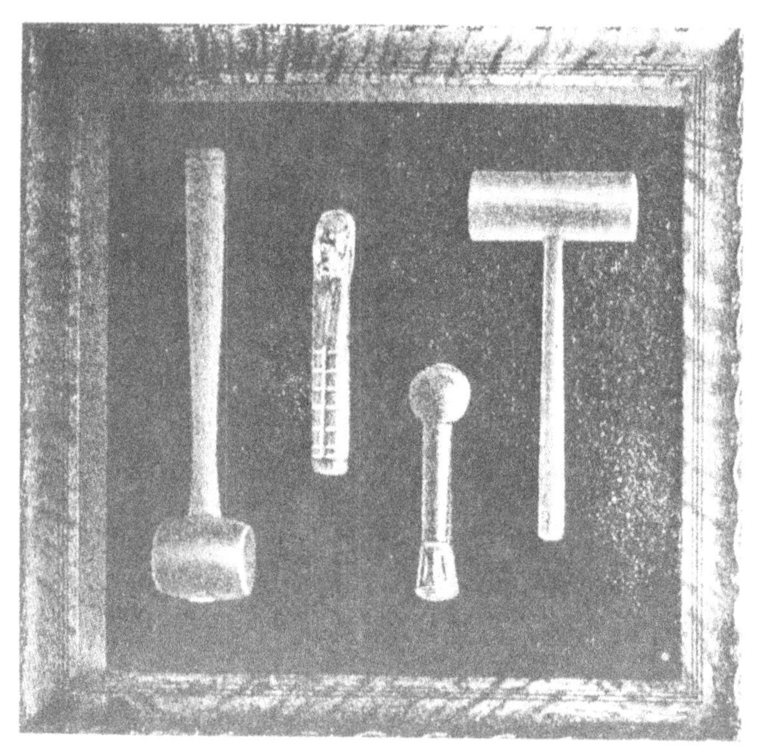

The above spine-sets and their drivers may be seen at The P. S. C. I do not approve of their use, as they do not come within "done by hand."

## INNATE NERVOUS SYSTEM.

"What is commonly known as the Sympathetic Nervous System and the 12 cranial nerves are but branches or portions of the Innate complete nervous system.

"This is a pet theory of mine, because of this peculiar fact in the development of the nervous system—we find that it develops into two systems. The Innate nervous system acts independently and alone, separate and apart, and is not a counterpart of the Educated nervous system; neither is the Educated a counterpart of the other, but while the Innate would be able to perform all its functions without the Educated, yet the Educated could not perform one action at any time without the Innate nervous system. It is because of this fact that we place such an importance upon the Innate direct nervous system—preceding the Educated at all times. If our Innate nervous system did not exist within our tissue cells, we could not live, and Educated could not control at will certain conscious actions. The minds behind those systems are conscious at all times."

Why not state that there are twelve pairs of cranial nerves instead of 12?

"This (the Educated and Innate nervous systems, distinct and separate, run by these two intelligences) is a pet theory of mine."

The writer of these quoted paragraphs, except the explanatory portion included in parenthesis, defines "theory" thus: "A theory is something which has not been proven." Then "what is commonly known as The Sympathetic Nervous System and the 12 cranial nerves are but branches or portions of the Innate complete nervous system," is only "a theory"—a "something which has not been proven."

This "theory," speculative scheme, ought by this time to have become practical and cease being theoretical. Why keep it as a pet; why not make it useful? This dividing the nervous system into two parts, one of which is run by Innate directing the functions of the vital organs, those essential to the life of the body, and the other by Educated, was first written upon by me about six years ago, in the early investigation of the principles which became a part of the science of Chiropractic. It has long since become practical and ceased to be a theory.

---

The late discovery is, that disease is the result of bone pressure on nerves, and that to remove that pressure is to relieve the cause, correct the wrong and bring relief, are statements which form the basis of the science of Chiropractic.

I have an eight-page Chiropractic booklet which will stand some Chiropractic corrections.

Because your "**spine is the casement.**" A casement is a window sash—not a spine. He may have read of the spinal cord being encased by bony segments.

"The **cord** which **carries** your nerve **food.**" The spinal cord does not carry any food of any description.

"The functions of the spine." The bones of which the vertebral column is composed, does not perform any vital phenomena.

"Nerve fluids . . . Vital fluids . . . The ill-fed or starved parts become irritated, much as a baby when hungry, and the cry they set up is the symptom pain. . . . Give a free nerve supply and you strike at the root of the trouble. . . . Give the starved organs their required motor force. . . . Excess of uric acid, which the kidneys have failed to filter out of the blood. This acid irritates the nerve ends and pain is the cry for relief. . . . Nerves give expression or impression of ease or disease. . . . To restore the nerve the cause must be removed. . . . My treatments are based upon an endeavor to aid nature to perform her work without the hindrance. . . . My examinations are made upon the spine and my corrections are mainly made upon it. . . . Specialist in nervous and chronic diseases." Students in The Adjuster class, please correct each sentence and send in your answers.

---

The following paragraph is on a Chiropractor's card. It is the combined effort of four persons who have a "Chiropractic Institute." Their education was received from a physician and a Chiropractor.

"**Chiropractic adjustments** remove the cause of chronic catarrh, asthma, bronchitis and consumption in its early stages, all diseases or troubles of the eye, ear, nose and throat, all stomach and liver troubles, rectal, kidney and bladder troubles, constipation and diarrhea, all forms of chronic sexual weakness and disease, female troubles and weakness, paralysis, headache, nervousness, sleeplessness, insanity, rheumatism; cancers, malignant ulcers and tumors, respond quickly and begin to heal after Chiropractic adjustments."

Why not say: "Chiropractic adjustments remove the cause of catarrh, asthma, bronchitis and consumption in their early stages; all diseases of the eye, ear, nose, throat, stomach, liver, rectum, kidneys and bladder. Constipation, diarrhea, female weakness, paralysis, headache, insomnia, nervousness, insanity, rheumatism, cancers, ulcers and tumors respond readily."

I have cut out 27 words; have said all in one-third less words.

## THE AXES OF VERTEBRAE.

All vertebrae have axes around which they revolve, performing parts of circles, arcs. The superior articular processes of a lumbar vertebra in conjunction with the inferior of the vertebrae above, perform a part of a circle as shown by cut 12, page 483.

Each vertebra has a certain portion of an arc to revolve or move in. Further motion is abnormal. It forces the articular processes out of alignment, creates a displacement and causes the exposed articular processes to infringe upon some spinal nerve.

The facets of the superior articular processes of the lumbar vertebrae are concave; they face inward, slightly upward and backward. Those of the inferior are convex, facing outward, slightly downward and forward. The superior surrounds in part the inferior of the one above, as an axle box does an axle.

The articular movement forms a curve—an arc—a portion of a circle. This deflection increases in size as we proceed down the lumbar vertebrae, the axis of which are posterior to the arcs and bodies, their position depending upon the size of the circles. Lines drawn directly from the two facets will converge until they cross each other. This intersection is the center, the axis of the circle formed by the rotary movement of the two contiguous surfaces.

In the lumbar vertebrae, the axes of the arcs made by their movements are posterior to the articulations, behind the bodies. In the dorsal and cervical region, the axes of the arcs made by their normal, or natural movement, are anterior to the bodies, instead of posterior, as in the lumbar vertebrae.

The axis around which the atlas revolves will be found anterior to the odontoid process; the arc, the portion of the circle or curved line being on the line of the posterior arch.

The facets of the articular processes of the dorsal and cervical vertebrae face in a different direction from those of the lumbar. By placing the same analysis on the dorsal and cervical, as we did on the lumbar vertebrae, we will find their axial centers are anterior to their bodies, whereas, the lumbar vertebrae are posterior. Therefore, the displacements and the racking of them into their natural position, would be to apply the force in an opposite direction. This is based on the fact that vertebrae are racked around their axial centers. All sub-luxations are made around a given center.

The Chiropractor will observe when he uses any one of the three processes as a handle or lever by which to move the vertebra into alignment, that the movement will be around the axial center, the axis of an imaginary cylinder.

Fig. 12 represents a lumbar vertebra showing the circle of the two arcs, also the axial center at the junction of the spinous process and the laminae indicated by a dot near the apex of the spinous process at its junction with the laminae.

The axial center of the atlas, around which it revolves, is anterior to the odontoid process.

The Chiropractor, using the spinous or transverse processes as levers, moves the vertebra around the axial point used as a fulcrum. It will be noticed that the axial centers of the arcs described by the movement of the lumbar vertebrae and atlas, are posterior to the bodies, while those of the cervical and dorsal are anterior, the fulcrum of each being at the axial center. Therefore, while we relieve an impingement in the dorsal and cervical by throwing the lever from the side where the nerve is impinged, we reverse the order of movement in the atlas and lumbar.

If the reader will examine the arthrodial articulations between the axis and the third cervical, thon will find a transitional change in their facial direction, the axial center of which is posterior to the spinal foramen.

The importance of the facts herein set forth will become more apparent as we proceed. The reader will bear in mind that the axial centers of the arcs formed by the lumbar vertebrae are posterior to the spinal foramen.

---

"To have pressure we must have a solid substance entirely surrounding a softer structure or substance—or have the soft structure compressed between two solid substances. There is only one place in the human body where a soft structure is entirely surrounded by a hard one, and that is at the intervertebral foramina, where the nerve may be compressed by the vertebrae becoming subluxated."

In order to cause pressure, it is not necessary that the substance pressed against must be surrounded by the object brought to bear against it; neither is it necessary that the nerve encroached upon must be between two bones. A nerve may be impinged upon, as shown in articles in this Adjuster. The reader will observe that a nerve may be impinged upon without being squeezed, pinched or compressed. An impingement consists of pressure on one side, pressure against; whereas a nerve must be between two substances to be pinched.

It has never been proven that subluxated vertebrae pinch, squeeze or compress nerves as they pass through intervertebral foramina.

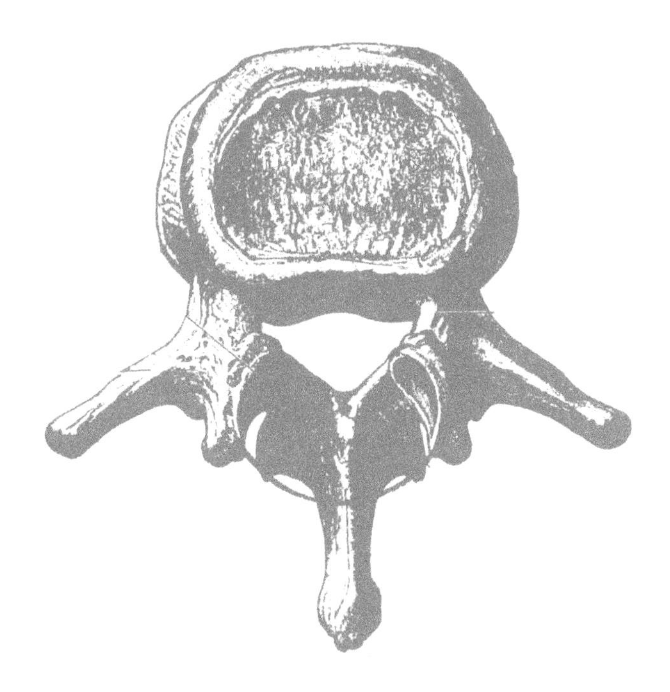

We shall be so kind in the afterwhile,
  But what have we done today?
We shall bring to each lonely life a smile,
  But what have we brought today?
We shall give to truth a grander birth,
  But how much advance today?
We shall feed the hungering souls of earth,
  But what have we done today?

—Nixon Waterman.

---

They say the world is round, and yet
  I often think it square,
So many little hurts we get
  From corners here and there;
But one sad truth in life I've found
  While journeying east and west,
The only folks we really wound
  Are those we love the best.

**Anomalies.**—If all bones were in regular position; if all nerves conformable to the regular rule; if the general growth of the body did not deviate from the specific type; if the four functions performed in a normal manner, our occupation as adjusters would be gone. It is the Chiropractor's business to be acquainted with the normal so that he may recognize irregularities; it is with the latter he has to deal.

If luxated bones retained their natural shape it would simplify the work of the adjuster. Displaced vertebrae gradually assume an abnormal shape, in all their parts, compatible with the position they occupy. To return them to their former position means that they will be required to resume their natural shape; to accomplish this may take the adjuster weeks or months. We occasionally find a vertebra whose spinous process is minus its epiphysis, making an apparent anterior luxation. Spinous processes are often bent to the left or right of the median line, showing an apparent curvature. There are many such anomalies which would be misleading to the adjuster, did he not have proper training. No inconsiderate student can fail to be appreciative and interested when he discovers so many variations revealed by the study of anomalies.

---

"When this controlling intelligence is able to transmit mental impulses to all parts of the body, **free and unobstructed,** we have normal action, which is health. By so doing, normal **transmission of nerve force is restored.**"

Nerves transmit mental impulses to the peripheral nerve endings, but nerves are never obstructed as the above infers. Nerve force is never transmitted over, thru, or by nerves.

Nerve force is the energy expressed by the nervous system in performing any of the functions. Nerve force is the power expended in performing the various acts of the body. The amount of energy or force used in performing any function depends upon the momentum of the impulse by which it performs its action. Vital energy, whether more or less, normal or abnormal, physiological or pathological, is inherent, its manifestation depends upon the force or power of the impulse. The motive power of impulses depend upon the impetus received while passing over the lines of communication. Organic force and muscular force correspond to the dynamic power within each. That which relates to the vital force is known as vital dynamics. The absence of this force is called adynamia. Dynamic diseases are those which arise from organic energy abnormally expressed. Vital activity is known as dynamia. Dynamization is the so-called potenizing of medicines by agitation and comminution.

## WHO DISCOVERED THAT THE BODY IS HEATED BY NERVES DURING HEALTH AND DISEASE?

"It will be of interest to 'The Chiropractor' readers to learn how Dr. D. D. Palmer discovered that the body is heated by nerves, and not by blood.

In the afternoon of July 1, 1903, in suite 15 of the Aiken Block, Santa Barbara, Cal., D. D. Palmer was holding a clinic. The patient was Roy Renwick of that city. There were present as students, H. D. Reynard, Ira H. Lucas, O. G. Smith, Minora C. Paxon, A. B. Wightman and M. A. Collier, in all eight witnesses.

"The patient, A. R. Renwick, had the left hand, arm and shoulder and on up to the spine, intensely hot. Dr. Palmer drew the attention of the class to the excessive heat condition of the portion named, the balance being normal in temperature. He then gave an adjustment in the dorsal region which relieved the pinched nerve on the left side, also the excessive heat of the left upper limb. But he had thrown the vertebra too far. He asked the class, 'Is the body heated by blood or by nerves?' He then left them for two or three minutes. He returned and asked them, 'Is the body heat by blood or by nerves?' The class unanimously answered, 'By nerves.' Thus was this new thought originated."

The above circumstance is substantiated by a letter written that evening to the doctor's son, B. J. Palmer, D. C., also by several following letters, which further explained that the caloric of the body whether normal or in excess, was furnished by calorific nerves. **These letters were placed with other original writings in one of the ten bound volumes in order to prove the autobiography of Chiropractic from its birth. Here are the original writings, which show beyond the shadow of a doubt who originated the principles of Chiropractic. The doctor's son anticipated that some sneak-thief would try to appropriate the credit of originality, and would desire to rob his father of the honor justly due him; thus, his reason for compiling his original writings."**

To more fully substantiate the facts related in the above, a cut of the class is given herewith, on page 487, and the classroom on 489.

Really—what did "this boy" discover in regard to the cause of disease? Who would then have thought that "this boy" would have proved to be a sneak-thief; that he would try to appropriate the credit of originating the principles of this science; that he would even desire to rob his father of the honor justly due him?

Since the writing of the above quoted article, I have advanced the science of Chiropractic. If I were to rewrite the above article, I would make two changes and bring it up to date. Instead of the nerve being **pinched** in the intervertebral foramen, it is **impinged** upon just as it emerges from the intervertebral foramen. As I previously have had occasion to explain, the spinal nerve trunk divides immediately upon leaving the intervertebral foramen into four branches. Two of these are somatic, that is, they go to the framework of the body and its covering and not to the viscera. These are pressed against, impinged upon, by the head of the rib and body of the vertebra being displaced. The ganglia lying close to and upon that joint, is impinged upon by its displacement. See cut on this page.

Instead of there being "calorific nerves," whose duty it is to furnish only heat; it is my present opinion that the same nerve fiber is used to convey impulses of various kinds.

The thought of nerves heating the body was new to B. J., therefore the necessity of writing several letters as stated. It will be seen that I was then, as now, anxious to give him any new ideas on Chiropractic.

The knowledge that the body is heated through the medium of the nerves instead of by the blood has materially assisted the Chiropractor in the explanation of the cause of many diseases.

A later development by me along this line, as announced to the Portland School on April 8, 1909, is that either a lack of, or too much, heat is the cause of each and every disease.

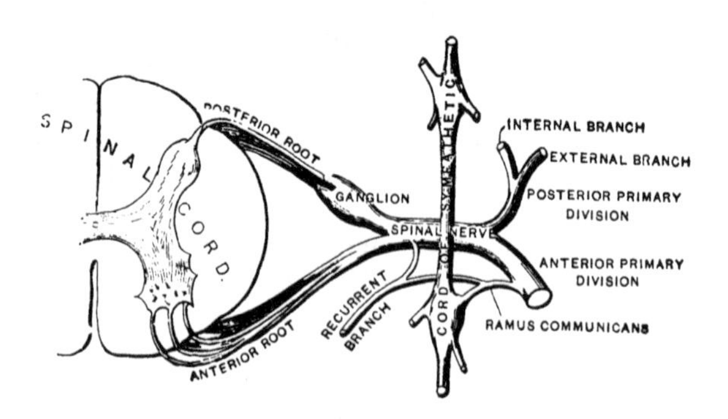

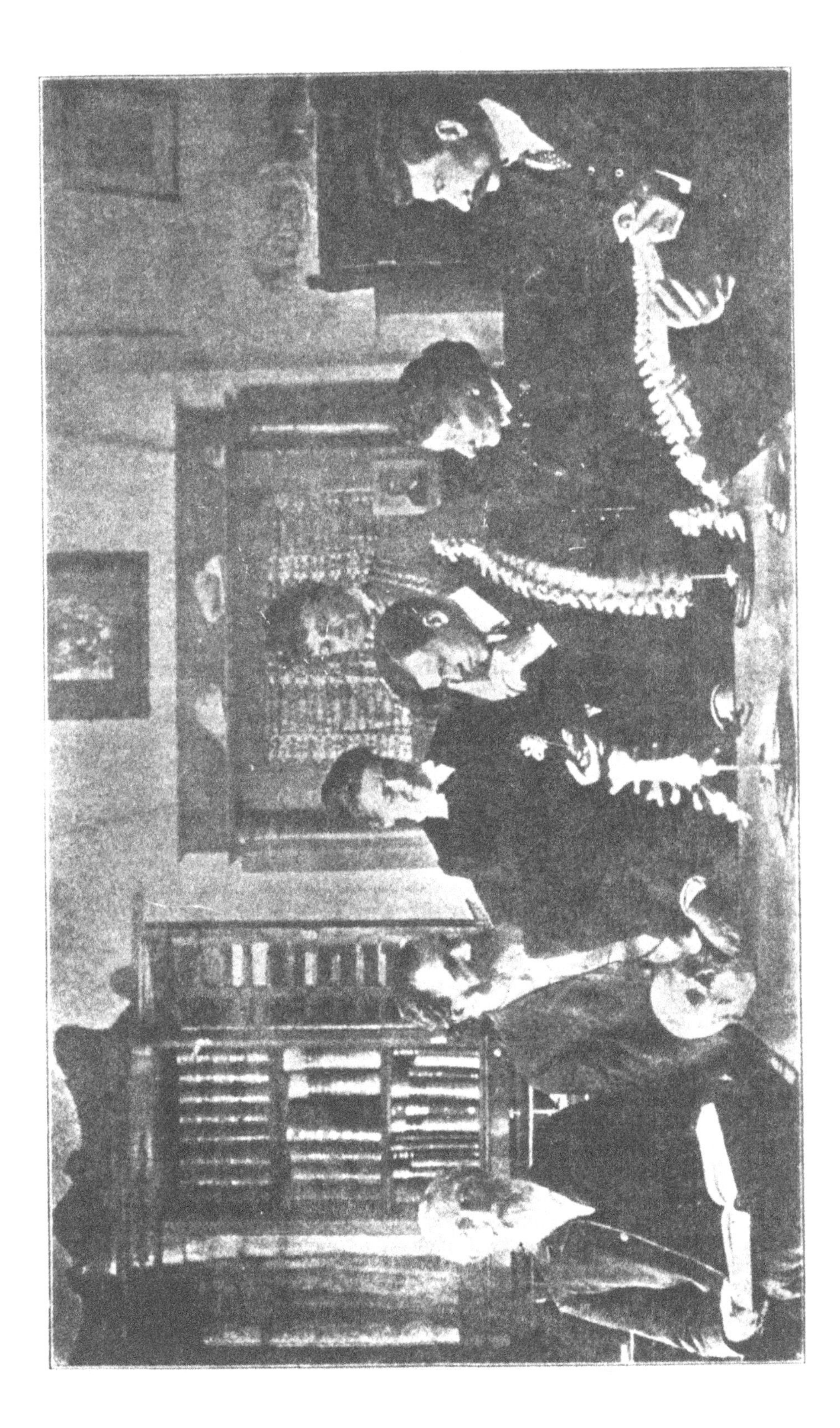

"Helpful for a Chiropractor." The requirements of one who already comprehends the science, and of one who contemplates becoming one, are quite different. To a practitioner of medicine books on Anatomy, Physiology or Symptomatology would be o. k. for reference. But for reading in advance, to prepare one's self for a Chiropractic education, they would be useless; they do not contain anything Chiropractic. Thousands have studied these branches for a lifetime, yet, did not find the principles named Chiropractic. If I had been educated in a medical college, there would not yet have been a Chiropractor. As a rule, we would rather have a clean piece of paper to transcribe our thoughts upon than one which has been used. I would rather take a layman to educate than one who is in ruts. Those who are already practitioners of some system, expect to add Chiropractic onto that which they already have. Therein they will have more trouble trying to add it on than they will in learning Chiropractic. A mind free from a therapeutical education presents a clear field for cultivation.

---

A book of 16 pages says: "Health is the result of functions performed in a normal manner, in the usual amount. All action, either vital or mental, depends upon the nervous system for its expression. When the physical and mental intelligences can so direct innervation along their pathways without obstruction we have health, functions performed in a normal amount. This vital force is what Therapeutics claim as Nature. The Chiropractor recognizes this power as mental impulses sent out by INNATE—BORN WITH.

Bones cause contraction of muscles. Contracted muscles impinge upon nerves by drawing them against bone, intensifying or decreasing the transmission of vital energy, creating too much or not enough functionating, known as disease."

Contrast the above with the following found in a booklet gotten out by O. G. Smith, D. C., and used by many Chiropractors:

"Man is a mill filled with machines and the product of this mill is either health or disease. These various machines, such as the heart, lungs, stomach, liver, spleen, bowels, kidneys, bladder, eyes, ears, arms, legs, feet, hands, fingers and toes are all operated by the same dynamo—the brain. By means of the nervous system, the brain sends the life current to the various machines of the body. When a certain machine in the body is out of order—sick—it is because the life current is either cut off or impaired. Under such conditions the human mill manufactures disease instead of health."

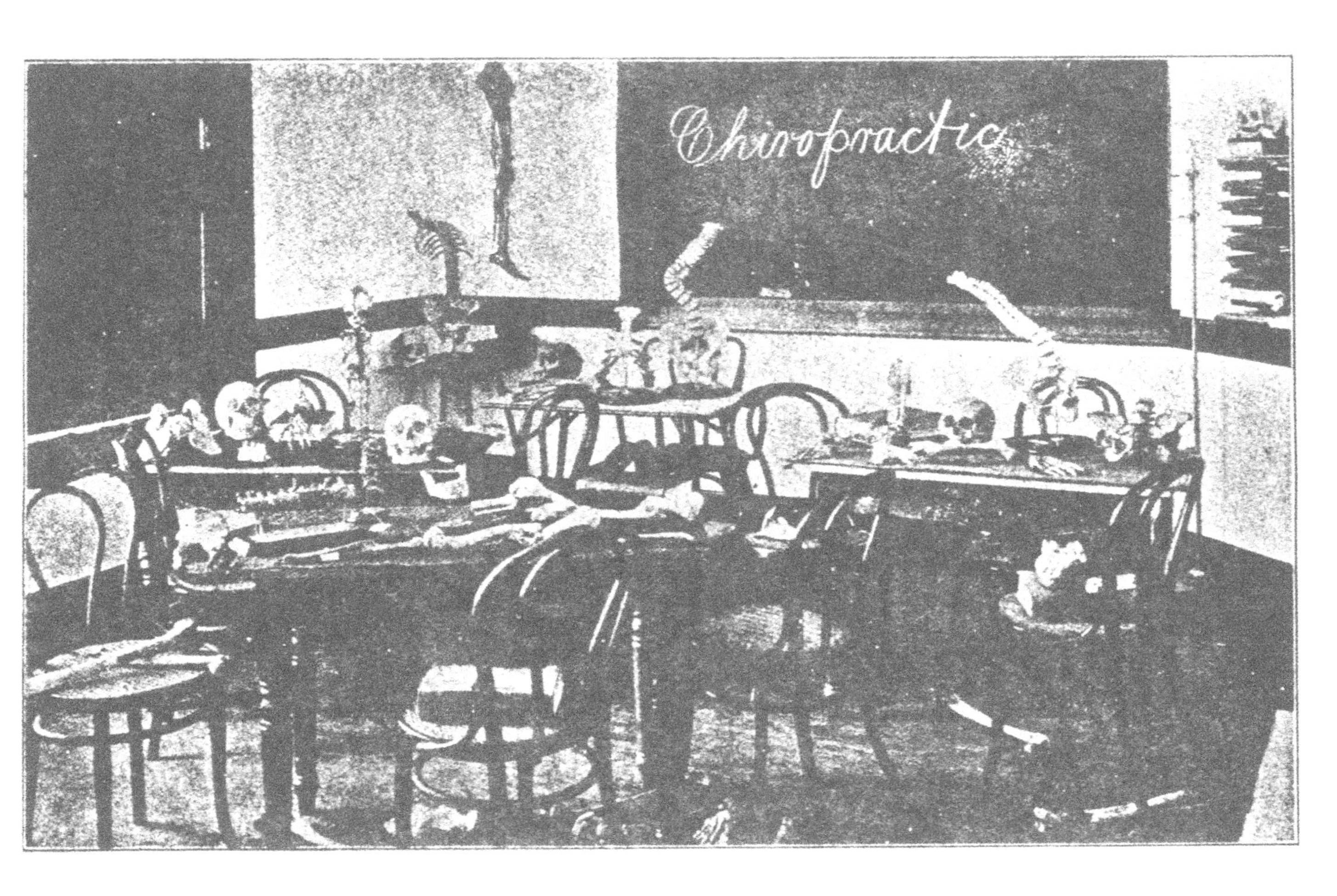
Chiropractic

**Chiropractic Luxation.**—A vertebra is said to be displaced or luxated when the joint surfaces are entirely separated. Sub-luxation is a partial or incomplete separation; one in which the articulating surfaces remain in partial contact. This latter condition is the one so often referred to and known by Chiropractors as sub-luxations.

A vertebra racked from its normal position ever so little, is rotated around its axis, thereby displacing all its parts proportionately. The relationship existing between bones and nerves are so nicely adjusted that any one of the 200 bones, more especially those of the vertebral column, cannot be displaced ever so little without impinging upon adjacent nerves. Pressure on nerves excites, agitates, creates an excess of molecular vibration, whose effects, when local, are known as inflammation, when general, as fever. Nerves are the conveyors of impulses which create functions; an increase of vibration causes an excess of function—local inflammation or fever—symptoms which are common to most diseases. These variations of the vertebral column should be duly noticed by students.

---

**A Chiropractor's Adjusting Room** contains a bifid table, used as a work-bench, on which he replaces displaced joints of the body. By so doing he releases pressure on nerves, so that vital energy may be carried in normal amount. If your building has sagged, so that the doors and windows are impinged upon, do not play the butcher by slicing off the seeming offending portion where it binds. Free the impingement by adjusting the portion of the building which has sagged.

You should not find any electrical apparatus to shock the patient; no vibrators or othopedical stretchers; no Osteopathic tables or instruments of torture; no microscopes to study tissue—just to kill time and put on professional airs; no pestle and mortar to pulverize nauseating drugs; no chemical laboratory to prepare pharmaceutical remedies to treat effects; no anesthetics or opiates to quiet nerves and lull the patient to eternal sleep. No corner cupboard used as an apothecary shop for powders, extracts, elixirs, tinctures, decoctions, salts, pills or ointments made from animal, mineral and vegetable substances; no praying to lord Jupiter to make this prescription efficacious; no individual idiosyncracies which may make a drug dangerous for one and safe for another; no antizymotic disinfectants founded on the morbific illusion of protecting us from evil; no keen-edged scalpel smiling with an insatiable desire to remove some portion of your anatomy; no operating chairs and tables to prepare the patient for the undertaker.

## INNATE.

What is life, disease, death and immortality?

These questions have been propounded by the savants of all ages and have remained unanswered until the advent of Chiropractic. This science and life are coexistant; it now answers the first three questions and in time will lift the veil which obstructs the view of the life beyond.

What is life? How did it create this human organism and continue its entity as a living being? What is this intelligent vital force? We are acquainted with the manifestations of life, disease and death. These are but the environments, the external conditions and influences which affect the human organism and thru it that intelligence which is eternal in its existence.

We possess an inherent craving, a longing aspiration, to know what there is beyond this life: what of the next step in our existence. As the discoverer of the principles of Chiropractic, the developer of its philosophy and the originator of the art of adjusting displaced vertebrae, I do not pretend to comprehend all there is of any one of these four questions, but Chiropractic has swung wide open the door which heretofore has stood ajar, exposing to our view the departments of life, disease and death. In time, the conditions of spiritual existence will be as well known and comprehended as are those of the physical world.

Man is a dual entity, composed of intelligence and matter, spirit and material, the mortal and immortal, the everlasting and the transient. These two entities are linked together by the bond of union—the soul—intelligent life.

The outward manifestations of Educated are patent to all. Its physical life is made evident by the five or more senses. Its functions are manifested in procuring food, raiment and shelter for the physical.

Innate intelligence, known, also, as Nature, intuition, instinct, spirit and sub-conscious mind, has duplicate senses in Educated Intelligence. While the former looks after the material corporal body night and day, as long as the bond of union—the soul—continues to exist, the latter cares for the outward needs; each has its special work to perform.

The physical body originates in the ovum which acquires life from the spermatozoon, and proceeds to form the embryo which by growth forms the fetus.

That which I named Innate (born with) is a segment of that Intelligence which fills the universe. This universal, All Wise, is metamerized, divided into metameres as needed by each individualized being. This somatome of the whole, never sleeps nor tires, recognizes neither darkness nor distance, and is not subject to material laws or conditions. It continues to care for and direct the functions of the body as long as the soul holds body and spirit together.

Innate's existence and consciousness are not dependent upon its body, no more than are we on the house we live in. It is invincible, cannot be injured or destroyed by material changes. It is invulnerable, is not subject to traumatic or toxic injuries, is not subordinate to material substance.

Science and art have need of technical nomenclature. Chiropractic is not an exception. In its development I saw the necessity of a suitable name to designate the intelligence manifested as the conductor of life—that intellect which superintends the vital and vegetative functions. The vital functions are innervation, circulation, transudation and respiration. These are essential to life. The vegetative functions are those relating to assimilation, growth and nutrition.

I observed a change of management of these functions at birth; that the one who took possession with the first breath of life was all-wise, as was the intelligence which had formed the embryo and assisted in the growth of the fetus. Nature was a term designating the world of matter, the creation, the universe, the usual order of events. Instinct referred to an unconscious prompting, an involuntary action without reason or meditation. The expression "subconscious mind" did not suit. Although the intellectual which controls the influence of vital force, is conscious of its acts, it is not sub-conscious, below normal; neither is it a consciousness beneath any other. It does not hold an inferior position or degree; its consciousness is not imperfect or partial; it does not serve under another. Therefore, it is not subordinate in any form or manner. None of the terms used by other investigators expressed the characteristic features I had in mind. Nature takes in the universe, whereas I wanted a term to express individuality. Instinct is an unconscious prompting; the individualized entity I desired to name is always fully conscious and needs no prompting. Intuition is a knowledge without reason; the manager of vital energy uses logical reasoning in conducting the functions at all hours and under all circumstances, as is instanced in the repairing of fractures and injuries. The personality I wished to name and designate correctly, was not an underling, but rather a master, in every sense, regarding the forming of bodily structure and employs its vital force. None of these terms embodied the characteristic qualities which this spiritual entity possessed, as the proprietor of a being possessing life. Each of the above terms had established meanings which did not belong to the spiritual entity I refer to. To express the individualized intelligence which runs all the functions of our bodies during our wakeful and sleeping hours, I chose the name Innate. Innate — born with. And so far I would not change it except to replace it with the name of that individualized entity which really is a part or portion of that All Wise, Almighty, Universal Intelligence, the Great Spirit, the Greek's Theos, the Christian's God, the Hebrew's Helohim, the Mahometan's Allah, Hahneman's Vital Force, new thot's Divine Spark, the Indian's Great Spirit, Hudson's Subconscious Mind, the Christian Scientist's All Goodness, the Allopath's Vis Medicatrix Naturae—the healing power of nature.

Innate becomes associated with the physical when the new being breathes the first breath of life. From this time, it is fully capable of running all the functions which constitute life, the growth, the replacing of worn-out tissue and the repairing of fractures and other injuries.

Innate is not transmitted from the mother to her offspring, but is an individualized portion of the All-Wise, usually known as spirit. Innate controls the movements known as involuntary, altho they are voluntary on the part of Innate. I now refer to metabolism, the circulation of the blood, the transudation of serum and lymph, and all the acts which create life or assist in its maintainance.

While the so-called involuntary movements are under the control of Innate, there are those which are voluntary, subject to the will of another; I allude to the movements of the muscle fibers which are the agents for voluntary movements.

Innate's knowledge is not acquired, is not gained by a life of experience, does not need years of observation. The Innate of each and every individual knows how and in what way to utilize vital force to the best advantage.

Associated with each individual is an intelligence which starts out as a blank, it learns to think and reason, its knowledge is gained by daily contact with its surroundings. This intellect I saw fit to name Educated, because without an education it would be a nonentity, it could not exist, and only does so in proportion as its growth is made by education. These two thinking entities exist in the same body; one is all-wise, knows all there is to be known in regard to the portion of matter it has under its control; the other knows nothing except as it is acquired.

These two intelligences reason from different premises. Innate has been thinking ever since spirit and matter began an existence; Educated commences with life and ends with it.

As I have said, Innate is the master, thè dictator. Innate lived long before the creation of the body it inhabits and will continue to exist as an individualized intelligence long after the soul ceases to be a bond of union between spirit and body. Innate will retain thruout eternity all the information obtained by Educated.

Educated reasons from the general to the particular; Innate from the particular to the general. Educated reasons by deduction; Innate by induction. Educated proceeds in a line of reasoning and deduces a conclusion from a general principle by an admitted instance. Innate, on the other hand, proceeds to reason from collated instances, thru attributes common to all, to a general principle from a general truth, seeking to connect it with some particular case.

Physical science, that which concerns life. actual existence, is learned from philosophical induction.

Innate has observed, with all individuals, that certain effects follow special acts, and, on the ground of analogy, extends what is known to others, thus arriving at a general principle—a law. Vital science is founded upon this law. The time is coming when Educated and Innate will develop an interchange of deductive and inductive reasoning; then, we will receive a true, direct, subjective diagnosis.

These two individualized entities, Innate independent of Educated, the latter dependent upon the former, look after the welfare of the body; one for the inner, the other for the outer well-being. Their wishes and desires should coincide, but on the contrary, from misunderstanding, they are often otherwise.

Educated and Innate assist each other, more or less; at times they are antagonistic—Educated with acquired experience during life, and Innate with experience obtained during a period that is co-extensive with the existence of invertebrates.

Educated may be limited in regard to its capacity to gather experimental knowledge because of some defect. Perhaps on account of a displaced portion of the osseous structure which presses against a sensory nerve causing the information received by Educated, which is transferred to Innate, to be abnormal.

Remember, all sensations or impressions are conducted inward over the sensory nerves; that motor nerves may be interfered with by pressure and the sensory be free and vice versa, or both may be deranged in their carrying capacity. For Innate to make the most of life—to be able to leave this existence and pass to the beyond with a life full of useful experience, a harvest of knowledge gleaned from the fields of observation and experiment, it is necessary that the nerve channels of communication be free to convey the recognition of surrounding conditions and influences by which living forms are modified in their mental and physical growth.

The universe is composed of the invisible and visible, spirit and matter. Life is but the expression of spirit thru matter. To make life manifest requires the union of spirit and body.

In nature we find many forms of physical force, but only one of the spirit. In this article we are interested in that of the spirit. Vital (life) force is spiritual, it cannot be used as mechanical, physical, mental or moral power, it is concerned in the expression of life. Energy may be physical or vital. Vital force runs all bodily functions. Normally expressed in matter it is physiological; more or less than normal is pathological.

To round out a life full of useful experience, it is necessary that Innate should have normal control of all bodily functions, for the intellectual is dependent upon the condition of the physical, but the latter is in no wise dependent upon the former. One might possess a physical, of which any man should be proud, yet have but little of the educated, or vice versa. Innate starts with a complete knowledge of its work, while Educated has a life-time to acquire its education; the length of which and its qualities pertaining thereto being dependent upon the relative position of its tissue. How necessary that we should look to the proper adjusting of the various parts of our physical structure.

All organized living beings are endowed with innervation, nutrition, digestion, motility, sensation, assimilation, absorption, circulation, transudation, diffusion, osmosis, calorification, secretion, excretion, respiration, reproduction and repairment. All of these are under the control of and are managed by Innate. The functions which perform all of these acts may be modified —increased or decreased—by the alterations of tissue. Such modifications need mechanical adjusting. Drugs may stimulate or restrain functions for a time, but they cannot change the position of tissue, or if so, it is accomplished as an antidote, a poison, which draws vertebrae into their axial alignment, as snake-bites. See index. Chemical analysis or combinations are out of the question for they cannot be considered in the realm of living tissue.

At birth there is a transition from the maternal Innate to that of the infant. In the mother the Innate of the infant began as a parasite and continued to prey upon its host until adopted. As a parasite it fastened itself to the walls of the uterus; the intelligence directing it thus is from the spermatozoid of the male; from its host is draws nourishment until it is cared for as her own. As an infant it becomes self-existent. Thon (he or she) no longer depends upon another for the performance of vital functions.

There is a radical change at birth. The functions are modified and substituted by others, which are suitable for its future environments; this exchange is made with the first breath of life. Innate makes this essential alteration as readily as tho it was an ordinary circumstance. From that moment until the close of life, all of the functions are performed in a normal manner, providing the functional channels are not interfered with. Being conversant with these facts, it becomes our duty to care for and keep this structure of bodily tissue in a normal condition.

The education of Innate has been continuous since the existence of the first vertebrate; that of Education during its lifetime. The education of Innate has been natural, cosmical; that of Educated is more or less fictitious, ascititious. Because of this difference in acquiring an education, these two thinking entities often differ greatly.

Innate is a segment of the All-Wise; Educated is an offspring of Innate, a servant for its life-time only. Educated continues with and lasts as long as life exists; Innate is eternal, always was and always will be.

Functions performed either in excess or insufficiently are pathological. Pathologically considered, drugs are disease producers. They increase or decrease the action of functions, and by abnormal muscular tension draw vertebrae in or out of alignment. They are given for the purpose of increasing or decreasing nerve vibration. If they do not excite or allay nerve action, they are considered useless. Innate desires to run functions normally both in manner and amount. Educated has been taught that inflammation and fever create physiological phenomena; that they serve a physiological purpose; that they are reactionary and reparative. On this mode of reasoning it is supposed that the escape of pus, edematous swellings, granulated tissue, and abscesses are phagocytic reactions on the part of the organism to free itself from irritants—a struggle between the phagocytes and the irritating agent; that the disturbances of hyperemia, characterized by pain, heat, swelling, discoloration and disordered functions are reactionary and beneficial. Yet it is known that crotin oil, calomel and turpentine will cause suppuration. These drugs, when externally applied, are rubefacients, produce redness of the skin—a division of the red and white corpuscles—leaving the red and expelling the white in the substance known as pus. Hyperthermia increases the red corpuscles and diminishes the white. Normal temperature produces an equilibrium of corpuscles each kind in normal proportion.

Thus, Innate would run functions physiologically, while Educated with a perverted mind would make them pathological.

In mythology, Somnus was the god of sleep, the son of Night, a twin brother of Death. Innate never sleeps, but makes favorable conditions for periodical rests for Educated. As far as possible all sense irritation is removed; the circulation of the cerebrum is lessened, a portion of the blood-stream is shunted to the skin and abdominal viscera, thereby lessening the physiological functioning of the upper and front portion of the brain. The eyelids are closed; the eyeball turned upward so that the pupil is under the upper lid; the aperture for the rays of light is diminished in size; the ear is protected against the reception of sounds by increased tension of the tympanic membrane; the mucous membranes of the nose and mouth are dryer, because of diminished secretion; thereby lessening their sensibility to odors and soluble bodies. The skin is made less sensitive to pressure; the pulse is slower; respiratory movements are fewer; the voluntary muscles are relaxed and the psychic activities are wholly at rest. These conditions give Educated an opportunity for repose, during which potential nerve energy may be recuperated. As the period of sleep termination approaches, the mental conditions return and the waking state is reestablished. During sleep the cerebral hemispheres are at rest, also the functions dependent thereon. The deeper the sleep, the less there will be of psychic activity and voluntary movements.

The cerebral hemispheres are the seat of all psychic activities. Thru them energy is transmitted for volition, sensation and thot. Microcephalic and hyprocephalic heads are deficient in voluntary functions—physiologic actions are decreased in force and volume.

Many theories have been presented to account for the cause of sleep—Chiropractors add one more—the all-wise provision of Innate for the recuperation of the physical; this includes the psychic, the soul, the living vital principle, the bond of union between spirit and body.

Dreams are involuntary combinations of confused ideas which present themselves to the mind during the period of sleep. A dream that would take hours for its real production, is completed in an incredible short space of time. For example; a railroad engineer told me that on one occasion when he was very much in need of sleep, as he passed the signal post, he blew the whistle for the crossing. He fell into a deep sleep and dreamed of being in a wreck, which would have taken an hour for its accomplishment. He awaked with the dream vividly on his mind and realizing the time taken for the wreck, thot he had passed the station which was miles ahead, but, to his surprise, he had not arrived at the crossing for which he had just blown the whistle. Dreams arise because of somnolence or renewed activity.

The Innate of the mother forms the embryo and develops the fetus.

Do not forget for one moment that every physical function of the body is managed by Innate thru the nervous system. Even nerve-sheaths and the walls of blood-vessels are covered by a complete net-work of nerves to facilitate the transportation of sensation, motion, transudation and circulation.

Some of my readers will observe that I am rewriting an article I wrote several years ago, which can be found in The Science of Chiropractic. I did not sanction its publication, as I then said, I did not know enough of Chiropractic to write such a book on the science, philosophy and art of Chiropractic as the subject demanded.

Every neuron—one of the countless number of units of which the nervous system is composed—is a separate and distinct entity. Those of mobility carry impulses outward; the sensory transport sensations inward.

Every vertebrate animal, at the beginning of its existence, is represented by an ovum or cell. After fertilization the ovum is carried into the uterus by the action of the cilia which line the fallopian tube. Upon arriving in the cavity of the womb, it becomes attached, as a parasite, to the mucous membrane. The villi penetrate deeply into the uterine mucosa like roots in a loose soil. These vascular tufts are hair-like projections on the surface of the ovum whose function is to absorb nutriment for the embryo from its host.

The portion to which it is attached develops into the placenta; thru this channel nutriment is supplied to the fetus by osmosis. The walls of the blood-vessels and nerve-sheaths are encircled with a network of nerve-fibers. Landois says that nerves are traced to within one to four inches of the naval. There is no doubt in my mind that by means of this bond of union the functions of the embryo and fetus are directed thru the nervous system of the mother by the intelligence I have seen fit to name Innate.

Innate is the body-builder before, as well as after, birth. Heretofore it has been supposed that the mother impressed her thots upon the fetus, but the facts are Educated directed Innate.

At birth there is an exchange in the management of the physical provisions; the fetus is severed from the mother; Innate, the metamere of Universal Intelligence, is segmented. Individualized spirit and a somite of matter form a new being. These are linked together by the soul, a living entity. Educated Intelligence looks after its environment in proportion to its development.

Osteological specimens have afforded me much pleasure and edification along this line of thot. While I am writing this article, a specimen of Innate's work is received from Gustavus Noque. Its extreme measurements are one inch by one and five-eighths. It is the osseous mending of the right 6th and 7th costo-cartilages, in the form of two united furls of bone. The circumference of the larger of the two is two and a half inches, that of the smaller is one and a half inches. The history, as read from the specimen before me, is that the owner received a costo-cartilage fracture. As cartilage has no internal nerves or blood-vessels for the distribution, reception and retention of cartilage or bone-forming corpuscles, the best that Innate, the intellectual which superintends the physicial functions during our sleeping and waking hours, could do, was to deposit osseous matter between and around the fractured ends of bone and cartilage, similar to the way in which a blacksmith would mend a wagon tongue which had received a transverse fracture. The intervening spaces between the ribs and cartilages were filled with callus. To produce this material a slight elevation of temperature was necessary; later a subnormal degree of heat hardened it. The function involved and the changes of temperature were physiological. The fracture and its mending were not pathological, were not departures from a state of health. This repairing of fractures was done by Innate without the knowledge of Educated, the man whom we knew as John Doe.

A description of a few of the many specimens I have picked up, I am sure will be appreciated. The study of them has done much toward my understanding of the workings of Innate. The intelligence manifested in the following specimens is truly wonderful.

It is interesting to notice the many displacements of osseous tissue, the resultant pathological conditions and the modifications resorted to by Innate to meet the exigencies which have arisen. Innate was not able to replace the displacements or prevent the diseased conditions resulting therefrom and had to adopt measures for self-protection.

A calvarium (the upper part of the skull), the inner table of which displays, when held before the light, two beautiful pictures, one on either side, of forest fires, as perfect as tho painted by an artist. The fire and smoke are of natural color. All bones in the recent state, when subjected to a high degree of temperature, are reddened, owing to an excess of the red corpuscles. The vimineous, arborescent interlacings are also pathological, produced by disease, not Innate.

The 4th and 5th ribs of the right side, a cut of which is shown on the next page, have eight healed fractures. The fifth has a comminuted fracture healed at an angle. Innate repaired these fractures, doing good work with all of them except the one in the center of the fifth rib. These fragments were not in proper position. Innate is not a surgeon; therefore, did not replace the displaced fragments. Educated should have done that part of the work. Innate did the best it could with the conditions imposed upon it. It filled the vacant space with osseous callus, but the fragments not being in proper position, the osteoanapleurosis was not perfect. The symphysis is not compact and is liable to refracture. To strengthen this weak place, Innate built a process from each rib toward and touching the other. The articulating surfaces were covered with hyaline cartilage, making a movable brace, similar to that which a carpenter would place to strengthen an unsound place in a joist, except that the ribs were capable of individual movement. The man, whom we knew as John Smith, knew nothing of this brace and had nothing to do with its building. This unusual joint showed architectural reasoning, judgment and skill in the means used to accomplish a certain purpose.

One set of ribs, which had received several costo-cartilaginous fractures, had osseous pegs which projected from the center of the elongated oval pits from which the cartilages had been loosened, and extended into the cartilages, thereby making a support such as is often used in the uniting of two pieces of wood.

The odontoid process articulates with the atlas on the anterior and the transverse ligaments on the posterior. Occasionally we find one whose apex articulates with the basilar process of the occipital bone, if so, it is provided with the ordinary requirements of an articulated process. Occasionally the processus dentatus is elongated for a purpose, with an aim in view. An axis shows two articular surfaces on the anterior of the odontoid, the lower facet was used in the earlier years of life and the upper in later years. An accident had displaced the atlas upward necessitating a new facet and the elongating of the odontoid to prevent the anterior arch of the atlas slipping upward, over backward and against the spinal cord, endangering life. These changes show judgment and skill on the part of Innate. The Educated knew nothing of this internal work. A Chiropractor would have replaced the atlas in its normal position.

Innate displays much and varied intelligence in the building of osseous abutments and piers in the spinal canal to prevent further displacement of luxated vertebrae, one of which is as nice a dovetail as any cabinet maker could have made.

Rachitic bones may present pathological and physiological variations. When the tibia and fibula are softened by excessive heat, muscular contraction and superincumbent weight increases the posterior concavity of the femoral shaft. Associated with these pathological conditions, we may find platycnemia, an increased breadth, and the linea aspera prominent. These physiological exaggerations of structure presents a pilastered appearance. In healed, incomplete, fractures of the femur, we may find the linea aspera built out in a pier to compensate for the extreme curve and the weakness created therefrom.

To say that this displayed intelligence made manifest by Innate is nothing but nature, instinct or intuitive force, does not meet my comprehension.

Monstrosities present a boundless field for observation and research. To designate those which are pathological, the result of deranged functions and those which are physiological, the product of Innate Intelligence, is instructive and worthy of our attention.

A part or all of the skeletal frame may become softened by hyperthermia, a portion of the bone substance oozing out of the vertebrae and remaining free, or depositing on the bone surface. During the second stage, the temperature becomes subnormal and eburnation, hardening, consolidation sets in.

Occasionally, when long bones are fractured, the fragments fail to unite because the callus material is not supplied. Many experiments are tried, but Innate fails to supply the osseous matter. The same accident which caused the fracture also displaced a vertebra. This displaced bone impinged upon the nerves which superintend the nutrient supply in the region of the fracture, thereby preventing the appropriation and use of needed callus. In such cases the vertebral pressure should be removed by replacing the displaced vertebra.

Innate is not a surgeon, does not reset displaced or fractured bones. It, however, builds osseous abutments and piers for self-protection, removes useless exostoses and temporary callus when no longer needed.

Hypnotism places the mind of Educated, that which understands and reasons, possesses consciousness, feels, perceives, wills and thinks—the sentient subject of all feeling pertaining to the material world, that of the physical—not of the spiritual or innerself—into a condition of sleep, or that of rest, and controls the spiritual mind, a condition known as sleep, by suggestion. All cures made by Christian Scientists, mental or mind healers, magnetics, suggestive therapeutists, metaphysicians, or charms, are made by Educated controlling the mind of Innate. The same condition is produced by auto-suggestion, self-hypnotism, in which expectant belief tends to cause harmony of disturbance of functions.

If you would comprehend physiological and pathological conditions, study the workings of Innate. The fads of vivisection, microbes, bacteria and the old blood delusion, do not explain any one of the four questions at the head of this article.

Innate Intelligence knows much more of functions than the medical world will ever know.

Dreams are of the Innate mind, more or less mixed with the memories of Educated which produce mental teratogeny.

All parts of the human frame which support and hold the nervous system in position should be properly situated; likewise, should the nerves which superintend all functions. Instead of removing diseased organs, would it not be better to replace any displaced bones which press against, impinge upon the nerve-fibers which conduct the nervous impulses?

---

Chiropractic is a philosophical science; it has solved one of the most profound and perplexing problems of the age, namely, what is life?

---

"(In other words the path of the nerve is 2-feet long. To try to cut in on the wire at the center of the nerve does not influence the periphery.)"

Some one has his wires crossed. He has the three nervous system on one line. He has a short circuit; a "direct" short-cut from brain to terminal cell and a "reflex" back to brain. This of itself is sufficient to give his readers a shock. His central fails to keep in touch with truth and veracity.

He has lost sight of two stations—the cranial and sympathetic. It is time for repairs. The Chiropractor's Adjuster calls attention to the luxations which disturb his equilibrium. It will aim to adjust and repair all luxations made by aberrated brain cells, and add resilence to his idea-producer.

## SPECIAL ANNOUNCEMENT.

I am pleased to inform the general public as well as our patrons past and present, that after a year and a half sojourning in Southern California, **where my father went for the purpose of curing Dr. T. H. Storey, of Duluth, Minn.**, of insanity, which cure was accomplished by one Chiropractic adjustment, **that we now have the pleasure of his** permanent **presence** in the **same offices in which he discovered the new adjustment cure** which he was pleased to call Chiropractic.

Dr. D. D. Palmer occupies the enviable position of being the president of The Palmer School of Chiropractic. Today we are pleased to state that he is president of a well organized Chiropractic School. He is not only president of this school but **also the discoverer and developer of the Chiropractic Science** that **he has unfathomed far beyond his expectations.**

He was born of humble parentage, reared in an atmosphere of independence and self reliance, never fearing to think or delve where others dared to tread. **Within him were combined the rare qualities of genius and hard work;** true, there were other men similarly gifted but **none possessed that peculiar quality that was needed to originate and develop** such a radically new system as this. A similar equal may be cited when we refer to Edison, for, as we all know, he has the peculiar qualities necessary to develop the Scienec of Electricity.

Becoming aware of the great importance of this new Chiropractic Science, his attention was turned to the problem of **how best to teach students** so that **they, too,** could do the same quality of work of curing the sick that .he was doing. Naturally the only solution was **genius, time and hard work.** Setting about his task with no thought but that of success, **this school has as a result of eighteen years of labor, a superior knowledge of Chiropractic, and is thus taught in this school.**

It is true that **no one can possess the same depth of thought** of a new idea, a new discovery, or a new system of healing **as the person who discovered and developed it. No one can possess the same peculiar ability to impart that knowledge** of Chiropractic, unadulterated, **as the man who is able to evolve and unfold Chiropractic from the depths of superstition.**

Dr. D. D. Palmer has personal charge of the classes in Anomalies, Chiropractic Orthopedy and Principles of Chiropractic. These branches are his special pride, his students getting the benefit of new ideas which are demonstrated by one or more Osteological Specimens; then the practical result of that idea is demonstrated on the living body in the clinic. **Those who know the value of getting their knowledge** of Chiropractic **first**

**handed, will appreciate what it means to study these branches under the founder and originator** of this drugless system of healing.

For instance, the study of anatomy is dry and uninteresting in the Medical Schools, but students of anatomy as taught in The Palmer School of Chiropractic are often heard to say, "It is very fascinating, the more we study the more interesting it becomes."

Too much cannot be said in regard to the benefits to be derived by students who have access to this Osteological Studio. **So much depends upon the fundamental principles being thoroughly demonstrated,** in this phase of the work, **that Dr. Palmer, Sr., has full charge of this class-room** and its magnificent collection, at the number and quality of whose pieces which every visiting physician or student in anatomy is surprised. No student can fail to be interested in the study of anatomy when it is so definitely explained by this immense, practical, illustrative collection.

B. J. PALMER, D. C.

---

Many a rich man, in bringing up his son, makes what Aaron made—a golden calf.

---

Heat is the essential agent of life. It is a kinetic force. Animated creation is dependent upon it for its origin, development and the invigorating influence by which functions continue our existence. It is created by a dynamic movement of atoms—molecular vibration.

The nervous system is intimately associated with the production, distribution and regulation of animal heat. By this function, the body in health is kept at the uniform temperature.

The heat of the body may be increased by electricity, poisons and bone pressure on nerves. Mechanical action excites; electricity stimulates; poisons increase or decrease molecular motion; impingement increases heat, rigidity and intensifies vibration. Normal nerve vibration is about 200 a minute; that of fever is often as high as 400. Extreme rapid vibration produces necrosis, softening of tissue. Excessive heat causes nerves to become enlarged, swollen, intense, rigid and very sensitive to the touch.

Neuralgia and rheumatism, in fact, every ache and pain are because of an excess of heat which expands the nerves and draws them tightly, lengthwise. The transmission of impulses is dependent upon vibration. The activity of functions is increased or decreased in proportion to the ratio of molecular vibration.

## THE CAUSE OF DISEASE.

The Chiropractor, on its first page, defines the cause of disease as follows: "Diseases are caused by a **lack of current of Innate Mental Impulse.** This is produced by a constricting force placed around nerves through accidents — vertebral subluxations. These displacements are **caused** by a concussion of forces, the external meeting the resistance of the internal, induced by traumatism."

The above is a sample of the 99 per cent of Chiropractic as developed at the P. S. C.

If a **lack** of Innate impulse is the cause of disease, then functionating would always be below normal in all ailments. The developer of Chiropractic has always maintained that disease is the result of too much or too little functional activity. He has always stated that "Disease is a condition caused by nerves being excited or depressed, deranging their functions." He finds that much the larger share of diseases consists of functions performed in too great a degree; instead of there being a **lack** of impulse, there is **too much vital activity.**

"Mental impulse." Mental pertains to the mind—the intellectual—the mental faculties. The intellectual functions do not run the vital functions. This first sentence should read "Diseases are caused by either an excessive or insufficient momentum or force of Innate's impulses." Vital functions are those essential to life. Animal functions belong to the encephalon; they are functions of the intellect—the mind. Mental impulses belong to the mind.

"This (lack of current) is produced by a **constricting** force placed **around** nerves through accidents—vertebral subluxations." Subluxated vertebrae—displacement of two bones—can only press against a nerve on two sides. In order to **constrict** a nerve, an organ or orifice, it must have something **pliable drawn around it.** A sphincter muscle, for example, surrounds a natural opening. By its constricting force (not a pressure on one or two sides) it closes the passage. Two bones closing together do not surround, encircle, draw tightly about, or cause a stricture.

"Displacements are caused by concussion." A concussion is **the effect** of two bodies striking against each other; the result of a collision. The consequence produced by a concussion is never a displacement, but a condition of agitation, a shaking or a shock.

What is that you say? Vertebral subluxations are displaced by traumatism? Traumatology is the science of wounds. Traumatism is a condition due to a wound. Displacements of vertebrae are not caused by concussions or traumatism. Traumatism is the **systemic condition following trauma.** Displacements may be traumatic—caused by a wound or injury.

The author of the above definition of the cause of disease either does not understand the fundamental principle of Chiropractic or he is unable to express himself intelligently.

It is no wonder that intellectual students of the P. S. C. are kicking. "This is not Chiropractic you are giving us. I came here to learn Chiropractic. I go home."

---

The first number of The Chiropractor, Dec., 1904, has on its first page a reminder which reads thus: "Historical: Chiropractic was discovered by D. D. Palmer, of Davenport, Iowa, in September, 1895. From that time he has **developed it into a well defined science** that has no resemblance whatever to any therapeutical method.

"All acts or movements of any or all parts of the body (including the circulation of the fluids), whether normal, in excess, or deficient, are due to the functional activity of nerves.

"Every act and thought is controlled by Innate and Educated nerves; they are the life of the body."

---

The following is copied from the August number of The Chiropractor of 1905, which in part reads: "Daniel David Palmer, Discoverer and Developer of the Principles of Chiropractic. A man of great personality and individuality. He is one of the few great thinkers, has the determination to advance a line of thought, continues to develop it, independent enough to make it recognized as a science." This was written four years ago and is in contrast to some statements made by the same author more recently. The same accusations can be made against Uncle Howard. The latter says that "Dr. D. D. Palmer by chance stumbled onto the basic principles of Chiropractic." Uncle Howard, there are hundreds who stumbled over the basic principles of Chiropractic and did not know enough to pick them up. But there chanced to be "one of the few great thinkers" who "advanced this line of thought" out of these basic principles which he stumbled on, stopped to pick them up, straightway reduced them to law and embodied them into a system and built thereon a "recognized science."

Although advanced in years and somewhat broken in spirit by acts of traitors, I have the same personality and individuality, and am still able to advance the Chiropractic line of thought, and develop the child of my genius, the science of Chiropractic.

## INNATE

Imagine, if you can, the feelings of the author of "Innate" when he read the following:

"The P. S. C. explains that Innate is in each being, next to which is the brain, this makes impulse, which passes through nerves and makes **mechanical** action, this movement is function. This stage is where man, with function, substance, or electricity, that is conveyed through pipes or wires makes action of machinery; it expresses the purpose of the machine. You have reached at fundamental, the basis of everything. From that can be elaborated all that Man's function has or may create. It is giving to man a unity that never existed before the advent of Chiropractic. No man ever linked the brain with the physical through a direct nerve system and gave to the brain the power of transforming or converting; of giving God the opportunity to express its quantities through man in that form of manner. It is not my purpose to express any opinion as regards religion, but we must take Life, step by step and show its bases, as it is. No matter what opinions each may have, it must have one basic truth. The alimentary canal, **alone**, is but a set of dead organs, but when analyzed through each successive step, and given an Innate, we have the physical canal philosophically complete."

When the writer of the above quoted paragraph had written two-thirds, he forgot that The P. S. C. was making an explanation of Innate and says, "it is not **my** purpose to express any opinion regarding religion," and yet, in the previous sentence he surpasses any potentate or clergyman on earth by "giving God the opportunity to express its quantities through man in that form of manner." We should unite the two (material and immaterial, as one, and we will do this in our study of theosophy as a foundation stone, the unity of earth (a concrete **thing**) with heaven (an abstract **thing)** which is accomplished by a third **thing**—God." "God being an intellectual thing." This kind of irreligious expression shows that he is no more fitted for a preacher of theology than for an educator of Chiropractic. The man who wrote the above quoted paragraph was not able to make an intelligent explanation of Innate, therefore started out to use The P. S. C. as a cat's paw.

This is the man of whom J. M. Loban says: "And I say to you that the world, when this man dies, will sustain a loss like unto the destruction of a nation—a loss which cannot be estimated. So here's to the real Force in the Chiropractic world—the underlying Source from which every Chiropractor, consciously or unconsciously, gets the best that he has—B. J. Palmer, D. C., Ph. C." This is the man who "linked the brain with the physical, through a direct nerve system." You might just as well make a direct, short cut from the stomach to the anus, by cutting out the small intestines, "including the duodenum, jejunum, ileum, Meckel's diverticulum and mesentery, cecum, colon, appendix and rectum, and make one straight intestine do the whole business, thereby saving about twenty feet of useless canal. Yes, it was he who made the "direct" short cut. It was (in his mind) quite an improvement upon man—cutting out the cranial nerves, and the entire sympathetic nervous system. Why not do as much for the digestive system as he has for the nervous system. He simplified the nervous system by reducing all to one brain system, branching from the spinal cord." Why not disencumber the human family from so much useless imaginary entrails by reducing the alimentary canal? Why will not one foot do as well as twenty? He has cut out the trunks, roots and rootlets of nerves by starting the branches direct from the spinal cord. Why not do as much for the digestive tube? He is the originator, discoverer and developer of this "direct nerve system." By these short cuts, the student is able to make comparatively the same short cut in time and labor. He will not now have to tax his ingenuity as to how the cranial and sympathetic are connected; for he has a direct route never dreamed of by former anatomists.

After filling 155 pages with such "jargonity," he appeals on the last page to the reader as follows: "The character of the science but expresses its creators. And if, after concentrated study you are pleased we shall be glad to hear from you or, if you desire to investigate further, remember it is our mutual interest to allow me to convert your interest to a practical possession of your own." This is the man who writes volumes of unintelligible "jargonity."

---

The January number of Vim contains four cuts of vertebra, copied from a Chiropractor's booklet. These are used to explain why vertebrae become luxated. The writer thinks that sitting cross-legged, resting the weight of the body on one limb, carrying heavy loads on one side, etc., cause the vertebrae to become displaced. "The parts affected by branches of the cut-off nerve," are reasons given why nerves are "pinched" and "squeezed." The writer concludes his three-page article by telling patients who have vertebral displacements how to replace them.

"The ill effects of these habits can be overcome by constant and determined efforts to shift the labor of the overworked limbs to the other limbs that have been neglected. Walk erect, and at all times, sitting, standing or walking, hold the body in a correct position, and, in time, with exercise and hygienic living the ill effects will be counteracted."

## NERVE PROPERTIES.

Nerves are capable of becoming tense or slack, firm or flaccid, expanded or narrowed, irritated or soothed, excited or repressed, lengthened or contracted, stretched or shrunken, degenerated or regenerated.

As I have said, in another article, nerves are composed of one or more nerve-fibers. The axis-cylinders of one or more of these filaments may become degenerated by pressure (injury) or poisons. They may be affected in part or in whole. Their medullary sheaths may become broken into segments and disintegrated. Their axis cylinders may undergo dissolution. Changes of a degenerative character occur as a result of poisons, which may be associated with such diseases as tetanus, diphtheria, septicemia, measles, smallpox and typhoid fever. The effects of poison on these neurones differ according to the rapidity of their action—depending upon the length of time over which it extends. As I have said, elsewhere, the same poison or injury does not affect the nerve-fibers in all persons in the same manner. This degenerative condition is one of necrosis, a softening of nerve-tissue, because of hyperthemia. The Chiropractor who knows the nature of nerves and their paths of distribution, is able to locate the vertebra on which those nerves and muscles are made to act abnormally. By replacing the displaced bone, even in an acute case of poisoning, he is able to prevent further abnormal functionating. Functions are performed normally when nerves are not interfered with by pressure, and abnormally when they are drawn out of alignment. Degeneration is pathological, regeneration is physiological. These two conditions may be simultaneously active in either neurotic or osseous tissue, or in peurones. Degeneration, of necessity, must precede regeneration. In chromatosis the degenerative process usually reaches its maximum in about three weeks—the length of time for self-limited diseases to terminate either in recovery or death. When the heat becomes sufficiently intense to necrose the nerve tissue, the degenerative process reaches its maximum, tonicity is lessened, the fever subsides, and the regenerative processes begin. These may progress rapidly or so slowly that it may take months to complete them. Or the necrosed neurotic tissue may never be fully regenerated without replacing the vertebrae and relieving the nerve impingements. Osseous tissue undergoes as perfect regeneration as any tissue of the body thru calcification and ossification of an embryonal tissue known as callus. Nerve degeneration is always accompanied by inflammation. Disease consists of modified functions and tissue. Inflammation of nerves is known as neuritis. An inflamed nerve will be found red and swollen and, perhaps, infiltrated with serum and pus.

The ability of nerves to conduct impulses and sensations depends upon their quality, and this is modified by heat. Efferent nerves contract muscles, supply energy for gland secretion, gauge the capacity of blood vessels; in fact, control every movement of the body. The power of afferent nerves to convey sensation is determined by their condition. For the proper performance of conducting impulses and sensations, they require a certain degree of tonicity, normal tension, and this depends upon a normal amount of heat. The variations of caloric modifies the quality of nerves.

**Nerves have but two functions—conveying impulses outward and sensations inward.** Their conductivity is said to be physiological when motor impulses and sensations are normal; pathological when abnormal.

A great amount of experimental work has been done by chemists and physiologists with a view to discover the why and the how of heat-regulation. This accomplished, the causation of fever—the distinctive characteristic of the larger share of diseases—would be explained and physiological and pathological metabolism would be understood. This is just what, by the discovery and development of Chiropractic, I have done.

Heat regulation is the most important problem which physiologists have to study. When it exists in a normal degree we have health; when there is too much or not enough, we have disease. The body—somewhere and somehow—possesses the ability to control the production of heat and to offset its loss. Exposed to zero temperature, there is of necessity a greater production. When the surrounding atmosphere is above the normal temperature of man, there is an all-wise provision to prevent its absorption. Perspiration is increased, preventing hyperthermia.

The production of heat is a nerve-function—functional activity of nerves, as well as that of muscles, requires nutritive support in the form of food. Involuntary heat production calls for involuntary muscular metabolism.

All functions, including that very essential one of heat, are under the control of Innate Intelligence. If all parts of the body are in normal position and the nerves free from impingement, all functions, including the production of heat, will be performed in a normal manner.

Chiropractors are able (so far as they know how) to regulate the heat of the body. They can create fever by luxating vertebrae, or decrease it by adjusting displaced bones.

Is not heat-modification concomitant with all pathological conditions?

## THE LIVER.

The liver is the largest gland in the body. It is from ten to twelve inches transversely, from front to back six to seven, and three inches thick. It weighs in the adult, in its normal condition, from three to four pounds.

A gland is an organ which secretes an essential specific fluid or excretes waste material. The largest glands are the liver, pancreas, spleen, testicles and kidneys. Some glands have excretory ducts, also reservoirs, in which their secretions are stored for future use. Others have neither ducts nor receptacles; their secretions being excreted by transudation and absorbed by nearby organs thru endosmosis. The splenic fluid passing from the spleen into the stomach is a good example.

The liver, like the pancreas and spleen, is very vascular.

The bile is a yellow, greenish, viscid, bitter, nauseating fluid secreted by the liver and excreted into canaliculi. These unite into larger ducts and finally end into two or more hepatic ducts, a larger one from the right lobe and a smaller from the left. The hepatic duct is joined by the cystic duct which is the size of a goose quill and from one to one and a half inches in length. The hepatic duct from the gall bladder and the cystic duct from the liver, form the bile duct which is about three inches long and one-quarter of an inch in diameter. The pancreatic duct makes a junction with the bile duct and together they enter the descending duodenum about three and a half or four inches below the pylorus. When the bile is not needed to aid digestion, it is stored in the gall bladder, a receptacle about three inches in length and from one to one and a quarter of an inch in diameter. The secretion of bile is constant; while digestion is periodical. It will be observed that the bile, which is held in the reservoir, is diverted from its original channel, the bile duct using the cystic duct as a diverticulum for the storing of the surplus bile.

The bile aids the action of the pancreatic juice. It emulsifies fat, promotes peristalsis of the intestines, and assists in the absorption of their contents. The bile reaches the duodenum partly directly from the liver, thru the hepatic duct, also, from the gall bladder thru the cystic duct.

The nerves of the liver are mostly non-medullated. They are derived from the left pneumogastric and the solar plexus of the sympathetic. They enter the liver with the blood vessels and are distributed to the walls of the blood vessels and bile ducts. They emerge from the spinal foramen of the central dorsal vertebrae on the right side.

The liver may be enlarged by inflammation (a surplus of heat). This enlarged condition includes tumors, cysts and abscesses. Its shape and position may be modified by curvature of the spine.

The liver, like other organs, is liable to variation of temperature above or below normal. When its temperature is above, a condition known as hepatitis exists. This inflamed condition may be acute or chronic. It is always acute before it is chronic.

McFarland says: "Inflammation of the liver depends upon the presence of micro-organisms in the hepatic tissue."

Belafield states that "Purulent inflammation in the liver almost always results in abscess. It is often due to the introduction of bacteria into the organ. Large abscesses of the liver may be traumatic (the wound or injury being the harbor or port of entrance to the inner portions), but are often due to unknown causes."

Stengel affirms: "In practically all, if not all cases, abscess of the liver is due to the action of micro-organisms."

An organism is a body consisting of an aggregation of organs having definite functions. Micro is a prefix, meaning small. How small? It is one-millionth part of the unit to which it is prefixed. If we knew the size of the organism referred to, then one-millionth of that would be the size of a microbe.

Stengel tells us how these bacteria (peace-disturbers) **may** gain entrance to the liver. He says, "The bacteria may gain access in several ways. In some cases penetrating wounds, or perforation of gastric or duodenal ulcers or of other pathologic lesions into the liver, occasion direct infection. In other cases the micro-organisms are carried in the circulation and enter the liver with the portal or hepatic blood, or by retrograde embolism through the hepatic veins from the vena-cava. Finally, infection may occur by invasion of the bacteria along the bile-ducts."

He tells us that wounds and ulcers may become pathologic lesions. If bacteria gain entrance into the system thru these wounds or ulcers and, thereby, cause disease, then these wounds become lesions, become causes of disease.

The pathologists are in a similar quandary as the boy was when he said that the bug got in the watch between the ticks. The boy's explanation is no farther fetched than are those of the pathologists.

Inflammation is a term used to express a local condition wherein there is an excess of heat, an obstruction of the blood currents, an increase of functional activity.

Atrophy, congestion, abscesses, scleroses, carcinoma and jaundice are abnormal conditions of the liver because of overheat, inflammation.

These conditions should be corrected as are inflammatory conditions of other organs; never forgetting that normal temperature means normal functionating—health.

---

"The more I practice Chiropractic, the more I study, the more I know about and think about this subject, the more I become convinced that if you will give me the five upper dorsals and the cervicals, you can do what you please with the rest of the body and I will bring the fellow through without them."

The more I practice Chiropractic, the more I am convinced that the displacement of any bone may impinge upon one or more nerves, more particularly those of the vertebral column, because of their close connection with the short compact bundle of nerves known as spinal nerves or trunks. These trunks start from the spinal cord by a series of root filaments, spread out vertically like a fan; there are two of these series, each forming a thread-like root. These two roots unite and form a trunk, which we speak of as a spinal nerve, and as such it continues until it passes from the spinal canal through the intervertebral foramen or groove. This mixed spinal nerve is quite short as shown in figure 8, where it is represented on the left as emerging from the foramen; but immediately gives off a branch to the sympathetic ganglia. The reader will observe that this branch to the sympathetic ganglionic chain is a part of the spinal cord; that it is composed of thread-like filaments which form two roots; these unite to form the spinal nerve. From this short trunk are three other branches, one of which is a recurrent branch, that is, it returns, after forming a junction with a branch from the sympathetic, to the spinal canal where it is distributed to the spinal cord and its membranes. The rest of the filaments of this short, spinal nerve-trunk innervate the skeletal frame, muscles and the skin covering the trunk and limbs. (The scalp is innervated by the cranial nerves, assisted by communicants from the spinal nerves.) The former are the somatic branches of the spinal nerve, in contradistinction to the sympathetic nerves which innervate the viscera.

This general distribution of the nerve branches from the short trunk is apparent in the lower seventeen pairs of nerves as well as in the thirteen for which only the author of the above has use. The more I study Chiropractic, the more I see that the displacement of any bone, projecting from the median line, is likely to press against and impinge upon adjacent nerves, thereby causing irritation if the pressure be light; if the pressure is heavy enough to **desensitize** this nerve, then its carrying capacity is nil.

We might think the above remark a joke, intending it as a rub on some one, if the author had not followed it with:

"Now, laying all jokes aside, there is no question but what the cervical region, and the five upper dorsal, is the field of battle in every affliction or abnormality, no matter what it is. And, by-the-way, it is the place which a good many Chiropractors have neglected."

"**Field of battle.**" He must have fancied that he was in a legal battle, fighting for the rights of his client; or opposing his opponent in securing a just claim; or else he had just that much of Allopathy left in him which had to be let out. There are very many diseases which are caused by displacement of the lower fourteen, true vertebrae.

---

"External injuries from falls, jars or bruises," do not cause subluxations. Injuries do not cause displacements. A sudden jar or fall unexpected may cause displacement of vertebrae, but bruises never.

---

Before me is a newspaper ad. "**Don't Commit Suicide With Strong Drugs.** If you have an acute or chronic ailment I can positively cure you by common sense and scientific methods, with the aid of Chiropractic, electricity and various other modern and scientific appliances."

A felo de se is one who deliberately and intentionally takes his or her own life. These are the ones he addresses in his ad. They are the ones he desires to cure by common sense. Drugs are substances employed in the cure of disease Persons desiring to commit suicide use poisons not drugs. **Strong** drugs is a misnomer—shows that the author does not know what he is talking about.

The man who advertises to "positively cure" **any** acute or chronic ailment by common sense, does not use common sense; neither is he honest, for he is not positive that he can cure any ailment that the suicide may have.

"Chiropractic, electricity and various other modern and scientific appliances," are used as an aid; they just help common sense and scientific methods.

Chiropractic is not an "appliance." If Dr. B. B. B. understood Chiropractic he would not need to use the various appliances as an aid to his common sense method.

## THE NERVOUS SYSTEM.

The spinal nerves emerge from the spinal canal. They originate in the spinal cord by rootlets which form two roots. These join as they enter the intervertebral foramen and pass through the opening as the spinal nerve. At its exit, the spinal nerve divides into two branches, the anterior and posterior somatic branches. Just before it divides, it gives off a small branch which returns inward. The anterior of the two divisions is joined by a branch from the sympathetic cord called ramus communicans. This latter gives to the recurrent branch a filament from the sympathetic. These two form one nerve which, returning through the intervertebral foramen, supplies innervation to the fibrous membrane which forms the outermost covering of the brain and spinal cord. It, also, sends branches to the vertebrae and vertebral ligaments.

After the spinal nerves issue and divide into branches they are no longer known as spinal nerves, although their fibers pass on and into other nerves.

The posterior, primary division of a spinal nerve divides into the internal and external branches; these are distributed to the muscles and skin behind the spine. The first cervical, the fourth and fifth sacral and the coccygeal nerves are exceptions.

The anterior, primary division of the spinal nerve supplies the parts of the body in front of the spine, including the four limbs. Each anterior branch is connected with the sympathetic by filaments named rami communicans. These are the spinal nerves. They are directed, with the sympathetic cord, inward from the intervertebral foramen, over the vertebral column, and becoming connected with the sympathetic cord, convey spinal fibers to the organs and tissues in the splanchnic area.

It will be seen from the above that the spinal nerve divides into four branches. Any one of which may become impinged upon, pressed against, by a displaced vertebra, or the head of a rib may be wrenched from its mooring, presenting an uneven surface against any one of these four branches of the spinal nerve; or such displacements may impinge the vertical, sympathetic ganglionic chains causing disease either in nearby or distant portions.

If the innervation of the recurrent nerve is interfered with by pressure, it becomes irritated, molecular action is increased, there is greater vibration, and the heat becomes more intense, causing pathological conditions varying from headache to that of brain fever; or spinal irritation, deviating from neurasthenia to vertebral caries.

If the bodies of the vertebrae or the heads of the ribs become luxated they may impinge upon the sympathetic ganglionic chain which reaches into the four cavities, thereby causing vegetative functions to be performed either in a greater or in a less degree than normal.

Impingement of the somatic nerves cause rheumatism and skin diseases.

---

Age makes a difference in the texture of nerve tissue.

The texture of nerves differ in individuals, which accounts for the difference in their makeup.

The number of nerve vibrations depend upon their solidity.

The amount of vibrations determines the degree of heat.

---

A booklet of a D. C. states: The body is nourished by fluid food carried through the nerves to all parts; that disease is due to the affected parts being ill fed, because of nerves being lessened in size by being squeezed; that this starved condition causes weakness, also an excess of uric acid which the kidneys fail to filter, this latter certainly being the cause of rheumatism.

Nerves are the lines through which intelligence, not fluid food, is received and sent. This impulse may be augmented or decreased. In either case, we have abnormal functions—disease.

Occasionally we relieve rheumatism in less than a minute. In such cases how about the kidneys filtering and discharging the uric acid in one-fourth of a minute?

---

"How and by what means could **abridged** nerve supply be produced?

"The organ, part or tissue is only affected or diseased in proportion to the **abridged** condition of the nerve supply to that part, organ or tissue.

"In 95 per cent of the cases we find this **abridging** of nerve energy is located in the spine, at the points where the nerve branches from the cord pass between the spinal segments, through the intervertebral foramina.

"Any pressure on a nerve alters its normal function; a light pressure, continued, will accelerate it to over-action, as is the symptoms produced in all inflammations, fevers, cancerous and goitrous growths, swellings, etc."

Abridge means to lessen, diminish, curtail, to make shorter. According to the above, "inflammations, fevers, cancerous and goitrous growths, swellings etc." are only five per cent "of the cases we find." A serious mistake in the **abridgment.**

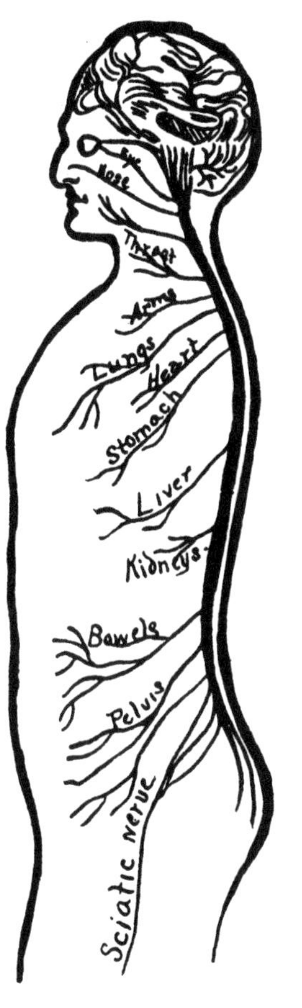


This cut "illustrates how the brain communicates with all the organs thru the nerve system."

"B. J. Palmer, in one of his addresses to his class in Portland this summer, aptly quoted, '**that he who tears down must rebuild greater,**' and said, 'when I saw there was **no use for a Sympathetic Nervous System, I threw it out,** and then just had to put something better in its place, so **I discovered Direct Mental Impulse.**' "

This same writer, a few months later said: "I wish to be clearly understood as saying that what has so many times been dissected as the Sympathetic Nervous System **is there—I do not question that for an instant**—IT IS THERE."

---

## THE NEW SCIENCE.

"By the **study** of the accompanying **cuts** and the following **reasons**, it will be easy to **comprehend** what causes disease, also how easy it is for Chiropractors, by **the most scientific method,** to reach the organs of the body **through the cerebro-spinal nervous system.**

"Chiropractors palpate the spine, locate vertebral displacements that pinch the nerves, which **reveal the diseased organs,** and thus

## "ANALYSE CASES.

"Nothing but an adjustment of the subluxated vertebrae will ever **properly** articulate these bones, **lift them off from nerves** and **allow life** and vitality **to at once proceed** to the diseased organs."

---

The medical profession is overcrowded; it is not so with Chiropractic.

---

Many patients imagine that they have tried everything. True, they have used many remedies, but they have never had the cause of their infirmity adjusted.

**Nerve Tracing.** Among the principles developed by me is the art of tracing sensitive inflamed, swollen, contracted nerves to and from the place of impingement and the organ or portion affected. This tracing, when made by an expert, is not only explanatory, but educational. Chemical analysis may determine the constituent qualities of urine in such diseases as nephritis, gravel, diabetes and Bright's disease, but it does not locate the cause. A Chiropractor by palpating determines the lesion in one or both of the kidneys, then follows the sensitive nerves of innervation to their origin in the vertebral column. By a unique movement he releases the impingement caused by a slightly displaced vertebra; the nerves freed from pressure, perform the function of innervation in a normal manner.

Several writers corroborate Dunglison's statement that, "Irritation is indicated by tenderness on pressure over the spinous process of one or more vertebrae or parts of the sides of the spine." He nor they ever mention that the nerves of innervation are liable to be impinged upon by slightly displaced vertebrae or other bones, a condition that is daily being demonstrated by Chiropractors. By nerve tracing we determine which one or both of the kidneys are not performing their normal function. This of itself would seem wonderful to the practitioners of other schools. But we do not stop here. By palpation, we determine the position of the vertebrae which to a Chiropractor is very important.

Chiropractors are daily demonstrating upon living subjects, without vivisection, that there are communicating nerve-fibers which have not been noticed by anatomists. We no longer have use for such statements as "sympathetic affections between two or more organs, so that the affection of one is transmitted to the other or others unknown." Chiropractors trace this "unknown" connection by following nerves from the same foramen to different parts of the body. We do not need such terms as reflex action, reflex function, reflex paralysis, reflex neurosis or reflex spasms. Nerve tracing explains this unexplainable explanation of vicarious commutation.

There is nothing more explanatory and convincing to the prospective student or patient than nerve tracing.

---

There are no two persons who have the same outside appearance; no two who are of the same age; no two who are alike in their osseous makeup; no two whose nerves are either sensed alike, or pass through the same foramina in the same manner, with the same amount of pressure. Therefore, we never find precisely the same combination with exactly the same symptoms.

## REFLEX ACTION.

To obliterate the spinal, cranial, or the sympathetic system of nerves, would blot out, not only reflex action, but all vital movements derived by and through nerves.

In animal life we have two forms of action, the voluntary and the involuntary, as they have been and are known today to all, except a few Chiropractors. I do not prefer the name sympathetic to designate a certain system of nerves, neither do I like the name reflex, which specifies action that we, as Chiropractors, consider under the management of Innate. But, to deny the existence of one or all of the three systems of nerves, or a certain combination of actions, because the name, to us, is a misnomer, would be equivalent to denying that there is such a sweet as honey-dew as it is not honey or dew, being an excretion of plant-lice; or to deny the existence of a tree named honey-locust, because it is neither honey nor a locust, being so named because of a sweet pulp found between the seeds in the pods. Christian Science is a misnomer, it is neither Christian nor Science, yet it would be foolish to state there were no Christian Scientists. Thus we might continue to give misnomers and homonyms.

A reflex action is regarded as one executed without volition or consciousness. We, as Chiropractors, should be able to give an intelligent explanation of such actions. To deny that which cannot be comprehended was not the method pursued by the one who discovered the fundamental principles of Chiropractic and founded thereon a science. We may consider reflex action a misnomer, but the fact remains that there are many conditions known as reflex—an involuntary movement.

The instantaneous closing of the eyelids when the eyeball is touched; the dilation or contraction of the pupil and iris to accommodate itself to the amount of light; the changes in the shape of the lens to secure perfect vision for objects at different distances, afford a few examples of reflex action. The spinchter pupillae is supplied by the third cranial nerve by way of the ciliary ganglion. The cervical sympathetic supplies the radiating fibers. The dilator pupillae is supplied by sympathetic fibers which have their origin in the superior ganglion; from thence we trace them back to the cervical vertebrae, into the spinal cord, and from thence to the brain.

The desire and act of defacation of the bowels, because of fecal deposit in the rectum, or because of a physic, are reflex actions to a medical man; to a Chiropractor it is a desire on the part of Innate to discharge waste material, or to rid itself of a poison which has been administered. It often happens that we cannot recall a certain portion of a poem without repeating the previous portion, each line suggesting another.

Railroad postal clerks tell me that when distributing mail matter to 25, 100 or more pouches, that the letter or paper often enters the pouch before the thrower has a mental conception of the address. Is that reflex action, or has the cuticle of the hand an **insight, an intuitive seeing with the inner eye?**

A reflex center is one in which a sensory impression is changed into a motor impulse; the transfer being made so quickly that it is certainly not done by our conscious intelligence. This all-wise intelligence we call Innate, is always on the alert to care for its incorporeal functions.

---

Among the wonderful achievements of this century, the discovery and development of Chiropractic is preeminent it is destined to replace all methods which treat effects. After centuries of untiring research by the medical world, it remained for me to discover the cause of disease and develop a method which removes nerve pressure by adjusting vertebrae, the displacing of which is the source of 95 per cent of all diseases.

---

To talk about "new nerves" is as foolish as to speak of a "new science," only it is more apparent. We may discover nerves which have heretofore eluded observation, but that does not make them "new nerves." So far as we know, the same number and kind of nerves ramify the body, perform the same functions, as they did a thousand years ago. We may discover by palpation or dissection some which have not been heretofore noticed, but that does not make them "new nerves."

---

A leaflet states under "Chiropractic and Vital treatment," "The methods employed are physiological Therapeutics, Thermo-Therapy (Hot Air) (Super-Heated Air), Electro-Theraphy, Massage, Hydro-Therapy, Mechano-Therapy, Mogna-Therapy, Suggestive-Therapy, and Vibro-Therapy. All these methods are used in treating disease."

As Chiropractic is not any one of the nine methods of treatment, we are led to believe that the nine methods are included in the Vital treatments. The first page, 8 by 10, is devoted to a picture of himself studying a spinal column, that is, in all probability, all he knows about Chiropractic. He uses "Appedictonomy" for appendicectony.

## FACIAL DIAGNOSIS.

There is much to be learned from the study of the face. We may obtain, recognize and determine therefrom much valuable information regarding disease. The lips of the patient may tell only one story, while the face is a correct tell-tale. Considering the many and varied expressions seen upon the face in health, it is not surprising that it reveals useful information to the Chiropractor who desires to know what functions are abnormal, that he may correct them. The true facial expressions of disease is seldom aped by the maligner.

To every practitioner, more especially the beginner, the question is, "How can I determine what ails my patient?"

The doctor who cares to read the face of his patient to learn something regarding thon's disease, should take such a position that he look the sufferer square in the face. If the patient, or thon's friends, should start to relate what previous doctors have said regarding his case the examiner should cut it short by saying: "Do not tell me what the doctors have said regarding your case; I would rather form my own opinion." Otherwise the knowledge of what previous diagnosis have been might prejudice and bias his opinion.

The complexion should be noticed. There may be pallor, yellowness, a lemon tint, an earthy bronze, blue or reddish color. An abnormal color of the skin is owing to degenerative pigmentation, an organic coloring matter concerned in the coloration of the skin. Pallor denotes anemia, bloodlessness, a deficiency of blood, a diminution in the per cent of red corpuscles; the serum containing a larger proportion of water than usual.

The general expression should be noticed. It may be one of anxiety and pain; animated or pathetic; intellectual or unconscious. It must be borne in mind that the general expression is affected by the mental condition, the habits, temperament, intellectual development, exposure to outdoor or indoor influences, avocation and pathological conditions. Age, also, must be taken into consideration. The intelligence of the face is readily recognized; it may be one which is keenly alert to the surroundings, including conversation. The difference between the face of the wage-earner and the professional must be considered. Is it full and smooth or drawn and wrinkled? Is one side placid and the other rough? Is the mouth drawn to one side or the face shorter on one side than the other? Is the face that of contentment and ease, or one of anxiety and distress? Occupation has much to do with the expression and movements of the eye. The farmer, sailor and business man has each acquired their characteristic manner and use of that organ. The eye has more to do with expression than any other portion of the face. The eyes may be restless and follow every movement of the attendant and doctor or they may stare vacantly into space; consciousness may be alert or dull. All peculiarities of the eye should be observed and studied.

In serious illness, owing to loss of muscular tonicity, the nose appears pinched, the eyes sunken and lusterless, and the chin and malar bones sharp and prominent.

The color, consistency, moisture or dryness of the skin **means much to** the observer.

The elated facial expression of the insane, the excited look of the maniac, the careworn features of nervous exhaustion and the hopeless forlorn countenance of the sufferer from melancholia, have each their place as a factor in our diagnosis.

This article deals only with what may be seen in the faces of those whom we are called to adjust.

In **acromegally,** the face has a full-moon expression.

Young persons with **adenoids,** an overgrowth of adenoid tissue in the naso-pharynx, have fishy mouths, kept constantly open to breathe.

The facial expression of paralysis **agitans** is that of distress, pathetic and somewhat intense.

In **anemia,** the lips are pale, livid and blue, showing a lack of red corpuscles; an opposite condition to that of hyperemia.

Unconsciousness comes on suddenly in **apoplexy,** the breathing is stertorous, snoring and hoarse. There is frequently a conjugate deviation of the eyes. The face is usually turned from the paralyzed side.

**Asthma** will be recognized by the inability of the patient to exhale the used-up air.

In **bleareye,** chronic conjunctivitis, there is a copious secretion of the sebaceous humor of the eyelids, rendering them gummy.

---

Variations of the osseous, nervous, vascular and muscular systems are of special interest to Chiropractors. That they do vary and their variations are continuous, should keep the adjuster from becoming stereotyped in certain set places for adjusting. Regional localization is safer and more scientific than by number.

Hare gives us much information on facial diagnosis. Hare's Practical Diagnosis is published by Lea Brothers & Co., Philadelphia. He says, "In the case of children, much information can be gained as to the state of the system by the facial expression, particularly while the child sleeps. If it is asleep and healthy and well, the eyelids are closed, the lips are never so slightly parted, the nostrils are practically immobile, and the general expression is very peaceful. If, on the other hand, the eyelids of a sleeping child are slightly parted so as to show the whites of the eyes, there is probably present some digestive or nervous disturbance, perhaps accompanied by moderate pain. If in the course of an illness the eyelids remain far enough apart to result in glazing of the conjunctiva from dryness, this is a sign of grave import. Again, twitching of the eyelids often indicate nervous irritation or the early stages of the convulsive state, and it is not uncommon for an expression to pass over the face of a child who, while sleeping, is suffering from pain, which begins as a smile and ends with a drawing-in of the corners of the mouth, an expression somewhat like that seen on the face of a waking child when it seems to be in doubt as to whether to laugh or to cry. Whether asleep or awake, a child in pain, if not crying, has a pinched look about its nose and mouth, and sometimes some idea of the seat of the pain may be gained by the part of the face which is drawn. When pain is in the head, the forehead is apt to be wrinkled into a frown; if the nose is pinched and drawn, it is said to show that the pain is in the chest; and if the upper lip is raised, pain is probably felt in the belly.

"When the skin of the entire body, the face being particularly affected, is of a livid or bluish-slate color, resembling somewhat the appearance of a person exposed to rays of light passing through blue glass, the condition is that of argyria or chronic silver poisoning. This discoloration is so characteristic as to admit of no difficulty in diagnosis, since the absence of any circulatory or respiratory embarassment excludes the possibility of its being due to cyanosis. Owing to the small amount of silver now given internally by physicians, chronic argyria is becoming rare. The discoloration is due to a deposit of oxide of silver in the rete Malpighii.

"The eye affords more information for diagnostic purposes concerning the condition of other organs of the body than any single part which can be examined. We gather from it not only a clear idea as to its own state, and the state of the nervous centers more or less intimately connected with the government of its movements and its special functions, but in addition we often gain positive information as to the condition of organs more remotely situated, as, for example, the kidneys. **The very fact that so many different tissues are found in this organ renders it susceptible to the many diseases affecting similar tissues elsewhere in the body.** The parts of the eye which give us the greatest amount of knowledge about changes in other tissues are the optic nerve and retina and its vessels and the ocular muscles. The crystaline lens, the conjunctiva, and the cornea often give additional evidence indicating the general systemic condition. Cataract should make the physician suspect diabetes, even if it appear in persons advanced in years. The eyelids, if puffy in appearance, may indicate renal disease, cardiac lesions, or the overuse of arsenic. An examination of the inner side of the lids may reveal a pallor due to anemia. Slight conjunctival hemorrhage may result from violent coughing, and when it is recurrent it should arouse the suspicion of renal disease with secondary vascular troubles. In old persons such a hemorrhage, if not due to injury, may indicate degenerative vascular changes."

In **blepharofacial spasm** there are paroxysmal spastic contractions of the obicularis palpebrarum and other facial muscles.

Fever **blisters** on the lip indicate "a breaking up of a fever."

Blepharitis, inflammation of the eyelids is known by their reddened appearance.

For **cancers** of the lips and face, see cancers in the general index.

**Canker** of the mouth; cancrum oris; see canker.

**Carcinoma** in any part of the body, when open, leaves a pigment of a straw or lemon color and an odor when once smelled will always be remembered.

**Cataleptics** have the expression of hysteria, except that, in the former it is a fixed one.

In **cataract** there is a pigmentary deposit in front of the retina.

**Chlorosis** is a disease which affects adolescent girls, usually those which have not menstruated. It is characterized by a pale complexion of a greenish tint, languor and listlessness. The blood of chlorotics is thin, light colored and deficient in red corpuscles; the clot is in less proportion to the serum in chlorosis than in health.

**Chorea** is expressed in the face by irregular and involuntary motions of one or more muscles. The spasms do not continue during sleep.

The face may be made to take on a gray or bluish **color** by the injection of coal-tar products. This color can be better noticed a short distance from the patient.

In brain **compression,** impingement upon the nervous center, the cheeks expand and the lips are passively blown outward at each expiration.

In brain **concussion** the patient can be roused to semi-consciousness; not so in compression for voluntary and reflex movements are in abeyance. The skin is cold and covered with perspiration. The pulse is slow and strong. The pupils are fixed, usually dilated, and do not respond to the light. Speech is impaired. In local pressure the patient does not lose consciousness, the symptoms depending upon the part of the brain which is impaired.

**Conjunctivitis,** inflammation of the conjunctiva, may be catarrhal, croupus, diphtheric, gonorrheal, phlyctenular or purulent in character and origin.

**Cranial cyanoses,** lividity from plethora of the venous system, is indicated by blueness of the skin.

**Cretinism** is readily recognized by the nose being broad and flat, the eyelids enlarged, the lips greatly thickened, the tongue lolling, saliva dribbling, mental dullness and constant stupidity.

**Cutaneous** eruptions are accompanied with fever. The diagnostic symptoms are varied, as are also the many febrile rashes. See catalogue for each.

Deaf persons seldom, if ever, smile or laugh.

**Death,** approaching dissolution, is recognized by sunken eyes, slightly parted eyelids, eyes glassily fixed on vacancy, a pinched appearance of the nose, drawn skin, drooping, and lack of muscular tonicity.

In **drunkenness** the pupils are usually contracted, but they dilate when the drunkard is aroused.

The **ears** may be illy developed, with a corresponding dullness of intellect.

**Ectropion** may be recognized by eversion, or the turning out of the eyelid.

The lower eyelids may be puffy, **edematous,** especially in the morning, a symptom of dropsy, from Bright's disease.

**Epilepsy** is known by distorted eyes and face, red, purple or violet countenance, grinding of the teeth and foaming at the mouth.

**Erysipelas** is characterized by superficial inflammation of the skin, with general fever, tension and swelling of the part. The surface is smooth and shiny, as if oiled.

Exopthalmia is readily recognized by the bulging or abnormally protruding eyes. Usually associated with goitre.

In **exophthalmia,** protrusion of the eyeballs is quite noticable. The eye is pressed outward and the eyelids separated. Goitre and heart trouble usually accompany this affection. All come from the same impingement.

**Facial hemiatrophy** is recognized by a wasting of the bones of one-half of the face and the subcutaneous tissue.

In **facial hemihypertrophy,** one-half of the face is normal in size, the other gigantic.

**Facial paralysis** is readily recognized. The affected side of the face is smooth and expressionless. The eye of the affected side remains wide open; the mouth is drawn to the healthy side, when the patient attempts to laugh. Such persons are unable to whistle or talk distinctly. It may or may not accompany hemiplegia.

**Fissures,** cracked or chapped lips are accompanied by inflammation; remove the pressure.

**Habit spasm** arises from an acquired movement.

**Hay fever** is known by sneezing, nasal and conjunctival catarrh.

**Headache** is expressed in the face as a frown.

In hectic fevers there is a bright blush over the malar bones.

**Herpes** of the lips is an inflammatory skin disease, characterized by the formation of small vessicles in clusters.

In **hydrocephalus** the skull is globular in shape, the forehead bulged forward and over the face which has an aged expression.

The facial expression of **hysteria** may be apathetic or that of devotion, rage or grief.

**Indigestion** in children is known by a whiteness around the mouth and flushed cheek.

**Insanity** is expressed in the eye.

In **iritis** the conjunctiva is pink and the vessels straight; while in conjunctivitis the color is brick-red and the vessels tortuous. Iritis is an inflammation of the eyeball itself; its cause lies in an impingement of the right fifth dorsal nerve; while that from conjunctivitis is from an impingement of the twelfth dorsal nerve.

In **jaundice** the conjunctiva is yellow where it covers the sclerotic. The skin is more or less of the same color, the depth of color depending upon the amount of bile pigment.

Tubercular **leprosy** is usually shown on the face. Ulceration and mortification usually occur. The face becomes lion-like in appearance.

**Malarial** pigmentation deposited in the cutaneous capillaries gives a peculiar tint to the skin.

**Marginal** conjunctivitis is indicated by inflammation of the edges of the eyelids.

The expression of **myxedema** is heavy and listless.

**Nictitating** spasm is indicated by a continuous and uncontrollable winking.

**Opium poisoning** is attended with drowsiness and the deep sleep which characterizes the effects of opiates. The pupils are contracted to a pin-point.

The face in **osteitis** is deformed and shaped like a triangle, with the base upward.

**Pain** in the chest or abdomen is expressed in a drawn condition of the lower portion of the face.

In **peritonitis** the upper lip is drawn upward, so as to show the teeth; there is an expression of anxiety and unrest.

In **pleurisy** the breathing is short, restrained and rapid.

**Pneumonia** is known by a flushed face, short breathing and a suppressed dry cough. The cheek of the affected side is usually flushed. Care will need be used to see that the patient has or has not been resting on that cheek.

Posture of the head may aid in diagnosis. Deafness in one ear causes the patient to turn the head.

**Pterygium** is a patch of thickened conjunctiva of a triangular shape, commonly occurring at the inner angle of the eye; from whence it extends over the cornea. Sometimes two or three pterygia occur on the same eye, covering the cornea with a thick veil, which totally prevents vision.

**Ptosis** is caused by paralysis of the levator palpebra superioris, which causes the eyelid to remain closed. The nerve fibers which supply motion to the eyeball and eyelids originate in the brain, pass down the spinal cord and emerge between the second and third cervical vertebrae; from which fibers go to the sympathetic cord by rami-communicants. From the sympathetic ganlionated chain the fibers pass along beside of the internal carotid artery and into the cranium thru the carotid canal where it forms a part of the cavernous plexus, from thence via the ophthalmic division of the fifth nerve to the eye. These convey impulses which cause dilitation of the pupil, the levator palpebra muscle of the upper lid.

**Pulmonary phthisis** is known by wide open eyes, a hunted expression, quivering nostrils, red flush over the malar bones and an eager, apathetic glance of the eye.

**Pyorrhea** is detected by suppurative inflammation of the connective tissue of the gums.

In **rickets** the skull is somewhat square, oblong, box shaped, owing to the development of hyperostosis on the frontal and parietal eminences and larger than usual. There is delayed closure of the fontanels and sweating of the head.

**Strabismus** is a squint, crosseyes, a lack of parallelism in the axes of the eyes. This may be due to paralysis or over action.

**Tetanus** is a contraction of the jaw muscles; the masseters and temporals are first involved in the tonic contractions.

**Tongue hemiatrophy** is of rare occurrence. One-half of the tongue is wasted away, shrunken, until it is only half of normal size.

In **typhoid fever** the face is dull and expressionless, the teeth covered with sordes, the lips move in a low, muttering delirium.

**Weeping** of the lachrymal gland is shown by lacrymation, excretion and effusion of tears.

**Worms** of the stomach and intestines may be readily known by an examination of the lower lip. If it is covered with red papillae the size of pin-heads, worms are present. The nerves of stomach innervation emerge between the fifth and sixth dorsal vertebrae on the left side. On the opposite side, between the same two vertebrae, nerves emerge which go to the mouth and lips. A displacement of the fifth dorsal vertebra is likely to impinge upon the nerves next below on both sides. The papillae present on the inside of the lower lip are the twig ends of fibers which emerge from the right side of the vertebral column, between the fifth and sixth dorsal vertebrae. The impingement causes an irritation which is present at their peripheral endings as noticed.

In wry neck, torticollis, the head leans to the affected side, the face and head is unequally developed.

---

The December number of the Chiropractor, page 4, under the head-line, "That 'Painless Adjustment' Question," says (?): "I have seen hundreds, yes, thousands, of 'new movements' come and go the way they all do, but I have seen the old stand-by (the one taught him by his father) still remain true to its post. "Old Faithful still continues at the old stand."

True; the movement devised and used by D. D. Palmer has not been improved upon. Many have been the departures, but the "Old Faithful still continues" to include the art of adjusting. To say, "**Hundreds, yes, thousands,** of new movements have come and gone," savors of prevarication.

---

Lynchburg, Va., April 21, 1909.

Dr. D. D. Palmer.

I read your suggestion of placing the patient's arms along the sides for adjustment, I find it o. k. A. R. ELY, D. C.

Bro. Ely:—I think the information you speak of is worth $10 to any Chiropractor, yet you are the only one who has appreciated it enough to even write me concerning it. I sometimes think that Chiropractic is not valued for what it is worth. Each single number of The Adjuster costs us for paper, printing and postage, 15 cents in cash; this does not include my time. Twelve numbers cost us $1.80, for which we get $1. I like to disseminate Chiropractic knowledge, but you are the only one, so far to appreciate the above suggestion enough to speak of it—**thanks.**

## SOME DISPLACEMENTS ADJUSTED.

"We have to the left a good skeleton. Let us study him as he was. In that skull was a brain. From that went downward and through the spinal foramen, where this steel rod is, a spinal cord. If you will notice closely, we have where these pieces of chalk are, small openings. Dr. D. D. Palmer is the first man, Chiropractic the first science, and The P. S. C. the first school that made these famous by calling especial attention to them, for at that point is the cause of all disease. Nerves branch from the spinal cord inside of the spinal foramen. Brain nerves emit through the intervertebral foramina."

Spinal nerves pass out from the spinal cord through the intervertebral foramina; they emerge from the spinal foramen. They do not **emit** anything; they do not send forth, throw out, eject or discharge heat, light, odor or steam. Nerves transmit the will of Innate for the purpose of performing functions. All nerves have their real origin in the brain, therefore, cannot be otherwise than "brain nerves." The cranial nerves do not "emit through the intervertebral foramina."

Nerves do not **branch** (divide) from the spinal cord. Spinal nerves proceed from spinal foramina. Each nerve arises from the spinal cord by two separate roots; these are composed of rootlets. These roots combine and form a nerve trunk; as such it passes through the intervertebral foramen (not foramin). It divides into four branches immediately after it leaves the foramen and not "inside of the spinal foramin."

"At that point is the cause of all disease." A point has no breadth, length, thickness or size; it is only an imaginary position. The reader will see that the writer refers to the intervertebral foramina, the openings between the vertebrae—these holes did not contain the shadow of a point, only pieces of chalk. The author referred to the foramina as being "the cause of all disease." They are not the cause of any disease. Their action expressed in displacements may cause a large portion of disease. Other bones than those of the vertebral column cause impingement by being displaced, for example, corns and bunions, also, the fractured ends of broken bones.

I was the first and only man to develop the science of Chiropractic. There was no second man to do that which had already been done by another. I, it was, who first made special mention of displacements of intervertebral foramina as the cause of 95 per cent of all diseases. Chiropractic is a name of a science; it did not name the two brains, any more than it named itself. I named that which I discovered and developed. The discovery of one principle did not make a science. It took the discovery of several principles and facts, mutually related and comprehended under a general law, to make a science.

"At birth the child has two brains. Chiropractic has respectively named these brains Innate and Educated." Why specify "at birth"? Is it not a fact that all persons at any age have two brains, even before birth? In the embryo six brains are recognized; the rhinencephalon (olfactory brain); diencephalon (inner or between brain); mesencephalon (middle brain); mylencephalon (after brain); metencephalon (hind brain); tetencephalon (end brain); these collectively are known as the encephalon (brain). Portions of these brains are exposed on the base of the encephalon (brain); all the cranial nerves emerge from this under surface. The olfactory and optic nerves originate in the rhinencephalon. Their apparent origin is between the two hemispheres of the cerebellum, however, they belong to the cerebral hemispheres.

Chiropractic did not name anything. I did not name the cerebellum Innate; neither did I name the cerebrum Educated. I did, however, in the early development of Chiropractic state that Innate controlled the vital functions through nerves which originated in the cerebellum, or back brain; that the cerebrum, front brain, was for the reception of knowledge acquired by Innate during life. Neither Chiropractic, nor its founder, named the two brains Innate and Educated. If I adjust all the dislocations in the next year, made in the science of Chiropractic, by the "Student, Author, Lecturer and Teacher on any Phase of Chiropractic Philosophy, Science or Art, Anywhere at Any Time," I will have to get busy.

It was I (not the school) who called especial attention to subluxations of vertebrae being the cause of 95 per cent of all diseases. This was done by my writings in The Chiropractor and other literature. Much of my hard work has been subverted by would-be arrogant fountain heads.

---

P. S. C. Announcement: "This is the pioneer school of Chiropractic . . . Was founded by Dr. D. D. Palmer (thanks), the discoverer of Chiropractic." Many thanks. "So that they may receive a diploma from the parent school, to hang in their office."

"Old Dad Chiro is the Daddy of Chiropractic."—Briggs.

To designate a school as the parent school, because it was founded by the parent (Father) of Chiropractic would make four parent schools—the four schools founded by me.

Why not get a diploma with the name of D. D. Palmer, the discoverer, developer and founder of Chiropractic upon it?

## WHAT IS A LESION?

The word lesion has been one of the most difficult for students under my personal instructions to comprehend. Dictionaries are not definite in giving the meaning of this word so much in use by medical writers, more especially by osteopaths. I presume that there are many of the Adjuster class who do not comprehend its full meaning.

A hurt, wound, injury or morbid structural change which causes functional derangement is a lesion. A hurt, wound or injury that does not cause functional derangement is not a lesion—is not the cause of anything. A lesion must be a cause, producer of some derangement.

Webster says of a lesion:—A hurt; an injury. Any morbid **change** in the **exercise of functions** or the texture of organs. In law: "Loss from another's failure to fulfill a contract; injury arising from failure of consideration in a commutative contract."

Lippincott: "A hurt, wound or injury of a part; a pathological alteration of a tissue."

Anders draws the attention of the reader to the fact that on account of the spinal cord terminating at the second lumbar, lesions may exist above or below this point, such as tumors, fractures or congenital anomalies and spina bifida.

Dunglison:—Derangement, disorder; morbid change, either in **exercise of functions** or in the texture of organs.

A rusty nail entering the foot may cause tetanus, lockjaw. If the nail was free of rust, the wound would not be a lesion. The rust (poison) is the lesion, the cause of the lockjaw.

The word **lesion** is frequently used by osteopaths. E. H. Laughlin, in his quiz, makes common use of it. The following quotations, out of many, show the meaning he attaches to it:

What may **lesions** of the upper dorsals **cause?**

What are the most common lesions? Ans., **Rib lesions.**

How many **lesions** in the lower dorsal or lumbar **cause cholera morbus**?

What may a **lesion** to the fourth sacral nerve **cause**?

What may **lesions** in the dorsal and upper lumbar regions **cause**?

How may a cervical **lesion cause** diabetes?

Where look for **bony lesions causing** diphtheria?

How might the **spinal** and **rib lesions produce** enteroptosis?

What are the most common lesions found in erysipelas? Ans., **Bony lesions** along the cervical region and **lesions of the first ribs and clavicle.**

How may a cervical **lesion cause** erysipelas?

How may **lesions** of the clavicle, first rib, or anterior cervical tissue **cause** goitre?

How may a **lesion** of the atlas **cause** insanity?

What kind of **lesions** are usually present? Ans., **Bony.**

How may splanchnic, rib and renal **lesions cause** insanity?

How may a **lesion** of a cervical vertebra **cause** insomnia?

What are the most common **bony lesions** found in neuralgia? Ans., Vertebral.

Vertebral displacement **is** a morbid change in texture and causes a modification in the exercise of functions. If the reader will bear in mind that a lesion is the cause of functions being deranged, there will be no trouble in comprehending the following use of the word:

McFarland:—The structural changes wrought by disease are known as lesions. They may be **initial**, or primary; **secondary**, or **tertiary.** The lesions caused by physical agencies are said to be **traumatic** and vary with the nature of the force.

Traumatic:—Pertaining to or **caused by a wound or injury. Traumatic fever** is a febrile phenomena **following a wound.** Produced by wounds, as, **traumatic tetanus.**

Gould:—An injury, wound or morbid structural change. Discharging lesion:—A brain **lesion** that **causes** sudden discharge of **nervous motor impulses.** Focal lesion:—A circumscribed **lesion** in the **nervous system, giving rise** to distinctive and localizing **symptoms.** Molecular lesion:—A very fine **lesion**, not discerned by the microscope or discoverable by chemistry, but **causing loss or excess of functional activity** and attributed to alteration of the molecular equilibrium of that part. Irritative lesion:—A lesion in the nervous system **exciting the functions of the part wherein it is situated.**

Dorland:—Any hurt, wound or local degeneration. Depressive lesion:—One that causes **diminution of functional activity.** Destructive lesion:—One which leads to the obliteration of an organ or the **abolishment of its functions.** Functional lesion:—One which leads to no obvious or discoverable change of structure, but which **causes disturbance of function.** Indiscriminate lesion:—A lesion **affecting distinct parts or systems** of the body. Irritative lesion:—One which **stimulates the functions of the part where it is situated.** Local lesion:—One in the nervous system **giving origin to distinctive local symptoms.**

**These lesions give origin to distinct local symptoms named disease. They excite functional activity—disease. They cause loss or excess of functions—disease. They stimulate, diminish or abolish functions, which is but disease.**

Webster:—Primary syphilis, the initial stage of syphilis,

including the period from the development of the original **lesion or chancre** to the first manifestations of symptoms.

Dorland:—Primary syphilis in its first stage; the **primary lesion (chancre)** usually appears between ten and forty days after infection.

Gould:—The earliest **lesion** of acquired syphilis **is the chancre.**

Second in the order of time or development, as the secondary lesions of syphilis.

Dunglison:—Syphilis generally makes its first appearance by a hard **chancre,** the latter being known as the primary or **initial lesion.** In the **second stage—secondary syphilis**—constitutional symptoms are developed, **as exhibited in lesions** of the skin and mucous membranes. **The chancre is an infective lesion.** The **lesions** peculiar to syphilis are the **chancre,** the **mucous patch** and the gumma. The **chancre is the primary lesion** of acquired syphilis. The chancre is an inflammatory lesion. The mucous patch is the most contagious lesion of syphilis. These mucous patch lesions in the **second stage** of the disease. The mucous patch is the most **contagious lesion** of syphilis, and as it makes its appearance about the genital organs, is probably that through which the disease is most frequently transmitted. The gumma is a characteristic lesion of syphilis; it may appear as late as twenty to thirty years after infection. Syphilitic bone diseases are common. Periostitis, ostitis and osteomyelitis occur. These lesions have a selection for the upper third of the tibia, the sternum and skull. They may become very destructive, especially when affecting the septum nasi or the bones of the cranium.

Lippincott: Chancre.—The primary lesion of syphilis. Syphilis.—The primary lesion originates by contact of an abraided surface with the virus. Lastly, meta-syphilitic lesions, such as locomotor ataxia and paresis appear.

From the above on syphilis we learn that **chancre is the** acquired original **lesion—the cause of secondary lesions,** the mucous patch; that lesions, the causes of other advanced syphilitic conditions, may appear as late as twenty to thirty years; **that a lesion may be the cause of another lesion.**

The most definite meaning and use of the word **lesion** I have found is on page 933 of Delafield and Prudden's Pathology. The item is not only valuable in explaining the meaning and the use pathologists make of lesion, but also on post mortem examinations. General considerations for the cause of death —post mortem examinations.

"The object in making a post-mortem examination may be to determine whether a person has died from violence or poisoning; to account for a sudden death; or to study the **lesions of disease.** In any case the examination should include all the important parts of the body, not merely a suspected organ, and the results should be recorded at the time the examination is made.

"Great care is necessary in endeavoring to ascertain the cause of death when the clinical history is imperfect or unknown. Mechanical injuries which destroy life by abolishing the function of one of the important viscera are relatively infrequent. Most of the **lesions found after death are rather the marks of disease than the cause of death.** We do not know, for example, how great a degree of meningitis, or of pneumonia, or of endocarditis, or of cirrhosis, or of nephritis necessarily leads to death. On the contrary, one patient may recover with an **extent of lesion** which is sufficient to destroy the life of another. So with accidents; there is often no evident reason why fractures of the skull or of the pelvis should destroy life, yet they usually do. In some of the infectious diseases, such as typhoid fever, **the visible lesions cannot always be called the cause of death.** Sudden death of persons apparently in good health are often **particularly obscure.** In many of them we have to acknowledge that we can find no sufficient **cause for the death.** This is, of course, due to our imperfect knowledge, but it is much better in such cases to avow ignorance than **to attribute the death to some trifling lesion.** The brain and the heart are the organs which are especially capable of giving **symptoms** during life, without corresponding **lesions** after death. Very well-marked cardiac or cerebral symptoms may continue for days or months and apparently destroy life and yet, after death, we find no corresponding anatomical changes. But it should be remembered that recent advances in our knowledge of the cell, which an improved technique in hardening and preparation has greatly fostered, have already shown that under various abnormal conditions the cells, especially of the nervous system, may undergo morphological changes of great significance without perceptible alteration in the gross appearance of the affected part, changes which even the microscopic examinations of the past have failed to disclose. So that, while there often appears to be a wide **discrepancy** between **symptoms and lesions,** with the increase of knowledge the **scope of this discrepancy is** steadily narrowing. It is the **novice in post-mortem examinations** who is particularly apt to **mistake for lesions ordinary post-mortem alterations** or the effects of embalming processes.

"The cause of death is not always to be found in the organ primarily affected or which **shows the most pronounced lesions.**

Thus chronic diffuse nephritis may exist for years with more or less marked symptoms of disease. But death may finally be due to a weakened heart which was secondarily involved, or occur in uremic convulsions, the **brain showing no lesions at all.** It is desirable, therefore, and in the majority of cases possible, **to differentiate between obvious lesions and the cause** of death."

"The bony lesion a cause of disease," in the November number of Osteopathy, is the head line of an article.

Dr. A. T. Still does not make use of the words, "bony lesion" or lesion in his work on Osteopathy, date 1892.

Dr. A. P. Davis, a member of A. T. Still's first class, in his masterly work on Osteopathy of 846 pages, does not use the words "bony lesion" or lesion.

Since the advent of Chiropractic, there has arisen a class of Osteopaths named "lesion osteopaths," who believe in displaced bones as the cause of disease.

A D. D. S. insists that a **lesion is the result** of a wound or injury, that **deranged functions is the lesion.**

That which causes a disturbance of functions is lesional because it is a disturbance maker. The damage done is because of a lesion.

---

Baker City, Ore., December 21, 1909.

Dr. D. D. Palmer:—

I note your description of the spleen—in your last Adjuster—and cannot understand where you find a description like the one you give in that number. Your multiple spleens and the thickness are exceptional, so far as my knowledge goes.

Fraternally, A. P. DAVIS.

Dr. Davis refers to my description of the spleen found on page 45 of number seven Adjuster. As his "knowledge goes," where he "understands," therefore, this adjusting.

Because the amount of energy which transmits an impulse and gives it force can be made to vary, causing functions to be performed in a degree either greater or less than normal, therefore, the spleen is subject to many diseased conditions. Stengel says on page 400, when referring to hyperplasia (excessive formation of tissue) of the spleen; the spleen is **large** in size and **firm.** The capsule may be greatly **thickened.** The **thickening** is either diffuse or circumscribed. Patches of cartilaginous **hardness** may occur. Dr. Davis can find more information concerning his question by referring to Prudden's Anatomy, page 457 and 458; McFarland, page 596; Hare, page 311.

The Doctor does not know where I got my information regarding accessory and multiple spleens, so I will tell him, as it may be new to others.

Prudden says on page 452: "Small, accessory spleens, from the size of a hazelnut to that of a walnut, are not infrequent. They usually lie close to the spleen, but may be at a considerable distance from it; thus they have been found imbedded in the head of the pancreas. Two spleens of about equal size have been observed."

McFadden tells us on page 595; "Frequently accessory or supernumerary spleens are observed. These are usually the size of a pea, or may be as large as a cherry. They may be single or multiple. They are readily recognized by their color and consistence. Marsh observed two quite well-formed spleens in the same person."

Stengel, on page 397, speaks of accessory spleens the size of a pea or a marble being very often found.

McMurrich corroborates other writers when he says: "Supplementary spleens are found near the hilus in the gastrosplenic ligament, or less often in the great omentum. From one to twenty of these small bodies may be met with. They are red and round, of the same structure as the spleen and vary in size from a pea to a walnut."

Gray's knowledge goes. He says on page 1355: "Accessory spleens vary in size from that of a pea to that of a plum; these are known as supernumerary or accessory spleens."

Cunningham is not in the dark. He says on page 1212: "Small globular masses of splenic tissue are not infrequently found in the neighborhood of the spleen. These are termed accessory spleens."

Even Gerrish knows of these supernumerary spleens. On page 795 he says: "Frequently accessory spleens are found. They are globular and small, but otherwise look like the principal spleen, near which they are situated."

The American Text-Book of Surgery is also aware of there being occasionally more than one spleen. "Supernumerary spleens are not uncommon, and are usually of small size. There are several cases recorded of multiple spleens. Cases of absence of the spleen are not unknown, and occasionally the spleen is of very minute size—not larger than a split walnut. Shepherd reports such a case which was otherwise perfect, having notch, hilus, etc., as in one of large size."

Cabrolius and Morgagni found two spleens in one subject. Cheselden and Fallopius reports three. Fatoni found four in one person. Guy and Patin saw five.

A case was shown at the Vienna Medical Society with a large number of spleens in the mesogastrium, peritoneium, on the messentery and transverse mesocolon and Douglas pouch. Every one of these spleens had a capsule, was covered by peritoneum and exhibited the histologic appearance of splenic tissue.

Bro. Davis:—You better get busy. There is much you may learn regarding spleens and Chiropractic.

---

The following is copied from the Annual Announcement of The P. S. C., Second Edition. **Copyright 1904, B. J. Palmer, D. C.**:

"**Chiropractic was discovered and developed by Dr. D. D. Palmer.**"

"**Dr. D. D. Palmer occupies the enviable position of being the discoverer and developer of the only system of adjustment** . . . Those who know the value of getting their information **first-handed** will appreciate what it means to study the different branches of Chiropractic **under the founder and originator** of this unequaled science."

"**Dr. D. D. Palmer, discoverer and developer of Chiropractic.**"

"The Palmer School of Chiropractic is presided over by **Dr. D. D. Palmer, the discoverer and developer of this science.**"

"The Palmer School of Chiropractic, and every student thereof, have good reasons to be proud of the large number of books that we have for their use.

"This library is composed of 897 volumes, which are in 32 sections of the Globe-Wernicke Book Case Units."

"This library also contains the only set, composed of nine volumes of original writings, of the autobiography of Chiropractic from its birth to the present date."

"**The origin and date of each article, when received by B. J. Palmer, were compiled in book form so as to prove in the future, without a doubt, the authenticity of the origin and subsequent development of the science of Chiropractic by that masterly and unique brain of its discoverer, Dr. D. D. Palmer.**"

"The cut on the left shows **a Chiropractic luxation, so named because D. D. Palmer, the discoverer and developer of Chiropractic, was the first person to bring such a sub-luxation to public notice.**"

"If Dr. D. D. Palmer had previously read in anatomies that it was almost impossible to move vertebra unless by very great force, he would not have attempted such an undertaking."

"So much depends upon this phase of the work that **Dr. D. D. Palmer** has special charge. **There is no one who has such an exhaustive knowledge in this line.**"

Before me lies a booklet of a Chiropractor. Much of it is copied, therefore, does not mix well with the author's expressions.

"Don't take drugs when Chiropractic will cure."

The science of Chiropractic does not cure. The adjuster relieves, removes the cause, then Innate can pass the impulses without hindrance.

"Chiropractic is a system of manual therapeutics."

Therapeutics consist of remedies. Chiropractors do not use remedies.

Chiropractic is a "hand practice."

Not by any means. Chiropractic is a science; it does not mean a "hand practice."

"Instead of treating disease by the effects, we adjust the cause."

A man who treats disease—the effects—knows nothing about Chiropractic.

"Effects can only be treated; causes must be adjusted, otherwise made right by replacing any structures that are not normal."

Pray, tell me, what you are going to replace—put in the place of these abnormal structures.

"When a nerve is impinged by pressure between two or more hard substances, as two vertebrae, the function of that nerve is decreased or rather there is a lack of ease, so the Chiropractor defines the term of disease of a lack of disease."

A nerve pressed between two bones is not impinged. To impinge upon a nerve is to press against it on one side. The impinging of nerves usually increases their functions, because of irritation. "A lack of ease" would be to make a person uneasy, because of irritation.

"We adjust the lack of ease."

We adjust displaced bones—not the effects.

"The nerve should be free from all abnormal pressure."

What pressure would be normal? **Any pressure** on a nerve **is not natural.** Why say "abnormal pressure"?

"Dorsal portion of the spine."

That would be the posterior side of the spine—the spinous processes. He should have said, a portion of the dorsal vertebrae.

"Imerging from the spinal canal."

Nerves emerge—never imerge.

---

The Chiropractor's Adjuster will give Chiropractors and the laity intellectual food and adjust any abnormalities found in Chiropractic literature.

## "THE CHIROPRACTIC IDEA."

"The Chiropractic idea represents the thoughts which originally led to the discovery of the basic principles of Chiropractic and later by other thinkers, to their further development."

He does not tell us what that Chiropractic idea is, perhaps he does not know.

The adjustment given Harvey Lillard for deafness led to the discovery and the development of Chiropractic as a science and an art.

The "basic principles" of Chiropractic were in that first adjustment; it was the embryo for three months; then the fetal growth; when born I had the pleasure of naming the boy Chiropractic.

The doctor tells us in six sections what "these basic principles are."

"That all nerves originate in the brain, converge at its base, forming the spinal cord, which passes out of the skull through an opening called the foramen magnum, into and through the center of the spinal column. From the spinal cord nerve filaments emerge. on each side of the spinal column, through a small opening between each consecutive pair of vertebrae, from whence they proceed to the parts and organs into which they severally terminate."

We are informed in this first quoted section that the originator discovered the basic principles. I am that originator. He emphatically states that, while all nerves (?) originate in the brain, all do not form part of the spinal cord; neither do all nerves pass through the foramen magnum.

The writer of this booklet is an M. D. If he ever followed the cranial nerves in a cadaver, he knows that the above statement made by him is far from being correct. He is wrong in his conception of **that** "basic principle." He **knows** that the olfactory and optic nerves **do not go toward** the foramen magnum, but proceed **direct to the nasal and orbital cavities.**

"Later by other thinkers, to their further development."

Space will be given in the Adjuster to the writer of this booklet, or any one else, to give the "further development" made by "other thinkers." The public would like to know who made the "further development" and what it consists of.

The above offer and request was made in the Adjuster of February, 1910; so far there has been no response. The same offer now holds good for the next edition of this, the Chiropractor's Adjuster. Perhaps the reverend gentleman who said "The man who is the foremost developer and propagator of the humanitarian science and art of Chiropractic," can name one. I do not ask for any more Chiropractic ideas, either of the science, art or philosophy which this foremost developer has developed.

The doctor further states that the "basic principles" which the "originator discovered are":

"That the vitality and activity of every organ, tissue and cell of the body is maintained and controlled by an inherent force and energy which is transformed or individualized by the brain and then transmitted to these respective parts in the form of mental impulses throughout the channels provided by the nerves."

That the "originator" discovered the "basic principle" of an "inherent force" which he named Innate, which furnished "energy to mental impulses," is correct.

He further states that the "originator" also discovered the following "basic principles":

"That when the transmission of mental impulses is normal both in volume and rapidity of delivery, or in other words, when 100 per cent of mental impulse reaches each organ and tissue in the body in a normal manner, all functions are perfectly performed with a result which is known as health. But when the normal flow of mental impulses is interfered with, in any manner, the vital activities of the tissues and organs which these mental impulses severally maintain is either increased or diminished according to the degree of interference, the result in either case being a condition which is recognized as some form of disease."

In this section he has mixed the idea of the "originator" with that of "other thinkers." I never made such a statement as "When 100 per cent of mental impulses reach each organ and tissue in the body." It is the amount of **energy** with which an impulse is transmitted that gives it **force; too much or not enough energy causes** functions to be performed in too great or too little degree.

**Per cent** is always applied to that which is capable of being divided into 100 parts. It must have the qualities of a solid, a liquid or gas. **Per cent** can only be applied to that to which the **gain may be added or from which the loss may be subtracted.** The **per cent** of gain or loss **can not** be applied to that which is psychical or mental. Therefore, to speak of a **per cent of mental impulse,** is not in accord with good usage of our language; it is incongruous, lacks intelligence and is not in accord with Chiropractic ideas.

The doctor also gives the "originator" the credit of discovering the following "basic principles":

"That the only place where interference with the flow of mental impulses to a degree sufficient to cause deranged functional activity, or disease **can** occur is at the intervertebral foramina, the little openings between the vertebrae on either side of the spinal column, already mentioned. At any of these places a slight misalignment or subluxation of a vertebra may so press upon the nerves passing out through it as to interfere, more or less seriously, with their conductive power."

Once more the doctor has the ideas of "other thinkers" mixed with those discovered by the "originator." If he will examine my writings which are locked up at the P. S. C., and which were written before I taught the science and art of Chiropractic to a living person, he will find the following: "Chiropractic is defined as being the science of adjusting by hand any or all luxations of the 300 articular joints of the human body; more especially the 52 articulations of the spinal column, for the purpose of freeing any or all impinged nerves which cause deranged functions. Ninety-five per cent of these are caused by vertebral luxations which impinge nerves."

The displacement of any bone may impinge upon, press against nerves, and thereby modify the amount of force used to propel an impulse. In the most of diseases there is too much energy, too much force; consequently, functions are performed in too great a degree.

The doctor further states as a fact that the originator discovered the following "basic principles":

"That Chiropractic affords an exact and scientific method of determining the location of any vertebrae which, on account of its misalignment, is responsible for nerve compression and also, an original, unique and most effective manner for correcting this abnormal condition by means of the hands alone, using either the spinous or transverse processes of the vertebrae as handles or levers."

The reader will bear in mind that "nerve compression" is not impingement; that there is a vast difference between **compressing a string, cord or nerve** (?) and that of impinging upon, pressing against. We do not **reduce the volume of nerves by compression; we do not make them more compact; nor do we condense their volume by compression.**

These five sections given by my friend as **the basic principles** discovered by the originator, with a few exceptions, constitute the science and art of Chiropractic as taught to my early graduates. Those "basic principles" are the basis of Chiropractic; in fact, they compose the science. I am now adjusting the abnormalities of metabolic Chiropractic literature—who has a better right to do so? You want "pure, unadulterated Chiropractic." If the originator does not give it to you, who will? If the originator and developer does not correct the incongruities of the science he has founded while he is alive, who will?

The doctor, whose letters to me display an eager desire to know all there is to be known of Chiropractic and that understandingly, correctly states:

"The discoverer of Chiropractic called this inherent power Innate Intelligence; Innate, because it is born with us and Intelligence, because it neither requires nor is susceptible of any form of education or training; its manifold and divers operations being carried on as perfectly and unerringly and with as much power, precision, indiscrimination and regularity in the helpless, newly-born babe as in the most robust and active adult."

In the early years of Chiropractic I used the terms Innate (Spirit), Innate Intelligence (Spiritual Intellect), Universal Intelligence (God), because they were comprehensive, and the world was not prepared to receive the latter terms just mentioned in parenthesis. It may be, even now premature to use them.

If it is a fact that I, the "originator, discovered" the "basic principle" for which Dr. Patchen gives me credit, and if this fact is substantiated and approved by the P. S. C. (B. J.), by offering to publish these booklets for general distribution at $2.50 a thousand, what was there left for "other thinkers" to discover or develop?

Dr. Patchen, when referring to the six quoted paragraphs, says:

"Such, briefly, are the principles upon which the science, art and philosophy of Chiropractic are founded."

If science is accumulated and established knowledge, systematized, formulated and embodied into a system, does not the six quoted paragraphs contain enough facts to constitute a science, or at least a good foundation on which to build one?

---

Chiropractic Principles. Nerves heat the body; normal heat is health; heat in a degree more or less than normal is disease. Pressure on nerves causes an excess of heat. Metabolism is normal when heat is natural—a condition known as health. These principles have been reduced to law expressing a rule of successive action of certain phenomena. They have been formulated into a system which constitutes a science.

The practical part of Chiropractic is the art of adjusting sub-luxations of vertebrae with the hands.

## NATURAL BONE-SETTERS.

A. J. Howe A. M., M. D., in his valuable Treatise on Fractures and Dislocations, on page 256, says of these Bone-Setters:

"A few individuals have gotten the credit of being natural bone-setters, but their merits, so far as they go, depend **more** upon **tact than skill**; and the prevailing credulity of the people has given them more reputation for ability than might reasonably be expected from the limited success.

"A family by the name of Whitworth, in England, and another by the name of Sweet, in Connecticut, have assumed to possess these wonderful inborn qualities. For two or three generations, one or more of the male members of these families claimed to possess a secret power for reducing dislocated bones; and not a few persons of average intelligence gave credit to these preposterous assumptions. Any uneducated man with a large endowment of boldness and self-assurance, claiming to be a natural bone-setter, could by giving every disjointed joint coming in his way, a severe pulling and twisting, accomplish some cures; the successes would be heralded far and near, and the failures would pass unmentioned and unremembered, consequently he would soon gain considerable experience in handling defective joints, and if he proved to be a good learner he would **acquire considerable skill** in his pretended art. Having received no lessons in anatomy and surgery, success even in a single case would be accepted by the popular mind as positive evidence of innate power. Love of the marvelous is so infatuating that every age will have to endure its quota of imposters. However, it is not to be denied that these charlatans have done some good indirectly. The fact that a dislocated bone could be reduced by manipulation, without the aid of pulleys and other instruments for multiplying force, led such discreet surgeons as Dr. Nathan Smith to put the manipulating plan into successful practice.

"**The Whitworths, Sweets and others of their order, studiously keep to themselves their plan of operation, though competent observers declare that it is not essentially different from the plan now followed by the most intelligent portion of the profession.** Being aware of their general incompetency in surgical science, these natural bone-setters preferred to keep secret the little knowledge they possessed, hoping to retain this meagre advantage over those who in other respects were their superiors. Probably a similar feeling actuated the Chamberlains to keep as a secret in the family a knowledge of the obstetric forceps. Such detested selfishness, by a law unvarying as that of gravitation, will taunt the name of those who in any branch of the healing art, withhold knowledge which accident or genius has placed within their power. Anything in medicine or surgery which will benefit our fellow men ought to be the common property of mankind; and he possesses a sordid spirit who from selfish motives will not promulgate a secret which will ameliorate the condition of the unfortunate. The dabbler in secrets is, by the common consent of all good men branded indelibly with the disgrace that cleaves to the quack and the charlatan.

**"It seems a pity that somebody before Dr. Nathan Smith's time did not take a hint from the Whitworth's or Sweets, and study out and put in practice a principle of reduction in dislocations which was demonstrated by those charlatans to have an existence. Perhaps the spirit of the profession was too arrogant to receive suggestions from such a source. Unfortunately for the world, good ideas are often kept from seeing the light on account of the illiberacy of the influential classes."**

Howe is the only author, so far as I know, who makes mention of the "bone-setters." Howe regrets that the medical profession are so slow to catch on and too arrogant to receive instruction from those whom they regarded as charlatans. Physicians thot it took great force to replace a displaced joint. It is a fact that joints are easily displaced and readily replaced when the subject is not resistant. If the subject is braced by muscular tension against an expectant injury, whether in displacing or replacing of bones, much more force is required; in fact, when the subject is well braced by muscular contraction, either the dislocation or reduction of a joint is almost impossible. In time Chiropractors will be given similar credit for ability and ignorance as are the "bone-setters."

The "Sweet Bone-Setters" live at Sag Harbor, a small town situated at the east end of Long Island, New York. The Old Doctor has been dead for several years, but his children, Steven, Charles and Mary, still follow the business of bone-setting. Many amusing stories are told about the Old Dr. Sweet. On one occasion he was asked by a physician where and how he got the knack or talent of setting bones. He replied: "Don't know; just came to me all of a sudden one day when I had caught a chicken and was about to kill it, and first thing I knew, I'd pulled a bone out of place. In putting it back I pulled another out of place, and I pulled another out of place in putting that back. Then, when I'd got 'em all back in place, I got an idea I'd learn how to set bones and give up farming. So, I practiced uncoupling and coupling up the bones of my dog until I learned the right twists for setting all the different bones. Guess I took that dog apart nigh onto a hundred times, on and off. He got so used to it that he seemed to enjoy it, and I do believe he missed the exercise when I let up on him."

Sweet always refused to explain to anyone, except his family, the peculiar twists that were required to set bones. The Old Doctor has migrated to a country where there are no bones to set, but his family continue the business with much dexterity.

A New York drummer, while at Sag Harbor, heard of the Bone-Setter and said: "Bet he's a fraud, and I'll prove it, too, if you fellows will bind up my shoulder so it will look as if it's broken and then call Sweet."

The shoulder was wrapped and Sweet was sent for. When the Doctor arrived, the New York man was groaning, as tho suffering intensely. Sweet examined the shoulder, smiled, and told him to raise his arm. The drummer could not raise his arm, and insisted that his shoulder was out of joint.

"You bet it is, stranger," said Sweet, "and you'll not get is back into place until you and your friends have paid me $25 for putting 'em back." The amount was finally raised; then Sweet gave the man's arm a jerk or two, which placed it in its socket.

This reminds me of two incidents, one of which was played on me as a joke, or rather to find out what there was in adjusting, or to expose me and my business. A certain physician, with an assumed name, called with his wife. He claimed to have neuralgia in his left shoulder and paid me my regular fee of $10 for an examination. I failed to find any neuralgia or displacement. He then told me who he was, that he had no neuralgia and wanted his money back. He threatened in vain; I kept the money and he the experience.

Rev. McCurdy, a Methodist minister of Davenport, had hemorrhage of the lungs, for which I gave him adjustments until he was well. At one call, he brot Rev. Smith, who did not believe that displaced vertebrae could cause disease. So, I asked him if he ever had rheumatism. He said "No." I offered to give him an adjustment, so that I might show him that vertebrae could be displaced and that such would cause disease. He gladly accepted the offer. I displaced a lumbar vertebrae, which then impinged upon the sciatic nerve. About two hours after he returned and said: "Rev. McCurdy says 'if you can make rheumatism, you can also remove it'." His rheumatism and skepticism was removed when the vertebra was replaced. It took one move to displace that vertebra and one to replace it.

The narrator of Sweet's bone-setting goes on to relate: A Fifth-avenue millionaire's mother, in her seventieth year, dislocated her hip by a fall. The best physicians of New York failed to replace the head of the femur. The man of wealth had heard of Steven Sweet and his bone-setting, while out hunting in the vicinity of Sag Harbor. So he sent for him.

A day later the door-bell of the mansion rang. The butler appeared, saw a large man with a long white beard and clothes that were well patched. The butler asked "Are you-ah-Mr. Sweet?" "I'm Sweet, the Bone-Setter," was the answer. The butler expected to see a different looking man and hesitated to let him in. Sweet became indignant and said: "I didn't come here to be kept waiting on the door step and what is more I don't give a d—— for the case."

The Bone-Setter started to return home. The butler told the millionaire of the tramp, who said that he was Sweet the Bone-setter. Sweet was overtaken and returned. Gently he handled the displaced limb; suddenly, before the onlookers knew what was being done, he gave it a twist and with a snap the bone was in place. "Now," said Sweet, as he turned to go away, "I'm no blundering doctor, thank the Lord; I'm just a bone-setter."

Fifteen minutes later Sweet left the house with a $3000 check in his pocket. He had asked $50.

I presume that Sweet's bone-setting was done by knack and a know-how, not by strength and awkwardness. The doctors watched him set bones, but failed to find the secret.

Alexander Wilder, M. D., of Newark, N. J., saw the above item and wrote me as follows under date of October 18, 1905:

In the paper which you recently published in relation to the "Natural Bone-setters," the Sweets, you repeated things that were not correct. Their origin was mis-stated and their methods hardly received justice. I care nothing for the authority to which you refer. I know something of what I am saying.

The ancestor of the Sweets had an office in the British army and taught his art to his children. They made their home first at Kingston, R. I. They were all carefully instructed in the art, but it seems to have been a rule with them that only one should engage in the business in the same town.

It may be that some of them were tricky and charlatans, but as a fact, they were simply country folk, hardly as wary and worldly wise as others. They were herbalists, as well as bone-setters and procured their own simple remedies in the woods and fields.

One of them lived and died in Newark. He was plain in manner, unpretentious, but diligent in his pursuit. When in his office he stayed behind the counter with his coat off and sleeves rolled up. His tact and perception, however, seemed almost superhuman and his probity could not be questioned.

Dr. Job Sweet represented the family at Kingston in the time of the Revolution when the French troops under Rochombeau were stationed at Newport; his services were employed with them as a surgeon. The daughter of Aaron Burr while yet a young girl had the misfortune to dislocate her hip. Col. Burr sent for Sweet to come to New York and replace the limb. He came by ship, but was with difficulty persuaded to enter Burr's carriage at the pier, lest there was some contagion. Coming to the house in Richmond Hall, now Varic Street, he greeted his patient and then applied a salve or ointment to the region of the injury. After some hours as he was about to go to bed, he asked to see her again. In a moment he had replaced the bone, then calling for a staff he made her walk. Next day many people and a score of physicians came to see the operation, but Sweet had returned to the ship and was on his way home to his blacksmith shop.

Perhaps I am visionary. I do not believe in a world beyond the present one, and in a power of perceiving what is not commonly known. There is somewhat of the mystic in my mental composition. I think that members of the Sweet family were "gifted." They were not educated in books any more than their neighbors and did not make vain pretendings. Old Job Sweet once visited Boston and a physician took him to the anatomical museum. Passing by a mounted skeleton he stopped and called attention to it. "I never saw a toiny before," said he, "but that bone in the foot is wrong side up." This was disputed, but he changed its position, knowng that he was correct. The late Thomas A. Hazard stated this in his History of the Hazard Family, and his veracity and intelligence are beyond question.

A son of Job Sweet was operating upon a patient with a broken thigh. A bystander, who knew him to be uneducated, asked him how he was able to replace the bones so exactly. He replied that he could not tell, but that he was as certain of the position of the bones when he was operating, as tho he saw them with the naked eye.

A grandson equally gifted made the following statement: "I see the bone that I am going to set just as plainly as if it had no flesh upon it."

Mr. Joseph P. Hazard of Peona Dale, R. I., having in some athletic exercise displaced the semilunar cartilage in one of his legs, applied to various surgeons, Dr. Hazard among the rest. He was told that to restore it was beyond the surgical art, that he must carry his leg bent up all his life. He visited John Sweet, a farmer at work in the hay field, and secured his promise to give him attention. At night-fall he came, well braced by a dram of liquor, as though nerving himself for a stubborn task. It need not be told that he hurt his patient mercilessly. But the crooked leg was made straight. Sweet gave a few directions and went away.

Some days later Mr. Hazard called to pay him for the operation. "I have to do a good deal for nothing," said he, "and I must charge you pretty high." The bill was two dollars. Such were the Sweets in Rhode Island.

In 1843, William Lloyd Garrison, the father of the anti-slavery movement and editor of The Liberator in Boston, spent the summer at the home of the Fourrerit Association at Northampton. Mrs. Garrison met with an accident, injuring her foot. After an unsatisfactory consultation with several surgeons, they repaired to Hartford, where one of the Sweets lived. He speedily adjusted the bones of the injured foot, as if by magic. Mr. Garrison was enthusiastic in praising his ability.

Some years ago, it is said, a Dr. Reid of Rochester, N. Y, obtained knowledge of the Sweet procedure and announced it to "the profession" as his own discovery. I have heard the late Dr. Morton Robinson of Newark describe it. He was a fellow townsman of the Sweets in Rhode Island himself, a descendant of the Hazard family and for years a partner of Dr. Jonathan Sweet in Newark. **His explanation was very simple. It was by first relaxing the tension of muscles** that were involved and then replacing the bone where it belonged, **following the same route which it had taken when fractured or dislocated**. In this way there would be no injury, and the torments to which patients had formerly been subjected would be obviated.

I have told a long story, longer perhaps than you have patience to read. It is at your service, in whole or in part, for publication, or the waste basket. But it is true to the dead as well as the living. (Signed)

ALEXANDER WILDER, M. D.

"Natural Bone-Setters" used natural means; that of relaxation and quickness, combined with the know-how made success, that which Dr. Howe calls "tact and skill." Dr. Howe says that they assumed to possess wonderful inborn qualities. If he refers to their knowledge and skill, they are certainly guilty. Howe, however, admits that these "charlatans" have done some good, that of teaching Dr. Nathan Smith and thru him the medical profession "that a dislocated bone could be reduced by manipulation, without the aid of pulleys and other instruments for multiplying force, the plan now followed by the most intelligent portion of the profession." "It seems a pity that somebody before Dr. Nathan's time did not take a hint from the Whitworths or Sweets, and study out and put in practice a principle of reduction in dislocations which was demonstrated by those charlatans to have an existence."

It is a pity that the medical profession are possessed of arrogance instead of liberality; that instead of encouraging and fostering advanced ideas, they stifle and discourage advancement; that they only adopt advanced ideas when they are compelled to do so by public opinion.

---

San Jose, Cal., July 14, 1908. James Gillman, a rancher, owning a small piece of grazing land on Mount Hamilton range and who, several years ago, became insane, has been restored to the full possession of his mental faculties by the bite of a rattlesnake. The marks of the fangs on the back of his hand bear out the tale. He was aware that he was not sound mentally. His mania has never been violent; he has lived peacefully on the ranch with his daughter.

About a week ago, according to his story, he was cutting wood back of the house, a rattler struck him on the hand while he was reaching for a stick. He ran into the house badly frightened. His daughter bled his hand, which had swollen, and showed the usual symptoms of snake bite. Several hours later, when the effects of the bite had passed off, Gillman found himself restored to saneness. His mind was as clear and active as it ever had been.

James Gillman was insane for several years. According to Chiropractic, a vertebra had been racked, or drawn out of alignment, impinging upon a nerve, causing mental aberration commonly known as insanity. Fortune smiled out of a seemingly unfortunate accident. Bitten by a rattler the venom acted as an antidote, as a counter poison.

Poisons act on sensory nerves; these affect motor nerves, which, in turn, draw vertebrae out of alignment. An antidote would be one that would exert such an effect upon the nervous system as to draw the vertebrae in an opposite direction to which it had been drawn, and to the median line, releasing the nerve which was impinged by the two movable walls of the foramen, through which it passed. In this instance it so happened that the snake venom acted on certain nerves which caused muscles to draw the displaced vertebra into its normal position. As a result the pressure upon the nerves was removed and their normal function was restored; accidental

Chiropractic. The effects of the poison passed off in a few hours. If there had not been a displacement to counteract the effect of the venom, the swelling would have lasted much longer.

A book of a dozen pages has a few mistakes, because of erroneous teaching. "The Chiropractic idea represents the thoughts which originally led to the discovery of the basic principles of Chiropractic." The discovery of these principles was due to an intelligent answer to the question, why?

"That all nerves originate in the brain, converge at its base forming the spinal cord, which passes out of the skull, through an opening called the foramen magnum, into and through the center of the spinal column." All nerves originate in the brain. The cranial nerves do not assist in "forming the spinal cord and do not pass out of the skull through the foramen magnum." "That the only place where interference with the flow of mental impulses to a degree sufficient to cause deranged functional activity, or disease, can occur is at the intervertebral foramina." This misconception will be fully answered and reinstated in this volume; do you want to know the latest development along this line by the discoverer and developer of every principle of Chiropractic?

---

Chiropractors correct the cause of diphtheria in one or two adjustments.

---

Many remedies are positively injurious, others harmless, some may be beneficial. Why not adjust the lesion which causes abnormal functions?

---

A leaflet of the National School of Chiropractic is before me. The first statement made is that Chiropractic is Nature's Greatest Ally. Chiropractic is not an ally, a helper or an auxiliary to Nature.

The personified power which produces existing phenomena does not need Chiropractic as an ally.

"The Howard System of Physiological Adjustment attacks the cause of Disease, not the symptoms." The Howard System of Adjustment was learned from The Palmers at Davenport. Chiropractic Adjustments do not attack, do not assail with unfriendly force; do not assault the cause of disease as we would an enemy; neither do we form an ally with Nature to fight an imaginary evil being.

## OSTEOPATHY.

As I have said, Osteopathy has advanced, at least as far as the definition is concerned. The January Journal of Osteopathy states, "The ideas held by Osteopaths as to the etiology of the various diseases may be summed up as follows: "Perverted mechanics: That is, mechanical derangement of the anatomic parts of the body. A very common cause of disease. Structure determines function. If the structural relations of the body tissues are all right, then the functions are normal, but if the structure is perverted in any way then the functions is also perverted, and this is what we denominate as the cause of disease. This is the Magna Charta of osteopathic declaration, the golden rule of osteopathic procedure."

"Bacteriology is alleged to be taught in every osteopathic school with the same exactness as in the best regular schools." The Osteopath has always held to the germ theory as the cause of certain diseases, and mechanical displacement as the origin of others.

The Osteopath believes that, if any portion of the body is infected with germs, by restoring a good circulation of **pure blood** the invasion of bacteria will cease. In other words, bacteria, germs and microbes, do not like, or cannot live on pure blood. They must have, according to the founder of Osteopathy, as given in his book, blood which has become bad because of stagnation and obstruction; impure, by being strangulated and detained; poisoned, by perverted circulation and a lack of drainage; diseased, by a shortage of blood supply, because of pressure on blood vessels. Why not state that germs, microbes and bacteria are scavengers; that they must have decomposing, putrid tissue to live upon.

We are told that Osteopathy is a system of medicine. Osteopaths study all branches of medicine except materia medica—and a considerable of that. Many claim to be physicians, yet do not give physic.

The founder of Osteopathy was educated in medicine; his followers cannot well evade his teachings. The February number of the Journal of Osteopathy states on page 134: "Osteopathy is a method of treating disease by manipulation. The underlying principles are: That the fluids of the human body contain all chemical substances, organic and inorganic, and hence a store of all drugs necessary for checking and destroying any disease; restoration of health by natural processes can only be prevented by the displacement of some bone or bones, which would naturally form some obstruction to the flow of the drug-saturated fluids, therefore, to cure disease it is only necessary to find the displaced bone and restore it to its normal position by the process of manipulation." This underlying principle, namely, that the body is a chemical laboratory, containing a store well supplied with all the drugs necessary for checking and destroying any disease, is well expressed on page 103: "The human body is a chemical laboratory, where are the acids, the salts, the alkalies, the solvents, etc., and how can we draw upon them with the certainty of a skilled marksman drawing bead upon his prey?"

"Pathological research will prove or disprove what we already are supposed to know and believe, but let us put up some further claims for advancement, that you and I can work out in our daily routine if we but observe and tabulate."

We find from the above that the leaders of osteopathy differ very much in regard to the cause of disease and the proper method of reinstating health. They are at sea without a compass—they do not know where they are.

A. T. Still states that the cause of disease is disturbance of blood.

A. P. Davis declares that the cause is interruption of the flow of blood.

J. R. Davis avers that deranged structure is the cause, and that they correct it by manipulating.

The Journal of Osteopathy sets forth that the human body contains a chemical laboratory, the fluids of which are saturated with organic and inorganic drugs, suitable for the cure of all diseases of the human body. Displaced bones obstruct the proper distribution of these drugs.

W. L. Harold affirms that the chemistry of inorganic matter is controlled by intelligent soul-forces.

Dr. Harold has opened his intellectual windows, allowing Chiropractic Rays of Light to shine upon his osteopathic curriculum.

Some osteopaths look upon the body as a machine; others as a chemical laboratory; and others still as inorganic matter controlled by an intelligent soul-force.

The Chiropractor looks upon the body as more than a machine; a union of consciousness and unconsciousness; Innate's ability to transfer impulses to all parts of the body—the coordination of sensation and volition: a personified immaterial spirit and body linked together by the soul—a life directed by intelligence uniting the immaterial with the material.

---

It is strange indeed, that a large number of typewriters use the capital letter I, instead of the figure 1. The Adjuster will adjust this luxation by saying to those interested, use the lower-case letter l for a figure 1. There now, take that.

## FEVER.

Fever is diffused inflammation. Inflammation is excessive local heat. Heat is a mode or rate of vibration or wave motion of ether, atoms or molecules. This vibration the sensation of which is known as heat, within certain limits, is essential to life and to all functions upon which organized beings depend for an existence. Above a certain degree heat is destructive to life and its organization. Temperature is a term used to denote the degree of intensity of heat or molecular vibration. The amount of vibration determines the quantity of heat.

Fever is that condition of the human body in which its temperature is raised above the normal limit of 99 degrees. Normal temperature has a slight variation, ranging from 98 to 99 degrees; this is not considered pathological.

The distinctive characteristics of fever are, an elevation of temperature, quickened circulation of the vascular system, a modification in the transudation of serum, chyle and lymph, increased catabolism — retrograde metamorphism, destructive metabolism, the passage of tissue material from a higher to a lower plane of complexity or specialization, tissue waste and disordered secretion.

When the temperature is above 99 degrees it is known as febrile or pyrexia, and hyperexia when above 107 degrees.

All diseased conditions are accompanied with deviations from a normal temperature. Temperature is subnormal when below 98 degrees. A collapse is an extreme depression and prostration because of lack of vital energy. The extremities are cold, the features pinched, and the skin is covered with a clammy sweat, accompanied usually with a sinking sensation and nausea.

A sudden rise of temperature from the normal is accompanied with chills and rigors in consequence of a contracture of the nervous system; this hypertension is relieved by the diametrical expansion of the nervous system which the heat causes. The human body is no exception to the rule of expansion by elevated temperature; this is more noticeable in the nervous tissue than elsewhere, as it is thru this system that heat is created and conducted. In chills and rigors the skin and nervous system are contracted.

When one of the bones forming a joint is displaced from its normal relation with other bones, it is said to be dislocated. Dislocations are traumatic when they are the result of violence; pathological, when they owe their displacement to destructive changes in the joint and toxic, when they are due to poisons which irritate nerves, causing contraction of muscles which in turn draw bones out of alignment. Dislocations may occur in utero as the result of any one of the above causes; if so, they are called congenital. A dislocation is traumatic; its displacement causes destructive changes in the joint or its surrounding tissue; such changes are pathological. The cause of dislocation may be predisposed, gradual or immediate. It is predisposed when the ligaments are lax; gradual, when the change is progressive and immediate when it occurs suddenly.

Pain is produced by bone pressure on nerves. Sprains refer to injuries resulting from impingements upon the nervous tissue by bone pressure.

Increased temperature indicates the presence of a nerve irritant. Irritants are traumatic or toxic. In fever, the tissues of the body lose more or less of their substance because of toxic irritation.

Toxicosis is a disease caused by poisons; a toxic or poisoned state; the conditions of disease induced by poison. Disease is an inharmonious action of functions due to structural change. Abnormal tonicity and the performance of functions in an unusual manner always accompany each other; it could not be otherwise. A toxicide is a remedy, an antidote, which prevents the usual effects of poisons.

Poisons affect nerves as irritants or narcotics. Every living organized tissue is capable of being irritated in response to a stimulus which may be normal, traumatic or toxic. Narcotic substances have a stupefying effect.

Those substances are poisons which, when introduced into the body from without, occasion pathological alterations of function and structure; these lesions are known as toxic in contradistinction to those which are traumatic. Poisons create nervous disturbances, modify functions and structure.

Some poisons, as chloroform, chloral, alcohol, digitalis and quinin cause a reduction of temperature. This is because they induce in the nervous system a pathological effect of sense depression. These substances render the nervous system, with which they come in contact, more or less lax, therefore the nerves possess a less degree of molecular action, less carrying force. In anesthetics, the sensory nerves are so affected that they fail to vibrate, do not carry sensation. A temperature below 92.3 degrees is nearly always fatal. The lowest recorded temperature terminating in recovery is 76 degrees in a profoundly intoxicated individual. Other poisons, such as strychnine, nicotin, picrotoxin, veratrum, laudanum, cause an elevation of bodily temperature. The highest temperature recorded by Wunderlich before death was 112 degrees Fahr.

## CARVER ADJUSTING VISCERA.

Carver's Analysis for adjusting displaced tissue says:

"**It is** not **the intention of this book** to discuss in detail all forms of abnormality, but only **to state the principles entering into all, with the discussion of a sufficient number to make the principles plain.**"

All right, you say you will now go ahead.

"**Adjustology is** a very **comprehensive** department of Chiropractic, and must be studied, **except** as to **its cardinal principles,** in clinic, and by demonstrations upon the living body. It consists in the principles, methods, processes, movements and forces which should be properly employed in restoring any character of displaced tissue to normal situ."

If adjustology is comprehensive, give it to your readers. Oh! It is very comprehensive, **except** the principles, methods, processes and movements employed. Leaving these out, what is there left on which to write a book? The principles of adjusting comprise the science, a very essential part to be understood.

He intended to use the word "situs," the Latin for site, situation, location or position.

If the cardinal principles of adjusting can only be taught in the clinic, why did you state in the preface that you would make the principles of Chiropractic plain by discussing a sufficient number of abnormalities?

"Visceral adjustment consists in replacing a displaced viscus in its normal position and relation, and having it remain in situ. This is accomplished by the art of adjusting, which consists in the position or positions of the subject, the position or positions of the adjuster, and the elements of the process employed in returning the viscus to its original position and relation. **This subject can only be taught by demonstration upon the living body.**"

In the first quoted paragraph, Dr. Carver refers to adjusting of any kind of tissue; in the last quoted he refers specially to the organs of the three lower cavities of the body.

"The manipulation for adjusting the sacrum and viscera for hemorrhoids **can only be taught by demonstration** and acquired by much careful practice."

Hemorrhoids may be internal or external. Chiropractically, they represent the same condition as a prolapsed rectum. All prolapsed viscera are so because of a lack of tonicity—their nerves and muscles are flaccid. Take off the pressure, relieve the lumbar impingement. There is no need of adjusting the sacrum or of replacing the prolapsed bowel. Hernia is nothing more or less than a prolapsed intestine, for the relief of which use the same principles and good judgment.

"Adjusting to replace the liver **must be demonstrated and cannot be described.**"

"Adjusting a floating kidney **cannot be taught except by demonstration.**"

Prolapsed kidneys, liver or stomach exist because of lack of tension—nerves and muscles lack tonicity.

"The manipulation, for sprains and bruises, where the tissue in the area itself is displaced, **can only be taught by demonstration.**"

If a joint, vertebral or otherwise, be wrenched sufficiently to impinge upon nerves or laceration of the ligaments or vertebral cartilage occurs, replace the joint by all means.

"After adjusting, to remove the occlusions of the first, second and third dorsal, it will be the duty of the Chiropractor to correct the displacements in the tissue of the thorax."

"Subluxated articulations may present a myriad of appositions which, of course, cannot be described and must therefore be left to the educated and delicate discernment of the Chiropractor acquired in clinic."

The apposition of adjacent articular surfaces, presents only juxtaposition of parts—normal articulation. Subluxations exhibit but few variations; but to discern and learn the knack of replacing them requires practice.

The Chiropractor will be surprised to learn that he has been neglecting a large share, and a very important part, of his work, namely, that of replacing viscera and tissue, other than that of the osseous frame-work. The student will be disappointed to find that that which he desired to know, that which induced him to buy the book, cannot be taught except by personal demonstration.

Dr. Carver has definitely stated that he cannot teach the adjusting of luxated bones or the replacing of organic tissue, except by clinical demonstration. He has given no information whatever in regard to adjusting, replacing, any tissue, altho the preface of his book reads: "It is no small task to evolve an analytical, logical, consistent and authoritative text-book which, **in its comprehensiveness, presents for the first time a newly constructed science; so that the student and practitioner may experience no difficulty in applying the same.**"

I fail to see where Dr. Carver has "evolved" anything logical or consistent. His dissertations involve rather than evolve the principles and art of Chiropractic. I trust that no one will consider his disquisitions as authoritative. The author lacks comprehension of his subject. His book will not assist the student or practitioner in applying the art of Chiropractic scientifically.

Prolapsus—a falling down—a displacement of the stomach, kidneys, liver, spleen, ovaries, uterus, vaginal walls, bladder, including hernia and internal and external hemorrhoids, is the result of the relaxation of their muscular supports. This slack condition, lack of tonicity, is owing to impingements upon nerves and muscles. Remove the osseous pressure.

The reader should understand that Carver adjusts vertebrae, as well as displaced viscera. Take off the pressure and allow nerves to resume their former vigor, normal tonicity. Do not forget that disease is either too much or not enough functional activity. The supporting tissue of viscera may be too tense or too lax in tension. In all cases of a relaxed, flabby, flaccid condition of the tissue, there will be found a corresponding condition of the nerves.

To each muscle of the body a nerve containing motor and sensory fibers is distributed. A few muscles receive two or more nerves. The action of a muscle is dependent upon the nerve of motion attached to it. The sensory nerves report the condition of laxity or tension existing.

---

"The Howard system of Chiropractic." I presume that The Howard system is more or less Chiropractic, as outlined in a booklet of 32 pages. What Howard knows of Chiropractic he learned of the Palmers. He opened an office with a drug doctor. He retained some of the drug system and at that time did not get all of Chiropractic. He must have imbibed some of it later while associated in business, although he states the Howard system is a "drugless healing system." The Howard system is one of the many **healing** systems. Chiropractic is not a healing system. All **healing** systems use remedies supposed to contain some inherent quality which acts as an antidote, or as an assistant in combating disease. Chiropractic is not one of the healing arts; it does not use remedies; it does not treat diseases. It is the only system that claims to, and does, adjust the cause of ailments. Chiropractic is a drugless system, but it is not a healing system.

We find several ear marks which belong to the medical profession, such as "a **powerful** factor in **aiding nature** to **throw off** disease; disease is **vanquished** and **completely banished.** He will **equip** his students to **combat** disease." He ends by saying, "What you have learned will not have to be learned again." A student of the above mixture of drug and Chiropractic principles will have to **unlearn** much before "embracing all there is known in the science." The same cranium cannot be filled with a drug education and that of Chiropractic. This booklet abounds with medical terms, such as: "other methods of treatment," just as though Chiropractic was one of them, which it is not. "Chiropractic system of treatment"; "other methods of treatment." Chiropractic is not a method of treatment. "Revolutionizing the various curative methods." We are not changing other methods. Chiropractic is peculiarly a method of its own; it is unlike any other; it is not built upon, or out of others.

"It cures where all else fails." This is copied from a stereotyped plate used by every advertising quack.

A general shortening of the spine by a contraction of the intervertebral cartilage, as occurs in old age, will not produce a luxation, a separation of articular surfaces. During a fever, the vertebrae and intervertebral cartilage adjacent to the impinged nerves, become softened by reason of excessive heat; the bodies of the vertebrae become thinner, owing to the contraction of muscles and superincumbent weight; the cartilage is deprived of a portion of the ground substance, leaving the fibrous portion intact. After the subsidence of the fever (excessive heat) the bodily temperature often falls, for a time, below the normal. During this period the bones and cartilage become hardened. Extreme conditions, **either way from normal,** cause disease.

---

Points of tenderness, on either side of the spine, do not always accompany sub-luxations. They will always be found where nerves are subjected to an over-amount of heat; but lacking where heat is below normal. The former condition enlarges, while the latter lessens their diameter.

---

The science of Chiropractic has given us the cause of disease, a knowledge for which humanity has been hungering since the dawn of civilization. It will, in time, do much to relieve poverty and crime, for they are largely diseased conditions. It will in time empty our jails and penitentiaries; it will give us a conscious connection with that unseen life which is believed in by all nations. In the near future we shall replace belief with a comprehensive knowledge.

When disease and crime no longer exist, and mankind live to a ripe old age, then the divide, known as death, will be passed with a knowledge equal to that we now have of disease. Then death, instead of being feared, will be welcomed because the life beyond the veil will be comprehended and known to us as we now know and comprehend this.

## HYPERMEGASOMA.

The following quotation is from the Seattle Times: "Hoy Walters, a young man of this city who has suffered the misfortune of being a hunchback, has, during the last two weeks, undergone a transformation by which the hunch of four inches or more has entirely disappeared from his back, and his height has increased fully one and a half inches. This phenomenal transformation has taken place despite the fact that the young man is 22 years old. The case is one of the most freakish that has come before modern surgery in all time, and has, so far as known, only one parallel. So far, the physicians who have the case in charge are unable to make a satisfactory explanation of the matter, but they are inclined to feel that it must be classed as what is known as Pott's disease. The suddenness of the change helps to substantiate this condition."

Several years ago I increased the height of a woman, aged 26, an inch a month, for three months, by Chiropractic adjusting. I wasted all her waists. Several of the vertebrae were wedge-shaped. By returning them to their normal position, they assumed their former shape.

We occasionally see, or read of, an accidental adjustment.

All deformities of the spine arise from injuries. Displacements may occur at birth or during infancy. A relaxed condition of the muscular system favors both displacement and replacement.

"Modern surgery classed it as Pott's disease." Pott's disease is a destruction of the bodies of vertebrae by osteitis. As this disease progresses, the spine bends forward where the bodies of the vertebrae are destroyed; thus, an angular projection is formed.

Before me is a vertebral column in which the body and pedicles of the first lumbar are absent. The last dorsal with which it articulated above, is uninjured. The second lumbar lacks three-fourths of its body; a portion oozed, covering its inferior intervertebral cartilage. The first and second are fused, ankylosed. This destruction and ankylosis were caused by hyperthermia—excessive heat—too much functionating. Later the temperature fell below normal and the bones hardened. Functions performed more or less rapidly, or vigorously than normal are pathological.

Gus Noque, from whom the specimen was obtained, writes me: "At death that part was a mass of decayed bone and flesh; one of the worst specimens I ever saw."

Excessive heat—pathological functionating—had necrosed, softened the osseous tissue and its surroundings. This was a case of Pott's disease. The one referred to above, which "is one of the most freakish that has come before modern surgery in all time," was one of spondylitis deformans, not Pott's disease. The vertebrae had grown wedge-shaped because of pressure on nerves and muscles; the bodies gradually assuming that form.

I have for many years taught and demonstrated that all kinds of curvatures are the result of one displaced vertebra. If so, and that one were replaced by the Chiropractor or by accident, the effect in either case being the same, the resulting condition would not be considered freakish; it would be a natural outcome from certain causes. This is specific Chiropractic. See article on rachitis.

"As far as known," this case has "only one parallel," which we give below. The reader will see that the "parallel" case is not an analagous one.

"The suddeness of the change" shows that it was not Pott's disease.

The following clipped from the same paper is the "parallel" case referred to:

"An inch a month is the average growth during the past seven months of Edward H. Whitley, of Antrim, N. H., who died at the home of C. F. Belcher, 148 Hawthorne street, Maldon, Conn., at the age of 21 years. From a boy Whitley grew very rapidly causing him to be poor in health most of the time. A short time ago he came to Malden, where he developed consumption. At that time he was six feet tall, but after being ill several months the young man died. Measurements showed him to be seven feet and one inch in height, having grown an average of an inch a month during his illness. The case has puzzled the medical world and, so far as known, this is the record for rapid growth."

The last quoted case is neither one of Pott's disease nor of spondylitis deformans. It is a case of hypergigantosoma, excessive height.

I have made many inquiries of hypergigantosomas and hypermicrosomas and find that giants and dwarfs usually have kidney trouble. It is the office of the kidneys to separate from the lymph and blood the excess of salts and thus maintain a normal balance.

Sodium chlorid—common salt—occupies a peculiar position among the inorganic constituents of our diet. Altho it exists in our food in relatively large quantities, we purposely add more. It is estimated that the average man ingests from 15 to 30 grains—one-third to two-thirds of an ounce—a day. This amount seems in excess of the actual necessities of the body.

When an excess is taken in, it is removed by the kidneys. In a diet free of salt, the amount of sodium chlorid—salt—secreted in the urine soon falls to a low degree, showing that the tissues are holding onto this constituent.

Sodium chlorid--salt—is of importance in furnishing material for the growth of the skeletal frame. This has been demonstrated by feeding experiments. Pups when fed on a diet poor in calcium salts—lime—fall into a condition resembling rickets, owing to a deficiency of lime salts in the bones. As in the case of all foods, there should be a definite amount of calcium and chlorid salts retained by metabolism. Most of the salts ingested pass thru the body without entering into its structure. They are eliminated, unchanged or unused. in the feces or urine.

Whitley's rapid growth was not the source of his poor health. The displacement which caused his abnormal increase in height was the origin of his poor health. The first mentioned case increased in height by straightening the abnormal curvature. The second, by regular growth made by increasing the length of the long bones, which takes place at the epiphyseal cartilages. The extremities—diaphyses and epiphyses—do not become joined until growth has ceased. In Whitley's case, at the age of 20, the epiphyses had not become solidified to the diaphyses. Functions performed physiologically means health; pathologically—above or below normal—disease. Giants and dwarfs are abnormal—the result of functions either excessively or insufficiently performed. If kidney metabolism is pathologic, there is either too much or not enough inorganic elements retained—the ossification of the epiphyses being hastened or delayed accordingly. Herein is the explanation of gigantism and dwarfism. The science of Chiropractic and its philosophy explains many heretofore unexplainable abnormalities.

---

Chiropractors are especially interested in bones and nerves, as the bones are the frame-work of the body, and the nerves the line of communication through which all sensations are conducted. They are more particularly interested with those of the vertebral column, for ninety-five per cent of diseases are caused by their displacements.

**Diagnosis** is the recognition or determination of the nature of disease and the pathognomonic signs of each. The act of recognizing a change in organs, functions or vital phenomena, in contradistinction to that found in health, deciding therefrom as to its character, is diagnosis.

Chiropractic diagnosis or analysis, is radically different from any other method; as much so, as adjusting causes is different from treating effects.

The physician makes his diagnosis from the subjective symptoms experienced by the patient; the objective signs perceived by himself; the chemical analysis of excretions; the microscopic examinations of morbid tissue; occular spectrum analysis; percussion; ausculation; pulsation; respiration; palpation and temperature. From these he determines the nature and progress of the affection and prescribes for the morbid conditions found.

The Chiropractor depends largely upon the subjective and objective symptoms, as his material to **locate the cause** of the ailment. Knowing the organ or part affected, he is able to **locate the impingement** which is the primary cause of deranged function. An examination of the region indicated, reveals to the educated fingers and eye that a vertebra or other bone is out of alignment, that the two articular surfaces have in a measure separated, causing one or both bones to be not only pressing against sensitive nerves, but, by their muscular attachment, the nerves are drawn tightly. The inclination of nerves to shorten when over-heated, affects joints, muscles, fibrous and serous structures, causing a great variety of diseases whose nature depends upon the structure involved. The fever, local swelling, distress, deformity and disability are dependent upon **nerve contraction,** and increased molecular nerve vibration. Dunglison says, "The morbid anatomy and etiology of rheumatism remain doubtful. The causes commonly ascribed are the presence of lactic acid, uric acid, or excess of fibrin in the blood, cold, and micro-organisms." The morbid conditions referred to as being probable causes are but effects the result of functions performed in an abnormal manner.

The medical man prescribes remedies for the treatment of effects. The Chiropractor adjusts the cause of deranged functions.

---

Two booklets entitled, "God has been misunderstood," and "God's witness to divine healing," state: "Divine healing is diametrically opposed to these (Christian Science, Metaphysical Healing, Hypnotism, Theosophy, Mind Healing, Trance Evangelism and Spiritualism) diabolical counterfeits which are utterly antichristian. These imposters are only seductive forms of delusion, which deceives many."

Mrs. Eddy pours out her execrations on all forms of the above mentioned list except her science.

They forget that the Great Healer said to his disciples, "Forbid him not; for he that is not against us is for us."

## NEUROPATHY—WHAT IS DISEASE?

On page 380 we are told that disease is an **organic or functional departure** in the system from a normal standard of the structure.

Page 116 says that disease consists in **affections differing from the normal.**

On page 669, the cause of disease is inharmony—**an inharmonious condition is disease.**

On page 16, Dr. Davis would have us understand that "**disease is a product**," from which we infer that health is also a product.

Pages 154 and 165 tell us that diseases seem to resolve themselves into **a mental ideality**—functional human ills, which may be dispelled, forced to get out of the body.

### The Cause of Disease.

In Neuropathy, page 257, we are informed that **inharmony** of the entire body **is the cause of disease.**

Page 202 says, Nerve strain, overuse of the nerves, cause, is **exhaustion**, and this results in what **is** dominated **disease.**

On page 33, Dr. Davis says, disease is the result of an **unbalanced condition** within one's own self and not generally due to something outside of the body.

Pages 17 and 513 enlighten us on this question. He says: It may be from cold contracting and closing the pores of the skin, a retention of the waste material which creates a **poison.** This is reabsorbed into the system, producing a **contamination of the blood**—disease.

On pages 201 and 204, we learn that it is a fact that all diseases are due to **nerve waste**, that by preventing this nerve waste, all ailments are cured.

On 669, we find disease is caused by **an excess of acid or alkaline** secretions.

On 14 and 257, we are notified that **nerve irritation** is the cause of disease.

Page 172 informs us that the blood is the life of the body, that blood is the product of food, that the kind of product—**disease** or health—**depends upon what we eat.**

Page 202: "Disease anywhere in the body is a result of **loss of nerve power.**"

On 402, we find the following instruction: The sympathetic nervous system directs and controls every action in the human body. **A modified or retarded suggestion,** executed, **produces all the pathological disturbances known as disease.**

On 137, we are told of Neuropathic causes adjusted by Chiropractic art: Inasmuch as all diseases are due to too much acid or alkaline elements in the body. There is no necessity of being sick with any chronic affection if the **spine is properly adjusted** daily, semi-weekly, or semi-occasionally.

On 163, **perverted nature** is given as the cause of all diseases; also, "as a man thinketh in his heart so is he."

Page 412: The letting down or the rousing up of the system, in any degree, is the result of **chemical changes** that take place in the body elements. If this is not understood, the comprehension of the meaning of disease has not dawned upon the mind of the reader.

On pages 207 and 213, the author tells us that "**nerve strain of the eyes** is the cause and source of all functional diseases."

On 257.—"So far as medicines are concerned those of homeopathic are more scientifically administered than those of any other medical system, as they supply the molecules with the element needed in a way that changes conditions and harmonizes the entire body with itself."

On 258, we receive the edification, that it is a fact, that **wrong living** is the cause of disease; therefore right living is the best means of restoring health.

On 209, we learn that **nerve exhaustion** is the cause of the various diseases to which we are subject.

On 401, we are told that **disturbed action** is the cause of all diseases.

On page 124, bacteria (bugs) is **not** the cause of disease.

On 208, **overuse of the eyes** is the reason given for disease.

On 377 and 480, he remembers his osteopathic text-book and says, that **the whole cause of disease**, in every part of the body, **is obstructed circulation.**

On pages 412 and 514, we are informed that **retrograde metamorphosis, chemical changes** in the body elements, are the cause of disease.

On 669, we are told that the **ununited** condition of the **two forces,** positive and negative, is the cause of disease.

Pages 28 and 122 state that impingment of nerves is the cause of disease, and all that is necessary to know is, what nerve is impinged upon. When the pressure is removed, all will be right.

On 401, we are told that certain results are brot about in the system by certain manipulations, how, is as **obscure** as the sun at midnight.

On 663, we learn that **disease consists of** three conditions, **invasion, retention and enervation.**

On 16 and 289, we are informed that the key to all pathological conditions is **nerve pressure.**

On page 513, we are admonished that if we would cure anything in the form of disease we must **take off the pressure.** It is downright cruelty to add more weight or pressure to the load by giving food before it is demanded. On 120, we find that all bodily complaints are **because of spinal trouble,** which must be looked after and corrected.

On 665 and 666, we find the **reasons given** for such a **diversity of causes and so many methods of treatment.**

"**In medicine, we have certain kinds for given conditions.** These constitute the curriculum of specifics. The routinist having tried his specific for a given condition and failed to obtain relief, his limit is reached and he improvises other means."

"**In the treatment of the various conditions called disease, it is well to have various recources to draw from** in order to meet the special demands at the time, so as to render the needed service for the given condition."

---

"**The Science of Chiropractic: It is written by Dr. D. D. Palmer, the discoverer and developer of Chiropractic.** . . .

"A hasty glance at its contents reveals to us that it is the **product of long experience, observation, and study by a man of penetrating intellect and originality.** . . .

"**The Science of Chiropractic contains,** moreover, **a thought of which no one else has ever dreamed.** Dr. Palmer has the key and has entered the secret of nature's laboratory, where he found the cause of human disease recorded. The efforts made by others have been all in vain suffering humanity has been the victim of experiments by those whose delusive hope was that man needed some external agent in order to correct his internal disorder by producing some chemical change in one way or the other, in the constitution. And the melancholy failure of this sort of experiments only increased pain, misery and death in the human family. **Dr. Palmer reached the conclusion that man can be diseased only when the mind failed to perform properly its functions. His ingenious and profoundly scientific theory is that the mind governs organic functions through the nerves connecting mind with body.** The brain impulse is generated by the brain under the command of the Innate mind, or the soul, and is carried along nerves to every individual cell in the living organism, regulating its functions. He states that the **brain impulse** in its transmission along the nerves **can be interrupted only when they are impinged upon** while leaving the spinal foramina, by sub-luxated vertebrae. When such a condition exists, in a living organism, the abnormal condition called 'disease' is manifested."

The fly leaf of the above volume of 413 pages—a compilation of the writings of D. D. Palmer, contains the following:

"With my kindest regards, I present you with No. 1 of the first issue of the first book ever published on Chiropractic.

"From son, B. J. Palmer, D. C., to father, Dr. D. D. Palmer."

The title page, date 1906, says, "**The Science of Chiropractic, its principles and adjustments by Dr. D. D. Palmer, Discoverer and Developer of Chiropractic.**"

The preface contains: "**B. J.**, the only son of D. D. Palmer, **cherishes and reveres with ardent fidelity any of his father's manuscripts pertaining to the development of Chiropractic.**"

Some inaccurate statements have been made in the above, regarding the science. As I shall not always be in the Chiropractic field, and desire to leave the science as free from dogmas as possible, I will correct all mis-statements that are in sight.

---

All nations have some form of home manual treatment.

---

Chiropractically: All functional and tissue variations from that of normal is disease.

Accidents may cause displacements of bones; if so, their pressure produces impingement upon the nerves with which they come in contact.

Poisons act on sensory nerves; irritation and contraction follow. By their action on muscles, bones are drawn out of alignment and they impinge upon sensitive nerves.

Pressure on nerves causes them to expand diametrically and contract longitudinally; to become more rigid and super-sensitive. Their carrying capacity of impulses is augmented. Increased energy enhances the vegetative and cumulative functions.

---

**The Clinic** should give the student an opportunity to put to practical use that which he has learned from lectures and the class-room.

A student learns the history of the case from symptoms and outward signs. From these he constructs his diagnosis locates the region where the lesion exists. He then examines the patient by digital palpation, locates the displacement, traces sensitive nerves to and from the parts affected. Important questions are answered. The adjuster should know what vertebra is luxated; how long and in which direction; the probable shape it has assumed; whether ankylosed or not; what nerve or nerves, and on which side or sides, it or they are impinged, and the movement required to replace it.

## LOCK-JAW OR TETANUS.

Definition:—This affection consists of a series of painful and violent contractions of the voluntary muscles, either of the jaw alone or of a considerable part of the body, while the intelligence and mental faculties remain unimpaired. In the majority of cases the disease occurs after a wound or injury, while in others there appears to be no exciting lesion.

The earliest symptom is usually a stiffness of the muscles about the neck and the back of the head, which is noticed upon awakening in the morning. This stiffness extends to, or begins in, the muscles of the lower jaw; the throat becomes dry and somewhat painful. At, first, the pain and stiffness may not attract attention, since precisely similar symptoms have been attributed to the position of the sleeper. But it soon becomes evident that this is something more than the stiffness following a cold draught or the position during sleep, for the jaws are found to be firmly closed by the spasmodic contraction of muscles. At first the patient opens his mouth with great difficulty and swallows imperfectly. It is from this feature of the affection that the disease derives its name of **Locked Jaw.** In some cases, these contractions remain limited to the muscles about the neck and face. The mouth, in many instances, cannot be opened either by the patient or by the use of force. Nourishment can be given only through the spaces which naturally exist between the teeth. Sometimes the muscles of the face, also, are involved in these contractions, occasioning the most frightful contortions of the countenance. Sometimes the muscles of the throat are so much involved that swallowing becomes quite impossible."

If the muscles of the trunk also become involved, the movements of the chest, necessary for breathing, are embarrassed, so that the patient, at times, seems to be in danger of suffocation. The abdomen is drawn inward and becomes very hard and stiff. Sometimes the limbs are similarly affected so that they are held as firmly as bars of iron. In such cases the entire body may be raised by a single limb, or even by the head, as if it were a statue.

In many cases, when the limbs and trunk are involved in this rigidity the body does not rest flat on the back, but takes the shape of a bow, the weight being supported by the head and the heels. Sometimes the body is bowed in the opposite direction, so that the patient can be placed with his head and toes on the floor while the body remains raised a few inches. It may be that the body is bent toward one side or the other.

The sufferer from tetanus is a most pitiable object. The remarkable positions which the body assumes during spasms, the fantastic and distorted countenace produced by spasm of the muscles of the face, the peculiar, sardonic grin caused by the contraction of the muscles about the mouth, and, withal, the evident pain and distress of the individual combine to render the sight an extremely painful one.

The muscles remain rigid continuously, but there occurs, at intervals, spasms whereby the force of their contraction is increased. It is during these spasms that the peculiar postures noticed are assumed by the body. These paroxysms occur at intervals, and vary extremely in duration; they are attended with extreme pain.

The mind remains unaffected; there is no delirium nor stupor in uncomplicated cases. The spasms are more apt to occur during the day than at night, presumably, because the influences which can excite the patient are more abundant by day. There is, usually, some fever; the skin is often moist with clammy perspiration. The disease usually terminates fatally in from two days to two weeks. This disease may occur in infants as well as in those half grown and in adults.

The convulsions of tetanus and those caused by strychnine poisoning differ. In tetanus the locking of the jaws comes first, while in strychnine poisoning it comes last. The convulsions of tetanus rarely, if ever, completely relax, while those of strychnine do have periods of complete relaxation.

Etiology:—This disease may occur from local lesions; if so, it is named traumatic tetanus, because it occurs as a result of the wound. It may be from poison which enters thru wounds or food. The infant may be poisoned by the mother's milk. Extreme anger will affect the milk while in the mother's breast. The poison causes muscular rigidity. The muscle is shortened, thickened and becomes somewhat denser; it is stiff, firm and solid, incompletely elastic and not extensible. In every case the lesion will be found to be that of a poison.

Pathological Anatomy:—The lesions will be found in local wounds or from poisons in the food.

Pathologic Physiology:—The rigidity of muscles is due to toxins which cause abnormal nervous action. The ganglionic chain is the distributing agency of this pathologic physiology. The toxin of tetanus is very poisonous, which accounts for its short duration and fatal ending. The spasmodic seizure first affects the muscles near the point of infection. In mild cases it may be confined to these muscles. The nerves are so extremely sensitive that a flash of light, a breath of air, or a sudden noise provokes a paroxysm.

Disease is a term which means any deviation from health. It may be defined as any departure from normal structure or functionating. By some, disease is applied to structural change and disorder to functional derangement.

It is a self-evident fact, that normal structure and normal functions are co-existent. It is also true, that change of structure and a corresponding change of functions must exist.

To have faulty secretion, absorption, circulation, respiration, digestion or bodily heat, we must have both disturbed functions and abnormal tissue.

---

Quality and price are what counts; we have both.

---

Peoria, Ill., April 22, 1909.

Dr. D. D. Palmer:

I like The Adjuster very much. Your adjusting is not any too severe. It will take systematic and heroic work to prevent curvatures becoming permanent. The backbone of Chiropractic literature needs close and careful attention during its infancy, so that it will not be disfigured in adult life.

I note that you say in regard to laying the hands and arms alongside of the patient, while giving adjustments, to prevent bracing. I know that I get better and quicker results since using this method Some adjusters are slow to see and use that which is for the patient's and the Chiropractor's welfare.

A. HENRY, D. C.

---

Dr. D. D. Palmer.

Dear Sir: I cannot express my surprise and delight in receiving No. 2 of The Chiropractor Adjustor. Its ring is just right; every page speaks the sanity of Chiropractic.

I am glad to note that The Adjuster is doing some adjusting along lines which is sadly in need of such. I hope to see these so timed and delivered that the very foundation of pseudo "Fountain Heads" will be severely shaken.

Coming back to The Adjuster, let me say, that your manner of handling the nervous system, is based on sound reasoning, and will surely appeal to the better element. This line of thought from The Fountain Head assiduously advanced in addition to other up-to-date ideas, will place all pseudos hors de combat.

## METASTASIS.

Metastasis is a term used by pathologists to designate the change in position, manifestation or character of a disease, as in mumps, where inflammation of the parotid gland is seemingly transferred to the testicle, resulting in a condition known as orchitis.

Metastasis is the transferrence of disease from one organ to another not directly connected with it, as in tumors and metastatic abscesses.

In the prolonged convalescence of typhoid fever, numerous, remote, suppurative lesions present themselves, such as periostitis, ostitis, parotitis and orchitis.

Metastasis, from a medical view-point, is a transference of diseasesd conditions, thru the blood currents.

All tumors are not limited to the part or region in which they first occur. Secondary nodules resembling the first may appear in nearby or distanct parts of the body; this change is called metastasis. The secondary tumors are known as metastatic. This seemingly, to blood pathologists, transposition of tumors, is accounted for by them, as transferrence of diseased cells thru the blood or lymph; others contend that micro-organisms escape from the diseased portion, find an entrance into other tissue and, because of a depressed vitality, succeed in establishing a footing.

Chiropractors hold that **all functions are the result of thot transference from the center to the periphery of the nervous system; that functional activity is increased or decreased according to the speed with which the impulse is carried and that momentum depends upon the volume of the vibration** which **transmit it.**

**Chiropractors recognize the various changes known to the medical fraternity, as metastatic, but do not concede that they are transferred thru the blood, lymph or any other channel.**

Closeby organs may become affected by diffused heat, as we have said elsewhere.

Other nerve-branches than those affected may become impinged upon by the same pressure which caused an over-excited or depressed condition of the trunk-nerve. Remember, the different filaments of a trunk-nerve reach various organs and parts of the body.

---

"Your policy has been one of consistent opposition to the administration."

"Yes," answered the agitator. "My motto is, 'Be sure the other fellow is wrong and then go ahead.' "—Washington Star.

## PRESSURE ON NERVES.

The backbone is known as the spine or spinal column, because of its projecting spinous processes. It supports the weight of the head, connects the bones of the thorax with those of the pelvis, and forms a basis of support and attachment for the ribs. Owing to its curves, intervertebral disks and its large number of slightly movable bones, it is prepared to lessen the effects of shocks. It furnishes a bony canal for the protection of the spinal cord and fifty-eight foramina and six grooves for the safe exit of the spinal nerves.

This column of bones form the backbone of the neuroskeleton. It sustains, gives firmness to and supports the splanchnoskeleton. It gives proper position and shape to the body thruout, and not only furnishes a support for the organs, but also for the nerves and vascular system.

The vertebrate endoskeleton is composed of segments, the skull and the vertebral column, which serve to protect the central nervous system from injury. The seven bones of the cranium, namely, the occipital, two parietal, frontal, two temporal and the sphenoid wedge form a bony envelope surrounding the enlarged portion of the cerebrospinal nervous axis. The brain fills the cranial cavity so closely that its impress is evident upon the cranial surface; whereas, the spinal cord occupies only a portion of its bony case. In no place does it touch the walls of its passage-way. The same intelligence which enveloped the brain in a solid covering, made ample room for the spinal cord and also provided for the safe exit of the thirty-one pairs of spinal nerves.

The bones of the upper expansion and the five of the lower, widened surface, become coalesced, while the twenty-four intervening segments remain separate.

The spinal cord is an outgrowth of the central nervous system. It occupies the spinal canal, composed of twenty-six bony rings, the upper and lower encircle the foramen magnum and the sacral canal respectively. Twenty-five vertebral foramina and the sacral canal compose the spinal canal.

Pressure upon any portion of the nervous system, whether of the brain, spinal cord, or its nerve branches, increases or impairs its carrying capacity of impulses, deranging the sonsory nerves, or causing too much or not enough functionating. An organ so delicate and sensitive refuses to perform its functions properly when encroached upon.

There are four kinds of nerve lesions: 1st, concussion, a shaking, jarring, agitation or shock caused by a collision of bodies; 2d, compression, to press together, to make more compact, to reduce in volume, to make narrower in one direction by expanding in another; 3d, squeezing or pinching by pressure between two opposing, hard substances; 4th, impingement, to impinge upon or against by pressure upon only one side of an object.

The brain is a soft mass of tissue, easily injured by concussion which is not necessarily accompanied by fracture. Fractures of the skull may result from falling bodies or personal encounters; they may be impacted, the fragments driven into each other, or partial, that is, the outer table may not be broken, yet the inner table may be fractured, the fragments pressing on the brain. Fractures of the skull may be compound or comminuted. If a depression takes place, there will be a hollow, the shape of which will depend upon the instrument by which it was made. There is no separation of the fragments, except that which is produced mechanically, as there are no muscles in the skull to cause displacement by contraction.

Fractures of the skull are healed as readily as those of other bones. On account of no separation, they require but little callus, consequently there is no thickening or deformity. The trouble may not end here, as a fracture may injure the brain by an impingement of the depressed portion upon the brain. Traumatism may lead to serious consequences. The outer table may not show any fissure or crack and yet the inner table be depressed; if so, grave consequences will result because of pressure. The fracture may be of the vault, the outer or inner table, or both. If pressure exists, inflammation is sure to follow, as an impingement upon nerves creates irritation and irritation produces an excess of vibration, and heat as a consequence follows.

There are three primary states of functional disturbance, arising from injury to which the brain is subject, namely, concussion, pressure and irritation. Any one of these may be followed by or be complicated with, inflammatory actions of various kinds that derive much of their peculiar characteristics from the conditions with which they are associated and the injuries by which they are occasioned.

Contusions of the skull, where there are no signs of a fracture, may affect not only the bones, but the membrane, pia mater, and the brain itself. The patient complains of malaise, headache, stiffness of the muscles of the neck, giddiness, chilliness, nausea and vomiting. The temperature rises and the senses of sight and hearing become very acute, as the result of too much functionating. Paralysis of some portion of the body may follow, the portion affected depending upon the part of the brain injured. If the pressure be local, the alteration or abolition of functions will be local, as paresis or paralysis of an arm or leg, or half of the face, alteration or abolition of speech, modified sensory or motor impulses. If there be an impingement upon the optic nerve or its tract, neuritis of the optic nerve will occur; if there is a displacement of a portion of the temporal bone, then an impingement upon the auditory nerve will be found and hearing will be interfered with.

The cranial nerves may be injured by pressure in the part of the brain which gives them origin, or along the pathway of the nerves themselves.

Concussion of the brain consists of an organic lesion and of necessity functional disturbance. Concussion consists of a stunning or shock communicated to the nervous system from the application of external violence, which produces commotion in the substance of the brain. As a consequence its functions become temporarily suspended, usually in a slight and transitory degree, but occasionally to such an extent that the patient does not rally for many hours, because of the depressed state into which he is thrown. In those cases in which death results from the continuance and severity of the concussion. the pathological conditions vary. In some cases the brain substance may exhibit no structural lesion; in others it may have been rendered soft and semi-diffluent by the shock to which it has been subjected, even tho no distinct rupture of its substance appears to have taken place.

Paralysis of one or more of the cranial nerves, after an injury, is evidence of pressure. Deafness and facial paralysis afford evidence of an impingement from a fracture or a displacement of osseous tissue. Pressure on the brain substance arrests or modifies function. The mass of nervous substance known as the brain is sensitive to pressure; its functions are easily modified by some portion being impinged upon.

The brain is well protected against injury by the hard bony skull, the thickness of which varies in different persons and in different regions in the same person; the density is modified by diseased conditions, the result of varied temperature. The bones of the skull are elastic; this elasticity diminishes from youth to old age.

Injuries of the head are important as they may involve the brain, the great nervous center. The treatment of fracture of the skull is based on the injury to the brain, rather than that of the skull. The prognosis depends almost entirely upon the brain lesion. Very little callus is used to heal a fracture of the skull; if great, it would cause pressure on the brain.

Cranial pressure on the tissue of the encephalon produces

encephalitis. Inflammation softens the brain tissue, produces focal necrosis and sclerosis. If the patient recovers, the temperature falls below normal and focalized or diffused sclerosis follows.

Encephalitis may be the result of a toxic or traumatic lesion. In many of the so-called infectious diseases, as diphtheria, typhoid, tetanus, lead poisoning and alcoholism, changes take place in the nerve-cells of the brain and spinal cord. Poisons irritate nerves, cause an increase of molecular vibration and an excess of heat. Traumatism may result from direct pressure upon the brain covering or an impingement on some one of the recurrent nerves which innervate the meninges of the spinal cord and brain. Poisons injure the brain tissue by irritation or by being lenitive.

The brain and its membranes are subject to inflammation followed by irritation which causes excitation of function. This alteration may apply to the intellectual, the sensory, or the motor functions of the brain, resulting in mania or coma, hyperesthesia or anesthesia, spasm or paresis, apoplexy or paralysis.

Inflammation of the dura mater, pia mater, the arachnoid membrane, cerebrum or cerebellum may be determined on the post-mortem table, but not as clinical instruction. The temperature may rise to 103 or 104 degrees. The pulse is at first full and heavy but afterwards light and weak. During life it is impossible to diagnosticate with any degree of certainty, inflammation of the membrane from inflammation of the brain.

Hyperplasia relates to the formative action of new elements; hypertrophy to an increase in bulk of already existing normal elements. These conditions, decreased or increased variation of normal functions, are pathological; each has its causes and is accompanied by hyperthermia or subnormal temperature.

Hypoplasia, arrested development of the brain, necessarily follows early union of the cranial bones; on the contrary hydrocephalus, water on the brain, separates the cranial bones by the pressure of the accumulated fluid. Hypoplasia of individual bones may occur from a local or general condition. General hypoplasia is found in cretans and dwarfs.

Microcephalia, advanced cranial ossification, may depend upon an intra-uterine condition, because of excessive heat on the part of the mother during gestation; or from an injury at birth or later in life, on account of which the temperature being subnormal, the production of the red corpuscles must lessen and that of the white increase, causing an early coalescing of the cranial sutures and a decrease of the diploe and consequently a compression of the encephalon. Altho the parts are smaller than usual, they may be properly proportioned. The convolutions are less numerous and abnormally narrower than in the normal brain, a condition known as microgyria. In rare cases the convolutions become membranous in character and so thin that they contain but little nervous tissue. Mycrogyria is not only a coarse, morbid lesion, but it affects the finer structure of the brain, being characterized by a loss of some of the cortical layers and a diminution or total absence of nerve-cells. The brains of such unfortunates may possess only one-third to one-half of the normal weight. The coalescing of the cranial bones is due to an impingement upon the sixth dorsal pair of nerves.

Cerebral localization is the determining of limited areas in the brain which preside over certain physiological functions, or are the seat of pathologic conditions which interfere with the proper functionating of these centers. Post-mortem examinations and animal experimentations have shown that certain parts of the brain are the seats of special physiological acts, and that pressure on such localities interfere with the proper discharge of functions. The cerebellum is supposed to regulate the vital and vegetative functions. That the cerebral functions are localized, has been proven and accepted only in the last few years, although cerebral surgery has been practiced much longer. The different parts of the brain differ in function as much as do the different viscera of the abdomen.

To trepan or trephine is to operate on the skull with an instrument of the same name; the trephine is an improved trepan. A trephine is used to excise a circular piece of bone from the skull. It consists of a cylindrical saw operated with a carpenter's brace. From the middle of the saw projects a center-pin which secures the saw; around the outer surface is a ridge to stop the progress of the saw as soon as the bone is perforated. The trephine is not placed on the fissure or crack, but next to the fracture. An opening seven-eighths of an inch in diameter allows the surgeon to raise the depressed fractured bone, thereby relieving any pressure it may have caused—just the thing to do. In many cases it is only necessary to introduce the point of an elevator underneath the fragment as a lever to raise the depressed portion.

From the mass of nervous material, known as the brain, there arise 43 pairs of nerves, 31 pairs forming a bundle or cord and finding a safe outlet thru the foramen magnum; the remaining 12 pairs are transmitted thru other foramina in the front and base of the skull. The 31 pairs of spinal nerves are cared for in the spinal cord which extends from the upper borders of the atlas to the lower border of the first or second lumbar vertebrae. The bundle of nerves which leaves the conoid, the distal end of the spinal cord and occupies the lower part of the canal, is designated as the cauda equina.

The spinal cord and its coverings are lodged in the neural canal. It does not occupy the whole cavity of the spinal canal, being separated from the inner surface of the vertebral arches by the contents of the extra dural space. The spinal canal is enlarged in the cervical and lumbar regions where there is the greatest amount of movement; the spinal foramen of the atlas affording more room than any other vertebrae, as it needs greater space because of more movement. A fracture of the vertebral column, at any point between the occiput and the third lumbar vertebra, produces an injury to the spinal cord; all the body below the fracture at once loses, completely, both motive power and sensation. The great nerve-center, being impinged upon or compressed, loses its functionating power, altho the parts depending upon it for nerve vitality are not paralyzed. The higher in the column the fracture, the greater the part of the body affected and the graver the consequences. Complete disorganization of the spinal cord is attended with entire loss of sensibility and motion below the point of injury, showing that the cord is the organ of communication between the brain and the external organs of sensation, and voluntary and involuntary motion. The degree of displacement without any symptoms of pressure is often considerable, owing to the absence of attachment of the spinal dura mater to the walls of the canal and to the relatively small size of the spinal cord.

Altho the spinal cord is protected in its jointed tube, it, nevertheless, is subject to injuries, fractures and luxations. Injuries of the spine, like those of the head, derive their importance from the extent to which the inclosed nerve-cord is implicated. Vertebral fractures are rare when compared with others, constituting only 3.3 per cent. The most common cause of fracture of the spine is forced flexion by the caving in of embankments, falls from scaffolding and railway accidents. As a rule there is associated with fracture of the vertebral column a tearing of muscles, laceration of ligaments, a crushing of the cancelated tissue of the body of the vertebra into the spinal canal and displacement of vertebrae. The portion of the spine above the fracture slips forward and pinches the spinal cord between the arch of the vertebra, immediately above, and the edge of the body of the broken vertebra. Owing to the squeezing of the spinal cord, there is more or less paralysis of motion and sensation or both. Rectification is secured by extension and counter extension, with manipulation, pressing the bones into position. If extension fails to replace the displaced vertebra, resection of the posterior arches or laminae is resorted to, for the purpose of removing the pinching and continued irritation and, moreover, the return of normal functions. Laminectomy is the name given to the operation of removing the laminae or posterior arch for the relief of pressure.

Concussion of the spinal cord is a condition which seems impossible, owing to the manner in which the cord is protected and held in the center of the neural canal, being free from the bones which surround it.

The symptoms of compression of the spinal cord, from fracture or luxation, are numbness, tingling and paralysis of the lower limbs and loss of control of the bladder and rectum.

Localization of the functions of the various segments of the spinal cord have been determined more accurately than those of the encephalon. Much has been determined, much is inferred, yet, there is more to be ascertained. The segments of the spinal cord correspond to those of the vertebral column, each segment consisting of the portion of the cord with which the several pairs of the spinal nerves are connected.

The spinal cord contains all of the spinal nerves; they cannot be encroached upon by the movements of the twenty-six segments of the vertebrarium. They find their exit from the spinal canal thru sixty-eight openings, of which eight anterior and ten posterior are in the fused sacrum, where there is no possibility of compression or pinching except by fracture. Six pairs pass thru wide, open grooves, the first and second pairs of the cervical and the last pair of the sacrum. There are many diseases arising from impingement of the first four spinal nerves; yet it is impossible to compress or pinch them in those wide, open gaps, called grooves, located between the occiput and the axis. Be it remembered, that the skull is the first vertebral section above the occipital nerves and that the nerves impinged upon are next below the displaced vertebra. For the relief of each pair of nerves, we adjust the next vertebra above the impingement. Who ever heard of anyone adjusting the skull for the relief of the first pair of cervical nerves? However, there are Chiropractors who, osteopathically, make use of the head as a lever, whereby to adjust cervical vertebrae. If there is no possibility of the first pair of nerves being compressed or pinched between the atlas and head, where can they be impinged upon? Please take your spinal column in hand. Throw the atlas to either side and observe that the sharp edge of the inferior articular process impinges upon the gangliated chain as it passes in front of the transverse process. Now, understand that this gangliated chain is a distributing agency consisting of nerve-fibers; that the ganglia are relays for the transmission of impulses from the region in which they arise to the tissues in which they are distributed; and that it reaches into the cranium thru the carotid canal, forms the carotid and cavernous plexuses, distributes nerve-fibers to several of the cranial nerves, noticeably to the fourth and fifth pairs. No Chiropractor has attempted to explain, with cuts or otherwise, how a displaced atlas compresses or pinches a nerve.

In adjusting the atlas, do so by striking it on the right or left side of the posterior arch, depending upon the direction you wish to move it, extending the hand, using the third joint of the little finger, being careful to place the hand between the occipital bone and the axis. The distinct click accompanying the movement, is caused by the striking of the transverse ligament tubercle against the odontoid process.

The brain is protected by its enveloping membranes and the close-fitting cranial bones. The vertebrarium is constructed thruout for the protection and safe transmission of the nervous system. The spinal cord has an abundance of room in the spinal canal, so much so, that the vertebrae in their normal movements do not touch the cord. The spinal nerves, also, have ample room to pass out thru the spinal column, without being compressed, squeezed or interfered with by pressure.

The spinal nerves originate in the brain, descend in the spinal cord and find their exit from the spinal canal thru sixty-eight openings. In the skull, the nervous tissue is liable to injury only by concussion and fracture. In the spinal canal the cord which contains the spinal nerves can only be impaired by complete luxation and fracture, which usually accompany each other. The spinal nerves emerge safely from the spinal canal thru intervertebral foramina and grooves. Sixteen of these foramina are in the fused sacrum and cannot be compressed or pinched therein, except by fracture. Three pairs pass out thru grooves. Of these the lower pair is in the sacrum and the other two are between the occiput and axis. Only because of fracture can any one of these nerves be compressed or pinched. Of the forty-six pairs remaining there are ten of the lumbar which make their exit thru large foramina, so constructed by the interlocking of the articular processes that compression or squeezing is out of the question except by fracture of the articular processes which, indeed, is a rare occurrence.

Fractures are accompanied with pain. It may be spontaneous when the part is at rest and is not always limited to the seat of injury. It is localized from external pressure or from the movement of the fractured ends. These sensations arise from pressure, known as impingements, against sensitive nerves.

The nervous system can only be concussed by jarring or shaking; impinged upon by pressure in the skull; and compressed, squeezed or pinched in the vertebral column and the intervertebral notches by fracture. By a slight displacement of bones, especially those of the feet and more particularly still those of the vertebral column, nerves may be impinged upon by bone pressure which contracts nerve tissue, causing an undue irritation, an excessive vibration and hyperthermia, with all its accompanying derangements.

Nerves are impinged upon or against by pressure; in no case are they compressed, concussed, squeezed or pinched except by fracture.

---

"You don't seem to have faith in Dr. Lance as an appendicitis expert."

"Why should I allow him to cut the appendix out of my dictionary?"

---

South Bend, Ind., March 19, 1909.

I think I have all Chiros beat on the youngest patient. Our daughter was adjusted when she was one day and two hours of age. That one adjustment corrected her of diarrhea.

DR. M. KUECK, D. C.

Dr. M. K., it is not considered good taste to place Dr. and D. C. both to your name. Either one is correct.

B. J.'s child was adjusted by his grandfather when he was four days old—you get the persimmon.

---

Every molecule consists of atoms. Ponderable atoms do not cohere, they are separated by spaces. Interposed ether prevents immediate contact of atoms. Solid bodies have fixed forms; their molecules are arranged in a permanent figure, an unchangeable relation to each other. Fluid bodies have a variability of shape, their molecules are constantly undergoing change of form.

Heat is the result of atomic action. There are three forms, or degrees of heat; animal heat, light and fire. These owe their different degrees to the number of vibrations in a given time. Vibrations are of a tremulous character. Deviations of heat have each their variation. Pathological changes are due to the modification of animal heat.

From page 105 I quote: "Dr. A. P. Davis, an Osteopathic author, of whom I have heard it said, was the real originator of Osteopathy instead of Dr. Still, has recently (1905) written a book called 'Neurology,' in which Chiropractic is taught as a part of Osteopathy and lauded as the greatest curative method known."

Dr. Davis does not state or infer in his book on Neurology, that Chiropractic is a part of Osteopathy. The following are brief extracts: Page 1, "We take up a method of application called Chiropractic, really what we call Neuropathy." Chiropractic is from two Greek words, which mean hand and done by—not a practice of the hand.

Page 6, "We evolved from Osteopathy and the Chiropractic system Neuropathy." Page 7, "Results of the application in the Osteopathic and Chiropractic sciences." Page 107, "We learned the fundamental principles of Osteopathy from Dr. A. T. Still, Kirksville, Mo." This does not read as though A. P. Davis claimed to be "the real originator of Osteopathy," as stated on the page we quote from. Page 142, "Evolved from the Chiropractic, the Osteopathic and Ophthalmic sciences a system we name Neuropathy. We hesitate not to state that our system of practice embraces all there is known in Chiropractic science as taught by its originator, and all there is in Osteopathy, and all there is taught in Ophthalmology." Dr. Davis means to state that Neuropathy does not "embrace all there is known in the three sciences—Chiropractic, Osteopathy and Ophthalmology."

Page 36, "No one is properly a scientific manipulator who does not understand how to adjust the spine, even if all taught by Osteopaths has been applied; for there is nothing comparable in Osteopathic manipulations which so effectually accomplishes the purpose as this does; for no one in Osteopathy has even known how to apply these treatments but those who have taken special instructions therein from what Dr. Palmer calls Chiropractic."

Dr. Davis took a course in Chiropractic of D. D. Palmer in October, 1898, and B. J. Palmer in 1902. Strange indeed, that the latter developed—see page 28—the science of Chiropractic and the art of adjusting four years after I taught it to Dr. A. P. Davis. Astonishing to read on page 29, B. J. Palmer, Chiropractic Fountain head." Surprising to find on page 40 that "Dr. B. J. Palmer . . . developed the philosophy, science and art of Chiropractic." However, when we know that he wrote that notice and caused it to appear in the Arenac Independent of Standish, Mich., the untruthful statement is accounted for. If you do not want the kinks straightened, stop twisting Chiropractic literature.

Page 94, "This method was discovered by Dr. D. D. Palmer in 1895. He found that all diseases were invariably accompanied by certain irregularities of the vertebrae, and became convinced that therein lay the cause, which was simply a pressure upon the nerves at the point of exit from the spinal column, and that this robbed the organs supplied or controlled by them, causing a diseased condition to exist. This science has further been developed by his son, Dr. B. J. Palmer, who was able to verify this by tracing the nerves to the parts affected and back to the place of impingement, and reasoned that if this pressure could be removed the disease would disappear of itself. He also argued that if displacements could exist, there must also exist a means to correct them. Thus was the principle established, but it took years of hard work and the assistance of many trained minds, to develop it into a success. In the last few years several schools have been established where it is taught, and the graduates have formed quite a strong association, but as yet it has not penetrated into the eastern states, to any great extent."

There are many statements in the above which are not correct and I do not know of a better time to straighten them than the present. It does seem to me that all Chiropractors should know what Chiropractic is, when and how it originated, and above all, be pleased to see luxations adjusted.

True, Chiropractic was discovered by me in 1895. But, it has taken me since 1895 to develop what there is of it, and yet the man who "evolved" it, has advanced it very much in the last six months. The Chiropractic method was developed by me, not discovered. I never stated that all diseases were caused by, or accompanied by irregularities of the vertebrae. I have always stated that about 95 per cent are caused by deranged vertebrae, the other 5 per cent by other joints which are displaced. I never claimed that pressure robbed the organs of their supply, that this robbery was the cause of disease. Impingement (pressure on nerves) causes too much heat, an excited condition. Excessive heat, known as inflammation and fever, expands the fibers which compose the nerve, causing too much tension and greater vibration. Too much or not enough functionating causes an abnormal amount of heat.

The tracing of sensitive nerves was practiced and taught to several students by me several years before I taught it to B. J. The principles spoken of were established by me years before B. J. graduated. Instead of there being one association of Chiropractors, there are several.

### "CHIROPRACTIC ADJUSTMENT.

"The graduates of The Palmer School think adjusting the most wonderful discovery ever made.

"As soon as Dr. (D. D.) Palmer had ascertained that any one or more of the 110 articulations of the spinal column were liable to be displaced and create diseased conditions, he set about to contrive some way of replacing them.

"If Dr. D. D. Palmer had previously read in anatomies that it was impossible to move the vertebrae **unless by great force,** he would not have attempted such an undertaking. He soon found that it took **nack, not strength.**

"This reminds the writer (D. D. Palmer) of a Chiropractor (O. G. Smith), who attempted to teach adjusting. He thought it **needed strength and muscle**; that no one should be taken as a student who weighed less than 140 pounds. He had exercising tables and was persistent for two months in drilling his students in physical culture, so that they might **develop the required strength** to move a vertebra; he had probably read some work on anatomy, which said, that it was impossible. (The original says "that it was almost impossible to move them.") His three lady students became disgusted and lost weight by such physical culture. **It needed a teacher who had a clear conception** (so, it does today) **of the movement. A knack was to be learned instead.** (The original, "A knack was to be learned instead of the use of great strength.") Persons of light weight make as good adjusters as those heavier. One lady student weighed less than 100 pounds. To learn to adjust is an important part of the work. **There is no one so well adapted to teach this unique movement** as the man who scientifically carried it into execution." (The original says, "**the man who conceived and carried it into execution.")** The above, even with the changes made by "**the developer,**" teaches the light, quick, elastic move.

It has just dawned upon me, that Dr. Finkelstein has read the above in The P. S. C. Announcement of 1909, and is in a quandary why he should have been taught to use great force in adjusting, when this item (which was written by D. D. Palmer and copied by B. J.) teaches light adjusting.

---

Ether fills the space of the universe. Through the vibration of its atoms, the light from the sun, moon and stars is made visible. Ether pervades all space; it penetrates the interstices between the smallest particles of ponderable matter. It is the medium of light and heat. Agitation of ether atoms transmits heat through space and bodies.

## THE SYMPATHETIC NERVOUS SYSTEM.

All nerves originate in the deep mass of the brain. Twelve pairs remain in the cranium; therefore, they are named cranial nerves. These do not pass into and down the spinal column. All others are known collectively while in the spine, as the spinal cord. This cord is, in fact, a large bundle of nerves some of which are responsilbe for the innervation of the skeletal muscles, while others go to the cuticle covering the trunk and limbs. The cranial nerves look after the cuticle of the face and scalp. Some of the spinal nerves — nerves of the spinal cord, in contradistinction to the cranial nerves—find their way to the interior of the four cavities of the body. Please return with me and know that the spinal cord is composed of several kinds of nerves, all of which form one harmonious bundle. This collection of mixed nerves are divided into thirty pairs, each a part of the spinal cord; therefore they are known as spinal nerves. They pass out of the spinal canal through thirty pairs of openings named foramina. Now watch closely. This cord or bundle of nerves is divided into sixty bundles or trunks, each containing innumerable nerves, filaments or fibers in a separate sheath. Remember that this bundle of nerves which forms the trunk and goes to and ramifies the body in its various portions, is being transported for convenience in one covering through the intervertebral foramen. As soon as this trunk, or bundle of spinal nerves emerges from the spinal canal, it divides into four branches. The first is a small one named the recurrent branch. It is joined by a branch from the sympathetic and re-enters the spinal canal by way of the intervertebral foramina. This recurrent branch is distributed to the spinal cord and its membranes or coverings. Very close to this branch is a second which immediately divides into two divisions known as the posterior and anterior nerves. The posterior branch is divided into two, known as the internal and external. These are called the somatic branches of the spinal nerve because they go to and provide for the frame-work of the body in contrast to those which go to the cavity organs, or viscera, by way of the vertebral ganglionic chains. We notice that the second branch is divided into anterior and posterior divisions. On the anterior branch, close to where it originates, its apparent origin, is an important branch to a Chiropractor. It is known as a communicating nerve — communicans of the sympathetic cord. The sympathetic chain of ganglia is almost wholly dependent upon this branch of the spinal trunk for innervation to run its various functions. At each spinal foramen it receives a branch communicans. In this way the organs in the cavities of the body, as well as the limbs, receive their innervation from the brain through the different branches of the spinal nerve trunk.

The above has been written especially for a P. S. C. graduate who asks, "Where is the sympathetic nervous system? How can any system be sympathetic? How can there be more than one system?" These questions remind me of a boy who, twenty years ago, persisted in using his left hand to figure and write. His teacher insisted that he should use his right hand. The boy was equally as persistent and determined to use the hand which the teacher said was his left, therefore, was not his right hand—it was the right one for him. This peculiarity in his make-up has always existed and is today a prominent feature. It took him years to learn that his right hand was the one on his right side. He was two years learning to understand the difference between **mis**placed and **dis**placed. He finally made such progress that he used the two words interchangeably. Knowing the boy, we excuse him for his perverseness and awkwardness in handling the nervous system. He will get his eyes open and see it all right in time; but in the meantime he will **develop** other vagaries to take its place. So, with this P. S. C. graduate; he has been frightened by the name "sympathetic." There is nothing in a name that should frighten him. If this one division of the three had been named the Splanchnic, he would not have been so terrified; he would have comprehended the true situation. Never mind the name; there are any number of names given to bones, nerves, muscles, ligaments and blood vessels which he and I do not like, but those parts of the body so named are there, just the same.

The subdivisions of the nervous system are called splanchnic, ganglionic nerve system, the sympathetic nervous system, the vegetative system, the involuntary nerves, those of organic life which act more slowly than those of the voluntary, those which are especially under the control of Innate, and are situated in the four cavities, head, chest, abdomen and pelvis. Any system of telegraph, telephone, or of nerves can be divided and subdivided. For convenience, the nervous system is divided into three systems; those of the cranium, those which are somatic, ramifying the walls of the body, and, the very important ones, the visceral nerves. "That is dead easy." The name sympathetic, or that of any one of the above, only designates a certain part of the nervous system. No Chiropractor or physician, so far as I know, now states that any nerve or portion of the nervous system is sympathetic in function. It was no great discovery to learn that a system of nerves, named sympathetic, were not sympathetic in feeling; one organ not expressing pity or sympathy with another. If it suits you better, just say the nerves of the head; the nerves of the four cavities, and the nerves of the walls. There should be nothing in a name to horrify you, more especially since your teacher now states, "I wish to be clearly understood as saying that what has so many times been dissected as the Sympathetic Nervous System **is there—I do not question that for an instant—it is there.**"

An extension to the main part of a house, that portion used as a kitchen, is named an L; it is a part of the house. Shall we say that the kitchen does not exist, just because it is named an L? The building may be divided into three or more parts; just so, the nervous system may be divided for convenience of description and study. Shall we deny the existence of a portion of the nervous system just because it is not named according to our conception? If you do not like the name of the L part of the house, or a certain described portion of the nervous system named the sympathetic, just call them by some other name. But don't show your ignorance of architecture or anatomy by saying that neither exists.

---

Gravitation, motion, heat, magnetism and electricity are only varying modes of manifestation of one and the same force—molecular, atomic action. Organic and inorganic force co-exist with atoms.

---

A Napravit booklet tells its readers of "a case of **headache** which **had fastened itself to the patient,**" and of "**curing female troubles** that **had** been a constant **drag** for **thirty years.**"

A headache that would fasten itself to the patient must have been a mean headache. Female troubles that dragged, must have been difficult to pull; equal to "a slow pull on a ligament is of no avail."

---

Those who contemplate entering a profession will find in Chiropractic a golden gateway to success. No work is more noble than that of alleviating humanity from suffering. There is no system of healing that begets so much interest as the study of Chiropractic; the affection is traced to where nerves are impinged upon and in acute cases the impingement relieved by one or two adjustments. Fever cases are returned to normal temperature in a few minutes.

## QUEER FREAKS OF LIGHTNING.

Perhaps the most surprising result of a lightning stroke is to be seen in those cases where no real harm is done, though the injury to the clothing makes it certain that the lightning did hit the person, as must have occurred in one instance in which a watch chain was fused without injury to its owner. It is, however, more common for temporary unconsciousness to be present, even if perfect health is regained. A very curious effect is sometimes produced. The person struck is killed and yet he remains in the very attitude in which he was at the moment of death. Eight farm laborers were resting at dinner time under an oak when they were all struck and killed by the same flash of lightning. When found they appeared to be still eating. One held a glass, another was carrying a piece of bread to his mouth and a third had his hand on a plate. In another case a woman was struck while picking a poppy. The body was found standing with the flower still in her hand. The most probable explanation of these occurrences is the instantaneous onset of **rigor mortis,** and it has been shown experimentally that in animals killed by electricity the onset of **rigor mortis** can be hastened by increasing the strength of the current.

Perhaps the most curious accompaniment of a lightning shock is the stripping off the clothes. This appears to be very common. Dr. G. Wilks, of Ashford, Kent, describes a case in which a man was struck by lightning while standing by a willow tree. Immediately afterward his boots were found at the foot of the tree and the man was lying on his back two yards off, absolutely naked except for a part of the left arm of his flannel vest. He was conscious, but much burned, and his left leg was broken. The field around was strewn with fragments of clothes, which were torn from top to bottom. The boots were partly torn.

Flammarion mentions a case in 1898 in which three women were standing round a reaping machine. One of them was struck by lightning and killed; the two others were uninjured, but they were stripped absolutely naked, even their boots being removed.

---

The spinal, cranial and sympathetic are nerves of distribution. The word sympathetic, when applied to a system of nerves, does not imply that they are in sympathy with any other system. Only by those who cannot comprehend how a word can have more than one meaning, can such an idea be entertained?

## FRACTURES OF THE VERTEBRAL COLUMN.

In this article I shall consider the cranium as a part of the vertebral column, because its six flat bones not only constitute the upper expansion and provide a protective covering for the vital portion of the nervous system, but because their displacement, in whole or in part, causes impingements upon the brain.

A fracture is the breaking of a bone by external violence or by the contraction of muscles; the former will be the only one considered in this disquisition. Fractures are applied to cartilages; they constitute a portion of the backbone.

There are many kinds of fractures, but I shall only consider those found in the spinal column.

A buttonhole fracture is one in which the bone has been perforated by a bullet; this may be incomplete, a piece of bone may be chipped off or punched out.

A comminuted fracture is one in which the bone is splintered, shattered or broken in several places.

A compound fracture is one in which there is an external wound.

A contre-coup (pronounced kontr koo), contra-fissure, counter stroke, is an indirect fracture, a cranial fissure or fracture produced by a blow upon the skull at a point distant or opposite to the fracture.

A depressed fracture is one in which a fragment of bone is driven inward, below its normal position.

An epiphyseal fracture is one confined to the union of an epiphysis to the shaft of a bone.

A diastasis is a separation of bones, more especially the bones of the cranium.

A gutter fracture of the skull is one in which the depression is eliptical, an oblong gutter-shaped depression.

A pong fracture is one in which the fissure circumscribes the radiating lines, causing a circular depression.

A stellate (star) fracture has a central point of injury, from which fissures radiate.

Fractures of the skull are of less consideration than the injury done to the brain substance and its membranes. A blow or other violence may leave no visible fracture, yet, the inner table may be splintered, depressed and impinged upon, press against the encephalon, or its substance may be concussed, causiug temporary suspension of functions.

Functional disturbance of the brain may arise from concussion or impingement. External violence may produce commotion of the brain substance, communicating a shock or shaking, an agitation of its makeup without a fracture, in consequence of which, functions may be suspended or modified. Where death is the immediate result from the severity of the shock or concussion, no lesion may be found, but the cerebral substance may be rendered soft, semi-diffluent, so as to be incompatible to life, even tho no distinct rupture of its substance appears. In the more severe forms of injuries to the head, the surface becomes cold and pale, the patient is insensible and motionless and only answers when spoken to in a loud voice, relapsing into insensibility or rather semi-unconsciousness. The pulse is feeble, the pupils contracted, the limbs flaccid, the muscular power lacking. Concussion of the brain may terminate in recovery or death. Post mortem examinations may show no visible lesions, only the morbid softening of brain tissue. If the patient has survived for some time and the temperature has become subnormal, there is hardening of the tissue, a condition known as sclerosis. Do not forget for one moment that, hyperthermia softens and hypothermia hardens tissue; that excessive heat increases the per cent of erythrocytes, and a decrease in temperature increases the leukocytes; that a normal number of red and white corpuscles is maintained by a normal temperature of 98 to 99 degrees.

Compression or impingement, arising from the pressure of a depressed piece of bone, is a common result of fracture of the skull. There will be more or less paralysis, depending upon the amount of pressure and the area involved. Care should be exercised in differentiating between coma, a symptom of some diseases and semi-consciousness as a result of traumatic injury.

Traumatic encephalitis--inflammation of the brain substance and its membrane from injury—causes the formation of more or less serous fluid and pus. The vascularity of the brain and its envelopes is greatly increased, the sinuses are distended and reddened with blood. The thoracic and abdominal viscera are liable to be affected, more especially the lungs and liver. These conditions point to a sub-luxation of the 6th dorsal or the next vertebra above; if this is the case, palpation will find those nerves taut, inflamed and tender.

Fractures of the skull are invariably the result of external violence, which may act directly in breaking and splintering the part struck, the fissures extending a considerable distance; or the violence may act in an indirect manner, producing a fracture at a part of the skull opposite to that which was struck. A person falling strikes the ground head-first or on his feet and fractures the base of the skull, or the atlas, by the force of the shock communicated to it. The fracture may be indirect, opposite to the part which is struck, named contre-coup, contre-stroke. A singular instance of contre-coup was shown in President Lincoln's skull after his assassination. The bullet pierced the left side of the occiput and passed to the cranial base below the right anterior lobe. The autopsy revealed a fracture in the roof of the right orbit, which had not been touched by the bullet. A person falling from a height, may strike some object on the way down with sufficient force to account for at least a portion of the counter-stroke injuries received. Muscular tension has more or less to do with fractures. If two bodies, one dead and the other alive, fall from the same height, the dead body will receive no broken bones or at least no counter-stroke fractures. The loose and passive condition of infants and the drunken seems to prevent fractures.

Fracture of the base of the skull may cause paralysis of the cranial nerves; especially of the optic, facial and auditory nerves. Deafness and facial palsy may be caused by fracture of the petrous bone. Pressure on the brain usually causes paralysis in some portion of the body. Dr. J. Thomson says: "In some instances of paralysis from sabre-wounds, as well as those made by gun-shot, paralysis was confined to the upper and in others to the lower extremity. In every instance in which it distinctly appeared that the injury existed on one side of the head, the paralysis uniformly manifested itself upon the other; but, we were unable to perceive any other fixed relation between the part of the brain which had been injured and the part of the body affected with palsy. A wound of the right parietal bone by a musket-ball was followed by palsy of the left arm and leg. In another case, a wound, penetrating the upper part of the right parietal bone, was accompanied with a slight paralytic affection of the left side of the mouth and complete palsy of the left leg. In a third case, a sabre-wound of the same bone, followed by extensive exfoliations, gave rise to a complete palsy of the left side."

A depressed fracture of the skull may be simple, that is, without a scalp wound, compound or comminuted. The external table alone may be depressed, especially over the frontal sinuses, where it may be broken into those cavities, or the inner table may be driven in without fracturing the outer table. In all depressed fractures, the inner table is splintered to a greater extent than the external. Fractures of the vault are usually the result of direct violence, while those of the base are from indirect violence, as by the weight of the body when striking on the head.

Fractures of the skull are of the vertex or vault and the base. The vertex includes all that portion between the orbital ridges in front, the occipital protuberance behind and the external auditory meatus on the sides. The base of the skull includes all below and beneath the lines making these points.

The surface of the impinging body determines the form of fracture. A narrow sharp body will pierce the cranium with less force than when the force of the impinging body is large, flat and smooth. The line of fracture usually follows the line of the striking object.

There may be fracture or splintering of the inner table without any sign of injury on the outer. This is accounted for by the elasticity of the skull, especially in youth.

Neurasthenia or neurosis may arise from concussion, a severe jarring or shaking of the contents of the cranium.

Skull-fractures in children are rare, owing to the thin, unsutured, elastic bones, which yield to direct violence without fracture.

It is surprising to witness death as the result of an apparently trivial injury to the skull and brain and yet more surprising to see persons survive an accident that seemingly must instantly prove fatal and yet retain in a large measure all their mental faculties. The following is copied from Gould and Pyle's Book of Curiosities and Anomalies, 968 pages, price $3.25, published by W. B. Saunders, Philadelphia, Pa. It contains more information for the money than any other book I know of.

"Head injuries with loss of cerebral substance:—The brain and its membranes may be severely wounded, portions of the cranium or cerebral substance destroyed or lost, and yet recovery ensue. Possibly the most noted injury of this class was that reported by Harlow and commonly known as 'Bigelow's Case' or the 'American Crow-bar Case.' Phineas P. Gage, aged 25, a foreman on the Rutland and Burlington Railroad, was employed September 13, 1847, in charging a hole with powder preparatory to blasting. A premature explosion drove a tamping-iron three feet seven inches long, one and a quarter inches in diameter, weighing thirteen and a quarter pounds, completely through the man's head. The iron was round and comparatively smooth; the pointed end entered first. The iron struck against the left side of the face, immediately anterior to the inferior maxillary and passed under the xygomatic arch, fracturing portions of the sphenoid bone and the floor of the left orbit; it then passed through the left anterior lobe of the cerebrum, and in the median line, made its exit at the junction of the coronal and sagittal sutures, lacerating the longitudinal sinus, fracturing the parietal and frontal bones, and breaking up considerable of the brain; the globe of the left eye protruded nearly one-half of its diameter. The patient was thrown backward and gave a few convulsive movements of the extremities. He was taken to a hotel, three-fourths of a mile distant, and during the transportation seemed slightly dazed, but not at all unconscious. Upon arriving at the hotel he dismounted from the conveyance, and without assistance walked up a long flight of stairs to the hall where his wound was to be dressed. Harlow saw him at about six o'clock in the evening, and from his condition could hardly credit the story of his injury, although his person and his bed were drenched with blood. His scalp was shaved, the coagula and debris removed, and among other portions of bone was a piece of the anterior superior angle of each parietal bone and a semi-circular piece of the frontal bone, leaving an opening three and a half inches in diameter. At 10 p. m. on the day of the injury Gage was perfectly rational and asked about his work and after his friends. After a while delirium set in for a few days, and on the eleventh day he lost the vision in the left eye. His convalescence was rapid and uneventful. It was said that he discharged pieces of bone and cerebral substance from his mouth for a few days. The iron when found was smeared with blood and cerebral substance."

"As was most natural such a wonderful case of cerebral injury attracted much notice. Not only was the case remarkable in the apparent innocuous loss of cerebral substance, but in the singular chance which exempted the brain from either concussion or compression, and subsequent inflammation. Professor Bigelow examined the patient in January, 1850, and made a most excellent report of the case, and it is due to his efforts that the case attained world-wide notoriety. Bigelow found the patient quite recovered in his faculties of body and mind, except that he had lost the sight of the injured eye. He exhibited a linear cicatrix one inch long near the angle of the ramus of the left lower jaw. His left eyelid was involuntarily closed and he had no power to overcome his ptosis. Upon the head, well covered by the hair, was a large unequal depression and elevation. In order to ascertain how far it might be possible for a bar of the size causing the injury to traverse the skull in the track assigned to it, Bigelow procured a common skull in which the zygomatic arches were barely visible from above, and having entered a drill near the left angle of the inferior of the maxilla, he passed it obliquely upward to the median line of the cranium just in front of the junction of the sagittal and coronal sutures. This aperture was then enlarged until it allowed the passage of the bar in question, and the loss of substance strikingly corresponded with the lesion said to have been received by the patient. From the coronoid process of the inferior maxilla there was removed a fragment measuring about three-fourths inch in length. This fragment, in the patient's case, might have been fractured and subsequently reunited. The iron bar, together with a cast of the patient's head, was placed in the museum of the Massachusetts Medical College.''

The sacrum is the lower expansion of the vertebral column; it is composed of five sacral segments. The uppermost is the largest, the succeeding ones become smaller until the fifth is only rudimentary. This bone is occasionally fractured. For the sacrum to be broken, the violence must be great, as it is a strong, thick, heavy, cancellated structure. Nevertheless it is fractured by falls and collisions. It would seem that the sacral nerves are liable to injury. While I have seen many fractured sacra I have not had a case of that nature. Much of the larger share of fractured sacra displayed a cicatrix in the lower third, with more or less displacement of the lower portion and a partial closing of the sacral foramen.

Malgaigne reports a case of oblique fracture of the sacrum; the violence was received upon the side of the bone; there were two incomplete transverse fractures. Two of the five cases mentioned by him terminated fatally.

Stimson says: ''In a case that came under my observation. there was extensive sloughing over the sacrum and denudation of the bone, apparently due to the direct violence that caused the fracture.

''The symptoms are: pain at the seat of fracture, both spontaneous and when provoked by pressure or movements of the trunk, or by the act of defecation, or by the act of coughing, and abnormal mobility and crepitus recognized by grasping the lower fragment between the thumb and finger.''

Howe informs us: ''The sacrum as a dry specimen, removed from its connection with the other pelvic bones, is not difficult to break, but in its normal state, wedged between the ossa innominata, and covered with ligamentous and other firm tissues, the bone is in little danger of being broken. A kick or a powerful blow, such as may be received in a fall, might cause a fracture of the bone at any point, the line of separation running in any direction. The processes of the bone may be broken off or a fracture may extend only as far as the central or spinal canal. In most instances, it is found that fractures of the sacrum extend through the lower third of the bone, and mostly in a transverse course.''

Agnew says: ''There will probably be present paralysis of the bladder and rectum, both of these organs receiving nerves from the sacral plexus.''

Lossen affirms: "When there is complete displacement of the fragment, paralysis of the lower extremities, bladder and rectum is never absent."

The os cocygis is less frequently broken than the sacrum, owing to its mobility. In elderly persons the different pieces are usually connected by ankylosis. A fall on the ankylosed coccyx may cause fracture. Coccygodynia—pain in the coccyx —is due to rheumatism, fracture or dislocation.

There is little or no difference in the opinions of anatomists in regard to the result of fractures of the cranium, sacrum and coccyx. They agree that any displacement of the osseous structure by fracture or otherwise may produce pressure upon nerves, inflammation and abnormal functions—disease; but, in regard to fractures and luxations of the true or movable vertebrae there is a wide difference in their views.

Stimson gives us 17 pages on fractures of the vertebrae, in which he says: "Fractures of the vertebrae have this in common with fractures of the skull, that most of their importance depends upon the associated injury of the nerve-centers and trunks contained within their canal.

"The spinal cord, occupying the centre of the vertebral column, is efficiently protected against any external violence that is not sufficient to break the bones that constitute the latter, or the ligaments and muscles that bind those bones together; and the column itself is constituted in a manner that combines elasticity and mobility with the necessary firmness and rigidity. Mechanically, therefore, the spine is exposed to fracture by direct violence, like other bones, and by direct violence through exaggeration or straightening of its normal curves.

"Fractures of the vertebra are relatively rare; fractures of the cervical and dorsal vertebrae are about equally frequent, while those of the lumbar vertebrae are much less common; the fatal cases of fracture of the cervical vertebrae are, however, considerably more numerous, actually and relatively, than those of the other two regions; that the fifth and sixth cervical, the last dorsal, and the first lumbar are more frequently broken than any of the others; and that it is common in fractures of the cervical and dorsal regions for more than one vertebra to be broken at the same time. They are extremely rare in childhood and old age, and relatively infrequent in women.

"Displacements narrow the antero-posterior diameter of the spinal canal and lacerates or compresses the spinal cord within it.

"The immediate causes are muscular action and external violence.

"As to the recovery of the cord after injury, with restoration of function, nothing definite is known beyond the fact that a number of autopsies made at various periods after injury have shown the cord more or less completely divided, or reduced to pulp at the compressed part, or replaced by fibrous tissue."

Stimson tells us that complete displacements of the vertebral column, those in which the articular processes of the upper vertebrae have slipped upward, forward and then downward, forming a lock, narrow the spinal canal and compress the spinal cord, dividing or reducing it to a pulp at the compressed part. It was needless for Stimson to add that when the spinal cord was compressed or pinched by displacements of vertebrae that all the functions below that squeezing was paralyzed. It would seem unnecessary for me to add that were it possible to compress or pinch nerves in the intervertebral foramina, that they also would be reduced to a pulp, or divided by the vice-like grasp of two bones, if it were not that such an idea is being advocated.

Samuel Cooper remarks: "Every kind of joint is not equally liable to dislocations. Experience proves, indeed, that in the greater part of the vertebral column, luxations are absolutely impossible, the pieces of bone being articulated by extensive, numerous surfaces, varying in their form and direction, and so tied together by many powerful, elastic means, that very little motion is allowed.

"The large surfaces, with which these bones support each other; the number and thickness of their ligaments; the strength of their muscles; the little degree of motion which each vertebra naturally has; and the vertical direction of the articular processes; make dislocations of the dorsal and lumbar vertebrae impossible, unless there be also a fracture of the above mentioned processes. It is certain that most of the cases mentioned by authors as dislocations of the lumbar and dorsal vertebrae, have only been concussions of the spinal marrow, or fractures of such bones.

"The cervical vertebrae, however, not having such extensive articular surfaces, and having more motion, are occasionally luxated. The dislocation of the head from the first vertebra, and of the first vertebra from the second, particularly the last accident, is the most common; but luxations of the cervical vertebrae lower down, though very rare, are possible.

"The os occipitis, and first cervical vertebra are so firmly connected by ligaments, that there is no instance of their being luxated from an external cause, and were the accident to happen, it would immediately prove fatal by the unavoidable compression and injury of the spinal marrow.

"As for the treatment of the preceding, experience has hitherto furnished little satisfactory knowledge."

Samuel Cooper considers compression of the spinal marrow (cord) must immediately prove fatal. What then would be the result of a similar compression of a spinal nerve in the intervertebral foramen?

Boyer further states: "As the mere concussion of the spine may occasion symptoms, which very much resemble those usually occurring when the vertebrae are fractured, the diagnosis is generally obscure. Perhaps an inequality in the line of the spinous processes may be observed."

Cooper further states: "A fracture of the upper cervical vertebrae, or of the processus dentatus, is always suddenly fatal. In such cases, the immediate paralysis of the diaphragm is said to be the cause of instantaneous death."

Some years ago I saw an axis, minus the odontoid process, which had been fractured at the neck; the fractured surface and the superior surface of the juncture of the laminae and the spinous process were worn smooth, evidence that its original owner had used it after the odontoid process had been separated from the axis.

Kirkland observes: "There are some luxations which are far worse injuries than fractures; of this description are dislocations of the vertebrae, cases which, indeed, can hardly happen without fracture, and are almost always fatal."

A. Cooper affirms: "In the spine, the motion between any two bones is so small that dislocations hardly ever occur, except between the first and second vertebrae, although the bones are often displaced by fracture. Young subjects rarely experience dislocations; their bones break, or their epiphyses give way much more frequently than the articular surfaces are displaced."

C. Bell refers to some cases of vertebral fracture and says: "Where palsy of the lower extremities comes on several months after an injury of the spine, owing to thickening of the membrane of the medulla, or disease of the medulla itself. Exposing the medulla to extract the fragments would so aggravate the mischief that inflammation, suppuration and death would be the inevitable consequences."

Erichsen says: "Wounds of the spinal cord may occur by the pressure of fractured vertebrae. In this form of injury the association is essentially the same as if the cord was divided.

"The local signs are usually pain at the seat of injury, greatly increased on pressure or on moving the part. In the majority of cases of fracture of the spine there is, however, such displacement of the bone as to compress the whole thickness of cord and thus to occasion complete paralysis.

"Fractures of the spine are inevitably fatal, death ensuing in the two different ways."

Gray's Anatomy states: "The main joints of which the spine is composed, together with the very varied movements to which it is subjected, render it liable to sprains, which may complicate other injuries or may exist alone; but so closely are the individual vertebrae articulated that these sprains are seldom severe, and an amount of violence sufficiently great to produce tearing of the ligaments would tend to cause a dislocation or fracture."

The physician's sprain is the Chiropractor's tension, the stretched condition of the nervous tissue, which causes not only pain, but functions to be performed in an unusual manner. A strain is caused by a strain; a physical tension. Release the tension by correcting the displaced osseous tissue. A fracture or dislocation so modifies the position of the supporting osseous framework, that the nerves are stretched, made tense.

Gerrish confirms Gray by saying: "The plane between any two vertebrae is interrupted by the upward and downward projection of the articular processes and other parts connected with the neural arch. Simple dislocation between two vertebrae is, therefore, almost impossible, unless perhaps in the cervical region, where the surfaces of the articular processes are more nearly horizontal. This is borne out in practice, where we find fracture-dislocation the common injury, the processes or neural arch being commonly fractured, if not the body itself."

McClellan's Regional Anatomy, Vol. 2, contributes to this subject by saying: "Dislocations and fractures of the spinal column are especially grave because of the damage to the spinal cord which usually attends them. A simple dislocation of any of the vertebrae can happen only in the cervical region, as the construction of the dorsal and lumbar vertebrae is such that a dislocation necessarily involves a fracture of some part of the bone. Even in the neck a dislocation is extremely rare, and when it occurs it is usually at the fifth cervical vertebrae —which can be accounted for by the degree of movement of this portion of the column, the comparatively small size of the vertebral bodies, and the obliquity of their articular processes. The usual deformity depends upon the displacement of the body of the vertebrae affected downward and forward upon the body of the vertebrae below, thus encroaching upon the vertebral canal and endangering the cord from pressure. The degree of displacement without any symptoms of pressure is often very considerable, owing to the absence of attachment of the spinal dura mater to the walls of the canal, and to the relatively small size of the cord. Fractures are produced chiefly by indirect violence, as in forcible bending of the spinal column forward, which crushes the bodies of the vertebrae together. In such cases there is always more or less laceration of the intervertebral fibro-cartilages and of the ligaments, with fracture of the vertebral arches, consequent upon the sliding forward of the vertebral bodies. Fracture due to direct violence usually involve only the vertebral arches, the bodies escaping unhurt.

Gerrish tells us that a simple dislocation, one unassociated without a wound, can only occur in the cervical. The construction and form of the five lower cervical and the upper eleven dorsal are the same. What can occur to the cervical can also happen in like manner with the dorsal.

Cunningham's Anatomy goes on record as saying: "Fracture-dislocations of the spine are commonest in the lower cervical and dorso-lumbar regions; that is to say, where the movable cervical and lumbar regions join the more fixed dorsal region. The spinal column above the injury is generally displaced forwards, so that the spinal cord is often severely lacerated or completely torn across by the upper end of the portion of the column below the fracture."

From the above quotations of standard authors, we can readily observe that they refer to complete luxations usually accompanied by fractures. They do not express their thots, if they have any, on Chiropractic luxations.

Herrick says: "It is impossible for any twist, jar, or shake-up of the body to have sufficient force to fracture any of the vertebrae or their processes. Considering the anatomical make-up of the spinal column, its numerous and well-padded vertebrae, its elasticity, its protection by huge bulks of muscle, it is easy to be seen that nothing less than a crushing force given externally upon it, or a violent flexion of the back could dislodge a fragment from the spine or separate the bone at the transverse process."

Beck has his opinion: "Fractures of the spinal column are subdivided into fractures of the vertebral body, the arch, and the spinous and transverse processes.

"Fractures of the vertebral bodies occur generally in the dorsal and lumbar portions. The place of predilection is between the twelfth dorsal and the first lumbar, and at the fifth or sixth cervical vertebra. It is generally caused by indirect violence (heavy weight falling upon the head or shoulder, fall from a horse or bicycle). Direct violence produces it but exceptionally.

"Infractions or fissures are also observed, but they are seldom diagnosticated on the living patient. Sometimes more than one vertebra is concerned.

"The most important sign is the traumatic kyphosis, produced by displacement of the spinous processes, whereby a prominence is caused. Naturally, there is always circumscribed pain. Crepitus and abnormal mobility are generally absent.

"In case of a crushing of the bone the spinal cord hardly ever escapes injury, the latter generally being of the nature of a severe contusion. Lighter injuries, such as commotion or compression, are of exceptional occurrence.

"If in fracture of the first and second cervical vertebrae the spine is compressed on account of much displacement, death is almost instantaneous. If the degree of displacement is very slight, the patient may live for a short while.

"If the phrenic nerve, which branches off between the third and fourth cervical vertebrae, is compressed in this region, its paralysis will be the consequence, and death will follow almost instantly.

"Frequent change of position, while necessary, must be done under great precautions, as it must be remembered that even a light torsion of the injured spine may cause instant death."

In my observations of several anatomical museums and a practice of fifteen years, I have found the twelfth dorsal the most frequently displaced and the cause of more ailments than any other vertebrae; the sixth dorsal comes next in frequency and the third cervical a close third.

The phrenic, the internal respiratory nerve, is chiefly from the fourth cervical nerve, but it usually receives a filament from the third and a communicating branch of the sympathetic from the fifth cervical nerve and, rarely, a branch from the vagus. Irritation of the phrenic nerve causes hiccough and persistent cough. Paralysis of the phrenic nerve as stated by Beck, causes death from paralysis of the diaphragm. Fracture-dislocation of the third cervical vertebra causes death from inability to breathe, which is one of the vital functions. To pinch, squeeze, or compress the phrenic nerve, or any of its filaments which emerge thru other foramina than the fourth cervical, in the vice-like grasp of the intervertebral foramina, would have the same effect as that referred to in the spinal cord. A displaced cervical or dorsal vertebra would impinge upon, press against, cause tension, rigidity, contraction of a nerve, and modified nerve-tissue produces modified functions. There you have it.

In diagnosis of the spinal column, I first glean from the patient by objective and subjective signs or symptoms the ailment; these give me the location and cause, which I announce to the patient as the one causing the nerve tension by an impingement or otherwise. Then I make an examination showing the patient that I am correct. By replacing the displaced portion of the supporting structure of the soft tissue, the impulse channels are returned to their normal tonicity.

I fully agree with the general trend of anatomists, that compression of nerve tissue, making narrow in one direction and wider in another, will cause paralysis.

Eisendrath observes that "True dislocations are most frequent in the cervical region, quite rare in the dorsal, and rarest of all in the lumbar region. We usually speak of the upper of the two vertebrae as the dislocated one. A diastasis is most apt to occur between the fifth and sixth or the sixth and seventh cervical vertebrae. It is often combined with a fracture."

Delafield and Prudden refer to this subject. "The spinal cord may be compressed or lacerated by penetrating wounds, by fracture or dislocation of the vertebrae, or by concussion without injury to the vertebrae. If life continues, the nerve elements may degenerate.

Helferich in a neat volume gives many colored and uncolored cuts of fractures. Under the head of "Fractures and Dislocations of the Spine" he says: "Fractures of the vertebral bodies, of which those of the fifth and sixth cervical vertebrae and of the lowest dorsal and upper lumbar ones are the most frequent, occur as the result of great violence. This great force is required owing to the extreme elasticity of the spine, which is due to the fact that one-fourth of its length consists of intervertebral discs. How mobile the spinal column can become through practice is shown in the so-called 'gutta-percha men,' who are able to bend to a sharp angle the cervical and lumbar portions of their spinal column. It is at these two points that fractures are most commonly observed, since the compressing force acts here at its greatest advantage.

"When the spinal column has been completely crushed we have paralysis of the lower and upper extremities (according to the site of the fracture), damage to the functions of bladder and rectum, sometimes a great rise of temperature if the lower cervical region has been involved, and speedy death from respiratory failure.

"In the dorsal and lumbar regions pure dislocation is excessively rare; in the cervical region it is of practical importance.

"The possibility of true dislocation in the region of the

dorsal and lumbar vertebrae has been provèd on the post-mortem table, but must be almost impossible to recognize in the living subject, i. e., it must be so difficult as to exclude fracture.

"It is a remarkable fact that this process (the formation of callus round a fracture) is the rule—alike in new-born children and in extreme old age, under normal conditions every fracture unites by bone."

Macdonald gives us some good pointers: "Injuries of the spinal column, like those of the cranium, receive their importance from the delicate nature of the contents of the strong bony canal. Fractures of the vertebrae are serious injuries, because the risk of compression, laceration, or contusion of the cord is great and the results of such injury are far-reaching. In the clinical picture of fracture of the spine the salient points are paralysis of motion and sensation, loss of control of the bladder and rectum, bed-sores, and a condition of utter helplessness.

"A case of fracture of the vertebrae comes under our notice of circumstances more or less like the following: A man falls from a ladder or is caught by a 'cave-in,' or is driving under a low arch which catches and doubles him up. He lies still, is in great pain, and cannot bear to be moved; there is more or less paralysis of motion or sensation, or both. The seat of the injury is painful to touch, and there may be evidence of displacement of the bodies of the vertebrae or of their processes. Later there is evidence that the bladder and rectum are paralyzed. The symptoms are, in the main, common to all fractures of the spine."

Howe describes vertebral fractures and gives an interesting case: "A fracture of the vertebral column at any point between the occiput and the third lumbar vertebra, where the cauda equina begins, generally inflicts injury upon the spinal cord; and all the bòdy below the fracture at once loses, more or less completely, both motive power and sensation. The great nerve center, being impinged upon, or compressed, loses its functions, and the parts depending upon it for nerve supplies, are paralyzed. The higher in the column the fracture occurs the greater the part of the body affected—in other words, the graver the consequences. The fracture of a cervical vertebra makes the case extremely dangerous, owing to effects upon the spinal cord high up, where the respiratory nerves arise.

"In a dislocation of a last dorsal vertebra, which occurred in a laborer engaged upon the government buildings in this city (Cincinnati), no reduction could be effected, and the patient lived twenty-seven days. The man did not suffer excruciatingly from the first, but was unable to move the pelvis and legs. He rode home and talked cheerfully all the way. He could not believe that he was seriously or dangerously hurt, and wondered why he could not move his legs. The urine was drawn with a catheter for ten days, and then it began to dribble, and flowed incontinently till death. The bowels were evacuated by means of enemas, except when profuse liquid discharges escaped involuntarily. Bed-sores formed upon the hips, and at length the flesh on the legs became gangrenous in spots. Death occurred from exhaustion and septicemia. An autopsy revealed the dislocation and a partial fracture of an articular process of the vertebra above the one displaced. The cauda equina was pinched by the dislocated bones."

Howe affirms that a fracture in the cervical is dangerous because it compresses the respiratory nerves. If the phrenic nerve is compressed or pinched in the spinal cord or the intervertebral foramen, the effect is just the same, viz., paralysis, loss of function, and thus it would be with any spinal nerve.

McGrath informs us: "Fractures of the spine usually involve the fifth and sixth cervicals, last dorsal and first lumbar vertebrae, and are usually caused by indirect violence, the curved parts of the spine being bent beyond the limit of their elasticity."

Gould and Pyle state: "Fracture of the lower part of the spine is not always fatal, and notwithstanding the lay-idea that a broken back means certain death, patients with well-authenticated cases of vertebral fracture have recovered. Injury to the spinal cord does not necessarily cause immediate death."

Wharton and Curtis are explicit on fractures and dislocations of vertebrae. "Vertebral column fracture and dislocation are almost invariably combined, the interlocking of the bony processes making it difficult for a dislocation to occur without fracture, and the dislocation is usually the more important part of the injury. To distinguish the two is often impossible. Simple dislocation is rare except in the cervical region, but there it presents a definite clinical picture.

"Fractures of the spine may occur in any part of the column, but are most common in the dorsal region, especially affecting the lower dorsal and first lumbar vertebrae. Fracture of the spinous processes or of the laminae are rare, the articular processes being usually broken or the bodies of the vertebrae crushed.

"In estimating the prognosis in injuries of the spinal column we must distinguish between the effect upon the column itself and that upon the nervous structure. Fractures in the cervical region are almost invariably fatal, and the large majority of the patients die within three or four days, while if recovery takes place a permanent paralysis usually remains. In the dorsal region the prognosis is better, and death is generally postponed for several weeks. In the lumbar region less than one-half of the patients die; if death occurs it comes later, and the paralysis may entirely disappear if recovery takes place."

The interlocking, referred to above, is the normal, the physiological; the pathological is where the upper vertebra is displaced forward. Take notice: The upper of the two vertebrae cannot be anterior to its neighbor below without a complete luxation. The lower of any two might be anterior to its neighbor above, but such a condition is altogether improbable, as the force to produce it must come against the ventral surface of the one which is superior. Now, my boys, if you will give this proposition due consideration, you will remodel your cuts.

The American Text-Book of Surgery states: "Dislocation of vertebrae are commonly associated with fracture, but a number of cases have been reported and verified by post-mortem examination in which uncomplicated dislocation has occurred.

"Crepitus and preternatural mobility are not always obtainable in fracture, and indeed cannot with propriety be sought for in the majority of such cases.

"The prognosis is, of course, more favorable in uncomplicated luxations which have been reduced than in fracture, but the injury in all cases must be regarded as a very serious one. Even after reduction paralysis often must be regarded as a very serious one. Even after reduction paralysis often persists, and death ensues on account of the injury to the cord."

An injury to the spinal cord, nerves or filaments occurs because the pinching or compressing, either expression meaning one and the same condition, is serious, paralysis being the result; whereas an impingement, pressure against the nervous tissues creates undue tension, a strain, a contraction, which intensifies the impulses passing over that channel, increasing functionating. A lessening of normal functionating is the result of lax nerves.

Hutchison and Rainy, edition 1910, give some good clinical advice along the line of this article: "The vertebral column and skull demand special attention. Observe in the former the presence of any local projection of the vertebral spines. If such there be, state which are the vertebrae involved, and at which the projection is most prominent.

"Note also the presence of any curvature of the spinal

column as a whole, or of one part of it, distinguishing carefully such general curvature from the local projections above referred to.

"Ask the patient to stoop down, and notice the degree of mobility of the vertebral column, and the occurrence of any pain during stooping, noting the exact site of the latter, if present. Then pass the hand down the vertebral column, and observe whether any tender spots can be made out. Such tender spots are not unfrequently met with in hysteria and in case of irritation of the posterior nerve roots. Their presence can often be more easily elicited by drawing a sponge wrung out of hot water down the vertebral column; the patient complains of pain whenever the hyperesthetic area is reached. To elicit more deep-seated tenderness of the vertebrae, it may be necessary to 'punch' the spines gently with the fist from above downwards, observing the point at which the patient complains of pain and verifying the observation by repeating the process from below upwards."

These gentlemen have touched upon the examination of the contour of the spinous processes and nerve palpation; but, what advantage to the practitioner or the patient these observations confer is not mentioned.

---

Disease, complaint, disorder, illness, indisposition, distemper, ailment, malady, sickness and affection are synonyms, that is, they mean the same thing.

---

When we see reddened eyelids, styes, blear eyes, granulated eyelids; when we find a clammy cold perspiration of hands and feet; when we see alveolar pyorrhea—the gums receding from the teeth, we should know that the nerves at K. P. are at fault. Thus we locate the cause of each disease; thus we make Chiropractic specific.

This in brief is what the Discoverer, Developer and Founder of the grandest and greatest science on earth sees fit to name specific Chiropractic adjusting.

---

Local death is proceeding at all times in all parts of the living body. Individual cells and elements are being cast off and replaced by new ones—a process essential to life. General death is of two kinds. Death of the body as a whole (somatic or systemic death) and death of the tissues. By the former is meant the absolute cessation of the functions of the brain, the circulatory and the respiratory organs; by the latter, the entire disappearance of the vital actions of the ultimate structural constituents of the body.

## IGNORANCE OF THE EIGHTEENTH CENTURY.

The proverb "The remedy is worse than the disease" must have been coined in the eighteenth century when physicians treated their patients with heroic treatment bordering on assault and battery. Sickness was thought to be some kind of a demon that must be overcome by pills, plasters, blisters and bleeding. Air and water were considered dangerous for a sick person to have; his desire for them was interpreted as a sign that he should not have them. The windows were closed and their curtains and those of the four-posted bedstead were tightly drawn around the unfortunate recumbent who was gasping for breath. If he was burning up with fever, blankets were piled on for fear he would take cold. A desire for cold water meant that he should have none, but, now, he is given all the ice he desires. A lack of appetite proved that he ought to be stuffed with food. A bath was positively forbidden.

The deadly results of breathing "night air" were censured by medical writers. All air was bad but that of the night was particularly dangerous. One bold medico recommended that a bedchamber should be ventilated in the day time. Another dared to suggest that consumptives might receive benefit from sleeping in the open air. The rule for ablutions were "hands often, feet seldom, head never." But a physician, far in advance of his age, said, invalids might bathe their feet in warm water once a week and, under special circumstances take a warm bath once a month.

The inefficiency and futility of medical practice at this period was truthfully expressed by the reply of the celebrated and convivial Dr. Garth when reminded, while tipping bumpers at the Kit Kat Club, that his patients needed his attention. " 'Tis no matter, if I see them or not. Nine have such bad constitutions that all the doctors in the world can't save them, and the other six have such good ones that all the doctors in the world can't kill them."

---

The pathology of therapeutics is not that of Chiropractic.

---

Our readers and the members of our class expect to have their corns stepped on, until they have learned that it is better not to have them—better to have the cause adjusted. They realize, to grow Chiropractically, their opinions must be changed by removing mental impingements. What if it does hurt a moment, if the result is O. K.

## THE SYMPATHETIC NERVOUS SYSTEM.

You will find my text on page 15 of Vol. 1 in The Science of Chiropractic; it reads: "The sympathetic nervous system, in name and functions expresses no intelligence to a Chiropractor." That depends entirely upon the intellect of the practitioner. The author of my text has sought to subvert the basic principles of the science of Chiropractic. My name has been made famous by giving to the world a knowledge which embraces not only the source of disease, but a method of adjustment which removes the cause of disease.

The originator of the above text was not satisfied to share the honors with The Fountain Head of the science. But because of an avaricious longing, the desire grew within him to possess the credit rightfully belonging to another, so that he might be IT. Therefore, to make such a change, to become notorious, not being able to advance the science he sought to destroy my fair name and the work I had accomplished; hence the assumed hypothesis in the text the author of which did not have intellect enough to comprehend the three nervous systems. He accordingly threw the cranial and the sympathetic systems out and placed in their stead "a direct brain system," not even counseling the Creator whether such would be satisfactory or not.

Fig. 9, page 41 illustrates five spinal nerve trunks and their branches as communicants. Communicating nerves join others and pass along with them in the same sheath, each filament retaining its own peculiar function.

Fig. 9 presents the spinal nerves as they emerge from the spinal foramina, each sending their branch to the ganglionic chain. We have first the brain, then the spinal cord, rootlets, roots, trunks composed of the nerves which pass into the sympathetic ganglionic cords and those which continue as spinal nerves. From the ganglia spring the sympathetic nerves which ramify the viscera. Some of these branches are shown in figure 8 to the right of the ganglionic cord. On page 57, Fig. 11, the spinal nerves are shown on the left as they enter the ganglion. The right and left ganglionic chains, with the nerves which emerge therefrom are shown in figures 10 and 11. These two chains of ganglia, with the nerves which emanate from them, constitute the ganglionic nervous system.

Fig. 8 presents the spinal nerves as they issue from the spinal foramina. These sympathetic ganglionic cords pass in front of the cervical costo-transverse foramina, traverse the dorsal vertebrae on both sides just in front of and against the heads of the ribs, lying close against the bodies until they arrive at the lumbar vertebrae, where they verge slightly toward the front until they reach the anterior of the sacrum. Here they pass in front of the sacral foramina, at which place they are connected by inter-ganglionic cords and unite on the anterior of the coccyx.

The Chiropractor will need to take into consideration the extreme sensitiveness of nerves to pressure. Remember, that there is no sensation in blood or serum; that in headache and toothache, the slight pressure of pulsation causes great distress; that sensation of aches or pains are because of sensation in nerves, made more so by the slight impingement occasioned by the pulsation of arteries.

Please return to the cervical portion of this sympathetic ganglionic chain; see Fig. 11. A portion of the superior cervical ganglion with the carotid and cavernous plexus extends into the cranial cavity where they communicate with the cervical nerves. The line of demarcation between the cervical and the cranial nerves is between the first cervical and the 12th pair of cranial nerves. The first single nerve represented on the left of the superior cervical ganglion is the first cervical. Opposite, slightly above, is the 12th cranial nerve—the hypoglossal with two branches. All the nerves above this line are from the sympathetic and are in the cranial cavity. They act as accessories to the cranial nerves. They originate in the brain, pass down the spinal cord, emerge from the spinal canal, pass out through the cervical foramina and into the superior cervical ganglion of the sympathetic. From thence they go to the cranial cavity through the carotid canal, join, and communicate with and by their presence add sensory or motor functions to the cranial nerves. These are the branches of the sympathetic nerves which are impinged upon near their emergence from the spinal foramina by the cervical and dorsal vertebrae being racked out of their normal position.

The sympathetic nervous system, although its functions may not express any intelligence to B. J., existed and had a name long before he had; and, in all probability, will continue to exist long after his name is forgotten. His excommunication of them will neither deprive them of their existence, nor lessen their functions.

---

Chiropractors are specially interested in bones and nerves. The bones are the frame-work of the body; the nerves are channels through which all sense and action are conducted. They are more especially concerned in the bones of the vertebral column, as ninety-five per cent of all diseases are caused by their displacement.

## SYMPATHY AND THE SYMPATHETIC NERVOUS SYSTEM.

"The genius that rapidly evolves new worlds of ideas constantly," does not comprehend the difference between sympathy, sympathetic, a fellow feeling, a feeling of pity toward one who is in distress and the sympathetic nervous system, one of the three divisions of the nervous system; that part of the nervous system which furnishes the innervation of the viscera and blood vessels; that portion of nerves which we do not control by the intellect, which is connected to the central nervous system by rami communicantes; that portion of the nervous system which presents a distinct contrast to the cranial and spinal nerves; the third division which does not include those confined to the cranium or those which emerge through the spinal foramina, except as a portion of the latter go to, and make up, the nerves of the sympathetic gangliated trunk; that portion which, after leaving the spinal system forms a separate system, named the sympathetic, is separate and distinct from the central nervous system, and yet, is permanently connected with and dependent upon the cerebrospinal system.

"This genius who rapidly evolves new worlds of ideas constantly," says: "I have reasons why it is impossible to have a sympathetic nervous system." I will not take the space to repeat the seventeen pages of ingenious twistings used in order to make a sympathetic feeling mean a system of nerves named the tri-splanchnic or sympathetic.

Dorland says of sympathetic: "An influence produced in any organ by disease or disorder in another part; a relation which exists between mind and body; the influence exerted by one individual upon another." The same author says of the sympathetic nervous system: "The system of nerve-ganglia situated in the cranium and spine and the nerves connected with them which supply the muscular and vascular structures of the viscera."

Gould says of sympathetic: "Effecting consentaneous activity or sympathy; and of the "Sympathetic Nervous System, a series of ganglia connected by commissural fibers, upon each side of the vertebral column from the base of the skull to the coccyx. It may also be traced into the head. It gives origin also to numerous plexuses, ganglia, etc. Lippincott, refers to the three meanings which this word has. "Sympathetic. Having or pertaining to sympathy; reflex; specifically, the sympathetic nerve or nervous system."

This man who "evolves new worlds of ideas constantly" says: "Anatomists do not state where the sympathetic nervous system starts or goes to." If he will turn to Gray's

Anatomy, page 1075, Morris 999, Dutton 331, McMurrich 654, Sobotta 244, 245, Gerrish 623, 642 and 645, Cunningham 707 709, 711 and 713, he will find cuts displaying the sympathetic chains of ganglia, the spinal nerves which communicate with this ganglionic chain. He then may add one more idea to his "worlds of ideas."

To assist "the genius that rapidly evolves new worlds of ideas," he will find these cuts have the spinal nerves numbered, showing from whence they come and where they go. Also by a glance he can see where the filaments branch off from the ganglionic chain to reach the various viscera. When those of mature age study the sympathetic nervous system, they do not consider the sympathy between mind and body, or that between persons, or the sympathy between one portion of the body and another as being the sympathetic nervous system.

The sympathetic and cranial nerves have their functions to perform in the human economy; vital energy cannot be transmitted without them. Chiropractors cannot afford to abandon and disown them.

This luxation must be adjusted, it must be replaced, even if it takes all Summer and then some.

---

Growing is inverse proportion to blowing.

---

Boston, Oct. 4.—"Operations for appendicitis should be classed as 'criminal,' and as such be prohibited by law," declares Dr. Chas. E. Page, one of the best known physicians of this city. Dr. Page states that he has for years kept a record of deaths traced directly to the appendicitis operations and the record is appalling. The deaths of Clyde Fitch and Governor Johnson of Minnesota he ascribes to the operation—not to the disease.

---

"Reaching the organs of the body through the cerebro-spinal nervous system" is the new short cut. "When I saw there was no use for a sympathetic Nervous System, I threw it out, and then just had to put something better in its place, so I discovered Direct Mental Impulse."

I see by The U. C. A. directory that the author of this booklet is endorsed by that association. The above pseudo Chiropractic is not endorsed by me, it does not strike the spot—the Chiropractic bulls' eye—and I want you to know and profit by it.

## OSTEOPATHY.

The July issue of The Journal of Osteopathy talks like Allopathy when it says, "**Combat** disease . . Blood is very quick and **powerful.**" That is not Chiropractic.

"**Blood** . . . constructs, nourishes and **keeps the whole nervous system** normal **in** form and **function.**"

"The kidney is a highly vascular organ . . . the **disturbance to the blood supply caused by straining and lifting is the cause of disease.**"

"Nature has built **the heart** so strong that it **is capable of sending the blood over the whole body.**"

Chiropractors would say that Innate constructs, nourishes and keeps the whole body in form and function **through the nervous system.**

Straining and lifting displaces bones, impinges and excites nerves, thereby causes the kidneys to perform their functions either excessively or deficiently; these abnormal amounts of function result in disease.

Innate directs, thru nerves, the energy, vital force, which gives action to the vascular system, heart, veins and arteries.

Too much functionating of the vascular system, is known as vasculitis, angitis; too much heat; inflammation. If this condition becomes extreme we have necrosis—softening of blood vessels—hemorrhage.

"We fully realize the broad gulf between the fundamental principles of the old school system of healing and that of Osteopathy, the former being medicinal and the latter mechanical. But that the one does not rely entirely on medicine nor the other entirely on mechanics surely cannot be denied.

"Osteopathy embraces primarily the medicinal adjustment of the various parts of the body, to secure free and harmonious action of its fluids and forces, but that it does not employ internal medication for the cure of disease.

"Then how can we, and why should we, declare it to be an absolutely drugless system of healing?

"We have been taught, in the same school, to employ to a moderate extent the use of antiseptics, antidotes, anesthetics and surgery."

These four paragraphs found on page 497, state the situation of Osteopathy today. The **principles of Allopathy and Osteopathy are identically the same.** The practice of the old school (Allopathy) and Osteopathy **differ only in degree.** The Allopaths are more medical and less mechanical; while the Osteopaths are more mechanical and less medical.

Osteopathy is not a drugless system of healing, for they

use antiseptics, anesthetics, and antidotes. They have found that massage and Swedish movements are not "powerful" enough to "combat" disease.

---

## PENSION FOR A MARTYR.

### Senate Committee Recommends $125 a Month for John R. Kissinger.

Washington, February 15, 1910.—The senate committee on pensions has ordered a favorable report on a bill to increase the pension of John R. Kissinger, of South Bend, Ind., from $24 a month to $125 a month.

Kissinger at the time of the yellow fever epidemic in Cuba, during the Spanish-American war, gave himself up to science and permitted the physicians to inoculate him with yellow fever germs in order that they might prove the correctness of a theory held by them.

It was contended by an eminent Chicago specialist that the fever would not attack a perfectly healthy man, or, that if it did, it would be of such a mild type as to be easily cured. He developed the disease and after several weeks' illness was pronounced cured, and apparently was as strong as before the attack.

It was not until several years later that the effects of the experiment made on him began to develop. He had returned to his home and married, when he was stricken with paralysis, which has left him a hopeless invalid. It was proved to the satisfaction of his physicians that the paralysis was due directly to the experiments and that Kissinger in fact was a martyr to medical science.

It was unanimously decided by congress that Kissinger's heroism was worthy of recognition, and that instead of $100 a month he should have $125.

If the above experiment proves anything, it is that inoculation with yellow fever germs, may cause yellow fever and later on, paralysis.

Chiropractically, poison draws vertebrae out of alignment, **causing, by impingement,** too much or not enough functionating.

---

On May 14, 1796, Jenner first committed the crime of vaccination by inoculating James Phillips who later died of consumption as did also Jenner's oldest son, Edward. Notwithstanding all this, the old scoundrel advised his professional brethren "to be slow to publish fatal cases of smallpox after vaccination."—The Ophthalmologist.

## CHIROPRACTIC.

In Vol. 1, 1905, Chiropractor, is the following, with corrections in italics, adjusting it to date.

Chiropractic was discovered in 1895 by Dr. D. D. Palmer. He developed this science, until he feels proud of it. Chiropractors find nearly all diseases are caused by subluxations of vertebrae which impinge upon nerves. When nerves are free to act naturally in their entire course, there is health. Chiropractors, definitely locate displacements **of osseous tissue,** the cause of disordered conditions. When these luxated joints are replaced, the impinged nerves freed, there are no abnormal **functions.**

The medical world has long recognized luxations of the spinal column accompanied **by** fracture, but have always insisted that it was almost impossible to displace a vertebrae. The M. D.'s wrenches and sprains of the back are Chiropractic luxations. These may be caused by a variety of accidents when asleep or awake.

Many a mother and her child have been injured at delivery by displacements of some one of the **117** joints of the spine. It is the Chiropractor's business to repair **sub-luxated articulations,** thereby freeing the impinged nerves, so that they may act normally.

The fundamental principles of Chiropractic are founded on anatomy, pathology, physiology and nerve tracing.

Four years after writing the above, I advanced **the principles of Chiropractic. Life is action governed by intelligence. Intelligent life, the soul, depends upon the execution of functions. Functions performed with normal energy result in health. Disease is the result of the performance of functions above or below normal. Impulses properly transmitted through nerves, result in functions normally performed which is health. The motive force may be exaggerated or decreased during its transit, because of the lines of communication being excited or repressed. The vegetative functions rely upon the amount of energy expressed by vital functions. The normal carrying capacity of nerves depends upon their freedom from pressure; the abnormal upon the force of impingement. Bones are the only hard tissue which can press against or impinge upon nerves.**

**Therefore, we state Chiropractic is founded upon osteology, neurology, and functions.**

Physicians, who give us 15 minutes' attention while we explain Chiropractic luxations by the use of specimens at hand, admit that there may be many diseases arising from displacements of the vertebral column. But being able to replace them by hand is very much doubted until demonstrated; one practical exhibition removes all doubt.

The spinal column is the central axis of the skeletal frame. It supports the head and ribs, and through them the weight of the upper extremities. The weight is transmitted downward through the bodies and the articular processes of the vertebrae to the osinnominata. The backbone is composed of bony segments, between which are interposed elastic fibrous cartilages.

Flexion, extension and rotation have a normal limit; to a certain extent they are permitted in all parts of the spinal column. These various movements are due to elastic cushions. Wrenches in many ways separate the intervertebral and articular cartilages and displace the vertebrae; **the projecting sides of the bodies of vertebrae press against, impinge upon the nerves, thereby** deranging functions.

When we study the anatomy of the spinal column, we no longer wonder at the many displacements or are surprised that we do not find more of them. Could we fancy the main shaft of a machine capable of the various movements, subjected to the many wrenches of the vertebral column, we would no longer be astonished when we find vertebrae **slightly displaced.** Is not the human frame much more liable to have its different parts racked out of their proper position and the resultant consequences **far more reaching** than that of inanimate machines?

The inevitable conclusion is, that the laws of natural philosophy apply to **the backbone, much more so, than they do to the main line on which mechanism depends for its workmanship.** Such being the case, why not use the same good judgment in adjusting the displacements of the central line shaft of the human body, which sustains and gives firmness to the skeletal frame? Why search the world over for antidotes? Why not look for the cause of our troubles within the **one affected,** then correct?

The above questions are answered by Chiropractors who locate and verify with definite precision the apparently slight **sub**-luxations which cause abnormal functions. This is done by an **anatomical** knowledge of the vertebral column, the finding of sensitive, swollen, inflamed nerves, which are traced by digital examination from its spinal exit to the parts affected. By hand adjusting we correct the wrongs which cause disease, we replace the vertebra in proper position, **relieve pressure which impinges.** These movements are done by the hands, using the transverse and spinous processes as **levers** for adjusting.

## TYPHOID FEVER.

### $50,000 for a Remedy.

Mexico City, Feb. 19.—The Mexican Academy of Medicine has offered $50,000 to the scientist who discovers a means of preventing typhoid fever. Of this sum $20,000 will go to the discoverer of a specific to cure the disease. A like amount will be paid to the person discovering a serum that will kill the germs in the blood, and $10,000 will be divided among those who give the most aid to the winners of the first two prizes in their experiments.

I wrote the Mexican Academy of Medicine in English, offering to go to their city at my own expense and relieve (cure) as many cases of Typhoid Fever as they desired, in their presence; the temperature to be reduced to normal, inside of an hour. I received an answer; their offer in Spanish print, appended by "On this subject it is necessary to write in Spanish language."

I accordingly went to A. R. Vegar, professor of languages and Mexican Counsel, who had studied medicine two years in Rush Medical College. He translated my letter into Spanish. My answer gave a brief explanation of what I proposed to do. So far I have received no answer and do not expect one. It would not be well for the medical profession to allow typhoid fever to be relieved (cured) by adjusting the cause. If typhoid can be relieved by such **means, why not other contagious diseases?** They dare not allow such an entering wedge. It would split the medical log wide open and expose the fallacy of their etiology. It would let in a flood of light on the causation of disease—the science of the causes of the phenomena of life and their relation to physical laws in general would become known.

The Mexican Academy of Medicine wants a REMEDY, a medicine, a serum, a poison, that will kill the germs in the blood. They desire to find a vaccine that will create the same disease in such a manner that it will destroy by excessive heat the germs within us, so that we may be forever immune. They desire "to find a means whereby the . . . deadly enemy . . . shall be robbed of its power to destroy." The M. D.s mission is one of warfare; not of peace. Disease is regarded as an enemy, not as a result of causes.

The Chiropractor finds that poison generated from decaying filth produces zymotic diseases. This poison affects sensory nerves by their sensing it. Traumatic injuries draw vertebrae out of alignment. Displaced bones irritate and excite nerves by their impingement; create an undue amount of heat—named fever. The Chiropractor would eliminate the primary cause by not allowing animal or vegetable matter to decay; then there would be no noxious effluvia to cause this specific poisoning of those who breathe its noxious effluvia. To remove the direct cause of typhoid fever, local inflammation, replace the displaced dorsal vertebra; remove the pressure on nerves, thereby allowing them to perform their normal amount of function.

In company with one of our students, Dr. N. J. Baxter, I called on the Secretary of the Health Board of Portland and laid before him what I had done for typhoid fever and thought to be able to do in future. The doctor listened attentively to us and treated us nicely. He gave us an answer by saying that he did not want to be mixed up in any advertising. I replied, "If typhoid can be relieved and the patient made well, you would like to advertise it; if I failed, you would like to advertise me."

We, as Chiropractors, should know just where to adjust for acute as well as chronic diseases. Acute ailments should be relieved by one specific adjustment, while chronic diseases may take weeks or months. We should not fail to relieve acute cases; to do so, creates lack of confidence in the Chiropractor and the profession. Recently a graduate Chiropractor had an opportunity to show his skill in a family of smallpox patients. He adjusted at 4th dorsal and k. p. instead of the 5th cervical. He, of course, failed—giving the M. D. much satisfaction and Chiropractic a black eye.

The medical fraternity consider that our bodies contain the germs of typhoid, typhus, smallpox, puerperal, fever, rabies; cholera. bubonic plague and other infectious diseases. Therefore they desire to find some method to excite an action which will destroy them by heat as an antidote, or to introduce harmless ones which will make a warfare on those which may give us no trouble—annihilate our foes, that we may have peace and be immune from our enemies. Therefore, as an experiment, on June 17th at Omaha, "eight men were inoculated with typhoid fever virus (poison), 800,000,000 germs having been injected into the left arm of each man." The reader will observe that medical men desire to make disorder, create a warfare among disease-producing germs, hoping that they may destroy each other.

Of late, the rat, mosquito and the fly are thought guilty of distributing typhoid germs.

Professor A. R. Sweetster, of the University of Oregon, says, "Every time a fly lights on a piece of bread or cake it may leave thousands and thousands of germs, a great many of which may be pathogenic or dangerous to man. When a fly drops into the milk or cream pitcher, even more germs and bacteria are washed off, and as milk is an excellent breeding ground, the common fly is a menace."

So strong was the campaign against the fly in one of the college courses this year that the students nicknamed the course "Swat the fly."

---

To discover means to uncover, to disclose, to lay open to view, to make visible, to make known what has been unknown or unseen. The discoverer is the one who is first to find out or ascertain. We discover what already exists, but is unknown.

---

"It is a great loss to the science for two of the greatest philosophers of Chiro to be separated."

As they now are, one can envelop as fast as the other develops; one's involution is equal to the other's evolution.

---

This science covers a field of usefulness, where the amount of work is unlimited. Chiropractors have the opportunity of making the world better for their having lived in it. Make yourself and others happy by learning a science which discloses the cause of disease and teaches how to adjust it instead of treating effects.

---

"You'll have to send for another doctor," said the one who had been called, after a glance at the patient.

"Am I so ill as that?" gasped the sufferer.

"I don't know just how ill you are," replied the man of medicine, "but I know you're the lawyer who cross-examined me when I appeared as an expert witness. My conscience won't let me kill you, and I'll be hanged if I want to cure you. Good day."—Philadelphia Inquirer.

---

When I was created, policy was not included in my make-up. I have as little use and respect for policy as I have for a plug hat. I am sorry that I am placed in a position wherein I must use policy—deceit. Chiropractic and honesty have no use for policy; either are good enough without it. I could slide through the world much more easily if I had more respect for policy and less for honesty. Instead of saying that "Honesty is the best policy," I would say that "Honesty has no need of policy."

## INNATE.

"Man can be diseased only when the mind fails to perform properly its functions." The **mind**, the intellectual, the rational faculty, the understanding, the intellect of man, is of the Educated. The functions of the mind, the intellect, are those of affection, voluntary motions, etc.

"His ingenious and profoundly scientific theory, that the **mind** governs organic functions." That boy is theorizing, speculating. He has not grasped the author's idea of Innate. No wonder that he says, "My pet theory." The mind governs the intellectual functions. Innate directs the vital actions, those of the vegetative functions of the animal economy.

"Connecting mind with body." The mind, like other functions, is dependent upon Innate and the condition of the nervous system. Innate is connected with the body; that union produces life—soul. Innate, the spiritual, has the power to conceive, judge and reason on matters, which pertains to the internal welfare of the body.

"The brain impulse is generated by the brain under the command of Innate."

The brain generates thoughts, produces the mind. The mind and thoughts are products of the brain—creatures begotten by Education. Innate's impulses, the energy which runs the vital functions, are not generated; they are not originated by any process, nor begotten, they always existed.

"The Innate mind, or the soul." Mind is a production of Educated, and not of the spirit of Innate. Mind and soul are not synonymous. Mind, as we have just stated, is a production of Educated. The soul is the life of the body—the breath of life. The life directed by Innate.

He used to cherish, revere and worship his father's manuscript; so much so, that he rummaged his father's waste basket in order to secure the articles blocked out, as written, corrected and finished manuscripts. These comprise quite a share of the "70 volumes of notes, copies of every idea that has been brought out and used in Chiropractic."

In strange contrast to the above is the statement made at the "Feast of the Buzzards," that "99 per cent of Chiropractic ideas are those of others than D. D. Palmer."

---

Two hundred years ago "superstition ascribed disease to evil spirits, or the displeasure of the divinities."

Today "scientific" medicine ascribes it to a bug and proposes to inoculate those who are well, so as to protect them from the entrance of the bug.

## "DIRECT MENTAL IMPULSE."

I have before me a Chiropractic booklet of 16 pages.

On the outside of the front cover is a cut of a spine. It represents the 5th cervical as being adjusted by the 3d and 4th fingers, instead of using the pisiform bone.

"The cause of disease and its **remedy.**" Chiropractors do not use remedies.

"The cause of disease is the **pinching** of nerves, as they **emerge** from the **spinal cord.**" "Pinching of nerves" is not the cause of disease. Nerves emerge from the spinal canal—not from the spinal cord.

"Kiro-prac-tic **brings** health without drugs, surgery or magnetic healing, but through the cerebro spinal system." Why did you cut out the sympathetic nervous system? Was it because your teacher did so? **Bringing health** through the nervous system is a "healthorium" method.

"Neural Chiropractic Healthorium." That is a triple affair. Chiropractic is the link which joins nerves to health. Yes, I see.

"We adjust the spinal column, **lift vertebrae** off **from trunk nerves**, and thus remove the cause of disease." Adjusting by lifting is a new way to me. How much strength is required to lift vertebrae, while in the spinal column?

"The nerves are the life of the human body." The nerves are not the life to or of the body. They may carry functions which pertain to life.

"**The very essence of life,** brain or nerve energy must be conveyed to all parts of the body through the nervous system." **The essence of life?** The extract of life. That is boiling it down.

"**All organs must be directly connected to the brain** through the nerves, **if they live** and properly perform their functions." They live if properly connected (see cut); if not directly connected they die.

"All cerebro-spinal nerves necessarily **emerge from the spinal cord** through the side openings of the spinal column." They spring from the spinal cord and emerge from the spinal canal.

"Vertebrae in the spinal column." "A bad taste in the mouth." Where else would you have vertebrae? Where else would you expect to find a bad taste?

"Shut off the nerve force." If nerve force was "shut off," they would be dead. The most of diseases are because of too much energy; not because nerve force is "shut off."

"The first ray of light leading to its discovery and development was **unknowingly stumbed onto** nearly fourteen years ago, when hearing was restored to a man by a **crude adjustment,** out of which process sprang the most scientific way of

**healing** nearly all **diseases.**" "Unknowingly stumbed onto." By diligently searching for 10 years I found the cause of disease. The ear-marks show from what literature you have copied many of your false statements found in your booklet. "Unknowingly." I knew what I had discovered, and straightway developed it a science. What Moore would you have me do? That "crude adjustment" was not a "process stumbed onto." Chiropractors do not handle diseases."

"The old way has been to doctor symptoms. Chiropractic doctors the cause." To doctor is to treat with drugs. Chiropractors **do not treat** the cause. They adjust.

"This little booklet will substantiate it with logical reasoning." The above is a sample of his and his preceptor's "logical reasoning."

"The nervous system contains the **principles of life.**" The nervous system does not contain the principles or the origin and source of life.

"The divine spark of life . . . first manifests this inexplainable power, which is the very essence of life, in the brain, acting similar to a dynamo giving off nerve stimuli." That "divine spark . . . inexplainable power . . . essence of life . . . dynamo nerve stimuli" must be the Chiropractic which I "unknowingly stumbed onto." I pity, rather than blame this copyist for repeating ignorance and falsehoods from a pseudo fountain head. He says in his letter of advice: "I enclose one of my booklets. I hope you will like it."

"The spinal cord is encased within a pyramid of hollow bones, of which there is twenty-five, **grown one upon another**, which **forms the very foundation on which our bodies are built.**" Just think of a teacher of Chiropractic telling his students of vertebrae "growing one upon another," and that our bodies are built upon the back bone; that the back bone makes a good foundation to build bodies upon. Wouldn't that jar your mother's preserves? This teacher of such rot, says to me, "I hope you will like it."

This booklet gives a cut (home-made) of the spinal cord with "Direct Mental Impulse," which we reproduce. The plan is simple; a child can understand it; the whole family should learn it. A direct nerve to the eye, direct from the spinal cord; another just as direct to the nose, one each to the teeth, throat, lungs, heart, stomach, liver, kidneys, bowels. You missed the spleen and pancreas, but no matter. Each and every organ has a direct nerve from the spinal cord. This "illustrates how the brain communicates with all the organs through the nervous system." No cranial nerves, no sympathetic; only "Direct Mental Impulse." There is much more I might copy, but I will close by reproducing the last page.

## SOME COMMENTS.

The Chiropractor states: "We have never intended to make this journal an instructive agent." It is unnecessary to remind your readers of that fact, but notwithstanding, we have found some items on Chiropractic in this number, upon which we take the privilege of making a few comments. This we have a right to do, as the Chiropractor's pages are for the benefit of the public. The Developer of Chiropractic thinks it judicious and beneficial to use the columns of The Adjuster for that purpose, so as to keep the science within Chiropractic lines.

Page 73: "To use the word treatment implies that something sick needs to be treated; that something which needs treating is something which is not normal, hence, disease. To treat, then, means to direct your attention, by any one of a thousand means to the diseased portions; to that place which is not normal; to that condition which is pathologically abnormal (1). Treatment, when resolved to its last analysis, means either stimulation or inhibition. Disease, resolved to its real analysis, means **too much or not enough function.** (2).

"Where we have too much function, as in Diabetes, Diarrhoea (3), Running Cold of the nose (he refers to cold in the head — coryza) (4), etc., Violent Insanity, and characteristic like diseases, the method of treatment always applied by any and every therapeutical school is to inhibit those conditions.

"On the reverse, in a case of Constipation, Bright's Disease, Melancholia, or any other disease where we have **a lack of function or not enough function**, that condition would need stimulation. In medicine there are stimulants; or in massage manipulation is designed and intended to stimulate; to excessively increase the present condition existing (5).

"To inhibit means where there is 120 per cent. of function at a specified locality; the intentions are to endeavor to compel that 120 per cent to reduce itself to the normal of 100 per cent. In a case where we have only 80 per cent. acting—a lack of function, the tendency of all therapeutical treatment is to make the 80 per cent. do the standard work of 100 per cent. (6). . . . . By a subluxation of a vertebra we are producing pressure upon nerves, or **reducing the calibre or carrying capacity of that nerve fibre**; by so doing, **interfering with transmission of** cylic **currents** (7). If this pressure upon nerves be light; be steady, **then function is excessive** at periphery. If the pressure be heavy and permanent, then we have a lack of function at periphery.

Page 75: "The question has been asked whether we can ever

have more than 100 per cent. of current or an excess of mental impulses, inasmuch as 100 per cent. is a standard. Have we more than 100 per cent. in any one given pathological condition (8)? We have always assumed (9) the ground that we could because we have recognized the pathological states or conditions wherein there was an excess of function. We know that 100 per cent. caloric mental impulses are equivalent to normal heat. When we get more than normal heat we have excessive heat. When we have an excessive effect, we must have an excessive cause. The cause of normal heat is a normal amount of mental impulses; the cause of excessive heat must be an excessive amount of mental impulses.

"Now, how to assume that we have an excess of current, and yet never more than 100 per cent. has been a problem (10). Let us assume the various states of excess of quantities or diminished quantities of electricity and see how the problem is deciphered. Let us go, in other words, from the known state of increased and diminished currents of electricity to the quantities that are present in excess or lack of in man.

Page 79: "The entire rub of the proposition is that after the body has gone through such a burning-out process it dies for want of enough of the reparatory impulses to adapt itself to that standard" (12).

(1) "Pathologically abnormal." Pathologically—pertaining to pathology—disease. Abnormal—not conformable to the general rule. Why not say, that condition which is pathological?

(2) The above definition of treatment, disease and function is truthfully expressed. I am pleased to see "disease is too much or not enough function," it being quite different from that found on page 78 of No. 4 Announcement, and second line of page 13, "We find the cause of disease, the **shutting off of the current,** as it were, of the mental impulses,"—disease is because of "functions shut off."

(3) In diabetes there is too much urine; over action of the kidneys. In diarrhoea, too much water with the stool either from a lack of function in the part of the kidneys, or too much on the part of the intestines. These abnormal conditions are because of nerve impingement—results of accidents or poisons.

(4) A running of the nose in coryza, is because of "the breaking up of a cold." The serum has been thickened and held from circulation because of local inflammation. The freeing of nerves from impingement, the resumption of normal heat liquifies the thickened serum; and a surplus existing, it is discharged.

(5) The author of the above lines does not have a clear conception of functions, or, he is unable to express himself intelligently. Therapeutical remedies are used to inhibit excessive action and stimulate those functions which are expressed below normal.

(6) To reduce the 120 per cent and increase the 80 per cent to normal, assuming 100 per cent to be normal.

(7) The carrying capacity of a nerve depends upon whether the nerve is excited or depressed. Vertebral impingement may produce either of the extremes, depending in each instance upon the amount of pressure as expressed in the remaining portion of this paragraph.

(8) That question was one of friction between B. J. and myself while we were in partnership. He asserted that water or steam pipes could not carry more than 100 per cent; consequently, disease was not because of an excess, or an oversupply of impulses. I then maintained, and do yet, that his pipes and tree illustrations are not illustrative of animal functions. The Chiropractic principle that disease is the result of either too much functionating, was enunciated by me, as may be seen by The Chiropractor, No. 1, page 1. The body has been likened to a pharmaceutical laboratory; to an electrical machine; to a gas machine; to an engine. But none of these express the action of functions directed by intelligence.

(9) He always assumed that there could not be more than 100 per cent. I am glad to learn that he is assuming Chiropractic ideas, that he has made this advancement, and trust that he will quit using the pipe, tree and other inanimate illustrations, which do not illustrate an intelligent creator of inanimate objects.

(10) That problem, that dilemma, the thought that disease is because of function expressed **above** or below **normal,** was difficult for him to grasp. Perhaps I was expecting too much of his youthful mind; possibly I should have had more patience. As it took two years for him to learn the difference between displaced and misplaced, I should have allowed him the seven years he has taken to discover the error of using the tree and pipe illustrations. But, better late than never; yet it is better to be never late. The last Chiropractor shows that he has now run off on another tangent—electricity, which cannot be used to illustrate functional activity, because it has no intelligence and no electrical amount which is considered normal.

(11) The above three lines is the summing up of deductions from two pages of electrical explanations, which do not explain the workings of the four functions—vital, vegetative; intellectual, and cumulative.

## INSANITY.

Insanity is disorder of the mental faculties, with or without consciousness and volition. Abnormal mental functions are always associated with diseased tissue. All abnormal functions, either vital or intellectual, depend upon structural change of tissue. Both diseased tissue and mental abberation may be congenital or acquired.

Insanity is characterized by any of one or more mental symptoms. The most common are change of character and habits, moroseness, confusion, elation, melancholia, mania, delusions and hallucinations.

Medical books recognize, according to their association, nearly 50 varieties of insanity.

As the vegetative function is subservient to the vital so the cumulative is subordinate to the mental. Normal **tonicity** of tissue performs absorption, assimilation and excretion in normal amounts, an equilibrium we name health. Likewise, the cumulative will accumulate normal thots. If the solidity and tension of nerves and muscles are not normal, too lax or compact, their intellectual and vegetative functions will be abnormal.

As the degree of tonicity depends upon the amount of heat, so, likewise, does the quantity of impulse transmitted.

The Chiropractor locates the impingement (to be specific, means one location and one adjustment; otherwise it is not scientific), which disturbs functions, mental or physical, relieves the pressure and restores normal innervation. There is no need of creating "dermameric, myomeric, osseomeric, visemeric, neuromeric, audimeric, olfameric, gustameric, sensomeric, omnemeric, unimeric or vertemeric forun, resistance current, quantity, capacity, power or work."

Chiropractic is a science just so far as it is specific. The ability to discriminate, to be precise, makes Chiropractic a science and an art.

---

Many physicians are willing that we care for the chronics, which they have failed to relieve; but think that we should not take the acute cases, as there is danger of losing them. They desire to have the disease develop under their care, so that they may know what ailed them and name the disease correctly. A Chiropractor steps in, takes charge of a case of fever before it has fully developed and consequently before he is able to tell which of the many kinds of fever it might result in. But he relieves the diseased condition and spoils the guess of the physician—is not that awful?

## NEUROPATHY.

Dr. A. P. Davis in the prospectus of his second book on Neuropathy says: "It describes the . . . safest and surest method of treatment that cures disease."

This would imply that there were other methods which were safe and sure; if so, how can his method be any more than safe or sure?

He truly says: "No disease can exist when the nervous system is **free** from pressure or irritation, and toxic poisons."

He talks Chiropractic. "The spinal nervous system is especially described and the best method of adjusting each vertebra to relieve pressure."

Neuropathy by A. P. Davis says: "How can an adjustment occur when there is no displacement? The word adjustment for treatment, is a manifestation of ignorance. We deny luxations being the cause of nerve impingements. To be effectual in arresting any complaint in the body it is essential that the two poles be united, this done, harmony at once supervenes. Recognizing the fact that two forces are to be considered . . . the application of this peculiar pressure has a far-reaching influence . . . this is done by the hands along the spine, so placed as to bear down suddenly at given places along the spinal column. It unites the positive and negative forces, which neutralize the acid and alkaline elements, and harmonize the system with itself.

"The best method of adjusting each vertebra to relieve pressure." The best method would imply that there were more than one. I do not know of but one unless he alludes to the mallet and chisel, which was popular among the Minnesota and Los Angeles Chiros a few years ago.

I am glad to see the advancement. There is a vast difference between "an adjustment can not be made where there is no displacement" and "the best method of adjusting each vertebra." I wonder if the forthcoming book will state, "disease is because of an unbalanced condition of the two forces, that a sudden pressure on the right vertebra will bring into accord the inharmony of the functions, thereby equalizing the acid and alkaline elements."

He further says of his future book. "It embraces the entire physical organism—the nervous system—and that means all there is involved in all diseases known to mankind. Right the nervous system and all disease ceases to exist—absolutely."

If this be a fact, "that there need be no difficulty in understanding how to apply each manipulation so as to relieve . . . easily-applied manipulations with the hands of some one of the family." If this be a fact, why give a department on "home remedies"? Why talk about correcting the eye-strain by wearing the proper lens? Why give special instructions in diet, deep breathing, bathing and suggestions? Why devote space for valuable recipes? Why tell your readers how Christian Science relieves its patients?

If, by righting the nervous system, uniting the two great forces by spinal adjustments—a new discovery found described in no other book—all diseases cease to exist, why give medical remedies, such as salt, lemon and kerosene?

---

Physicians give drugs because the patient is not content with out them. By giving medicine at regular specified times, the patient in made aware of how time flies. Prescribing is an experiment with the doctor who gives, and the patient who receives. The giving and taking is a gambling speculation.

---

The doctor, it would seem, is not in high repute with Paddy. A man in Limerick went to the undertaker to order a coffin for Mike Connell. "Dear me," said the undertaker, "is poor Mike dead?" "No, he's not dead yet," answered the other; "but he'll die tonight, for the doctor says he can't live till morning, and he knows what he gave him."—Massachusetts Medical Journal.

---

An advertisement states, "The only Chiro-paths. Dr. Blank, originator and founder of the Chiro-pathic system." He has two "regular graduates."

Chiro means hand; path, disease; therefore, this doctor is a hand-disease kind of a fellow. He is the originator and founder of the hand-disease system. He has two "regular graduates." How many irregular graduates he has hand-diseased he does not state.

---

A certain would-be teacher of advanced Chiropractic tries to illustrate the possible per cent of impulse which can be passed through a nerve, by using a pipe for an illustration. He wisely states there cannot be more than 100 per cent pass through the pipe and yet he tells the class of "excessive heat." An "excess" is more than normal, more than 100 per cent. Impulse cannot be percented; neither can steam. Why talk nonsense? Inanimate objects do not illustrate animate living vital beings.

## COPYRIGHT.

The above is a copy of the title page of a book compiled, published and copyrighted by the last named person. On the next page is a copy of a portion of the title page of its reissue.

The party to whom I am indebted for a copy of my mutilated articles says: "Vol. 1 is a dandy compilation of gall and usurpation of another's labors and ideas."

But few have any knowledge concerning the laws on patents and copyrights. The following may be of interest to those who are inclined to plagiarize the ideas and language of others:

Portland has one of the best law libraries in America; from a volume on copyright I have copied the following:

A work in order to be copyrighted must be original, in the sense that the author has created it by his own skill, labor and judgment, without directly copying or evasively imitating the work of an auther.

It must contain something meritorious from the author's own mind, which would not have found existence in the form presented but for the distinctive individuality of mind from which it sprang.

To constitute a person an author within the meaning of the copyright laws, he must by his own intellectual labor and skill produce a work new and original in itself.

An employer is not an author. A person who hires another to write a book and gives him the description and scope of the work is not the creator of the work for which protection is claimed.

Penalties for inserting or impressing false notice. The false insertion or impression of a notice of copyright in or upon any article, whether such article be subject to copyright or otherwise, or knowingly to issue, sell, or import any article bearing such false notice of copyright, is prohibited under a penalty of one hundred dollars, recoverable one-half for the person who shall sue for such penalty and one-half to the use of the United States. The circuit courts of the United States sitting in equity are authorized to enjoin the issuing, publishing or selling of any article marked or imported in violation of the copyright laws.

So too, an author may maintain an action at law for the injury to his reputation as an author arising from false representations as to his authorship of a work or from the publication of his work in a mutilated form.

About one-half of the 432 pages of the reissue were original with me, created by my own skill, labor and judgment. The articles (40 of them) are meritorious; they would not have found existence in the form presented, but for the distinctive individuality of my own mind from which they sprang.

The party mentioned as the second person in the first title page, and as being the author and copyrighter of the reissue, as evidenced by the second cut, has given a false notice of copyright. He has knowingly issued and sold such copyrighted articles as his own production, containing a false notice of copyright for which there is a penalty of one hundred dollars for each and every article bearing such false notice of copyright.

The above mentioned plagiarist has injured my reputation as an author by falsely claiming that he is the author of 40 articles which were written by my own hand, created by my skill, labor and judgment, and their mutilation by his hand has damaged my distinction as a writer as well as the science I originated and founded.

An explanatory page in the reissue reads: "He (B. J.) has shown indomnitable will and courage in preserving the science of Chiropractic from corruption." No one Chiropractor has done as much to vitiate, deprave and pervert the principles and philosophy of the science and art originated, developed and founded by his father.

The historical page states: "Mrs. Weed and daughter took Chiropractic adjustments in 1896 and were much benefitted, after which Mr. Weed also received adjustments for sciatica and was relieved. About this time he was asked to suggest a name for the science and art. He simply translated the description of it, 'done by hand,' into Greek and thus originated the name Chiropractic."

B. J. being the author and copyrighter of this book, the reader would naturally think that he was the man who did the adjusting referred to and that he was the one who asked Rev. Weed to suggest a name for the science and art. The facts are, in 1896, B. J. was 14 years of age. Six years later he graduated under his father as a Chiropractor. Mrs. Weed and daughter took adjustments from me, after which Rev. Weed also received adjustments from me. It was I who asked Rev. Weed to cull from the Greek a word meaning done by hand. Rev. Weed presented me two words, from which I selected the word Chiropractic. Rev. Weed will verify my statement. His address is Monmouth, Ill., R. F. D. No. 7.

A photo cut of Rev. Samuel H. Weed appears on the following page.

There are 10 articles, written by my own hand and original with me. which have been garbled, mutilated and copyrighted by B.J.Palmer and sold as his own production. Not knowing his

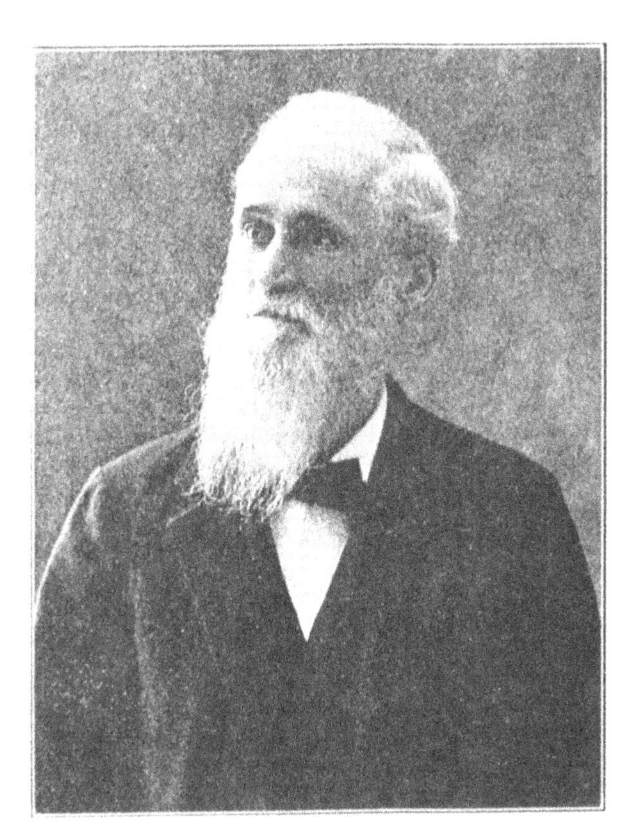

REV. SAMUEL H. WEED, Monmouth, Illinois.

unstable slippery position, he says: "Woe be unto those who see fit to copy any part or parcel of them. Infringements are as bad as bold copying. We shall proceed without mercy to relative, friend or foe."

Any one reading my article in his reissue, "The First Chiropractic Patient," would be led to believe that B. J. Palmer, when he was 13 years of age, was the one who gave that first adjustment to Harvey Lillard on September 18, 1895. He failed to cut out, "Magnetic healing was, for nine years, the forerunner of Chiropractic," which dates the author's practice back to when he was three years of age.

The purloiner has prefaced my lengthy article, "Chiropractic Rays of Light," with the head-line, "Chiropractic founded on principle," and nine paragraphs, which have no natural connection with the subject matter in my article. This unprincipled act would justify me in maintaining an action at law for injury to my reputation as an author, arising from false representation as to the authorship and the publishing of my articles in a mutilated form.

The heading of my article, "The body is Heated by Nerves," which was written by my own hand, created by my own skill and judgment, which relates the details of my discovery that the nerves and not the blood are concerned in the heating of the body, is so mutilated as to give the compiler of my writings all the credit of one of the greatest discoveries of this or any age.

The original article, as written by me, contained in the first four paragraphs, the following:

"It will be of interest to learn how Dr. D. D. Palmer discovered that the body is heated by nerves, and not by blood.

"In the afternoon of July 1, 1903, in suite 15 Aiken block, Santa Barbara, Cal., D. D. Palmer was holding a clinic. The patient was Roy Renwick of that city. There were present among the rest as students, O. G. Smith, Minora C. Paxson, in all told eight witnesses.

"The patient A. R. Renwick's left hand, arm, shoulder and on up to the spine, was intensely hot. Dr. Palmer drew the attention of the class to the excessive heated condition of the portion named; the remainder being normal in temperature. He then gave an adjustment in the dorsal region which relieved the pinched nerve on the left side, also the excessive heat of the upper limb; but he had thrown the vertebra too far, which had the effect of pinching the nerves on the right side, and immediately causing the upper right limb to be excessively hot. He asked the class, "Is the body heated by blood or by nerves?" He then left them for two or three minutes. He returned and asked, "Is the body heated by blood or by nerves?" The class unanimously answered "Nerves." Thus was this new thought originated."

The above circumstance is substantiated by a letter written that evening to the doctor's son, B. J. Palmer, D. C., also several following letters which further explained that the caloric of the body, whether normal or in excess was furnished by calorific nerves. These letters were placed with other original writings in one of the 30 bound volumes in order to prove the autobiography of Chiropractic from its birth. Here are the original writings which show beyond the shadow of a doubt who originated the principle of Chiropractic. Dr. B. J. Palmer anticipated that some sneak thief would try to appropriate the credit of originality and would desire to rob his father of the honor justly due him; hence his reason for compiling his original writings.

Little did I then think that B. J. Palmer, my only son, would prove to be the sneak thief who would try to appropriate the credit of originality and would desire to rob his father of the honor justly due him. Little did I think then, that my only son would play the Judas, put me in prison, rob me financially and of credit justly due me. The reader is referred to page 165 of The Science of Chiropractic, for the original from which I copy and to pages 179 and 180 of the revised edition for the verification of the following which shows the mutilation and the purpose thereof.

The headline was changed to "The Body is Heated by Mental Impulse."

The above four paragraphs were replaced by the following two: The first and last were omitted for obvious reasons, as was also the paragraph inserted and the mutilation.

"It will be of interest to learn how the body is heated by mental impulses which creates combustion of chemicals arterially and serously deposited, and not by blood, and therefore the blood acts as one of the attributes in preference to performing all the calorific duties thereof.

"The patient upon whom the first tests were made (July 1, 1903) A. R. Renwick's left hand, arm, shoulder and on up to the spine, was intensely hot. Dr. Palmer drew the attention of the class to the excessive heat condition of the portion named; the balance being normal in temperature. He then gave an adjustment in the dorsal region, which relieved the pinched nerve on the left side, also the excessive heat of the left upper limb; but he had thrown the vertebra too far, which had the effect of pinching the nerves on the right side, and immediately causing the upper limb to be excessively hot. He asked the class, "Is the body heated by blood or by mental impulse?" He left them for two or three minutes. He returned and asked, "Is the body heated by blood or by mental impulses?" The class unanimously answered, "By mental impulses.' Thus was this new thought originated."

The added spurious paragraph reads: "The patient upon whom the first tests were made." In this case of A. R. Renwick, there were no test paper, no test spoon, no test glass tube, no test types, such as are used by occulists, no test solution, no test culture nor any chemical tests made; it was not a test case. I know all about it, as I was there, in Santa Barbara, Cal., and the would-be discoverer was in Davenport, Ia. The Dr. Palmer referred to was myself, and not B. J. Palmer. "Nerves" have been changed for "mental impulses" in order that the incorrect statement made in the first paragraph might be braced by a false statement. "Thus was this new thought originated by myself, in Santa Barbara, Cal., and not by B. J. Palmer in Davenport, Iowa.

The lengthy article "Chiropractic Rays of Light," written by my own hand, has been mutilated by the purloiner who has given it a new heading and prefixed it with nine paragraphs, which have no natural connection.

The one page item on "Typhoid Fever" has been copied and alterations made. The first line of the original as written by me, reads: "Mrs. M. E. Kale, of Milan, Ill., allows me to say:" has been changed to "Mrs. M. E. K. allows me to say." The cure was made and the article written while B. J. was in his teens, before he had ever given an adjustment.

A similar alteration and mutilation has been made with the one page article on "Diphtheria." The original was written by me read, "Mrs. J. H. Murray and her two children, of 412 West Bijou Street, Colorado Springs, was visiting at her mother's home, Mrs. Mary Kale, 702 Second Avenue, Rock Island, Ill.

Mrs. Murray had set a day to return west. But as her daughter, Morine, age nine years, was taken with diphtheria in an aggravated form the home trip had to be deferred. I was called on September 23, 24 hours later. The neighbor's house had a "diphtheria" card on it, and the usual quarantine regulations. The article written by me has been changed and mutilated to "Mrs. J. H. M.—— was visiting at her mother's home in Rock Island. She had set a day to return west. But as her daughter, Morine, aged nine, was taken with diphtheria in an aggravated form, the home trip had to be deferred. I was called on September 23, twenty-four hours later."

The "I" who wrote this item was myself and not B. J. Palmer as represented. The same can be said of each and every cure mentioned in this revised edition.

I have written the above so that my readers may understand who is entitled to use and revise those articles many of which appear in this issue.

---

You may think Chiropractic is like Osteopathy. If so, go to an Osteopath for a treatment and afterward take a Chiropractic adjustment. You will then not only know there is a difference between them, but you will know just what that difference is.

---

We are indebted to the Journal of Osteopathy for the following, which reaches 133 years farther back in medicine than several books in our library:

"Some light is thrown upon the state of things herefrom resulting by a work translated from the German in the year 1561, and entitled, 'A Most Excellent and Perfect Homish Apothecarye or Physicke Booke, for all the Grefes and Diseases of the Bodye.' The first chapter is 'Concerning the Head and His Partes. Galen sayth the head is divided into foure partes; in the forepart hath blood the dominion; Cholera in the ryght syde, Melancholy in the left syde, and Flegma bareth rule in the hindermost part. If the head doth ake so sore by reason of a runninge that he cannot snoffe hys nose, bath hys fete in a depe tub until the knees and give him this medicine * * * which riseth into hys head and dryeth hys moyst braynes. Galen sayth he that hath payne in the hindermost part of hys head, the same must be let blood under the chynne, especially on the right syde; also were it good often to burn the heyre of a man before hys nose. The braynes are greved many wayes; many there are whom the head whyrleth so sore that he thinketh the earth turneth upsyde doune: Cummin refraineth the whyrling, comforteth the braynes and maketh them to grow agayne; or he may take the braynes of a hogge, rost the same upon a grede yron and cut slices thereof and lay to the greved parts." The reader will note from the above the nature of Galen's theories and conceptions of disease and the cure thereof. King also states * * * "in medical works of the middle ages we meet constantly with such prescriptions as these: Take the right eye of a frogg, lap it in a piece of russet cloth and hang it about the neck; it cureth the right eye if it be enflamed or bleared. And if the left eye be greved, do the like by the left eye of said frogg.' Again, The skin of a raven's heel is good against the gout, but the right heel skin must be laid upon the right foot if that be gouty and the left upon the left,' etc.' "

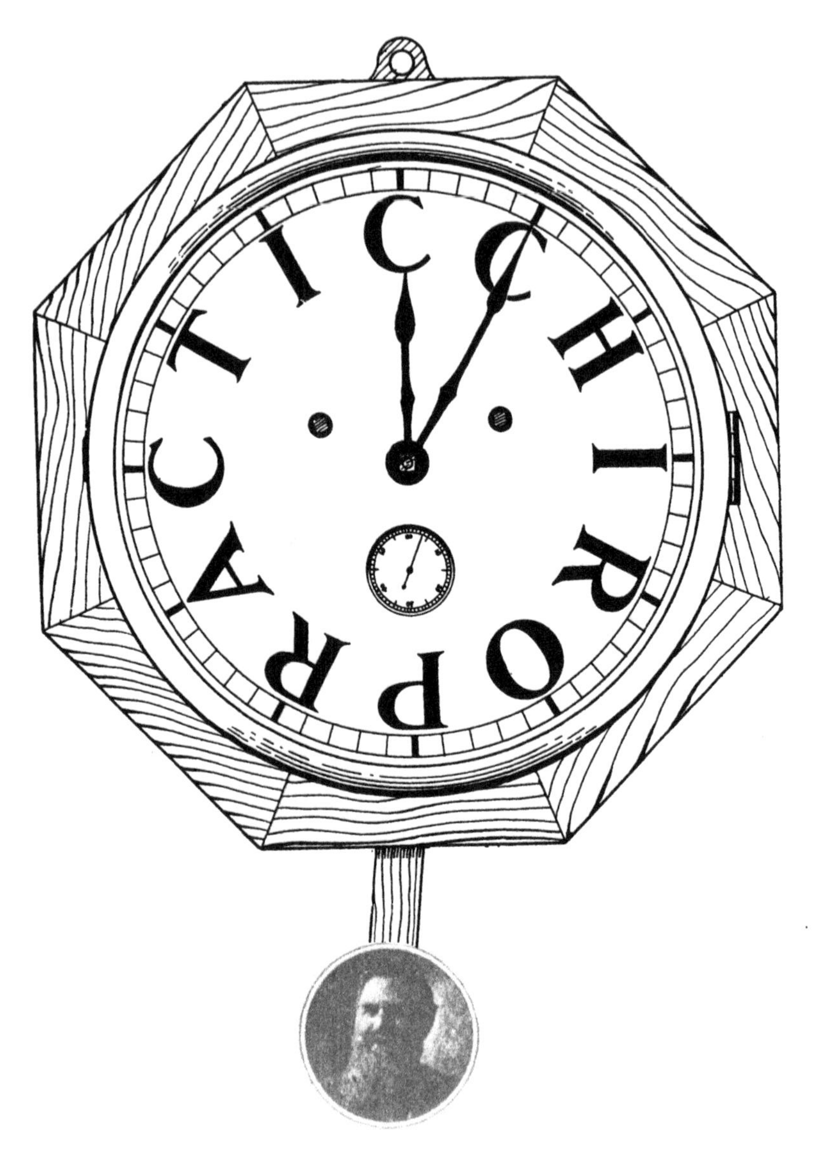


As Chiropractic marks the hours of the day by encircling the face of the clock, so, tone, by its elasticity and renitency forms the basis of the science of Chiropractic. Tone is the foundation upon which I built the science, reasoned out its philosophy and created the art of adjusting luxated vertebrae.

## MONSTROSITIES.

Under this head I shall confine myself to the human embryo and fetus. The fertilized germ is known as the embryo up to the third or fourth month. After the quickening period it is known as the fetus.

A monster is an organized being which has an extraordinary conformation of one or more parts.

A monstrosity is one which has **great** congenital deformity.

There are many kinds of malformations. It is in the province of this article to notice only those with an excess or a deficiency of structure; anomalies of volume, form, color and structure; monstrosities by defect appearing at birth.

The cause of monstrosities has been shrouded in mystery. The science of Chiropractic is slowly but surely clearing up this obstruse question.

Chiropractic can only be developed on Chiropractic lines. To annul a portion of the nervous system in order to discover a direct mental impulse, is not advancing the science. Such teaching lowers it and brings in into disrepute.

Chiropractors have so far been content to correct postnatal deformities. The adage that "An ounce of prevention is worth a pound of cure" is as good in Chiropractic as in any other business. We now want to take another step forward—prevent vegetative functions being performed abnormally before birth, as well as after.

If it be a fact that functions may be performed as excessively or as deficiently in the embryo or fetus, as in the adult, is it not possible that where functions are not performed there would be an absence of parts corresponding to those which would be atrophied by the same impingement? If so, functions in the fetus which are performed either with excessive or deficient energy may account for all forms of monsters, whether the abnormality consists in deficient or excessive tissue.

Among the many hypotheses entertained concerning the origin or the cause of monsters, may be mentioned the influence of the maternal imagination upon the embryo or fetus in utero; changes made direct by accidents; defects in the germs or ovum.

If the growth of the embryo and fetus is accomplished through vital and vegetative functions, and of this there is no doubt, then, is it not a fact that they are performed in accordance with functional activity? Disease is but an **alteration in** function or **the structure** of some organ or part of the body. Normal parts are the result of functions performed in a natural manner. Defects in structure are the result of too much or not enough functionating. May we not state that lesions in the mother's vertebral column, while affecting nerve-fibre functions, would also affect her unborn? Would not that which produces abnormalities in the mother produce the same in the embryo or fetus? Innate directs and controls the nutritive activities of both the unborn and the mother through the nerves of the latter.

I have said that the science of Chiropractic is founded on osteology, neurology and functions. I include arthrology under osteology. The Chiropractor needs to make special study of these two branches of anatomy and that of physiology. These treat of the phenomena of living organisms as expressed by vital and vegetative functions, as these two have to do with the building and growth of the physical. The intellectual and cumulative functions have to do with knowledge of external things, of our environments.

While embryology, myology, and angiology are instructive, they are not so essential to a Chiropractor as are the branches of osteology, neurology and physiology. While Chiropractors make a specialty of these three branches, they study them for quite a different purpose than do other schools.

We have just stated that we have four kinds of functions: the vital and vegetative, the intellectual and cumulative. If these are properly performed, there can be no disease or monstrosities, physically or mentally.

The Innate of the mother runs all the functions of the embryo and fetus until delivery. **The breath of life** is evidence of the union existing between spirit and body, the intelligent life, known in the Good Book as the soul, the symphisis which makes a triplet of spirit, soul and body. The vegetative function, guided by intelligence, constitutes life—the soul. The cumulative function is accumulating an aggregation of likes and dislikes; angelic or fiendish; humane or brutal; polished or rude; sensitive or unfeeling; conscientious or cruel, which may continue through life and in a great measure determine thon's mental characteristics. The vegetative function is forming a body, that may be regular or deformed; comely or monstrous; attractive or hideous, depending upon the vital function for the energy which directs the vegetative, the builder of mind and body.

How necessary it is, that we should understand the laws of our mechanism which govern our functions. Chiropractic has a great work to perform, one that is far reaching; it begins before conception and should continue as long as the soul holds spirit and body together.

Knowing that our physical health and the intellectual progress of Innate (the personified portion of Universal Intelligence), depend upon the proper alignment of the skeletal frame, prenatal as well as postnatal, we feel it our right and bounden duty to replace any displaced bones, so that the physical and spiritual may enjoy health, happiness and the full fruition of our earthly lives.

The vital and intellectual functions perform the vegetative and cumulative, the building of the body and growth of mind in a normal manner, if communication is not disturbed.

The principles discovered and promulgated by me are as effectual before birth as after. The elements upon which I founded the science are as immutable today as when I discovered them. Those who seek to advance the science, must do so with these as a basis.

The construction of the embryo and fetus is performed by Innate, as much so as that of the mother after birth. The component parts of the mother and her offspring are the result of functions performed. Club feet, prenatal and postnatal, are formed by the same law; a displaced lumbar vertebra impinging upon the posterior primary division of the spinal nerve trunk which passes dorsalwards between the arches or transverse processes of the two adjacent vertebra. It then divides into the medial and lateral branches, which show a general tendency to run caudalwards. Fibers of these nerves go to and innervate the feet. Club feet are because of bone pressure on these nerves, causing contraction. These nerve functions are reciprocated, normal or abnormal, to the fetus, the same as in the mother. Remember that the principles laid down by me during the early history of Chiropractic—disease is too much or not enough function—is true before birth as well as after. Thus it is with the embryo and fetus. Parts that are disproportionally large, small, or entirely lacking, are because of functions performed accordingly. Each nerve-fiber has its separate and distinct function. Its administration, prenatal or postnatal, depends upon its freedom from impingement.

Therefore to prevent monstrosities, and produce the beautiful, mentally or physically, we should see that the bones of the skeletal frame of the mother are not impinging on the conveyors of impulses, which are behind vegetative functions. **Remember,** that the same law which governs the functions of the mother operate in a like manner in building the unborn.

## MEASLES.

This disease is also known as morbilli and rubeola. It is not dangerous to life, but the sequelae embrace morbid phenomena in the form of various chronic affections, due to medication or the vertebral lesion. The onset of the disease resembles a severe cold or an attack of influenza. The individual sneezes repeatedly, there is an acrid discharge from the nostrils, the eyes are red, inflamed and watery. There is a soreness of the throat and a dry, hoarse, painful cough. There is usually a chilly sensation, but rarely a distinct pronounced chill. There is fever, but it is commonly less intense than that of scarlet fever. The appetite is impaired, nausea and vomiting may occur. There are wandering pains in various parts of the body, especially in the head and limbs, general debility and languor. Convulsions and bleeding at the nose may occur. The eruption of the skin is the visible evidence of a moderate dermal and subdermal inflammation. The liver in acute cases may show focal necrosis resembling those found in other inflamed organs.

The disease affects principally the young. The medical dictionaries and pathological books assert that one attack confers perpetual immunity. The principal reason is that it is a disease of childhood; a period in our lives that never comes but once. but once.

The following complications often follow measles: Pneumonia, bronchitis, phthisis, otitis media, diphtheria, croup and deafness. These lesions are secondary affections, whereas the primary lesion was a poison which drew a dorsal vertebra out of alignment. In the primary affection or any one of the secondary named there will be found a displaced dorsal vertebra in the upper dorsal, and on its right side an enlarged nerve, very sensitive to the touch. If the adjuster will examine this rigid nerve previous to adjusting and again immediately after, he will find a vast difference in its texture. Before adjusting it will be found contracted lengthwise, enlarged diametrally, rigid and tender; immediately after it will be lax and not sensitive to the touch. The fever will rapidly subside.

---

There are two kinds of doctors—the dispensing and the prescribing doctor. A dispensing doctor is one who carries his medicine and gives it direct to the patient. A prescribing doctor is one who carries no medicine with him, but writes a prescription, which is taken to the drug store named on the prescription tablet, for which he usually gets a percentage.

## THE SYMPATHETIC NERVOUS SYSTEM.

The sympathetic system consists of the nerves of organic life which control the vital functions and the vegetative processes. The vital consists of the energy, the vegetative includes that which is accomplished.

The cerebro-spinal nerves are those of animal life, they look after the somatic portions and the environments of the body.

The sympathetic portion of the nervous system consists of nerves, ganglia and plexuses.

The nerves are tubular cords, filled with nerve fibers, which extend from the nerve centers to every part of the body, supplying a means of communication between two or more parts of the body. They communicate frequently with each other. They may proceed alone, or accompany blood vessels for convenience, economy or safety, through foramina or channels of bone. They convey impulses and sensations to and from the nerve centers.

There are three kinds of ganglia (nerve centers): glandiform, vascular, such as the spleen, thymus, thyroid and suprarenal, the lymphatic, lymph ganglions or glands, which form and circulate lymph; the nervous ganglia, those especially concerned in this lesson. These are known by an enlargement in a nerve; they are confined to the sympathetic system. One exists on the posterior root of every spinal nerve. It seems that every sympathetic nerve fiber passes through a ganglion; ganglia are especially connected with the nerves of organic life.

In addition to the ganglia (dispensing locations) of the two vertebral chains, we have sporadic ganglia (also distributing localities) situated along nerves which have left the two vertical nerve chains. They are the ciliary, Meckel's, otic and sub-mandibular; these are connected with the cranial nerves by junction with them, become a part of those nerves, and thereby convey certain functions. The ciliary one of the smallest ganglia of the body, is also known as the ophthalmic or lenticular ganglion. Ciliary, hairlike; ophthalmic, pertaining to the eye; lenticular, having the form of a double-convex lens. It is a small, reddish body about the size of a large pin-head. It lies back of the orbital cavity. This orbit is formed by a junction of the frontal, sphenoid, ethmoid, nasal, lacrimal, superior maxilary and palatal bones. The ciliary ganglion is supplied from the nasal branch of the ophthalmic, the third cervical nerve, the cavernous plexus and Meckel's ganglion. Those from the cavernous plexus are from the sympathetic; the superior cervical ganglion is supplied from the 1st, 2d, 3d and 4th cervical. Chiropractors, by actual test, supply one from the lower dorsal. This ganglion, by the above names, sends to the sclerotic coat, encircling around the optic nerve, 12 to 18 fine filaments which supply sensation and trophic functions to the eyeball and sphincter iridis and sympathetic nerves to the dilator fibers of the iris. These nerve fibers, which give energy to the vital functions of the eye and perfom the vegetative function, pass from the cranial to the orbital cavity by way of the sphenoidal fissure, optic foramen, orbital foramina and the spheno-maxillay fissure. Thus we might trace all the cranial nerves and their accessories which communicate functions. If it requires 12 months to study "direct mental impulse" as shown by a cut in this issue, how long would it take to study neurology as just touched upon in this article?

A plexus is a network of nervous filaments, which may be cerebro-spinal or sympathetic in its makeup; from these proceed branches to other plexuses or organs.

From the base of the skull to the coccyx there are two series of ganglia, which are to the sympathetic system what the spinal system is to the general nervous system; therefore, they are sometimes called the vertebral nerves.

The sympathetic nervous system, as a functionating distributing agency, presents a distinct contrast to the cranial and spinal nerves. It is dissimilar to the central nervous system, inasmuch as it includes mainly the visceral and vascular nerves. Although it has manifold communications with the cerebro-spinal system, it represents, to a certain extent, an independent system. It is most intimately connected with the cerebro-spinal system and, with it, has the same developmental origin. From the sympathetic system fibers pass to the various viscera of the head, chest and abdomen, where they again form plexuses from which fibers endowed with varied functions pass to the different organs.

The system under discussion consists primarly of two chains of ganglia, lying one on each side of the spinal column. The cervical portion passes in front of the transverse processes. The thoracic part of this sympathetic trunk is situated in front of the ribs and at the sides of the bodies of the vertebrae covered by the pleura. The lumbar and sacral portions converge toward each other, uniting at the coccyx.

---

In the near future Chiropractic will be as much valued for its preventative qualities as it now is for adjusting and relieving the cause of ailments.

## INNATE.

I quote: "This (Innate and Educated Intelligence) is a pet theory of mine because of this peculiar fact in the development of the nervous system, we find that it develops into two systems. The Innate nervous system acts independently and alone, separate and apart and is not a counterpart of the Educated Nervous System, neither is the Educated a counterpart of the other, but while the Innate would be able to perform all its functions without the educated, yet the educated could not perform one action at any time without the Innate Nervous System. It is because of this fact that we place such an importance upon the Innate direct nervous system—preceding the Educated at all times. If our Innate Nervous System did not exist within our tissue cells we could not live and Educated could not control at will certain conscious actions. The minds behind those systems are conscious at all times."

He says, "This is a pet theory of mine." The Chiropractic principle of the two intelligences may yet remain a **theory** with him, a scheme which may terminate in speculation. Is it possible that he yet holds Innate. the source of functional energy, only as a tentative conjecture of vital phenomena?

"This is a pet **theory of mine.**" Innate and Educated Intelligences were among my earliest Chiropractic conceptions. They were to me a vital fact, a condensed proposition of important practical truth; one of the basic principles of the science of Chiropractic. That boy should long ere this have received it as such and not continue to hold it as a "pet theory." Among my writings of five years ago, was one on "Innate Intelligence." It can be found in Vol. 1 of The Science of Chiropractic, commencing on page 109, covering five pages It is "Copyright, 1906, B. J. Palmer, D. C., Davenport, Iowa, U. S. A." It is included in the revised edition without giving due credit, thereby assuming ownership, and making the author liable to a "penalty for inserting or impressing false notice. The false insertion or impression of a notice of copyright in or upon any article, **whether such article be subject to copyright or otherwise**, or knowingly to issue, sell or import **any article bearing such false notice of copyright, is prohibited under penalty of one hundred dollars, recoverable** one-half for the person who shall sue for such penalty and **one-half to the use of the United States. The circuit courts of the United States sitting in equity are authorized to enjoin the issuing, publishing or selling of any article marked or imported in violation of the copyright laws.**

"So to, he may maintain an action at law for the injury to his reputation as an author arising from false representations as to his authorship of a work **or from the publication of his work in a mutilated form.**'' See sections 925 and 930 of Law and Procedure.''

There are forty articles which have been falsely copyrighted. Each of which stand liable to a penalty of $100, also damages for mutilation and injury to my reputation as an author.

If I should authorize the circuit courts of the United States sitting in equity to enjoin the issuing, publishing or selling of any such article marked in violation of the copyright laws, the penalties would be sufficient to blow up that pseudo fountain head.

I have been lenient, knowing that if I should deprive the thief of my property, that it would **dispossess him of nine-tenths of all the literature he has which is characteristic of the science, art or philosophy of Chiropractic.**

Inasmuch as Innate controls all the vital functions, it forms one of the basic principles of Chiropractic. And whereas, it is stated on page 10 of the twelve feet of knocking, ''I can stand before you and say that 99 per cent of these are ideas of others than D. D. Palmer.'' I am not satisfied with such small favors, being only allowed the credit of one per cent of what is now known as the science of Chiropractic.

On page 91 of August and September number, 1908, of The Chiropractor, I find, ''Dr. B. J. Palmer, the developer of this wonderful science and philosophy.''

In the June and July number of The Chiropractor, 1908, page 37, ''It has long been proclaimed that D. D. Palmer was the discoverer of the fundamental crude principles and that B. J. Palmer, D. C., Ph. C., was the developer of this science. It is up to you to disprove that if you can. You have never made any efforts in that direction, for its basis is too well established.''

It has been proclaimed for fourteen years that I was the discoverer and developer of the science of Chiropractic. The honor of being the developer of the science was not self-appropriated by another until within the last two years. Even up to 1907, page 35, of the Chiropractor states, ''What little you (O. G. Smith) know of Chiropractic was taught you (in 1899-1910) years ago, by D. D. Palmer, as **original principles, the product of a masterful mind that dared to conceive, teach and prove** the efficiency of that which you are today trying to give to others in a jumbled scrap pile. I know and have been with both for years.'' So, that **long proclaimed,** consists by his own statement, of **one year.**

''The fundamental, crude principles,'' were the ''original principles'' ten years ago. These ''original principles'' cover a hundred pages as recorded in Vol. 1 of the Science of Chiropractic. We are told that they were "the product of a masterful mind." These are the basic principles which "Uncle Howard" said at the "Feast of the Buzzards," "D. D. Palmer stumbled onto by chance."

The Chiropractor tells us that these original principles of Chiropractic were conceived—not "stumbled onto by chance" —by me. "Uncle Howard," when addressing the "Feast of the Buzzards," said, that they were all acquainted with the facts regarding the discovery of Chiropractic. The Chiropractor states that he was with O. G. Smith and D. D. Palmer for years and **knows** that **the master mind of D. D. Palmer conceived and originated the principles of Chiropractic previous to ten years ago.** It is now too late in the day to attempt to steal these discoveries.

Yes, I see by your letterhead that you established it in 1885, when you were three years of age, ten years before it was born.

It seems that it is about time that I should get a move on myself and make an effort to disprove that falsehood or otherwise the basis "Established in 1885," by the pseudo "fountain head" may become history.

The article on "Innate Intelligence," written over six years ago by me, contains the one-hundredth per cent referred to by "Uncle Howard," of that which has been developed as Chiropractic. It also contains the Chiropractic principles of which we are told, on page 4 of February 5 of the P. S. C. weekly output. "It was only a matter of two years ago that this physiology was first thought out."

Since then the possessor of those notes has not added one single thought to the science that is worth picking up.

"The reason for the recent progress in the **last two years** was because man has been analyzed as he is; man has been resolved into his component elements; he has been found out to be a thinking and an active product. He has been found to be alive with thoughts; dead without them. This shows the necessity of the joint composite condition of anatomy and intelligence--that they should be studied together. The keynote of physiology, then, as it stands today, is anaylsis and observation, rather than experiment."

"It is up to you to disprove that if you can." We will disprove the negative proposition by proving the affirmative.

"The true status of physiology today has been worked out by **one** who has never performed a torturing experiment on any living animal." That **one** is myself.

If any there be, who has a doubt as to who wrote the following article on Innate Intelligence, they can find the original manuscript at 828 Brady Street. It was written by my hand. As stated on page 10 of the "Feast of the Buzzards," which is not copyrighted, "I do not know that I have ever stated to you that we have on file in the 70 volumes of notes which we have, copies of every idea that has been brought out and used in Chiropractic and even before Chiropractic began—I can give you the date and origin of every step."

These "70 volumes of notes" are silent witnesses and will show when inquired for, that I was the originator of every idea in Chiropractic up to the time I left Davenport.

Innate Intelligence embodies the religious plank of the foundation of Chiropractic. I am the man who hewed out that plank and fitted it in the framework of Chiropractic.

The reader can judge, from the following article written by me and now copied from Vol. 1 of The Science of Chiropractic, whether the philosophy of Innate Intelligence "is two years old" or more than five. Thon can learn who was the originator of the theosophical philosophy of Chiropractic by reading

**"Innate Intelligence."**

"Each individual has two distinct and separate intellects, the Innate and the Educated. These thinking forces existing in the same body are very closely associated and influence each other."

Innate retains its education acquired in past ages. Educated starts in life without any knowledge of the past.

---

We aim to give free rein to Chiropractic thots and expressions.

---

Innate is that vital principle, the heretofore unknown intelligence which, associated with matter, controls the manifestations and properties of organized bodies, thereby distinguishing organized from inorganic matter.

---

Localization of functions in certain portions of the brain is adhered to by an overwhelming preponderance of present-day scientists. So is it, too, with localization of sensation. An overpowering, predominant portion of scientists of the present day are agreed that all functions and sensations have their origin in certain localized portions of the brain. It follows logically that what is called crime and evil are nothing more than an abnormal combination of function and sensation, or better, perhaps, an abnormality of function that produces a monstrous sensation.

## SPRAINS.

In pathology **a sprain is an undue tension or stretching of nerves** and other fibers, **caused by strains.** A sprain is the result of a wrench, a violent strain or twist of the soft parts surrounding a joint. **The neuro-skeleton,** in its normal position, **supports the vascular and nervous systems and affords them normal tonicity; any displacements thereof causes tension or relaxation of the filaments or thread-like structures.**

A sprain is usually regarded as an incomplete luxation. It is accompanied with more or less inflammation and pain.

Dorland says: "The signs of a sprain are rapid swelling, heat and displacement of the joint. The pain is usually great and is much increased by moving. If recovery be slow, immobilization is indicated."

An examination of the spine will reveal a corresponding luxation in all chronic sprains and nerve impingements, which cause a weakness in the joint at their peripheral endings. If the sprain is confined to the joint of a limb, it will be of short duration.

Carver affirms: "In sprains and bruises, adjusting to remove occlusion of stimulus to the area should be followed by adjusting the displaced tissue in the area itself. This manipulation, however, must be performed with great care. After that of securing normal relation of tissue parts, the primary object to be attained by the manipulation is to aid in every possible way the restoration of normal circulation through the area affected. This manipulation can only be taught by demonstration."

In using the word "occlusion" Dr. Carver means, the suppressing, checking, hindering, retarding or lessening of nerve stimulus. Webster defines occlusion as "the transient approximation of the edges of a natural opening, as of the eyelids." Gould says it is "a closure, blocking or shutting up of a normally patent aperture, as of the anus or ear."

Stimulus is a word frequently used by Dr. Carver meaning thereby "the energy or force which acts through the brain and nerves, constructing and maintaining the body and controlling all of its functions."

The **controlling intelligence** which acts thru the brain and nerves, directing the construction and maintenance of the body by functional activity, **is not energy or force**; it is the **communicating impulses** which **direct energy or force.** Energy or force is the power displayed by an organ or organism in the performance of functions. Energy or force is the capacity for doing work, not the directing of such work. Energy or force does not act thru the brain and nerves, but impulses do.

Vital force is inherent in the organization. Energy is the expenditure of vital force, vigor or action. Function is the special action of an organ. Vital force is the power which gives action to the organ. Energy is the sum total of the amount of power expended in the performance of function.

Dorland says of stimulus: "Any agent, act, or influence that produces functional or trophic reaction in an irritable tissue."

Dunglison defines stimulus as "An agent capable of causing demonstrable changes of dynamics in the tissue or organ on which it acts."

Gould informs us that stimulus is "Anything exciting the animal economy, or any part therof, to increased functional activity."

According to the above three standard authors and the following from Webster, **stimulus is an over amount of force, not a normal amount**, as assumed by the Analyzer.

Webster referring to physiological stimulus says: "Any substance or agent capable of evoking the activity of a nerve or irritable muscle, or capable of producing an impression on a sensory organ or more especially on its specific end-organ. Of the stimuli applied to the sensory apparatus, physiologists distinguish two kinds: Homologous stimuli, acting only on the end-organ, and for whose action the sense organs are especially adapted, as the rods and cones of the retina for the ether vibrations; and heterologous stimuli, mechanical, chemical, electrical, etc., acting on the nervous elements of the sensory apparatus along their entire course. For example, causing the flash beheld when the eye is struck."

Under the head-line of Strains, the Analyzer claims: "In connection with sprains and bruises, it is necessary to mention another form of tissue injury, which we usually refer to as strain. Unquestionably, many persons think that a strain and sprain are the same. Strained tissue is the condition resulting from an overuse of a part, which need not, in any sense, come within the scope of a sprain.

"The occlusion is produced by the motor reaction and constriction which result from the irritation."

A strain is not a tissue-injury. A sprain is produced by a strain; the former is the pathological condition, and the latter is a disease producer. Sprained tissue, not strained, is the condition resulting from an overmovement of a part. Nerves or muscles have simply been overdone, overstretched, not overcome by overuse. A bruise or contusion is not the result of a sprain; it has no relation to it. An author, lawyer or Chiropractor, ought to be familiar with and comprehend the meaning of words which he freely uses; or, at least, not be backward in the use of a dictionary.

The occlusion of a sprain, bruise, tissue injury, strained tissue or displaced tissue, Dr. Carver avers, is produced by the motor reaction and constriction which result from the irritation.

My reader, can you analyze and comprehend the above sentence, which contains the words occlusion, motor reaction, constriction and irritation?

Moullin wisely remarks: "It has been said, and not untruly, that in all probability half the crippled limbs and stiffened joints that are met with every day, date their starting point from the occurrence of some apparently trivial accident of this description."

If Moullin had been acquainted with Chiropractic, he could have added, "which could have been relieved at once by adjusting the slightly displaced osseous tissue."

"Erichsen maintains that "when a joint is twisted violently so that its ligaments **are** either **much stretched** or partially torn, though there is no displacement of the osseous surfaces, it is said to be sprained. These injuries are exceedinly painful and troublesome in their consequences, they most frequently occur to the wrists and ankle joints. The pain attending them is very severe, and often of a sickening character, and the sprain is rapidly followed by swelling and inflammation of the joint and investing tissues, often of a very chronic and tedious character. As the inflammation subsides, stiffness and pain in using the part continue for a considerable length of time, which, in some cases, give way to a kind of rigidity and wasting of the limb. In others again, a rheumatic tendency appears to be set up by injuries of this description, and occasionally it happens that in strumous subjects destructive disease of the joint is induced."

These injuries of limb-joints ultimately become chronic and one of four forms of affection follows; stiffness and pain, rigidity and wasting, rheumatism or destruction of the joint, and they continue without any displacement of the osseous surfaces. They have their causes in what are known as Chiropractic luxations of the vertebral column; displacements which have been heretofore overlooked.

Whitman asserts: "The ankle is, from its position, especially liable to injury, in fact the term 'sprain' is popularly associated with this joint.

"A sprain is most often caused **by an unguarded movement**, by which the foot is turned suddenly inward or outward, with sufficient force to rupture some of the fibers of the muscles, to strain tendon and tendon sheaths and even to rupture ligaments. If the foot is twisted inward, the injury is most marked on the outer side of the joint; if outward, on the inner side of the ankle. In the slighter degree of sprain, the injury may be confined to the tissues about the joint, but in most instances there is effusion within the capsule, even hemorrhage when the injury has been severe.

"Many of the so-called sprains of the ankle are simply injuries of a weak foot and are examples of the rigid or inflamed, weak or flat foot."

Moullin correctly says: "A sprain and a fracture may occur in the same limb from the same accident, and owing to the great amount of attention paid to the one, the other may be altogether overlooked."

I will add: A sprain or fracture may happen to a limb, and, from the same accident, **a vertebra may be wrenched**, slightly displaced, impinge upon nerves, and **create tension or atony with associated affections.**

Cooper remarks: "It is a curious circumstance that when the functions of a limb are obstructed by disease, the bulk of the member generally diminishes, and the muscles become emaciated. Nearly as soon as the least degree of lameness can be perceived, the leg and thigh have actually wasted, and their circumference has diminished."

**The functions of a limb may be diminished but not obstructed. Impulses will be lacking in force, momentum.** Therefore, the functions lack energy; they are not performed with the usual amount of vigor. The functions of a limb depend upon impulses. Impulses originate with Innate, the spirit. The same impingement which modifies the motor functions, impairs the trophic function. The universe consists of intelligence and matter. All phenomena are the result of matter modified by intelligence.

Some persons are continually complaining of a weak ankle or a sprained wrist; in such cases there will be found luxations in the lumbar and dorsal regions.

The American Text-Book of Surgery claims that "by far the most common joint is sprain. This is produced by a sudden wrench or twist of the articulation, and is experienced most frequently in the ankle and wrist, in the former because of a misstep or a fall upon the foot, in the latter because of a fall on the hand. The accident is most common in young and middle aged adults, is most likely to affect a joint that has been previously sprained, and is much more easily produced in a deformed limb or one in which the muscles are feebly developed and the ligaments relaxed; hence its frequency in the weak-ankled."

The predisposing cause of chronic sprains in the joints of

the legs and arms, when they are feebly developed or deformed should be looked for in the spine.

Moore affirms: "The ankle, owing to its location, is peculiarly liable to sprain—**a condition which will often tax the surgeon's skill** to the utmost, in both its early and late stages.

"It is a common belief among the laity that **a 'strain is worse than a break.'** "

It is not altogether owing to its location that makes the ankle liable to sprains. It is partly due to the location of the area from which it derives its functional impulses. The nerves of the lower limbs emerge from the lumbar vertebrae which are liable to be wrenched from their normal location. The surgeon, not comprehending this fact, his skill, not knowledge, is taxed to the utmost. It is no wonder that the laity consider a sprain worse than a break. A break is repaired, but the displaced bone with its attending thread-like filaments of nervous, muscular, cartilaginous and tendinous tissues, remain uncorrected.

One year before B. J. graduated and had the degree of D. C. conferred on him by his father, the founder of Chiropractic, J. M., a farmer, about 60 years of age, entered my office on crutches. In answer to my question, "Well, sir. what is the matter with you?" he said: "Three years ago a cow kicked me on the ankle. I managed to walk to the house, but have been unable to bear any weight on that foot since. I have tried several doctors and many remedies, but nothing has done me any good."

An examination of the ankle showed no displacement, no local injury, the subjective symptoms pointing to a sprained ankle. By pressure above the ankle I discovered a hypersensitive nerve which I traced to the lumbar region. I tried to explain to him that the instant he was kicked he jerked his leg away from danger, wrenching a lumbar vertebra of his backbone; thereby placing a pressure upon the nerve which reached to, and had its ending in, the affected ankle.

He did not accept my explanation. In about six months he returned; he was yet on crutches. I remembered him and his case. I found the affected nerve at its exit in the lumbar region and again followed it to the ankle. He insisted on my treating the ankle, saying his back was all right; that the ailment was in the ankle. He insisted that the kick of the cow was the cause, not a displaced bone in his back. I refused to touch the ankle, telling him I did not want to rob him of his money nor fool away my time.

In about three months he again returned, walking on one leg and two crutches, as on the two previous calls. He threw down a ten-dollar bill, saying: "I might as well fool my money away here as elsewhere."

After one adjustment of a lumbar vertebra, he walked out of the adjusting room and said: "See what I can do. I can bear considerable weight on that foot." In time he was able to discard the crutches.

This case is reported by B. J. in his volume of "new matter, cut and torn to pieces" from my writings, as one of his cases.

Moullin gives the diagnostic symptoms of a sprained joint thus: "Creaking or grating, as the surfaces move on each other, is always present in these joints. It may be but the faintest sensation of friction, only to be perceived by pressing the hand firmly on the part, as if two smooth silken surfaces were being rubbed together; or the noise produced as the fluid is squeezed from one side of the joint to the other may be distinctly audible to those around. This, of course, depends upon the condition of the lining membrane of the cavity, whether it has merely lost the polish from its surface or is covered over with folds and fringes, which project from all round the margin into the interior."

The above symptoms will also be found in rheumatic joints.

Inflammation is usually present in diseased joints. The conditions are known as synovitis, inflammation of the synovial membrane; thecitis, inflammation of the sheaths of the tendons; syndesomitis, inflammation of the ligaments; arthritis, or osteo-arthritis or pan-arthritis when all the structures of the joint are involved.

Herrick states: "In sprains of the back some difficulty may be met with in managing the cases satisfactorily. As remarked in another chapter, it requires quite a force to produce a true injury to the spinal cord, with which condition a sprain of the back is most liable to be confounded. The history of the injury and the appearance of the individual, as well as the position the patient assumed when first seen, or even thereafter, will serve to lend aid in making the diagnosis. The patient always favors the muscles of the back, and is careful not to put these in contraction, yet he is perfectly able to use them. In associated spinal trouble local tenderness is not always prominent, while disturbances of sensation and motion are to be observed."

There is no difficulty in handling sprains of the back satisfactorily if the adjuster knows what vertebra is displaced, and how to adjust it. A sprain is usually caused by a strain in an unguarded moment, when tension is relaxed. As Astley Cooper remarks, "**It is only possible for dislocations to take place when the muscles are unprepared for resistence;**

otherwise the greatest force would hardly produce the effect." A sprain of the back, partial displacement of vertebrae, affects the spinal nerves. When we speak of the spinal nerves being impinged upon, we include not only the four branches, but their filaments. The patient always favors the nerves and muscles of the back, they being already unduly contracted, so as to not place any more contraction upon them. Local tenderness is always present in spinal diseases, except when nerves are paralyzed; they then are devoid of sensation.

MacDonald says: "A forcible twist of a joint, as when a person 'turns his ankle,' is liable to cause more or less laceration of the tissues. The ligaments may be stretched or torn across, and may detach a thin scale from the bone, the synovial membrane may be rent, the muscles may be lacerated or overstretched, and their tendons thrown out of their grooves. In severe sprains the bones themselves are wrenched asunder, but slip back into place. Between a sprain of this kind and a dislocation the only difference is that in the one case the bones return to their normal position, while in the other they remain dislocated. It is a common saying that a bad sprain is worse than a fracture, and to a certain extent this is true."

Ashhurst maintains that "when a joint is twisted violently so that its ligaments are either much stretched or partially torn, though there be no displacement of the osseous surfaces, it is said to be sprained. These injuries are exceedingly painful and troublesome in their consequences. They most frequently occur to the wrists and ankle-joints. The pain attending them is very severe, and often of a sickening character, and the sprain is rapidly followed by swelling and inflammation of the joint and investing tissues, often very chronic and tedious. As the inflammation subsides, stiffness and pain in using the part continue for a considerable length of time, which, in some cases, give way to a kind of rigidity and wasting of the limb. In individuals of a rheumatic or gouty habit of body, the inflammation set up in the joint as a consequence of the strain is often of a most tedious and chronic character, and will only yield to appropriate constitutional treatment; and occasionally it happens that in strumous subjects destructive disease of the joint is induced."

The twisting of joints, the stretching of interosseous and articular ligaments, displaced osseous surfaces impinge upon nerves, creating tension, nerve-strain, results in great pain which is increased by moving. **The neuro-skeleton gives the proper amount of tone to the nervous and vascular systems; their displacement modifies tension, vibration, heat and the motor and sensory functions.** To adjust, replace, the displaced osseous framework, is to **reinstate normal tension, vibration, heat and normal momentum to impulses and normal functions.**

Ashhurst continues to assert: "Twists, sprains, or wrenches of the spine, without fracture or dislocation of the vertebrae, may occur in a variety of ways.

"These wrenches of the spine are, from obvious reasons, most liable to occur in the more mobile parts of the vertebral column, as the neck and loins; less frequently in the dorsal region.

"In railway collisions, when a person is violently and suddenly jolted from one side of the carriage to the other, the head is frequently forcibly thrown forwards and backwards, moving as it were by its own weight, the patient having momentarily lost control over the muscular structures of the neck. In such cases the patient complains of a severe straining, aching pain in the articulations between the head and the spine, and in the cervical spine itself. This pain closely resembles that met with in any joint after a severe wrench of its ligamentous structures, but is peculiarly distressing in the spine, owing to the extent to which fibrous tissue and ligament enter into the composition of the column. It is greatly increased by to-and-fro movements, however slight, and especially by rotation; also by pressure, and by lifting up the head, so as to put the tissues on the stretch. In consequence of this, the patient keeps the neck and head immovable, rigid, looking straight forward.

"If a joint, as the shoulder or ankle, continue to be weak and preternaturally mobile, in consequence of elongation of the ligaments, or weakness or atrophy of the muscles, beyond this period, it will, in all probability, never be so strong as it was before the accident. The same holds good with the spine; and a vertical column which has been so weakened as to require, after a lapse of several months, in order to enable it to maintain the weight of the head, will not, in all probability, ever regain its normal strength and power of support.

"One great prospective danger in strains of the spine is the possibility of the inflammation developed in the fibrous structures of the column extending to the meninges of the cord. This I have several times seen to occur. It is particularly apt to happen when the strain or twist occurs between the occiput and the atlas or axis. In these cases a rigid tenderness is gradually developed, which is most distressing and persisting and evidently of an inflammatory character. Or the paralysis may remain incomplete, being confined to the nerves that are connected with that part of the spine that is the seat of the wrench, one or other of their roots either having suffered lesion, or the nervous cord itself having been injured in its passage through the intervertebral foramen. Lastly, a twist of the spine may slowly and indidously be followed by symptoms of complete paraplegia, and eventually by death from extravasation of blood into the vertebral canal."

Ashhurst says: "Twists, sprains, or wrenches of the spine, without fracture or dislocation of the vertebrae." I assert that twists and wrenches displace, more or less, the bone levers of the body; that **it is impossible to tip a vertebra, or change the position of any two corresponding articular surfaces without causing an extra stretching, a tension, on the surrounding fibers.**

The pain is greatly increased "by lifting up the head, so as to put the tissues on the stretch." That sentence expresses the basic principle—tone—of Chiropractic. Increased tension—increased pain. Tension above normal—tone—not only causes pain, but abnormal functionating—disease.

Whenever tissues are put on the stretch, they become tense, rigid, have a greater vibration and consequently more heat. These conditions are accompanied by pain and abnormal functionating of the organ or part to which the nerves extend.

Ashhurst refers to "elongation of the ligaments." Why not also include the nerve-fibers. He is also aware of inflammation being developed, extending to the meninges of the cord because of strains of the spine. Remember that what a physician calls a sprain is a Chiropractic subluxation. It persists because of slightly luxated vertebrae which perpetuate tension.

In closing this article I cannot do better than quote, altho somewhat at length, but, nevertheless, quite interestingly and instructively, four paragraphs from The American Text-Book of Surgery: "Sprains of the spine are of all degrees of severity. The structure of the vertebral column is so complex and its relations are so numerous and varied that a greater variety of symptoms may follow a sprain according to the extent of the damage which is inflicted. In the mildest degree of sprain the muscles alone are involved, and we have then merely a temporary stiffness and a little local tenderness over a limited area. In more serious accidents, as those occuring during railway collisions, the ligaments may also be involved and are sometimes actually torn. When this happens in the case of the ligamenta subflava, there may be immediate and severe extradural hemorrhage, followed by temporary paraplegia. The symptoms which are never absent are pain and stiffness. Occasionally there is a little local swelling, but this is not constant. The pain is referred to the extremities of the injured nerves, sometimes shooting down the limbs, occasionally, when the injury is at the lumbo-dorsal junction, being referred to the pubic region. The skin over the injured part is apt to be exceedingly tender. The stiffness produces a degree of rigidity of the spine which resembles very much that seen in Pott's disease, the patient involuntarily immobilizing the vertebral column and avoiding rotation and flexion as carefully as possible. When the injury is unilateral this muscular rigidity is very marked on the injured side, and is a valuable means of distinguishing real from asserted injury, especially in medicolegal cases, as it cannot be simulated.

"The diagnosis of severe sprains followed by great helplessness and by some degree of paralysis will sometimes be difficult, as the conditions may closely simulate that of fracture. In the latter, however, the paralysis is more absolute, the disability more complete, the tenderness over the spine less diffuse, and there is often an irregularity in the line of the spinous processes which will serve at once to indicate the more serious character of the injury.

"These symptoms are very common, and are often associated with those belonging to traumatic hysteria, which Thoburn describes as a functional affection of the nervous system resulting from an injury, due probably to a change localized in some portion of the cerebral cortex, and manifested by well-defined and localized symptoms. He adds that it has no known basis, is not reflex in origin, and is neither shock nor neurasthenia.

"The symptoms may be either psychical, including epileptiform attacks and hysterical insanity; motor, including paralysis and contractures of the limbs and special effects upon such organs as the larynx and the bladder; sensory, in which case there is anesthesia, hyperthesia, or paresthesia of the general or special sensory nerves; or lastly, there may be vasomotor, secretory, orthropic nerves."

The pathological conditions attributed to sprains by the above writer, I refer to as subluxated impringements. More than this, I relieve the same by vertebral adjusting; so, I am led to think, that much of what has been associated with sprains, should be imputed to vertebral luxations. Nerve-tension superinduced by impingements, or nerve relaxation from atony, want of tone, a loss or diminution of vital force, is accountable for all diseases.

Bad sprains are those which have their source or origin in luxations of the spinal column. They would not be considered any worse than others if their etiology were known and the art of adjusting vertebrae comprehended and followed.

While reading the following from Moullin, I could but wonder WHY, he had not caught onto the principles derived from nerve-tension, known as Chiropractic. "Sprains of the back and neck are sufficiently common and important to deserve a certain amount of separate consideration. The structures concerned are exceedingly complicated; there is an immense number of separate joints of various shape and size, and in addition there is the spinal cord running in a canal down nearly the whole of its length, and giving off the nerves which pass out on either side between the bones. Nor do the injuries themselves vary less in character and severity. In some they are exceedingly slight; in others the consequences are as serious as any that occur in surgery. Some, too, have gained a most enviable notoriety from their connection with railway accidents; for whatever may be the truth as regards many of these cases, whether they are deceptions or not, there can be no question that sometimes very considerable injuries are produced by the way in which the backbone, and the structures in connection with it, **are strained and wrenched** when the body is thrown violently backward and forward as it is in collisions.

"**One of the most singular features in connection with these sprains is the way in which the backbone itself, and the muscular and ligamentous structures around it, are overlooked and ignored.** Even in the ordinary accidents of every-day life there is a great tendency to lay everything that is serious or lasting to the credit of the spinal cord. In railway cases there is no hesitation at all; if any serious result ensues it must be the consequence of damage this structure has sustained, or of inflammation following it; little or no attention is paid to anything else. Yet it is difficult to see why the other structures should enjoy immunity. **The vertebral column may be strained,** especially in the cervical and lumbar regions; the ligaments torn or stretched; **the nerves bruised or crushed; the smaller joints between the segments twisted and wrenched.**

"**Sometimes** a certain amount of hyperthesia or **increased sensitiveness** of skin **may be detected** over a small area immediately above the seat of injury, but **the general tenderness all down the spine, which is such a common symptom in sprains of the back,** whether they occur in railroad accidents or elsewhere, and the strange sensations, such as crawling, creeping, or tingling, experienced in the limbs, are probably due entirely to other causes. They are certainly met with in cases in which there is no reasonable ground for suspicion that the cord itself has been hurt in any way.

"Sometimes the strain falls on the smaller joints between the vertebrae, though it must be admitted that it is rarely possible to find any direct evidence of their being hurt. There are so many of them; they lie so close to each other; and the amount of movement possessed by each is so slight that unless the injury is extremely localized its effect is spread too widely to strain any single one. **It is not improbable, however, that**

**they suffer more often than is generally suspected; only the injury, owing to the depth at which they lie, and they way in which they are covered in by muscles, is not correctly diagnozed.** At least, evidence of past mischief is sometimes found post-mortem, long after all history is forgotten.

"In the milder cases (of sprains in the back) merely local treatment may suffice, but **it is so common for an outbreak of some complaint** (the existence of which may hitherto not have been suspected) **to follow strains**, that practically in all general treatment adapted to the particular constitution of each patient is essential. Just as an injury to the foot is often the apparent cause of the first attack of gout, so many of the muscular strains of the back owe at any rate their persistent character to the presence of some similar complication. It is for this reason that careful attention to diet is necessary; and that such drugs as colchicum, iodide of potash, chloride of ammonia, the carbonates of the alkalies, and others prove so useful. Only, **it rarely happens that any indication as to which of these internal remedies is likely to prove most beneficial can be derived from the condition of the back itself.** This is only to be ascertained by carefully inquiring into the previous history of the patient, and thoroughly investigating the other symptoms that are present. In other words, local measures should be employed to relieve the pain and stiffness, and to restore the condition of the muscles as soon as possible; but it must not be forgotten that the general state of the patient in most instances needs quite as much attention.

"A very favorite application in Germany, known as Hoffman's balsam of life, consists of an alcoholic solution of balsam of Peru and seven of these aromatic oils mingled together. They may be either painted on the skin, and left exposed, or dissolved in spirit in various proportions, and covered over with oiled silk to prevent too rapid evaporation. Menthol is one of the most convenient, and acts especially well when mixed with camphor or croton-chloral, so as to form a thick oily liquid. Probably in this instance, too, relief is in no small measure due to the effect produced upon the cutaneous nerves."

If, as Moullin says, "The vertebral column may be strained, the smaller (articular) joints between the segments twisted and wrenched," why would not this disarrangement account for much of the diseases following numberless accidents? Moullin should remember that there is a ganglionic nerve chain, on either side of the vertebral column, which serves as a distributing agent for motor and sensory impulses of normal as well as abnormal force. This accounts for "the general tenderness all down the spine, which is such a common symptom in sprains of the back."

In addition to the above "favorite applications" and "most beneficial remedies," I will add others, which are "highly recommended." Hot and cold water applications, hot air, hot fomentations; vapor, steam, douch and Turkish baths; bandages of plaster; elastic bandages; adhesive plaster strappings; a Paris plaster jacket for sprains in the back; belts of flannel or silk to be worn around the body; elastic stockinetts; counter irritants; rubefacients; liniments; poultices; cauteries; hypodermic injections of morphine; acupuncture by thrusting a needle thru the skin and deep into the muscles; dry cupping; kneading and rubbing with embrocations; massage; elevation; rest; fixation; traction; special diet; friction with the hands or brush; ironing of the muscles of the back with a hot iron; turpentine; morphine; belladonna; veratria; static electricity; electric brush; galvanism; thermic hammer; electro-magnetic apparatus and quack remedies.

Many remedies, none of which are satisfactory, show plainly that the pathology and etiology of sprains are not understood, that the "most beneficial remedies" and " favorite applications" are worthless.

---

Knowledge of a single fact does not reach the meaning of science.

---

Dr. Carver, the Analyzer, tells us: "In order to intelligently discuss this form of displacement, it will be necessary to explain that visceral is here used in its more limited sense as applied to the internal organs of the body, or viscera, remembering that this word is also applied to the soft tissues of the body generally."

Webster says of viscera: "The internal organs, especially those of the cavities of the body or trunk, as the heart, liver, intestines, etc."

Viscus is the singular of viscera, of which Dorland says: "Any large interior organ in either of the four great cavities of the body, especially the abdomen."

Dunglison: "Viscus—Any internal organ of the body, especially one of the larger abdominal organs."

Lippincott: "Viscus—Any organ contained in a body-cavity, especially within the abdomen."

Gould: "Viscus—Any organ enclosed within either of the four great cavities, the cranium, abdominal cavity or pelvis; as the brain, intestines, spleen, bladder, uterus, lungs, liver, etc."

No medical or other dictionary, outside of Carver's Analysis, considers the "soft tissues of the body generally" as viscera.

"He compared Chiropractic to electricity."

The two sciences of Chiropractic and electricity have no resemblance, have nothing in common, have no similarity whatever.

"Elimination of disease."

To eliminate is to expel from the system; the kidneys eliminate urea; the lungs eliminate carbonic acid; poisons are eliminated from the system. Eliminanting medicines are those which increase the excretions. Disease is not an entity, a something to be expelled; it is a condition.

"Supposing we have a subluxation at the atlas, it can produce a cancer at the stomach, a bunion on the toe, insanity and constipation."

A subluxation of the atlas never produces a cancer of the stomach, a bunion on the metatarso-phalangeal joint of the great toe, or constipation. Such a statement is a mere supposition.

"A subluxation cutting off currents."

Currents flow. The blood flows, it has a current, the only current in the body. An impingement by a subluxated bone might impede the venous current and thereby cause varicosity.

"Displacements are caused by a concussion of forces."

"An adjustment is a concussion of forces."

Is that so? Displacing and replacing, either one or both, are caused by a concussion of forces?

In biology, force is known as the physical strength, the vigor of a living being.

A concussion is the jar or shock received from a collision of bodies, or the morbid condition resulting from a fall or blow.

A luxation, or displacement, may be the result of a concussion of bodies—not forces, and an adjustment may replace that which is displaced by a concussion of bodies—not forces.

An adjustment is not a concussion or the result of a concussion.

The fundamental principles of Chiropractic are physiological tone, normal tonicity: the state of healthy tension, or normal contraction of nerve and muscle fibers while at rest; and pathological tension, too much or not enough nerve tension. **The source or origin of Chiropractic principles is tension.**

---

The Medical Trust Health (?) Board of Minnesota, angry because the people opposed vaccination, refused to even quarantine. The result has been, no spread of "smallpox" and the Trust is disconsolate.—The Ophthalmologist.

## PHILOSOPHY AND SCIENCE.

I have just learned the difference between the philosophy and the science of **heat production as taught at the P. S. C.**

In "The Philosophy of Chiropractic, Vol. V, Palmer, 1909," on page 549 I find the philosophy of the "**Serous Circulation in Animals.**

"Animals have **blood** but it **is utilized to make heat** (internal heat), the same as animals have internal digestion, or internal digestive apparatus which plants have not."

In "The Science of Chiropractic, Vol. I, Palmer, 1906-'10," I find on page 179, "**The body is heat by mental impulse.**"

"It will be of interest to learn how **the body is heat by mental impulses** which creates combustion of chemicals arterially and serously deposited, and not by blood, and therefore the blood acts as one of the attributes in preference to performing all the calorific duties thereof."

We are told in "The Philosophy of Chiropractic" that the "Serous Circulation in Animals" in the condition of blood is utilized to make internal heat; that animal heat is derived from the blood.

In "The Science of Chiropractic" we are told that the body heat is created by "Mental Impulses"; that heat is created by Mental Impulses depositing chemicals in the serum and arteries, that this creates combustion, a chemical process accompanied by the liberation of heat. The depositing of chemicals and combustion—the burning of these chemicals—is "not by blood." The blood only acting as one of the **attributes,** it does so in preference to performing all the calorific (heat production) duties—you read it, and determine, if you can, what he says the "calorific duties" are and what "the attributes" of the blood are, as I do not understand him, cannot comprehend what he means.

The P. S. C. explanation of how Mental Impulses heat the body is an addition to an article which I wrote July 1, 1903, while in Santa Barbara, Cal., relating the circumstances under which I discovered heat production. In this article, see Vol I, date 1906, page 165, I state that heat is the production of nerves. An explanation of this plagiarism and mutilation is given in The Chiropractor of February, 1910, page 62, which reads, "The entire book has been torn to pieces. Much has been 'cut'—much 'new matter' added—in fact the body is so new that, if it wasn't for a few of the old articles and the old volume number, we could have announced it as a new book."

This false notice of copyright and mutilation of forty of my articles is a violation of the United States copyright laws, punishable by a stipulated fine—see index for copyright laws.

The above two self-contradictory, would-be explanations, of the origin of animal heat is made by B. J. Palmer, the enveloper. As may be seen in the following pages, either explanation of his is far from being correct.

---

A circular from a Chiropractic college reads: "The principles of Chiropractic are true—the cause of disease is specifically removed by a purely scientific process of skeletal adjustment and health is the inevitable result.

"The science of Chiropractic removes the cause of disease which is superinduced by disobeying the Laws of Health.

"Its principles teach the Laws of Right Living."

Prof. E. B. Warman delivers a series of lectures to this school on "Right Living."

The above seems paradoxical. We are told that the principles of Chiropractic are the laws of right living. That the cause of disease is disobeying the laws of health. That skeletal adjustment removes the cause of disease.

The promoters of the above school would make **poor** signs for a boarding house. They are certainly disobeying the laws of health, not living right, or do not understand scientific specific adjusting.

Chiropractic teaches that disease is caused by accidents and poisons, which wrench and draw vertebrae out of alignment. That displaced vertebrae impinge upon nerves by protrusion; that pressure on nerves creates abnormal functionating; that disease is the result of functions performed excessively or deficiently.

The promoters of the "Health College" may envy the savage who knows nothing of the "Laws of Health" their well-rounded out bodies, their ability to endure hardships, and their freedom from disease.

Chiropractors say "eat and drink what you desire and all you want." It is not how much or when you eat and drink that causes disease, but displaced vertebrae pressing against nerves.

"Purely scientific process." Chiropractic adjusting is not a process, or at least should not be made so; it is an art acquired by skill and practice and the know how. Chiropractors should be specific in their adjusting and not make it a reversible process—every other vertebra today and the alternate ones tomorrow. It is not specific when we make it a process. Yes, "the principles of Chiropractic are true," but the writer of the above does not comprehend them, as shown by his attempt at mixing. It is not "purely scientific" when mixed with Warmanism or any other system

## TONE.

The **basic principle** of the science and philosophy (not the art) of Chiropractic **is tone,** a word of four letters, yet it comprises a whole thot, a complete sentence; grammatically it is entire, inasmuch, as it expresses a complete thot.

Basic, is pertaining to the basis, the fundamental or foundation.

**A basic principle** is the foundation, **the source, the origin,** that from which other **principles** may proceed, or **are derived.**

**The science and philosophy of Chiropractic is built on tone. The source of every Chiropractic principle, whether physiological or pathological, is founded upon tone.** That one word means much to a Chiropractor who desires to comprehend the basis of Chiropractic in its scientific or philosophical phase.

Tone is that state or condition of a body, or any of its organs or parts, in which the organic or animal functions are performed with due vigor.

**The tone or tension of muscles and organs depends upon the tonicity of the nervous system.**

**Tone,** in biology, **is the normal tension or firmness of nerves,** muscles or organs, **the renitent, elastic force acting against an impulse.** Any deviation from normal tone, that of being too tense or too slack, causes a condition of renitence, too much elastic force, too great resistance, a condition expressed in function as disease.

Tonicity, or tone, is a quality belonging to solids; it is normal when the tension, or partial contraction of nerves and muscles is at rest.

**In botany,** a plant is said to be in **tone,** when the relations of light, heat and moisture are evenly balanced, that **is, when conditions are such as will produce a normal tension of its fibers.** Too much or too little heat causes the plant to wilt, its fibers to become lax.

**In music and acoustics,** the science of sound, including its production, transmission and effects, stringed instruments, bowed as in the violin, plucked as in the harp, guitar and mandolin, struck as in the piano and dulcimer, or blown upon as in the aeolian harp, **are said to be in tone when the vibrations impress the ear in a relation of harmony.**

**All life,** vegetable or animal, **depends upon tone,** for its normal or abnormal existence.

**Tone is the basic principle upon which I founded the science and developed the philosophy of Chiropractic.**

---

A Chiropractor should be well versed in osteology.

**Orthopedia** is the surgical and mechanical correction of deformities in children.

From the earliest psychological history, congenital aberration of the human form has invited the serious consideration of the most conscientious and wisest men. Prenatal, bodily deformity is one of the most deplorable misfortunes that can be conceived, not only to the unfortunate malformed child, but to the parents. The subject of congenital and acquired distortions has been enveloped in obscurity; former investigation has only resulted in speculation and probable surmise as to the nature of the unfavorable influence that impressed the enciente, culminating in conjectural and seemingly plausable solutions of the cause of these lamentable occurrences. Even now, mental and physical impressions are usually considered as the producer of these abnormal conditions in the fetus.

The developer of this science aims to deduce a rational theory, founded upon physiology, regarding the primary, formative process of the embryo.

The encircling of the limbs during fetal life by the umbilical cord, which varies from one inch to five feet in length, has resulted in congenital amputation.

The formation of the embryo and the development of the fetus depends entirely upon the nervous functions of the mother, she being the matrix of that which is to be. To insure perfect formation of the embryo and a uniform development of the fetus, the functions of the mother must be normally performed. A curtailment or increase of functionating, in any part of the body of the mother, results in either a correct or abnormal development of its counterpart in her offspring. The relative evolution of the embryo and the development of the fetus proceeds in strict ratio with the nutrient supply. Consequently, atrophy, imperfection, or absence of any portion is attributed to lack of functionating. To insure perfect form and development of the fetus, we must have material functions performed in a normal manner in the mother and imparted by her to her offspring.

It will be observed that I have made great innovations in orthopedy, as in other branches of the healing art, by adjusting the cause of deformities instead of treating the distortion.

It is of the greatest importance that we comprehend that mental and physical deformities are because of abnormal functionating, and that by correcting functionating we remove the cause of malformation. It is the purpose of this science to emphasize this phase of orthopedy.

## CHIROPRACTIC.

In Vol. 1, 1905, Chiropractor, is the following, with corrections in italics, adjusting it to date:

Chiropractic was discovered, in 1895, by Dr. D. D. Palmer. He developed this science, until he feels proud of it. Chiropractors find nearly all diseases are caused by subluxations of vertebrae which impinge upon nerves. When nerves are free to act naturally in their entire course, there is health. Chiropractors definitely locate displacements **of osseous tissue,** the cause of disordered conditions. When these luxated joints are replaced, and the impinged nerves freed, **functions** are no longer abnormally performed.

The medical world has long recognized luxations of the spinal column accompanied with fracture, but have always insisted that it was almost impossible to displace a vertebra. The conditions which physicians call wrenches and sprains of the back are Chiropractic luxations. These may be caused by a variety of accidents occurring when one is either asleep or awake.

Many a mother and her child have been injured at delivery by displacements of some one of the 117 joints of the spine. It is the Chiropractor's business to repair **sub-luxated articulations,** thereby freeing the impinged nerves so that they may act normally.

Four years after writing the above, I promulgated the following principles of Chiropractic: **Life is action governed by intelligence. Intelligent life, the soul, depends upon the execution of functions. Functions performed by normal energy is health. Disease is the result of the performance of functions above or below a normal degree of activity. Impulses properly transmitted through nerves, result in functions being normally performed, a condition which results in health. The motive force may be exaggerated or decreased during its transit, because the lines of communication are excited or repressed. The vegetative functions rely upon the amount of energy expressed by vital functions. The normal carrying capacity of nerves depends upon their freedom from pressure; the abnormal upon the force of impingement. Bones are the only hard tissue which can press against and impinge upon nerves.**

The fundamental principle of Chiropractic is tone. The science and art of Chiropractic is founded on anatomy, physiology, pathology, nerve tracing and adjusting.

Physicians, who give us 15 minutes' attention while we explain Chiropractic luxations by the use of specimens at hand, admit that there may be many diseases arising from displacements of the vertebral column. But being able to replace them by hand is very much doubted until demonstrated; one practical exhibition removes all doubt.

The spinal column is the central axis of the skeletal frame. It supports the head and ribs, and through them the weight of the upper extremeties. The weight is transmitted downward through the bodies and the articular processes of the vertebrae to the ossa innominati. The backbone is composed of bony segments, between which are elastic fibrous cartilages.

Flexion, extension and rotation have a normal limit; to a certain extent they are permitted in all parts of the spinal column. These various movements are due to the interposed elastic cartilage. Wrenches in many ways separate the intervertebral and articular cartilages and displace the vertebrae; **the projecting sides of their bodies press against, impinge upon, the nerves, thereby** deranging functions.

When we study the anatomy of the spinal column, we no longer wonder at the many displacements. On the contrary, we are suprised that we do not find more of them. Could we fancy the main shaft of a machine, capable of the various movements possible to the spinal column, subjected to the many wrenches received by the vertebral column from time to time, we would not be surprised to find some portion of it out of adjustment. Why, then, should we be astonished to find vertebrae **slightly displaced?** Is not the human body much more liable to have its different parts racked out of their proper position than those of an inanimate machine? And are not the consequences far more reaching?

The inevitable conclusion is, that the laws of natural philosophy apply to the **backbone much more so than they do to the main line upon which mechanism depends for its workmanship.** Such being the case, why not use the same good judgment in adjusting the displacements of the central line shaft of the human body, which sustains and gives firmness to the skeletal frame? Why search the world over for antidotes? Why not look for the cause of troubles within the **one affected** and then correct it?

The above questions are answered by Chiropractors who locate and verify with definite precision the apparently slight sub-luxations which cause abnormal functionating. This is done by an **anatomical** knowledge of the vertebral column and the finding of sensitive, swollen, inflammed nerves which are traced by digital examination from their spinal exit to the parts affected. By hand adjusting we correct the wrongs which cause disease, we replace the vertebra in proper position, **relieve the pressure.** These movements are done by the hands. using the transverse and spinous processes as **levers.**

## PHYSIOLOGY AND PATHOLOGY.

Physiology is the science which treats of the functions of organic beings. Pathology is the study of abnormal functions —functions modified by diseased tissue.

Pathologic physiology may seem to be antonyms, of opposite meaning; but they are correlative, of reciprocal relation. While physiology refers to normal actions of functions, pathologic physiology points to the disturbance of functions, to diseased conditions which disqualify tissue for the normal amount of energy.

Physiology treats of the functions of living bodies. Morbid physiology, or pathology, considers functions as we find them modified by disease. While physiology relates to the functions of living forms, pathology has for its object the study of life as performed by abnormal actions; changes of organization and functions differing from those which are found in health.

Health exists when normal tissue performs functions in a natural manner.

Physiology is the science which deals with normal energy and its results. Pathology is the science that deals with disease in all its aspects. It includes the study of causes, manifestations and results. The symptoms of disease are the expressions of abnormal functional activity or lassitude.

Physiology may be hygienic or morbid. It may accord with the laws of health or consist of conditions inducing disease.

Pathology may be divided into three divisions, namely, etiology—the cause of disease; morbid or pathological anatomy, the study of structural changes and pathological physiology, the study of disturbed functions.

Disease is abnormality in structure or of functionating, or both.

Alteration in functionating cannot occur without modification in structure. This is made apparent by our previous articles on functions and molecular vibrations.

Chiropractors are demonstrating the existence of this heretofore obscure, structural change which causes functional aberration. All functions performed are the result of impulses forwarded thru the nervous structure. Palpation demonstrates that nerves which end in diseased structure are sensitive, rigid, enlarged in diameter and contracted longitudinally. Postmortem examinations do not show these conditions, because of the muscular rigidity manifested in rigor mortis. Cadaverous rigidity appears in man in from ten minutes to seven hours after death, the difference in time being due to the manner of death. The duration of rigor mortis is from one to six days. During this period the heat of the body is above the surrounding atmosphere. It may even raise above normal. This continued heat is because of the tension and rigidity of the tissue; an increase of tension and rigidity increases molecular vibration — heat. Decomposition — dry or liquefactive necrosis, depending upon the surrounding humidity—sets in as soon as rigidity ceases. Tetanus is a more or less persistent tonic spasm of nerves and muscles. Dorland says of this affection: The temperature usually rises and may obtain a remarkable height (113 degrees F.) and continue to rise for a time after death.

The determining producers of disease, the agencies which cause functions to be performed in too great or too little degree, are poisons and traumatism. Heat, cold and parasites constitute a very small factor in the causation of disease.

Disturbed metabolism, the auto-intoxication of medical authorities, the self-poisoning, intestinal putrefaction, caused by an unequal activity of the processes of assimilation and dissimilation, is nothing more or less than the result of too much or not enough heat.

Normal heat is 98.5 degrees. If the temperature of the digestive tract be increased or decreased from that which is normal we have fermentation, decay, putrefaction of its contents. The equilibrium between absorption, assimilation and secretion, named metabolism, is deranged, all because of the function of heat being abnormal.

Animal or vegetable food which is on the road to putrefaction, when used as ingesta, acts as an irritant to the nerves with which it comes in contact; therefore, it is a poison. Bodily temperature, above or below normal, changes the character of the tissue of the various organs and the mucous and serous membranes which control metabolism. Marked changes are found in the lymphatics and even the bones are changed in color and texture. Thus we have disturbed metabolism as the result of abnormal temperature. Exposure of healthy or unhealthy tissue to X-rays causes cellular degeneration because of excessive heat.

By the principles of Chiropractic we learn that auto-infection, auto-intoxication, is caused by an excess of heat and not, as taught by medical schools, that auto-toxemia is the cause of febrile disturbances and ferment intoxication.

Traumatism, mechanical injuries, the displacing of any part of the osseous framework, causes pressure upon the channels of impulse communication, thereby deranging the quantity of functionating, which results in conditions we name disease. The kind of disorder—functional disturbance—is determined by the portion of the osseous framework displaced and the functionating channels of communication which are subjected to impingement; so that life and health depend upon the extent of the injury and the part of the body affected.

---

"Modernized Chiropractic" states: "I do know this, that every fundamental Chiropractic original idea (with meagre exceptions) was gained—either borrowed or stolen—directly from the Bohemians."

The editor of "Modernized Chiropractic" must seriously regret not having known of Napravit nine years ago, for his city and the surrounding country contained many Bohemians. It would have saved him going to Davenport to me, to have his spine adjusted and $500 and a year's time, for he could have learned the whole thing in a few hours of his Bohemian neighbors for a thank you.

The above stupidity, ignorance and myopic vision is equaled by the following, which is copied from the same journal. "Dr. Lorenz is a scientist of world renown. I am told that while he was in Chicago a girl was treated and cured of paralysis by him. It cannot be supposed that this was done by his 'hip operation.'

"How, then, was it done—certainly not by any of the ordinary accepted methods. Could it have been done by means of Bohemian Chiropractic, which perchance he employed, but for reasons best known to himself preferred to not exploit or explain. It would not surprise me if this were the case."

The Armour girl referred to had a dislocated hip, not paralysis, and, as I well remember, the operation was not a success. The case and the Lorenz method was freely written up in the public press and talked of by Oakley G. Smith, Miss Minora Paxson and myself when we were in Chicago, as the operation was performed at that time. How short-sighted and foregetful one can be when he desires to replace truth with falsehood. O. G. Smith does not need to send Dr. Faust to Bohemia to inquire of Lorenz as to his method, for by turning to page 653 of Dunglison's Dictionary he may read: "Dr. Lorenz operation. For congenital dislocation of the hip; the displacement is reduced by manipulation, the knife not being used, and the head of the os femoris is then held in the ascetabulum by means of an immovable apparatus until a new socket is formed for it."

For a more complete description of the Lorenz method, see page 386 of Orthopedic Surgery by Whitman; page 342 of Orthopedic Surgery by Moore, and page 474 of Fractures and Dislocations by Stimson.

## "BRACE YOURSELVES."

"**Brace yourselves**; I can't help you." Thus spoke E. W. Melendy, a motorman on a Seattle street car loaded with 80 passengers, on the 24th of September.

The motorman had lost control of his car; the speed attained was 30 miles an hour when it careened, left the track and crashed into a one-story building. The motorman retained his presence of mind and gave his passengers the best of advice while facing danger—"**Brace yourselves.**"

Do you remember while descending a stairway in the dark, how you thot you had reached the floor and found to your surprise that you had made a miscalculation of one step? You were **not braced,** you were not prepared for that unexpected step down. How well you remember the shock you received; how it hurt you all over. Do you not remember when walking on the highway and unexpectedly stepping into a hole, how that unexpected drop shocked you, because you were **not braced** against danger?

How well you recollect after you had "retired as well as usual" that you were awakened in the night with a "stitch" in your side or back, and unable to take a full breath or turn over. Do you recall sending for the family physician and how he injected morphine in your side to deaden the pain—treating the effects? He would have adjusted the cause had he known where and how.

In going down the stairs, you thot you were at the bottom and unconsciously took off the **brace.** During sleep we rest because of our **unbraced** condition, our **lack of tension.** We have a dream, it may be remembered or not; we are **not braced** against impending danger. In this relaxed condition, our bones, more especially those of the spine, are easily displaced by some sudden move.

How easily the Chiropractor replaces displaced bones when the patient is relaxed. How difficult, how impossible, when the patient **braces** himself against him.

To make an adjustment, to move a vertebra, the patient should be relaxed.

That motorman could not have given his passengers any better advice than "brace yourselves."

Quite a large share of our vertebral displacements are occasioned during sleep, when we are fully relaxed and unprepared for danger.

---

The man who bangs his head against hard facts, feels his bumps of approbation.

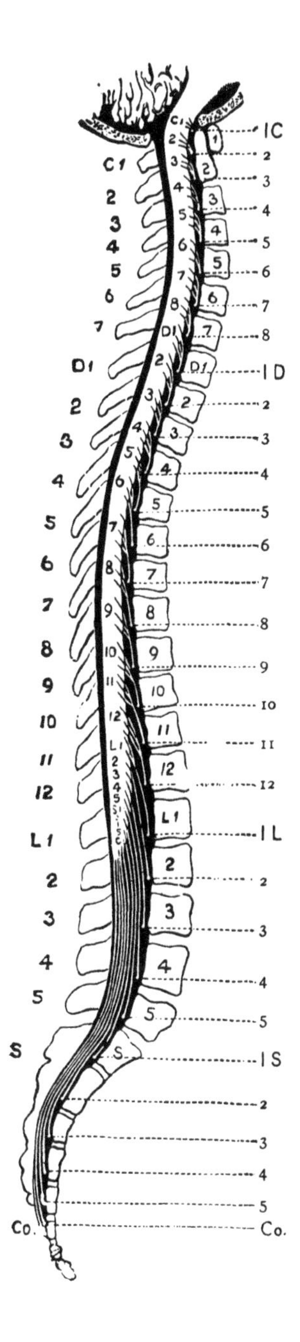


Cut of vertebral column, sawed in half, lengthwise, showing the spinous processes and their relative position at the exit of the spinal nerves; the vertebrae numbered on their bodies; the origin of the spinal nerves in the spinal cord and their relative emergence.

The pons varolii is situated at the base of the brain, behind its center; it connects the cerebrum, cerebellum and oblongata.

The medulla oblongata is the cerebral protuberance, the upper, enlarged part of the spinal cord. It extends from the pons varolii, downward, to the lower surface of the foramen magnum. The foramen magnum is occupied by and surrounds the medulla oblongata.

The spinal cord, in the adult, extends from the lower surface of the foramen magnum down to the first or second lumbar vertebrae; it is an extension downward of the medulla oblongata.

The cauda equina is a brush of nerve-roots which, as may be seen in cut, extends downward from the terminal cone of the cord.

Indebted to P. Blakiston & Co., Philadelphia, for this cut.

A twelve-page booklet written by Oakley G. Smith, in common use by many Chiropractors, who are unable to write original advertising, states: "Chiropractic is a distinct and complete drugless and knifeless system and has nothing in common with Osteopathy, Massage, Swedish Movements or any other system."

From page 3 of this booklet we copy the following:

"The Human Mill. Man is a mill filled with machines and the product of this mill is either health or disease. These various machines such as the heart, lungs, stomach, liver, spleen, bowels, kidneys, bladder, eyes, ears, arms, legs, feet, hands, fingers and toes are all operated by the same dynamo—the brain.

"When a certain machine in the body is out of order—sick—it is because the life current is either cut off or impaired. Under such conditions the human mill manufactures disease instead of health."

Why not include the twenty finger and toe nails as being machines, each tooth and hair a machine?

A mill may contain one or more machines, or be a machine in and of itself.

A machine is a mechanical contrivance. Mechanical pertains to the quantitative relations of **force and matter as distinguished from mental, vital, chemical and catabiotic force.**

A machine is an inanimate mechanical contrivance operated by and designed to produce some mechanical effect; whereas, metabolism consists of a group of phenomena, which convert foodstuffs into tissue-elements (assimilation), and complex substances into simple end-products (dissimilation).

A human body is not a mill or machine. Health or disease are not manufactured products, they are conditions. When any of the above mentioned organs or parts of the body are "out of order," they are said to be diseased, not "sick." they cease to perform their natural functions.

"The life current is either cut off or impaired." Most diseases are because of **too much** "life current," instead of being impaired or cut off.

---

G. H. Patchen, M. D.; "Impeded currents of mental impulse are the cause of disease."

In disease, mental impulses are **not** inpeded, hindred, stopped, obstructed or "cut off."

The conductibility of nerve tissue is normal when we have normal temperature. If bodily heat is above or below normal, then impulses which direct functions are correspondingly carried too forcibly or too freely.

## PAINLESS ADJUSTING.

A student of the Bohemian thrust writes: "I lay awake at night searching the depths of my creative ability for a painless thrust. For the last three years I have clinked each vertebra of the entire spine without pain or discomfort to the patient. With this thrust I cannot jump about here and there in the spine, but must start at the sacrum and end at the occiput, and I have the satisfaction of knowing that I have set every vertebrae where it belongs, plumb against the facet of its neighbor."

While the above statement seems to me to be incredible, but it is not any more so, than my statement, made fifteen years ago, was to others, that I could displace or replace any vertebra with my hands, thereby cause or relieve disease.

A correspondent writes me of this "painless adjustment." **Dr. Arnold adjusts ribs and tarsals, etc., out of joint, as well as displaced vertebrae.** I am sorry to say, however, that while she has displayed considerable liberality in permitting the boys to see her in action and is pleased to answer questions, I have not yet been able to master even the rudiments of her system, and I know none, save her students and assistants who have labored under her for a time, who have been able to properly execute the work."

Another correspondent writes: "**In regard to Dr. Arnold's painless adjustment, I am satisfied by much personal experience and observation, that her vertebral adjustments are painless as compared with those given by any other Chiropractor** I have seen. **Her adjustments would hardly waken a sleeping child.** To me it is wonderful. She uses a straight bench, with a small pillow under the hips. **There is no thrust, and no perceptible downward pressure.**"

I was interested, and wrote to headquarters for information. Under date of June 21, 1910, Dr. Arnold says: "**I do use a strong pressure from one pound on an infant to 125 pounds on a strong back, when the muscles and ligaments are obstinately stiff, and my skill is shown by the fact that I give no more pressure than is needed to move the vertebrae. I give pressure rather than thrust.**

"**Your correspondent is wrong in saying 'she claims to adjust vertebrae without any pain whatever,' for I know that my thrust is not entirely painless,** except on nearly normal spines. **Old, chronic luxations, I must hurt to some degree, but my work is as nearly 'painless' as is possible to make an adjustment of spinal luxations.**"

**She begins at the sacrum in all cases, no matter what the affection, or what vertebrae are displaced.** She makes a distinction between her method of "**re-construction of the spine for constitutional correction** as opposed to the usual method which is specific and remedial."

Under date of New York, July 20, 1910, Dr. Arnold writes me:

"Dear Doctor: Your letter received, and I will gladly give you an explanation of my work.

"I doubt not when you started this great work, you knew that it could not stand still; you knew, also, that development was not likely to come from one brain alone. Others would see lines along which it could grow and being a big man, you would give credit where it belongs.

As you know, I studied with Dr. Langworthy after he had cured me of a twenty-year invalidism. **The work** as he gave it, **was severe beyond expression**, especially **to a highly sensitive nervous system**, and it took all my courage, and I might say lack of love for life, to go through it. Later, as I studied, and watched others adjusted, the thought took possession of me that something could be **accomplished in the line of skill** and ease. After years of work, I found that pressure upon the spinous processes, rather than thrust, moved vertebrae without shock to the most delicate constitution. But this pressure had a disadvantage, viz.: **When I moved one vertebra I dislodged its neighbor below.** Then I reasoned, why not move each vertebra beginning at the sacrum, which I did, and immediately I knew I had the 'ne plus ultra' of healing illness. My experience with a practice of fifty patients daily confirms and strengthens with each year I am in the work, and my success as a practitioner is unquestionable.

"**This method of putting the whole spine right by resetting each vertebra** plumb against the facet of its neighbor **re-constructs the entire spine** in most cases, and thus removes the cause of the present distressing symptom as completely as does the specific adjustment, but **in addition, it puts the constitution into such shape that it can resist disease in every other region, and thus corrects tendencies which usually lie dormant until late in life.**

"I practice with this complete adjustment, a system of dietetics to make good the nerve matter so newly released from impingement. and to build the intervertebral cartliage which holds the reset vertebrae in place.

"I consider my work a step in the advance that this great work must continue to make, and if you ever come to New York I know I can convince you.

"Thanking you again for your just inquiry into the work at first hand instead of accepting the criticism of casual observers, I am, very sincerely yours, with every wish for your success and prosperity. ALMA C. ARNOLD."

From other informants I learn that Dr. Arnold's "adjustments would hardly waken a sleeping child"; and that they are "painless." I would think that "a strong pressure from one pound on an infant to 125 pounds on a strong back" would be liable to waken a sleeping babe or a sound sleeper. As to her adjustments being painless; she does not "claim to adjust vertebrae without any pain whatever." She states in the above letter that her adjustments are "not entirely painless," but as near so as possible.

Her "thrust is not entirely painless, except on nearly normal spines." Ninety-nine per cent of Chiropractor's adjusting is of the former, therefore, ninety-nine per cent of Dr. Arnold's adjustments are more or less painful. The facts are, Dr. Arnold's adjusting is like mine, as near painless as she can make them. When compared with the "pile drivers," they are painless. "Old chronic luxations I must hurt to some degree."

I find the acute inflammatory cases are the most sensitive, painful cases. And, they are like the boy who had a tooth extracted, "Just as it was killing me, it came out." I think twenty-five per cent of my patients say, "Is that all? That don't hurt." Yet, I had not thot of saying that my adjusing was painless.

I am well aware that the majority of Chiropractors think an adjustment requires great force. It is not necessary to use a sledge hammer to drive a nail, or a pounder on the keys of a piano to create music, nor the jamming down on typewriter keys to write a legible letter. There is an elastic touch which may be acquired and used on the piano and typewriter in order to create melody in music and neatness in writing. There are piano pounders, typewriter thumpers and Chiropractor jammers. There are many Chiropractors whose adjustments are "severe beyond expression" as I have often witnessed and have repeatedly told by those who have taken adjustments of these heavy adjusters, when comparing their former treatments with those being received from the originator of the art of adjusting. I have had children cry for adjustments and others scream when being adjusted. I have had some persons who were nearly killed, judging by the uproar made while being adjusted, some of which were hurt so bad that they commenced yelling before I touched them, "but my work is as nearly painless as is possible to make when adjusting spinal luxations."

A knowledge of the normal and the unusual position of vertebrae; comprehension of the construction of vertebrae and just what you want to do with practice, skill and knack will make adjusting easy for the adjuster and the patient.

There is no more necessity of "clinking each vertebra of the entire spine, because one vertebra is displaced, than there would be in replacing every joint of the appendicular portion of the skeleton because one joint was luxated.

Dr. Arnold starts at the sacrum and ends at the occiupt, adjusting each and every vertebrae. Very many Chiropractors commence at the atlas and adjust (they either pretend or think they do) each and every vertebrae to the coccyx.

Dr. Arnold, so I am told, adjusts ribs and tarsal bones, as well as vertebrae, with the same ease as a Chinese laundryman plays with the balls on his abacus, counting rack.

It is evident that Alma C. Arnold has been misunderstood, for there is a vast difference between "there is no thrust, and no perceptible downward pressure," and that of one pound to 125 pounds administered at each thrust. She uses skill, which is commendable, a stranger to many Chiropractors. Knack, skill and the know-how are the essential principles of success in the art of adjusting.

Dr. Arnold "gives pressure rather than a thrust," a sledge hammer with a light stroke. While I use but little pressure with a forcible thrust, a light hammer with an energetic, quick stroke.

Dr. Arnold "makes re-construction of the spine for constitutional correction," adjusting the entire spine instead of the usual specific adjusting for a spinal ailment. She manipulates each and every vertebra, regardless of the disease. There are many Chiropractors who are doing the same. To do so, is easy to learn; no need of recognizing one disease from another; the adjuster is not required to know one vertebrae from another; no necessity for knowing from which side of the spine the nerves emerge, which innervate the throat and other special portions, the liver, spleen, stomach, pancreas or appendix "alie same;" uncouple each vertebrae, then link them together in their serial order, being sure that the segments are homologous and that the metameres are of the same organism, being careful to "reset each vertebrae plumb against the facet of its neighbors." It is useless to learn the "six words" around which a "jargonity" has been arranged.

"When I started this great work." The doctor must have read: "Twelve years ago D. D. Palmer had certain youthful principles that he based Chiropractic around. Its early years was simple, yet accurate and homely. The present day philosophy of adjusting vertebrae is practical yet so unmixed and pure that it is technically scientific. The application, today, is equal. This is now laid down in 2x2 exactness, reasons given for all deductions and conclusions. The stupendous development of the past two years in this respect alone marks another era in accord with Chiropractic's early teaching.

"Today we have the best; that which it does seem cannot be improved upon—the outcome—The Science of Chiropractic.

"This book is based around six words. The aim has been simplicity in preference to a jargonity that has no semblance to anything. It is absolutely plain, unadorned, undesigning and its art portrayed in detail. This book will deliver that which is simple fundamental principles for adjusting, show how to palpate for each and every one and how to give adjustment. Every move taught at 'Chiropractic's Fountain Head' is given.

"The basis of the book, in writings and illustrations, are mechanical. Its thots are clear and in accordance with such lines as make mechanics a true science in any factories line shaft or that of man. All thots, ideas and half-tones are thus based. No theory enters its composition. Each detail must be characteristic and proven or it will remain absent. Chiropractic is a practical art and as such is capable of easy illustration."

It was not surprising to me to read under date of Nov. 4, 1910, "I invested in your son's five books and could make nothing out of them at all." I have not known of any person who could.

"When I started this great work" I did not intend it to stand still, yet, I was careful to not give an idea to the world until it was well proven. I trust the contents of this volume will give this great work another start, in the right direction, as effective as was the one referred to. I am pleased to know that other brains than mine are developing (not enveloping) this great work. So far, there is only two developments from other brains than my own; those are the bifid table from the fertile brain of Dr. T. H. Story of Los Angeles, Cal., and Dr. Henry's idea of placing the hands and arms along the sides of the patient's body to prevent "bucking," being rigid, getting their backs up, just at an unappropriate time. Thus I personally and willingly give credit where due.

Dr. Arnold states: "When I moved one vertebra I dislodged its neighbor below." If this is a fact, as she states, of which a practice of fifty patients a day for three years ought to substantiate; I say, "If the moving of one vertebra displaced its neighbor below, how does she get all the vertebrae in place by commencing at the sacrum and proceed upward?" If I figure her adjusting right she would only have the last one in place and all the rest "dislodged." She may be like the boy who was very late on his arrival at school one winter morning. I asked him why he was late. He replied, "It was so slippery, when I stepped forward one step I slipped back two." I then asked "How did you get here?" He replied, "I turned round and went backward."

When adjusting, I have never known that while replacing one vertebra, "I dislodged its neighbor below." If that is a fact, why not do, as many Chiropractors are doing, commence at the top, instead of the bottom, then, dislodging its neighbor below would be immaterial; for the dislodging could be continued until the sacrum was reached and displaced, then, it being replaced, would drive out the coccyx, which can be displaced and replaced segment by segment until the last bone is reached, then by a little ingenuity it can be passed off on the unimportant coccygeus muscle.

Adjusting the whole spine "puts the constitution into such shape that it can resist disease in every region."

Really, that is a new thot and an important one for Chiropractors. Diseases are the result of vertebral displacements. These luxations are caused by direct traumatism, poisons or auto-suggestion. That thot of Dr. Arnold's beats Chiropractors out of a future job or jobs, as adjusting the whole spine puts up a constitutional defence, a fortified fortress, against traumatic accidents, toxic poisons and over tension by auto-suggestion.

I am satisfied that Dr. Alma Arnold has been innocently and grossly misrepresented.

---

If you do not remove the cause, how can you expect the patient to recover from the effects?

The November number of The Chiropractic, page 39, "A. P. Davis, D. C. (P. S. C. man)." A. P. Davis graduated in 1898, receiving his Chiropractic education and D. C. from me four years before B. J. graduated under the founder of the P. S. C. B. J. was 16 years of age at the time of A. P. Davis' graduation.

From the above we find that the P. S. C. was in existence in 1898, four years before B. J. graduated, that it was founded by D. D. Palmer.

---

On many occasions I have been able to enumerate on my own person the number of nerve pulsations to be 200 per minute. By a little practice I could count every other beat.

Is not the carrying capacity of nerves in ratio to the number of their pulsations? Are nerve beats increased in the same proportion by inflammation, as are those of the arterial circulation? Who can throw any light on this?

## MIRACULOUS CURE, BUT DOCTOR DIDN'T MAKE IT.

New York, June 7.—At a recent meeting of the County Medical Society, in Philadelphia, says the Medical Times in its publication today, Dr. De Sajous related how a man brought his daughter to him for treatment. She had lost her voice.

"I tried the battery on her," said the physician, "and her voice returned perfectly in a short time. The father was in such glee that he hugged me. When they had gone I happened to look at the battery, and observed that the current had not been turned on."

---

"This specimen carries necrotica, represents abnormal action of chemicals, poisons. 'Poison' has been allowed to gather through the inability of the tissues to transfer it onward to other tissues and they were unable to remove it from the body because of a lack of power which was due to a subluxation of one or more vertebrae."

Webster does not know such a word as "necrotica." I find necrosis, the death of bone, and necrotic, affected with necrosis.

I cannot comprehend how a bone carries necrosis. A bone may be affected with necrosis. The teacher handling this specimen states that "necrotica" is caused by "abnormal action of chemicals." Chemicals do not act on substances. The nature of a chemical is to **react.** The ineraction of two or more substances result in chemical decomposition. A compound composed of chemicals is not a chemical; its ingredients are. **The reaction** (not "action") **is always normal—could not be otherwise.**

Necrosis is the result of inflammation—too much heat. Chemicals have nothing whatever to do with it. Necrosis is the death of bone during the life of the individual—not after death. A chemical combination could only be used on a bone outside of man. Chemicals are only used in chemistry to produce chemical changes, either of analysis or of combination. The enveloper uses chemicals and poisons as synonyms, meaning one and the same thing. Poisons are not gathered in the tissues or cavities of the body. A poison is any animal, vegetable, or mineral substance which, when applied externally, or taken into the stomach, or injected into the body by a physician or reptile, causes such a change in the animal economy as to produce disease or death. A chemical may be poisonous or otherwise. Chemicals and poisons have entirely different uses.

## GERM PROOF.

One time the charming Widow Wise was feeling all run down,
So she went to Dr. Antigerm, the best M. D. in town.
"A wondrous microbe specialist," they said, "and handsome too.
Who knows, my dear, but he might prove a splendid match for you?"

The Widow found the doctor in his germ proof office, where
He listened to her symptoms, seated in a germ proof chair;
And as she told her fancied ills the doctor, for his part,
Began accumulating an affection of the heart.

Said he. "You know bacteria abounds in every place;
I really must be watchful in so serious a case.
You need most careful treatment, so I'll call each day at two
And take you for a little drive to see what good 'twill do."

So their acquaintance ripened. and the Widow liked the way
He watched her case so carefully and kept the germs away.
Why, when she'd go to dine with him, in hopes 'twould do her good.
They'd go to special restaurants which served but germ proof food!

One day he sent her roses, and she said, "How odd they smell!"
"Ah, yes," said he, "I've had them boiled and nicely smoked as well;
For microbes lurk in roses and you must take care, you see."
"Ah," thought the silly Widow, "how my doctor thinks of me!"

And then he started hinting of how much he'd like a wife,
For whom he'd build a germ proof house and lead a germ proof life.
"Now," thought the Widow with a thrill, "he'll next propose, I guess.
He'll offer me his germ proof heart and I shall answer yes."

He did, and she accepted him; then raised her blushing face,
Her ruby lips all ready for the kiss and fond embrace.
"Back! Back!" he cried in wild alarm, "There's suicide in this!
No microbes are so fatal as those lurking in a kiss!

"Ere we enjoy that labial treat advance your lips, my dear;
I'll spray them with the contents of this atomizer here!"
"Away!" cried she, and glared at him with anger in her eyes.
"TRUE LOVE IS NOT AFRAID OF GERMS!" exclaimed the Widow Wise.

**Paul West.**

## SOME LUXATIONS ADJUSTED.

We were recently handed some questions with their answers. Being the discoverer and developer of Chiropractic I feel like taking the liberty of correcting them.

The teacher states that the **function** of the left lamina of the axis is to unite the anterior arch with the posterior. Functions are either vital or intellectual; they perform vital acts and intellectual acts. A bone, or a part of one, does not assist in performing any of the vital phenomena either of the body or mind. The laminae and pedicles constitute the arch, the atlas being the only vertebra that has two arches. Therefore the laminae do not unite the two arches of the axis.

Again he says: "The lack of current is the cause of any disease in any person." A large per cent of diseases while in the acute stage have too much heat, an excess of function, too much activity, are hypersensitive, have a hypertrophied condition, as does cancer in its growth.

In his disertation on sunstroke he looses sight of one of the principles of Chiropractic, namely, that disease is but the result of functions performed in too great or too little degree. He says: "A person could not have sunstroke unless there was a subluxation." An exposure to the sun's rays may cause either extremes of activity. Remember that disease is either too much or too little functionating. The patient may exhibit symptoms of asphyxial insolation, with coma, a feeble pulse, coldness of the skin and diminished temperature, or that of hyperexia with full rapid pulse, hot skin and a high temperature.

Of all backward steps the following is the greatest: "Every step from one (advancement) to the other has been a continual fight. For instance, I was talking only the other evening with a man who was a graduate from this school four years ago. He graduated when we **did** teach the sympathetic system (nerve system). Today when I tell him there is no such thing, he battles me; fought me until 7 o'clock last night—for three solid hours we chewed the rag on that, and he left just as determined as when he came. He is but a practitioner, but here is a school starting out, making a standard of its own, which it thinks is the only one there is, and we give them credit for thinking so, although they have (or take) no means of comparing their work with what the other fellow has."

There is a system, one of the three sub-divisions of nerves, which anatomists have seen fit to name sympathetic or trisplanchnic. The nerves of this system originate in the brain, pass down and in the spinal cord, leaving the spinal canal by way of the intervertebral foramina, and so far they are known as spinal nerves, subject to impingement, as are all nerves. Those of the sympathetic leave the sheath, proceed to and enter one of the ganglia of the ganglionic chain, from which they emerge and proceed to their respective organs to perform vital functions under the instruction of Innate. The balance of the fibers which help to make the bundle go to other parts of the body and are under the control of Educated.

When a teacher of neurology tells you that there is "no such thing" as the sympathetic nervous system controlled by Innate, it is foolish "to battle with him three solid hours" or that many minutes. He might as well deny the existence of the spinal and cranial nerves. With such vagaries he has turned Chiropractic backward into the ignorance of the past when it was asserted by the medical men that the sympathetic was an independent system. The writer "chewed the rag" for two years with the same teacher, in a fruitless effort to show him the difference between displaced and misplaced.

It is no wonder that he writes of himself, "His every thought is a gem, and when compiled in this fashion are treasure houses of knowledge." It would be nearer the truth to say that his thoughts are frequently the outburst of egotistical ignorance, filling his cranium and others with a lot of rubbish that retards Chiropractic.

If it is the name, sympathetic, he objects to, why not change it. He could use splanchnic as referring to the three great cavities of the body. But, instead, he says there is no such thing as the sympathetic system. Why not leave him in his determination to build a standard of his own founded on ignorance of bones and nerves, as shown by the above quotations?

This teacher uses illustrations in demonstrating which of themselves are incorrect. For example, "A cloud letting out water." Does he not know that a cloud consists of watery particles suspended in the atmosphere sufficiently dence to be visible?

Again he says: "In a disease of the urinary system, what would you say was the cause?" His answer is, "A shutting off of impulses to that system." All there is of disease is either too much or not enough functionating. If the kidneys receive too much nerve force we have over action, more than a normal amount of urine; if there is a lack of functionating the flow of urine is scanty and dropsy is the result. When functional activity is less than normal we have a condition known as paralysis, paresis or atrophy.

"Urinary system."

A system is a group of organs similar in function, irrespective of their structure. There is no "urinary system," nor a group of urinary organs. "Urinary" relates to the urine, as the urinary bladder, urinary calculus, urinary canal, the urinary apparatus, the kidneys, ureters, bladder and urethra. Anatomists mention many systems, but no "urinary system."

Again he says: "Suppose one had a sub-luxation which cut a nerve off entirely. In that case would it not be a disease of the nerve?" His answer is yes. A sub-luxation was never known to sever a nerve, excision is not produced by an impingement; what is the use of supposing what never happens? A nerve may be severed by an instrument. In that case, whatever sensation were produced by pressure will continue as long as that pressure exists, although that part of the body in which the nerve ramified was removed.

"The Educated Intelligence is wholly acquired—learned by experience. The Innate is not acquired. It is born within and with us, is just as capable of running all functions of the body at birth as in adult life. It is not obtained by experience, but is inherent, and does not depend upon years of observation."

Today we assert, that the knowledge possessed by Educated Intelligence is acquired during life, in one generation; that possessed by Innate was obtained during the life of the vertebrata.

"Some have but little of the Educated, but Innate performs all functions of the body in a manner which the inventors and philosophers would be glad to enjoy."

The education of some persons is limited; that of Innate is comparatively perfect, having had untold ages of adaptation, knowledge and skill in running the vital functions.

"Nature, instinct, subconscious mind and intuition are terms often used to express this idea of intelligence, but they do not bring forth the sentiment."

By Innate, I refer to that **intelligence** which is born with and within us, and which continues to **furnsh vitality** to our bodies as long as life lasts. **Nature** does not include that ever present **intelligence which exists as a separate entity. Instinct** is an inward impulse **without reason**; it prompts our actions. **Subconscious mind** is a **product** of Innate, vital **phenomena occurring without consideration. Intuition** is an apprehension or recognizance **without reason.** None of these terms expressed the precise meaning I wanted to convey. I therefore chose the word Innate, meaning born with.

"The mother, whether human or of the lower order of mammalia, transmits the Innate to her offspring, but it takes a lifetime to educate the voluntary mind."

The mother bequeathes to her offspring that intelligence which I have seen fit to name Innate. This is as true in the vegetable kingdom as in the animal. The willow and orange transmit their qualities through and by their own individualized lives, each to its kind. The Educated takes cognizance of its external surroundings and this collected education becomes a part of Innate.

"In all organized living beings endowed with sensation, innervation, assimilation, circulation, nutrition, caloricity, reparation, excretion, secretion, and respiration are under the control of and managed by Innate, except where the action of Innate nerves are affected by pressure upon, causing abnormal functions. Such need mechanical adjustment, not chemical changes made by drugs."

In all animated nature, the functions are ordered by an intelligence, named Innate, which has had a lifetime experience (measured by the time its kind has existed.) Its commands are expressed in vital functions; their quality depending upon the condition of its channels of communication. The nerves are Innate's lines of intercourse; the ability to convey intelligence depends upon their freedom from impingement. Bones may be displaced, their projecting surfaces irritating the nerves which they strike against. It is the business of the Chiropractor to replace these bones in their natural position, thereby freeing nerves from impingement, and allowing Innate to perform her work normally.

"Innate comprehends that birth is a transition from mother-dependence to self-existence, that thon (he or she) no longer depends upon the mother for the performance of vital functions; thon must breathe, take nourishment, digest and assimilate the same and pass the refuse out of the body. These various functions are performed as natuarally and with as much intelligence on the first day of existence as in after years."

The future graft, or scion, which is about to be severed from the parent tree, is a part of and dependent upon the functions of that plant for an existence; when separated and suitable conditions furnished, it becomes a tree with all the functions of the parent and is like unto it. The Individualized Innate and the physical become independent, and yet the material is dependent upon the immaterial for life and its continued existence. The first breath confirms the fact that all functions are established—"breathed into his nostrils the breath of life and man became a living soul," a living being. Innate is as much an individualized intelligence as the physical is a living form.

"Often Innate and Educated differ in their opinions of the same subject. For example, in a normal condition the bowel actions are under the control of Innate, but because of luxated vertebrae the nerves of bowel innervation are inactive, being pressed upon in the intervertebral foramina, consequently there is a lack of action, usually named constipation. Innate would like to have Educated relieve that pressure and restore innervation, but because the latter's senses have been warped by years of training, he proceeds to give a physic, compelling Innate to collect water and wash the intruder out by way of the bowels. Innate finds an undesirable drug forced down the throat and into the stomach, much against his sense of right, and proceeds to get rid of the objectionable dose. The poison does not act upon the stomach and bowels—Innate acts upon the poison or drug."

Subluxated vertebrae disarrange the costo-central articulation—the juncture of the head of the rib with the vertebrae. These projecting surfaces press against and impinge upon one or more of the four branches of the spinal nerve.

The time is coming when these two intelligences will converse freely with each other, for their mutual benefit, upon subjects pertaining to their common welfare.

"Innate Intelligence never sleeps. It runs all the vital functions of our bodies night and day, by and through nerves. If these were free to act in a natural manner, we would not know an ache, pain or any of the symptoms of disease; the life power and force would be unobstructed and normal."

Innate is not controlled by physical laws; it never sleeps, knows neither night, gravitation, distance, heat nor cold. It is not subject to disease, yet its intellectual advancement depends upon the physical condition of its body.

"Innate is the body builder before as well as after birth. The Educated directs the thoughts that are above and outside of the material body."

Innate looks after the vital functions of the mother and her unborn. The Educated impresses its thoughts upon Innate, directing its functions more or less.

"The prospective mother, seeing abnormal sights, transmits thoughts of the spectacle to the Innate builder, which constructs a portion of the unborn just as the mother has strongly impressed it to do. This is commonly known as naevus, marking the child, material imagination of the foetus in utero."

The more I study "mother marks" in connection with Chiropractic, the more I find natural, explainable causes for abnormal shapes and developments. The same cause which produces club feet after birth, does so before birth. Contracted nerves draw the different parts of the feet into unnatural positions. The varying number of ossifying centers, their failure to unite because of a lack of psychological and physiological co-ordination, is the cause of many anomalies. The occasional inclination to "sport" when Innate, for many and varied reasons, sees fit to make a change from the ordinary, with a view to co-ordinate its environment is accounted for in the same way.

"Heretofore it has been supposed that the mother transmits her thoughts directly to the unborn, but the facts are that the Educated directs Innate to form the child not only in its physical make-up, but also in its sensational likes or dislikes. If the mother is strongly impressed with vivid ideas, they are transmitted to Innate who is never at rest and who develops the new being as it is impressed."

The mother transfers to her offspring during gestation, certain physical and intellectual peculiarities. Innate and Educated influence each other, more or less, through intellectual communication. Physical characteristics and mental inclinations may be changed in after years.

"If the mother is acquainted with this law, she will exclude all suggestions that are not to her liking, and direct aright the future physical and mental inclinations of her offspring."

The expectant mother may create the unborn, make thon's physical and mental what she longs for, by impressing her desires upon Innate, the builder, the creator of the new being. These physical and mental conditions may be modified in after years. For example, the color and texture of the hair is often changed by sickness, fright or old age.

"Remember that these two separate and distinct intellects, whether sane or insane, good or evil, stamp their thoughts, more or less, upon each other."

Therefore, how necessary it is, that to have harmony they should understand each other. Innate should have a perfect physical through which to receive impressions of its environments and be able to express itself correctly. Neither of these can be accomplished if bones are displaced, impinging upon the carriers of expressions and impressions.

"We can see and study much of the work of Innate intelligence by an examination of osteological specimens. An examination of such specimens was truly wonderful to D. D. Palmer. A calvarium (top of a skull) shows on both sides of the inner surface beautiful pictures of forest fires as perfect as though drawn by an artist, the fire and smoke being of natural color. This building of vimineous arborescent exostoses was due to an excess of functionating on the part of Innate."

Sometimes it requires close discrimination to distinguish between the work done by Innate and that resulting from disease. The superior bisected portion of the above cranium cerebrale, the skull cap, has grooves for the meningeal arteries and veins which are much more clearly defined than usual, hence their resemblance to the artistic delineation spoken of above.

"The unique monstrosity is an extraordinary piece of work. To be fully appreciated it must be seen and explained."

This monstrosity is a vertebral column of seventeen vertebrae —if we consider each vertebrae as having one body—fifteen true and two false. Seven cervical, eight dorsal and two lumbar vertebrae, sacrum and coccyx. It has the usual number of ribs, intervertebral foramina, spinous and transverse processes. The last four lumbar vertebrae are coalesced into one centrum, which has seven intervertebral foramina, four spinous and eight transverse processes. There are fourteen ribs, seven spinous and fourteen transverse processes clustered around the first dorsal body. Innate must have been advised by Educated to make a hunchback.

"The fourth and fifth ribs of the right side are shown to have eight healed fractures. The fourth has two, the fifth a communicated fracture at salient angles. Innate repaired these fractures, doing the best it could. The one in the center of the fifth rib and its mate were not in proper apposition. Innate not being a mechanic, could not adjust the displaced pieces. Educated should have done that; nevertheless Innate did the best it could under the conditions imposed upon it. It filled in the vacant space with interposed callus, but the pieces not being in right position, the osteoanapleurosis was not perfect. The symphysis was weak and liable to refracture. To strengthen this weak place, it built a pier (exostosis) from each rib toward and touching the other. The ends of these piers were covered with hyaline cartilage making a brace similar, with a very ingenious exception, to that which a carpenter would make to strengthen a weak place in a joist. This exception was that the brace, instead of being immovable, as the carpenters would be, was united to each rib by a joint. This arrangement gave to the connected ribs the benefit of a movable joint as well as a brace. The man himself (the educated) knew nothing of this brace built between the two ribs by Innate who did the repairing. It showed intelligent architectural reasoning and judgment and skill in adapting means to accomplish the purpose intended."

Innate is acquainted with the laws of equilibrium and motion known as animal mechanics. Eduacted has a knowledge and makes practical application of the laws of matter and motion in constructing machines and buildings.

The osseous formation of human frames, while similar, are no more alike than our features. Any one vertebrae will not fit in the place of another. Many unusual additions are found which display an intelligent adaption of means to a definite end.

"The first two vertebrae next to the head, the atlas and axis, show Innate's Intelligence and ability in coping with existing difficulties. By an accident the anterior arch of the atlas was displaced upward, causing Innate to make a new facet on the odontoid, for articulation. This facet was so near the apex of the processus dentatus that there was liability of the atlas slipping up and over it and backward against the spinal cord. Such an accident, we are taught, would cause instant death. Innate showed reason, judgment and skill in elongating the process to prevent fatality; yet, the Educated man knew nothing of this internal work, although he no doubt suffered from the imprringement of nerves. A Chiropractor would replace the atlas to its normal position."

The intelligence which made these repairs was back of them directing nature, instinct and sub-conscious mind. This intelligence, I choose to call Innate, will in time develop more than the recognized five senses. Educated will be informed of the precise condition when nerves are impinged upon and the best means for their relief will be suggested. A kind of telepathy will be inaugurated.

"It is interesting to a pathologist to note the various changes in the shape of different parts of the vertebrae resulting from its adaption to some displacement which Innate was not able to adjust, and which the physician did not discover. Innate displays much intelligence in the formation of many locks found in the vertebral column to prevent further displacement of an already subluxated vertebrae. One of these is as nice a dovetail as any artificer could make. Very many times we find vertebrae ankylosed by an osseous symphysis for the purpose of preventing any further displacement. Innate is not a mechanic, therefore cannot replace them. These osseous unions are removed after Chiropractors replace the luxated vertebrae to their former and natural position."

Nature, instinct, or the mind does not manifest the intelligence herein shown in the uniting of fractured bones. It requires action, guided by intelligence. A mechanic is one who is skilled in the laws of motion and force, as applied to construction. Therefore Innate is a designer. There is this particular difference, however; Innate does not use tools or instruments to build or construct.

"Four rachitic specimens of tibia and fibula, bent while softened by excessive heat, show the effects of superheat. In bow legs we find a corresponding flattening (Platycynemia) of the fibula to compensate and strengthen its fragile mate. In femurs which have been weakened and curved by greenstick fracture, we find the linea aspera built out in a pier to compensate for its frailty."

In Vol. 2 of The Science of Chiropractic, page 61, referring to me, it is stated: "His actions and thoughts are sharp, alert and ahead of the times. His every thought was why? He would study two bones, and by comparison, would find one normal and its opposite very much abnormal. Why? would be the first question. The destination **was to place behind these actions an intelligence.**"

Up to the time (1904) this treatise was written, B. J. had not written an article, a paragraph or a sentence on Innate, **the basis of the science** of Chiropractic, and now only alludes to it as his "pet theory."

"To say that this intelligence displayed by Innate is nothing but nature, instinct, or intuitive force, does not meet our comprehension."

The reader will notice that I am quoting from my own article, which was written over six years ago, a paragraph at a time. How strange to read, "B. J. Palmer was the developer of this science. It is up to you to disprove that if you can. You have never made any effort in that direction."

"The immense variety of monstrosities which are created or built by this Intelligence, opens a boundless field for observation and research."

To emphasize and make more emphatic that I am the author of this article and the originator of the idea contained therein, the compiler of my writings placed in the midst of this, my treatise on Innate, a page cut of the author, with the words: "Dr. D. D. Palmer, Discoverer and Developer of Chiropractic," a copy of which may be seen on page 917.

"Different kinds of work in various parts of the human body are performed by nerves which have various functions. Occasionally, when long bones are fractured, the fragments do not unite, the callus material is not supplied. Physicians try many expedients to make a union, but they experiment in vain, for they do not know why the osseous matter (symphysis material) is not supplied. Chiropractors who have studied the morbid anatomy of nerves would know why they did not supply the necessary material for uniting these fractures, and would be able to assist these useless repair nerves to their normal condition and usefulness."

May not the same nerve transfer orders for various functions at the same time, as telegraph wires convey several messages at one and the same moment? The delivery of the messages and their condition would be determined by the conductibility of the transferring tubes.

"These conditions referred to, showing intelligence, do not include deformities, abnormal growths, exostoses caused by overheat, excessive nutrient supply by deranged functions. A part or all of the skeletal frame may be softened by superheat (fever), a portion of the bone may ooze out, be deposited on the surface, causing morbid enlargement and ankyloses. When heat becomes less than normal, we find the third stage, that of hardening, consolidation, and eburnation; functions are performed in a less degree. Disease is but the performance of functions in either an excessive or deficient amount."

All diseases shorten life by deteriorating the quality of the tissue; they also hamper the intellectual progress of Innate. Knowledge is gathered through the physical according as Innate is able to co-ordinate the spiritual with the material body. It is therefore necessary, in order to enhance our present and future existence to keep our bodies in proper condition.

"Some diseases are due to the morbid conditions of Innate nerves, while others are the result of an abnormal sensibility of the Educated; the distinction being determined by perceiving whether the abnormal conditions that exist are produced when asleep or awake."

The involuntary jerking of muscles when awake, ceasing in sleep, is the distinction referred to above. Some nerves are entirely under the control of Innate—the involuntary. The voluntary are controlled by Educated, while others are more or less under the management of both.

"Hypnotists put Educated in a condition of sleep and control Innate by suggestions. All cures made by Faith, Christian Science, Metaphysics, Charms, Mental Healers, Magnetics and Suggestions are produced by the Educated controlling Innate. Many persons in whom Innate is prerogative, assert themselves in thought over and above the Educated, compelling the mental to believe the possessor is ailing. It is a poor rule that won't work both ways."

The unfoldment of the soul—intelligent life—is only begun. Here and there we find unexplainable mental wonders—attributes of the soul. Herein is the latent undeveloped progression of the human race. Persons quite illiterate, by auto suggestion—self-hypnotized—will give a discourse on any given subject or compose poetry as fast as they can talk. Psychometry leads us into an undeveloped field of soul-life; it also explains first impressions on which fortune-tellers depend.

"If you would comprehend diseased conditions of the vital organs, study Innate nerves. The old blood delusion of disease, the present fad of microbes, bacteria and bugs, do not explain the unpleasant sensations of nerves."

If all parts of the body were normal, so that Innate could express its thoughts in a natural manner, we would have health. Why not study nerves—the conveyors of impulses—and bones, the frame-work of the body, which, if disarranged impinge upon nerves and cause deranged functions—too much or not enough action. The time is coming when Innate will analyze its own condition and Educated will recognize that determination.

"Dreams are thoughts of Innate nerves, afterwards remembered, varying more or less, according to the impressions made upon it."

Dreams are seemingly imaginary transactions, which occur during sleep. They consist of impressions taken in by Educated during our wakeful hours. It is said that those who never had sight never dream of seeing; those who were always deaf never dream of hearing. The transactions which make the deepest impressions, or those which occupy our minds the most, are the ones remembered when we awake. It is probable that only a very small part of our dreams are remembered when we rouse from sleep. I presume Innate is ever busy handling impressions received through the physical, as much so, as it is with the management of the vital functions. Circumstances dreamed, which would take many minutes or hours to accomplish, pass before the mind in a remarkably short space of time, as is proven by persons who were asleep but a moment or at the most a quarter of a minute; yet they dreamed of incidents that would have taken hours to perform had they really occurred. Occasionally dreams are of importance and systematic, giving us information upon subjects of which we were very much in need. This mysterious intercourse between Innate and Educated will in time be made more clear and taken advantage of.

"Innate does not study laws of animal mechanism, does not set displaced or fractured bones, but after the bones are replaced, it will unite fractures, remove temporary callus, a temporary protection which is no longer needed, and put to natural use those nerves which were useless or deranged."

Innate makes use of the mechanical principle of the lever. The bones form the arms of the levers, the contracting muscles the power, the joints the fulcra or points of support, the weight of the individual limbs or parts to be moved—the weight or resistance. The Chiropractor—the Educated—uses this principle when adjusting displaced portions.

Nerves are never deranged. Their fibres may become tense because of impingement by bone; their diameters may be increased, they may become stiff, rigid and over-heated, or become lax, feeble and unable to carry impulses with normal force.

Innate does the best it can, adapting itself to conditions under which it exists. We can see this intelligence displayed in all animal and vegetable life. A duality of the spiritual and physical—spiritual beings and mortal existence.

"If all parts of the human machine are in their normal position, if not, they should be made so, Innate can use them in a natural manner to perform the various functions of different organs. But the physician's present fad is to remove any diseased organ that they think can be spared. Too often the patient's friends find, when too late, the removal is a fatal mistake."

While the human body has been compared to and called a machine, it differs from it very materially. Yet there is some similarity. The harmonious working of the human body depends upon the condition of its lines of communication—the nerves. Their ability to carry messages, without augmentation or diminution, to the various parts, insures that the work will be performed in a satisfactory manner, as Innate desires. The carrying capacity of these lines of intercourse depends upon their freedom from contact with the osseous frame-work. If any of the bones composing the skeletal frame should be out of alignment, rubbing against, impinging upon the tubular lines of transit, they will need replacing to their normal position, thereby releasing the pressure against nerves. This important part of the work has been named adjusting. Chiropractors should have a thorough knowledge of bones, nerves, the principles of Chiropractic and the art of adjusting the displaced portions to their natural position.

"Innate Intelligence knows much more of the normal workings of the stomach, liver, kidneys, pancreas, spleen and appendix than the medical world."

Medical men have experimented for hundreds of years and yet know but little of physiology—nothing of the source of energy which runs the bodily functions. Innate has devised and built the different parts, each adapted to their respective work, and therefore, knows far more in regard to their functions than man will ever know, unless he becomes associated with and a student of Innate.

I cannot refrain from using the language of T. J. Owens, D. C., which will be found in The Chiropractor, August and September numbers, pages 23 and 24.

"The child (Chiropractic) being born and christened, it became the duty of its father to enter upon a course of training and development which would prepare the child for the duties and demands that might be made upon it.

"Some there are, I am sorry to say, those who have vilely attempted to disparage the parentage of this child, but the records of his birth are too well authenticated to admit of any success of such vile traducing by the ungrateful beings who have profited most by reason of his birth. They have not even stopped at this, but have given additional evidence of their base ingratitude to their benefactors by attempting to kidnap the youngster, rechristen and raise him as their own. Failing in this, they have tried to claim relation with him, when the facts are, they hardly have a speaking acquaintance with him."

I have now made an effort to prove that I originated the idea of Innate and all wherein Chiropractic is connected with it; that I wrote the first article upon Innate, the philosophy of the science of which I have the honor of being the developer. If the party in question, who has tried to rob me of the credit of being "the developer of this wonderful science and philosophy," will mail me any manuscript, or a sworn copy, that antedates this article on Innate which I have quoted, I will give it free publication in The Adjuster.

I understand since the publication of number two Adjuster, that the kidnaper, the pseudo fountain head, the would-be developer, has entered his private office, muffled the bell, hung up the receiver and shut himself up like a clam. He knows I am fishing for him. The adjuster has his sleeves rolled up to his shoulders, pen and ink at hand, his Underwood typewriter oiled and a 32 c. p. to furnish light by night. If you have any more dares, just throw them out. "The man who is right and knows he is right," cannot afford to allow another to steal his belongings and lie him out of his property rights.

---

The following are opinions of members of the science circles of Osteopathy:

"On examination he found the three lower dorsal vertebrae so far anterior, that he could place his three fingers in the concavity to bring it level with the other vertebrae."

The fingers are three-fourths of an inch thick. This would make an anterior displacement of "the three lower dorsal vertebrae" three-fourths of an inch forward of the vertebrae above and below. The spinal canal in this region is a half-inch in diameter. If there was a displacement anterior equal to the thickness of the fingers, the spinal cord would be compressed to a quarter of an inch less than its normal diameter, which would amount to a complete division.

This apparent displacement was due to the absence of the spinous processes which had been removed by accident, as shown by a specimen in the writer's possession. These detached portions were absorbed. He does not say that he replaced them.

"The chiros, mechanos and neuros are multiplying outside of the schools faster than inside and he thinks the proposed law will not stop them. They advertise flashily and get as good a class of patients as he does, and they openly boast that they give all there is in osteopathy and more, and they are doing more business than any D. O. in town. The general public don't know the difference between them and Osteopaths and don't seem to care."

"The general public . . . don't seem to care." All they want is health.

A D. O. "thinks Osteopathy is too hard work to have to compete with all the fakes in the country."

Learn Chiropractic—do less work and more good.

"He is opposed to licensing any one to practice any method, who has not put in as much time as we have in preparing for their method."

"Their method" may not require as much time to equal or surpass other methods. If so, why put in as much time?

"The treatment given by the chiro of his town is nothing like osteopathy, as he gives a treatment in five minutes, by placing the patient on his face on a bench and gives him a thrust opposite each vertebrae from one end of the spine to the other and then pounds them with his fist over the same area and tells them that is all, come again tomorrow, and charges them one dollar."

I am glad to learn that the treatment given by the chiro is nothing like Osteopathy. I am sorry to learn that the chiro is not specific—has not learned Chiropractic as a science or an art.

"The mechano-therapy is simply a combination of massage and Swedish movement."

And so was Osteopathy previous to their learning medicine and Chiropractic.

Charley Still says, "We are specialists." He does not want a strictly medical course. He wishes to remain a specialist.

"He says the druggists in his town give him the regular physician's discount and patronize him besides."

Chiropractors get the regular discount from druggists if they ask for it, and many patients from druggists' families without asking.

The Journal gives me the credit of composing the famous Boston poem, "The Path the Calf Made." I have never claimed to be a poet—I never composed a verse of poetry.

Number 4 Adjuster contained the essence of the following, but as I found the class under my personal instruction unable to grasp what it contained, I was assured that it would have to be spread out, so that the Adjuster class could see the substratum upon which Chiropractic was founded. To be sure, Chiropractic may be practiced without the knowledge contained in the following, but, why not know what your business is founded upon?

The triad.

Innate—Soul—Body.

Innate—Intelligent Life—Body.

Immaterial—Vital—Material.

The life directed by intelligence is the soul (the life) of the body.

The Soul (the life) is the symphysis which unites Spirit and Body.

Without the connecting link, the Spiritual and Physical are separate and distinct from each other.

Man is a part of Creation.

Innate is a part of the Creator.

Innate is the Creator of man before as well as after birth.

Mother Innate builds before birth—the individualized, personified Innate after birth.

Innate is a part of The All Wise.

Innate (Spirit) is a part of Universal Intelligence, individualized and personified.

Innate desires to assist the Chiropractor in making a correct diagnosis.

The Universal Intelligence, collectively or individualized, desires to express itself in the best manner possible. It has been struggling for countless ages to improve upon itself—to express itself intellectually and physically higher in the scale of evolution. Man's aspirations should be to advance to a superior level, to make himself better, physically, mentally and spiritually.

This marvelous existence of many systems, harmoniously associated and controlled by the I AM, constitutes the duality of man.

The spirit was a living intelligence before it was united with the body. It will continue a living, intelligent entity after it is separated from it.

---

Future copies of anatomies will contain a section on subluxations and the results therefrom.

## CERVICAL RIBS.

The transverse processes of the seventh cervical vertebrae are broad and flattened vertically. They project considerable more than the sixth and are equal in extent to the maximum width of the atlas. Its vertebraterial foramina vary in diameter and are frequently absent on one side; the vertebral artery passing in front of, instead of through the vertebraterial foramen.

The transverse processes are composed of the costal and the true transverse process. The costal element is occasionally found separated from the posterior half and constituting a cervical rib. This is because of the independent centers of ossification in the anterior and posterior roots.

The interval between the neck of the rib and the front of the transverse process, forms an arterial passage which corresponds to the vertebraterial canal in the transverse processes of the cervical vertebrae; the anterior bar is homologous with the head and tubercle of the thoracic rib, whilst the posterior part corresponds with the thoracic transverse process.

The cervical rib is, therefore, due to the independent development of the costal root of the transverse process of the seventh cervical vertebra.

Cervical ribs, as a rule, are of small size; they seldom exceed an inch in length, but may reach the sternum as do other ribs. The head always articulates with the body of the seventh cervical vertebra. Its tubercle is large in comparison with its length and forms a sharp angle. Between it and the first thoracic rib there is a well-marked intercostal space.

A cervical rib may possess only a head, neck and tubercle; its shaft may end freely and join the first thoracic rib, or the sternum; this union may be by bone cartilage or ligament.

A spinal column recently came into my possession which had twenty-five ribs, the extra one being a right cervical of two and three-quarter inches in length. Its head and also that of the right first thoracic were small. The tubercle was comparatively large and one inch from the head. The shaft was small. The distal end was comparatively large and articulated midway on the upper surface of the first thoracic rib, but articular cartilage was lacking.

The twelfth pair of ribs in this specimen were each one and a half inches in length.

The eleventh and twelfth vertebrae were ankylosed and wedge-shaped, making a sharp kyphosis. The bodies of the third and fourth lumbars had oozed out a portion of their substance, which was loose—not attached to the vertebrae as usual.

## MEDICAL PRIESTHOOD, BY A LONDON PHYSICIAN.

Some thirty years ago, a distinguished woman of letters published a small book entitled **The Age of Science**, which began by announcing as the greatest discovery ever achieved by man, the invention of the new **Prospective Telegraph**, which enables the obstacles of time to be effectually conquered as that of space has been by the electric telegraph.

**The Age of Science** purported to give extracts from the newspapers of 1977, which referred with pride to the consciousness of its readers that they live in a period of the world's history "when science reigns supreme over human affairs, and has altogether superceded most of the pursuits of mankind in under ages, such as war, the chase. literature, art and religion."

The idea was not new. Jules Verne's wonderful books foreshadowed the submarine warships, the flying machine, and many marvels that have since become familiar to us. Other works of fiction have occupied our attention in more recent years with notions that are very likely to be realized in the near future.

The great poets of the world have ever been its prophets, and imaginative writers have often substantiated their claims to foretell the future.

**The Age of Science** dealt chiefly with the time when the churches would all be abolished, and their buildings devoted to the use of the medical profession, and for physiological and other researches, "for which the vaults beneath offer peculiarly interesting specimens." And so in the journals of Monday, January 1, 1907, we read that His Grace the Lord Archphysician of Canterbury presided over a congress of Right Reverend Lord Doctor's of Medicine in Henry VII's chapel, called to prohibit the laity from daring to peruse Medical Guides and Treatise on Domestic Medicine, which have pretended to direct the multitude how to cure or prevent disease without the aid of a physician. "Doctors," said his lordship, "were the appointed Ministers of the Body, and the man who imagines his health could be saved without them would find out his error when it was too late."

Then we read of the proceedings of the Lower House of Convocation, assembled in the Nave of Westminster Abbey, under the presidency of the Very Eminent Archdoctor of Cheltenham. Amongst the Schedules of Gravamina and Reformanda the inadequacy of the fees to be legally claimed by doctors was dealt with. These were concerned with certificates of Vaccination, Equination (inoculated with the virus of horsepox), Porcination (inoculated with the virus of the hog), and especially for the certificates of those having died under due medical care and supervision, and consequently admissible for cremation. The laws relating to Medical Heretics were considered, and it was arranged that a solemn protest, carried by 50,000 doctors in procession, should march down Witehall to demonstrate against the interference of the Secular Power in Things Medical.

In police reports we have accounts of the flogging of a number of men and women for neglecting to send their children to the new Science Classes in the Tower that they might learn the rudiments of Astronomy and Paleontology.

At the Middlesex Session we are not surprised to read that five noble ladies and gentlemen were sentenced to the extreme penalty of the law after being found guilty by a jury of doctors for having deceived the officers of Domestic Inspection respecting their own and their children's Canination (inoculation with the virus of the dog) and Porcination. "It was shown that all the defendants had been vaccinated according to law four times during the last year, and equinated twice during the late prevalence of glanders, but though rabies and measles were both known to be raging in London they had not only neglected to present themselves and their children at the Canine and Porcine Stations in Queen's Gate, but had deceived the inspectors as above stated by exhibiting the former scars for the latter. Mr. Justice Draco sentenced all five prisoners to be vivisected for the instruction of the students at the magnificent new School of Physiology in Carlton Gardens. Some sympathy was expressed for an elderly nobleman in feeble health, who seems to have feared being inoculated by the saliva of mad dog. Lady Clara Vere de Vere implored that she might even be Ratified sooner than given over to the experiments of Dr. Blacksmith on the Nervous System.

Several medical heritics, who had contumaciously refused to take medicine according to law, were ordered to be burnt before the doors of the London University. Two homeopaths were ordered to be burnt alive in Trafalgar Square after hearing a lecture delivered by the King's Medical Confessor in Ordinary, Dr. Torr Quemada, under the Dome of St. Paul's. These are but a few specimens of this brilliant brochure, and as I read it many years ago I confessed to myself that I saw no reason why it should not ultimately be no satire but a record of awful doings to come. The world, which has complacently witnessed the tortures and persecutions of the past in the interest of theologians—speculative as were the doctrines concerned—may tolerate in an age when materialization has dethroned God, and science has abolished religion—a medical domination equaling, if not surpassing, in tolerance the cruelties of a theological epoch.

We may take the recent riots about "The Brown Dog of Battersea" as a **ballon d'essai** of medical feeling relating to interference with the rights and privileges of medical men and boys. Could we see anything in these demonstrations but the determination of medical students to make their profession dominant? The toy dogs they carried in procession were the emblems of their laboratory researches. Their ribald songs were their defiance of the humanitarians who try to impede their cruel work, and the whole spirit of the riots meant the claim of orthodox medicine to rule the public in the interests of their craft.

Those who cannot see in these disturbances, and in the spirit which animated them, the warning of what will come when science rules us unchecked by a nobler spirit must be deficient in the ability to discern the signs of the times. To me the demonstration is a potent of evil.

Dominated by a medical priestcraft the world will be worse off than it was under the rule of the clerics.—**Herald of Health, England.**

---

A Chiropractor sent me his leaflet saying: "Dad, if this is not **pure** Chiropractic, adjust it."

He is a subscriber for this book, therefore, he and you will see this adjusting.

The composition is good; however, there are a few mistakes which need adjusting.

"**Pure Chiro.**"

To be pure is to be separate and free from any extraneous or heterogeneous matter or material; as pure air, pure water, pure food. To say that you have pure Chiro. is to infer that some one else has an **impure Chiro. To be impure is to be foul, unclean, filthy, unwholesome, adulterated.** "Pure Chiro." **A pure science and an impure science. A science can not be impure, foul, dirty, unclean, filthy, unwholesome, adulterated.**

"Chiropractic and Naturopathic Physician."

A physician is one who gives physic, a medicine man. A Chiropractor or a Naturopath does not give physic. To use Chiropractic and Naturopathic as adjectives, to qualify physician, a man who gives medicine, is to misqualify what is already qualified, by using opposite meaning terms. If Chiropractic and Naturopath mean anything, they signify no medicine, no physic. Why say physic is no physic? To combine those three words is to use terms which are **counterterms**, words which are opposite in meaning. It is like saying I have a good, bad taste.

"Read the following pages and you will be convinced that Chiropractic furnishes what suffering humanity needs.

"A prominent place must now be given to a newly-developed and accurate method of securing health—the science of Chiropractic.

"Chiropractic is the most advanced and by far the most thoroughly developed system of replacing displaced structure. Chiropractic takes off the pressure. Chiropractic is successful in all forms of disease.

"Through an elaborate system of spinal analysis and the use of palpation in a manner and to a degree of accuracy not approached in any other system of therapeutics, sub-luxations are located and exactly defined as to their nature and extent.

"Cure of disease follows Chiropractic adjustment because Chiropractic removes the cause.

"We use the only method of treatment that can really cure."

Notwithstanding all that this D. C., D. O. says of Chiropractic, it is an "accurate method of securing health. . . . It furnishes what humanity needs. . . . Is successful in all forms of disease. . . . Cure of disease follows Chiropractic adjustment" because it is accurate and exact in locating subluxations. He says, "Our combined system has proven irresistible." This "combined system" includes Chiropractic, Osteopathy, Magnetic Healing, Chromopathy, Hydropathy, Thermal Steam Baths, Swedish Movements, Manipulatory and Vibratory Massage. If Chiropractic is all that he says it is, **why use all the above adjuncts?**

From expressions found in this booklet, I am satisfied that the author has copied Chiropractic expressions which he does not comprehend. They looked well in other literature, why not use as good judgment in compiling his reading matter as he did in furnishing his treating rooms?

"Prolongations of the brain extend outward through openings in the skull to organs in all parts of the body, by far the longest being the spinal cord which gives off thirty-one pairs of nerves, each controlling some **functions** of the body. . . . Nature is thus again free to make right whatever is diseased in the body **functions.**" And yet this C. D., D. O., was not able to inform me how many kinds of functions there are, or what a function is.

"Man is a mill, filled with machines." The "heart, lungs, stomach, liver, spleen, bowels, kidneys, bladder, eyes, ears, arms, legs, feet, hands, fingers and toes are machines. operated by the same dynamo—the brain. . . . When a certain machine in the body is out of order—sick—it is because the life current is either cut off or impaired. Under such conditions the human mill manufactures disease instead of health." How does this mill racket work as an adjunct to the science of Chiropractic of which he speaks so highly?

"Cut D (copied from other literature shows the spinal nerves **pinched** in the spinal **window.** The **free** flow of nerve **is cut off,** the **nerves are shriveled up** and disease of the organs to which these nerves lead is the inevitable result." This D. C., D. O. remembers having his fingers **pinched in the window,** therefore considers that if the **free flow was cut off, his fingers would become shriveled.** These finger machines would manufacture disease. How is that for Chiropractic?

"These handles I use in adjusting **mis**placed vertebrae.

"There must be a reason why they (the organs) cease doing their duty. This reason we find in the cells and tissues themselves. The awakening of this power of Nature in the cells . . . arouse the quality of Vitality, known as spontaneity, in the cells involved in the luxation." That is certainly a mixup.

"Chiropractic is a system of manual therapeutics." Chiropractic is not therapeutical, it does not use remedies.

"The body itself heals a fractured bone; it will do the same with a disordered liver or an inflamed appendix, if the nerves are free to do their work. . . . We know that Nature always works along the lines of health and that it is Nature that cures." This D. C., D. O. knows nothing of the fundamental principles of Chiropractic. He is a brother Chiropractor. I will make it possible for him to advance along Chiropractic lines. These criticisms should set him to thinking; if so, there will be a good show for improvement, inasmuch as he is now a subscriber for The Adjuster. But for the man or woman who will not think, there is but little show for advancement. These unthinkables will be found in all classes of all schools—are you one of them?

P. S.—Since writing the above, I have the booklet from which this was copied, and this, I am told, was copied from another. This D. C., D. O. received this instruction as Chiropractic. No wonder such teachers are unable or unwilling to learn Chiropractic as a science. They look wise when the first question is asked, flounder on the second, and shake their heads on the third. Those who receive such pseudo-Chiropractic education are not to blame for thinking it to be Chiropractic. The Adjuster fills a long-felt want. Shall we advance in Chiropractic or retrograde?

---

The goat is not the only animal that is given to butting in.

"The object of this leaflet is to briefly **outline the basic principles of the science** of Chiropractic."

To outline is to give the outer limits of an object or figure, to give a boundary, an exterior line of something. How can you outline a principle, a source or origin, that from which anything proceeds? I have read this leaflet thru very carefully and **do not find the basic principle of Chiropractic, or any of the principles derived from the fundamental principle.** When the writer of this leaflet reads this, **I want him to** reread the leaflet and **underline the principles** of Chiropractic **which he has outlined.**

"Chiropractic signifies hand practice."

Not by any means. It means just what the two Greek words signify, cheir the hand and practos done—**done by hand.** From what he writes me, **he does make the art** of Chiropractic **a practice. He makes a systematic exercise of his adjusting; he makes of it a practical exercise of practice. He writes me, "I am working in a regular course of adjustment correcting a number of subluxations for the drink habit." He does make a "hand practice" of Chiropractic.** This book will teach him specific adjusting, for I know he is willing to learn.

"As applied to the healing art."

Chiropractic is not one of the systems of the "healing art." It is not related to it in any shape, form or manner. We do not heal by first, second or third intention, by adhesion, by scab or by granulation. We are not healers; we are fixers, adjusters.

"It is the science of analyzing the specific **physical causes of disease.**"

Disease is any departure from a state of health. Physical pertains to the body in contradistinction to the mental. There are those who believe that all diseases originate in the mind by wrong thinking. This Chiropractic Naturopathic Physician believes that disease has a cause in the body, that **the cause of diseases is physical and not mental,** whereas, **"Dad Chiro" says the causes are traumatic, toxic, or auto-suggestive.** The doctor says, disease is specifically physical, specially of the body and not of the mind. So, he **analyzes the body causes of disease and not those of traumatic, toxic or auto-suggestion.**

"The **nerve systems** are the mediums over which the Innate mental impulses, or currents of motive power, are transmitted to every part of the system."

**Nerve** is never used as an adjective; it is always employed as a noun or a verb. The author should have used the adjective, **nervous.** The forepart of the above sentence should have read, "The nervous system is the medium," as there is only **one nervous system,** which for convenience **is divided into the cranial, cerebro-spinal and sympathetic.** The word Innate is used several times in this leaflet and is misspelled each time.

"Inate mental impulses."

The impulses of Innate are transmitted over the sympathetic, ganglionic, nervous system, the nerves of organic life which ramify the viscera of the four cavities of the body; whereas, the mental impulses are of the mind, under the control of Educated; they go to the somatic portion of the body over the anterior and posterior branches of the spinal nerves. It will be seen that the impulses of Innate and those of Educated (the mind) have different origins, are each transmitted over their special nerves, the splanchnopleure to the inner or visceral portion and the somatopleure to the body wall. It will be readily seen that these two classes of impulses, destined for different portions of the body, over entirely different divisions of nerves, the one voluntary, the other involuntary, the former devoted to animal life, the latter to organic, ought not to be thrown into one indiscriminate lot, as Innate mental impulses.

"Currents of motive power."

**Impulses do not flow with the current. They are transmitted by nerve vibration.**

"Motive power."

The power to act, to perform voluntary or involuntary functions, **is not transmitted, it is inherent** in the organism as a whole, or in each individual organ. In biology, motitation is the quivering motion, nerve vibration, which carries impulses of thots; motive and power are quite different entities.

"Distribution of motive power or nerve energy."

**Energy is inherent in the organism, or individually in the organs; it is not produced in some portion of the body and then distributed from a special center.**

"The developers of the science of Chiropractic have demonstrated by a careful system of nerve tracing and analysis that a very large per cent of the nerve channel impediments are the result of displaced spinal vertebrae."

"Careful system."

I would infer that some others have "**uncareful systems.**"

"Nerve channel impediments."

An impediment is an obstruction, that which impedes or hinders. The obstructing or **impeding of any of the vital functions means death.**

"The developers of the science."

**There are envelopers and developers.** Altho they are as

dissimilar, or more so, than the different nerves and their functions, they are liable by some readers and students to be confounded. **The developer of the science, art and philosophy of Chiropractic never writes or talks about impediments or obstructions being placed in the channels** (?) of nerves or blood-vessels. It is the enveloper who does that kind of talking.

"The human spine is composed of a column of movable vertebrae, interspersed by cushions of cartilage on which they articulate or rotate. Each vertebrae has a normal orbit within which it may rotate without friction or discord."

"Each vertebrae" should be each vertebra. Each vertebra could not be more than one. I was not aware that vertebrae were discordant, disagreeing, at variance with each other; that they were quarrelsome, clashing, inharmonious, discordant; neither was I conscious that there is any friction, rubbing of one against another. In anatomy the orbit is the eye socket, the cavity of the skull in which the eye is located. I learned fifty-five years ago that the path described by a heavenly body in its revolution around another body was its orbit. I cannot comprehend how a vertebra can have an orbital cavity, or revolve around another body, normal or abnormally. To rotate, is to turn as a wheel around an axis. **The atlas is the only vertebra which rotates around an axis,** namely the odontoid.

"Cushions of cartilage on which they articulate or rotate."

There is a vast difference between rotating and articulating. The intervertebral fibro-cartilage serves as the chief bond of union between the vertebrae to which it is firmly attached. The bodies of the vertebrae may twist, tilt or incline in any direction, but **they do not rotate.** The vertebrae are articulated, joined, united by cushions of cartilage, **not on.**

"The spinal cord, the main trunk nerve or power line of the body. Like a cord it is not a nerve but a bundle of myriads of nerves, smaller bundles of which branch off between each pair of vertebrae, to ramify all parts of the system."

The author of this leaflet tells us that the spinal cord is a nerve, is not a nerve, and is a bundle of nerves.

"Between each pair of vertebrae."

When did that happen? At what age are the vertebrae paired off, arranged in couples? This pairing of vertebrae is new to "Old Dad Chiro."

"The cartilage is impinged and flattened or rendered misshapen, the shape and size of the **spine windows becomes altered,** thus producing friction, irritation or impingement of the nerves passing through them."

What hard substance is there in such a position, that it

may impinge upon, press against the intervertebral cartilage? I **was not aware that the spine had windows, that it was a graded observatory with openings at each landing for observation, light and air, protected by glass for the admission of light, closed by shutters to keep out the cold, heat and storms.**

"All forms of acute attacks of fevers and diseases in whatever part of the system they may occur."

The author does not designate what group of organs similar in function, whether the nervous, the arterial, the lymphatic, the alimentary, the cerebro-spinal, the dermoid, the glandular, the muscular, the osseous, or the sympathetic system is referred to. Fevers are not located, neither do they occur in different parts of any of these systems. The author no doubt refers to inflammation, which is localized, excessive heat. Diffused heat, fever, is not localized.

"Where the displacement is sufficient to partially shut off the flow of nerve impulses, a deficient functional action results, but by our method of careful, accurate adjustment may be restored to health."

I would not think the "**working in a regular course of adjustment correcting a number of subluxations for the drink habit" was a careful accurate method of adjustment. Nothing specific in adjusting a number of luxations for one disease.** Nerve impulses do not flow, are not shut off. The saying so of the enveloper does not make it so. Nerve impulse and the blood pulse are the wave movements which pass along the nerves and blood vessels. Nerve impulses are transmitted by vibration; the blood pulse by the muscular action of the vascular walls.

"The theoretic principles of Chiropractic."

The basic principle and other principles which originate from the basic principle are now comprehended, they are fundamental Chiropractic truths, they are no longer theories.

---

The man who had the intellectual capacity to comprehend the displacement of vertebrae; the mental ability to grasp the significance of nerve impingement; the power to conceive and discriminate between normal and abnormal positions; the foresight and wisdom to discern the outcome; the genious of originality to create such a unique science; the judgment needed for the occasion; the brain caliber capable of reasoning on this heretofore perplexing question —the cause of disease; the sense of touch required to discover a racked vertebra and the skill and tact to replace it, was the one destined to discover and develop the science which he named Chiropractic.

"Historical—The first accidental, crude Chiropractic adjustment of a vertebra was given in September, 1895, by D. D. Palmer. Neither the art nor the science was formed at this time. Its growth remained practically dormant till 1903. Since which time his son, B. J. Palmer, D. C., Ph. C., has developed it into a well-defined, non-therapeutical philosophy, science and art, that has no resemblance to any therapeutical method."

"Accidental adjustment." When Harvey Lillard told me that he felt something give way in his back and at that moment he became deaf; when an examination of his spine showed one spinous process projecting where he had felt something give way; when I thot I could replace it, and proceeded to do so so with some expectation; when I had a foresight directed with reason, and had a certain purpose in view, was that "accidental"? I understand that an accident is that which occurs without a design, without anticipation, a transaction unlooked for, something "stumbled upon." If so, **that adjustment was not "accidental."**

That first adjustment may have been "crude Chiropractic"; but **it was specific,** as shown by results—a man very deaf for seventeen years—so much relieved by two adjustments that now, fourteen years later, he hears as well as the man who says the adjustment was an accident. Crude as it may have been, the man who would belittle that quick relief of deafness has never equaled it.

If such false statements were made while I am alive, what would be said were I not able to defend the truth and myself?

"The child (Chiropractic) being born and christened, it became the duty of its father to enter upon a course of training and development which would prepare the child for the duties and demands that might be made upon it."

"D. D. Palmer, the scientist of Chiropractic," proceeded to do so, for there it reads:

"**D. D. Palmer simplified the replacing of vertebrae. He discovered a simple method of using the processes as handles.** Instead of finding a few rare cases of slipped vertebrae, that had been wrenched from their natural position, he found them very common; indeed, it was the rule instead of the exception. Others who had preceded him allowed that a vertebral displacement might occur, that such might cause diseased conditions. D. D. Palmer said, in print and person, **that 90 to 95 per cent of all diseases were caused by displacements of the spine.** He it was who first described how and why luxations were the cause of disease. **He has created a science of vertebral adjustment.** True, there were others, perhaps thousands, who had replaced joints of the backbone, but none had knowingly used the spinous and transverse processes as handles."

"Its growth remained practically dormant till 1903." Is it not strange that the discoverer, the father of Chiropractic, should allow this grand science, when he had nothing else to do but develop "the child of his genius," should allow it to remain dormant for eight years, more especially in view of the fact that during that time he graduated many of the leading Chiropractors; and moreover, that there was not a Chiropractic principle upon which he had not written more or less before 1903? It is true that he did not forbid fevered patients having ice when they begged for it. It is a fact he did not develop the human body so that it had no use for the sympathetic and cranial nerves. This developing of idiosyncracies made a philosophy (?), but did not make Chiropractic.

"Historical—Chiropractic was discovered by D. D. Palmer in September, 1895. **From that time he has developed it into a well-defined science** that has no resemblance whatever to any therapeutical method."

Since the teacher of The P. S. C. has developed the sympathetic nervous system and the cranial nerves into oblivion, there has been but little said of them except in their excommunication. But I am pleased to notice on page 2 of February 11, nine inches devoted to the cranial nerves. He says: "**Either our scope must broaden or it must restrict. Facts in the past have told us which to do—we have broadened.**" "These fibers are commonly known as the twelve cranial nerves—**we are willing for them to be so called.**"

I am glad to know that "we have broadened." He would not now refuse water to the woman who was "burning up" with fever, crying: "Give me some ice. Go, get me some ice." He now says the sympathetic nervous system **is there** and the cranial nerves **are there.** I think the Adjuster, with friendly assistance, is doing valuable adjusting.

"It is a chain without a head, without system." That is not the first chain he has seen without a head. If he has ever seen one with a head, he is ahead of me. "Without system." The sympathetic nervous system is the most wonderful, the most economical, the arrangement the most complete for the purposes intended that Innate could devise, and to think of intellectual man knowing better than Innate what was required to run the vital economy. Just think of the arrangements to supply the cranial nerves with communicants, those from the spinal cord going upward in the spinal canal; those from the superior cervical ganglion, by way of the carotid and cavernous plexus and those from the sympathetic nervous system.

"When I illustrate the Innate brain being two-thirds larger

than the Educated, I do so to show you its greater importance.'' This statement does not correct the mistake: ''The Innate brain (cerebellum) is larger'' than the Educated—the cerebrum. Why not say you were mistaken? Why say you made the mistake just to illustrate? You did not make the mistake large enough; for the cerebrum is ten times, instead of one-third as large. Own up to the whole mistake; you will feel better. If you don't, I will give that atlas another adjustment, and take the impingement from the sympathetic nerve.

''Pressure on a nerve never stimulates.'' It certainly does, or else its carrying capacity could never be above normal. In all fevers, or local inflammation, there is an excess of function, which is owing to the excited, over-stimulated condition of the nerve. The giant and dwarf are samples of too much or not enough functionating.

---

Chiropractic is founded upon the relationship of bones, nerves and muscles.

---

A distinguished surgeon of France declared that operations were the ''opprobrium of surgery''; and an equally distinguished physician of England declared: ''It is our ignorance that renders operations necessary. Doubtless but for ignorance, the entire healing art would become obsolete or be merged in a general and universal education.''

---

The word surgery is a contracted form of the obsolete word chiurgery, and signifies ''hand work,'' or manual operations.

The ''setting'' or adjusting of broken bones and dislocations belongs to surgery; but **surgical anatomy** treats only of the **structure of parts of the body**, where manual operations are more frequently required.

---

By the way, the man who discovered and developed Chiropractic, never studied phrenology. I fail to see whenein phrenology has anything to do with Chiropractic or vice versa. They are two entirely different sciences, in no way related to each other. Either science has not been advanced by the other.

The skull is not the first four vertebrae according to Gray or any other anatomist. Some consider the occipital, the two parietal and the frontal as the **upper expansion** of the vertebral column. There are 22 bones of the skull, but only four constitute the upper expansion as the five of the sacrum do the lower expansion.

## NEUROPATHY BY A. P. DAVIS.

"Some people want medicine (page 664) and to such we recommend getting the best and the least harmful, and the most effectual for meeting the emergencies and curing certain conditions. That there are agencies in the way of medicine which are useful we hesitate not to say and believe that common sense should be exercised in all things and nothing should be withheld which is harmless, that will ameliorate the conditions of suffering humanity. **We cordially recommend all that is needed to relieve suffering humanity.**"

This kind of sophistry is used by every dispenser of drugs. This fallacious reasoning is given for using every substance, no matter of what nature, for the cure of disease.

Why not unite the two forces (preface)—the positive and the negative—to harmonize the acid and the alkaline secretions, which cause disease?

"We have at the first lumbar (page 60), **a set of nerves** that control the peristalsis of the intestinal canal, including the colon, and **thereby are instrumental in producing** that condition called **constipation, an adjustment at that particular part of the body relieves the difficulty.**"

A set of nerves which produce constipation. Is that Neuropathy?

"Constipation of children (page 665): **to cure without medicine.** Apply olive oil all the way down the spine, repeating it three times a day and also apply the oil around the posterior and sides of the body. This is usually **effective in a few treatments.**"

Webster tells us: "Any substance administered in the treatment of disease is medicine. Gould says: "Any substance given for the cure of disease" is medicine. Is not olive oil a substance? Is not the patient treated with it? Is is not prescribed and administered for the cure of disease? Is not olive oil used as a medicine? Does not Dr. Davis give this prescription in the "Medical Department" of his book "Neuropathy?" Adjusting the vertebra for constipation would be "without medicine."

"Foreign substances (page 2), in the way of medicine, are not needed." Then, why advise their use? Why write for the "Medical Department" and elsewhere in Neuropathy, over 100 prescriptions for external and internal use? Dr. Davis aims to answer this last question in the preface. "The domestic department . . . is replete with many valuable home remedies for treatment which will be extremely useful to know about and how to use to relieve many pains and save expense and much suffering."

This book, "Neuropathy," contains Osteopathy, "**Chiropractice** (page 1) really **what we** (A. P. Davis) **call Neuropathy,"** Ophthalmology, Magnetic, Suggestion, Hypnotism and Medical.

"In the use of either method (page 8) of treatment mentioned in this book, the one object aimed at is that of **freeing the nervous system."**

Greasing the backbone three times a day is found in the "Medical Department." How does this lubrification free the nervous system?

"Unobstructed circulation" (see introduction, page x) of fluids to and from the heart, in all parts of the body and uniting the forces and removing the pressure, constitute the basic principles of this (Neuropathic) philosophy."

Does greasing the backbone remove the obstruction to the circulation? Does it unite the two forces—the positive and the negative? Does it harmonize the acid and the alkaline secretions? Does it remove the pressure? Or does it do all these? Is backbone greasing a part of Neuropathy? We would like to be able to comprehend the "philosophy" of Neuropathy. You certainly include olive oil as one of your "many valuable hints." Or, does the author of Neuropathy hold to the "basic principles" of superstition—disease is an entity, something that must be gotten rid of—the grease opens the tubular prolongations of the cutis glands and hair follicles, so that this something may find an easy exit? Such seems to be the idea, for we read on pages 16 and 17: "We would have the reader to understand, once for all, that disease is a product." "Disease as the product." "Disease being a product." "Disease usually becomes seated in some weak part of the body." Is disease a product that becomes **seated in some weak part** of the body, where it holds possession because of being the stronger of the two? Is it a manufactured product that must be eliminated, gotten rid of, the greasing making its seat unstable, or does it aid in its escape?

Does Dr. Davis hold to the same idea of disease as do some Chiropractors, viz.: "Man is a mill, filled with machines and the product of this mill is either health or disease." If greasing the backbone three times a day disencumbers the product, gives liberty to and permits the escape of disease, is there not danger of health escaping also?

Dr. Davis seems inclined to believe that disease is an entity, an ideality, a something that may be talked to, suggested to, eliminated, dispelled.

"Diseases (page 154) of all kinds seem to be influenced by suggestions and if repeated often enough so as to become fixed and a part of the life thought of the individual, the results will be as desired by the suggestor, so that **diseases seem** to resolve themselves into a mental ideality, which may be **eliminated by intense thought** in the direction indicating such a desideratum. **Many diseases have been** permanently **dispelled** by this means."

Dr. Davis, from many years' experience with medicine, wisely remarks on page 50: "The whole catalogue of theories of the various so-called medical sciences, are certainly unreliable and are not founded on actual facts, nor in any theory or so-called system of medicine to be depended upon in any case of disease. The idea of a foreign substance, taken into the system, being a cure for any special condition is preposterous."

I think Dr. Davis knows whereof he speaks in regard to medicine, for he has studied all methods and is a graduate of all or nearly all.

If the so-called medical sciences are a catalogue of theories; if they are not founded on fact; if they are unreliable; if there is no system of medicine to be depended upon; if the idea of any foreign substance curing any disease is preposterous, please tell me why you have used 43 pages of Neuropathy to give your readers over 100 prescriptions, to be taken inwardly and applied externally for 70 diseases. Remember that "Science (page 50) means to know, hence what is not known is not science. No theory can lay any claim to science, for theories are simply suppositions—the vagaries of the imagination, unsupported by actual demonstration."

"With medical men (page 18), we find they use one remedy for many so-called diseases; many of them use not over a dozen remedies for the six or seven hundred diseases named in the books—and have better success than those who use the seven or eight hundred remedies."

Dr. Davis prescribes 100 remedies (often several for the same disease) for 70 diseases; for "seven hundred diseases," in this proportion, he would use 1000 remedies.

"Medicines (page 126) are based largely upon supposition, the effects are doubtful under the most favorable conditions, for they may injure rather than benefit."

"Medicines are uncertain (page 48) and dangerous in many instances and doubtful in all conditions. There is no relationship between causes of disease and the remedies taken as medicines to the cure of the affection, hence unphilosophic and irrational to say the least; and their known uncertainty and harmfulness, in many cases where used, is prima facie evidence that they are not the thing to use and, being a foreign substance, renders them incompatible in all cases and conditions."

If medicines are uncertain, **dangerous** and doubtful in all conditions, if there is no relationship between the cause of disease and the supposed remedy; if they are uncertain and harmful; if all medicines are foreign and incompatible; if they are not the thing to use, the theory is unphilosophic and irrational. "That medicines (page 33) are foreign substances, no one with an idea will question. That medicines are indicated in any case as hypothetical, to say the least of it, and hence questionable, whether it ought to be taken into the human system at all." That "Medicines (page 51) under the ban of curatives, have produced more misery and premature death than famine, pestilence and sword combined." I say: If all this is so, why continue to prescribe medicines for the sick and ailing? **Why?**

If "Every known **disease** (page 50) in the body **is a result of nerve irritation,** and this nerve irritation produces a contraction of muscular fiber and pressed upon the vessels passing through the muscle and interferes with the nervous and circulatory systems," and if "**There is no uncertainty** (page 49) **in this method,** inasmuch as there can be **no disease when the nervous system is unimpinged** and the elements of the nervous system are in their proper proportion, it is evidence incontrovertible that when the system is diseased in any way and its functions are disturbed, **all we are required to do is to adjust everything to rights, to take off the strain or pressure** which caused the difficulty and harmony is established and nature performs her normal function," and "Our treatment (page 68) at the first lumbar relieves torpid conditions of the intestinal canal and especially the lower portion of the colon, and the outlets of the body."

If it is true, as you state, that every known disease is the result of nerve irritation; no disease can occur when the nerves are unimpinged; that at the first-lumbar is a set of nerves which control peristalsis (the vermicular movement of the bowels) of the intestinal canal; that an impingement of these nerves produce constipation; that an adjustment at this particular place relieves the difficulty by removing the pressure which caused constipation; and if of this there is no uncertainty, I ask in the names of common sense and rational reason, **why not quit the practice of medicine and use "Chiropractic (page 1), really what we call Neuropathy?"**

"The Chiropractic cervical adjustment (page 142) in upper area on side of cervix is not to be neglected when indicated by drawn, deep, muscular rigidity.

"**The above treatment surpasses all gargles and stupes and local applications** in diphtheria, scarlet fever, malignant sore throat and enlarged tonsils that were ever used.

"The one who fully comprehends the philosophy of this treatment will need **no medicine, but simply use the brain and direct the fingers and hands how to remove the pressure.**"

---

"Dr. F. C. Lathrup, Neuropathic Physician."

A physician is one skilled in physic; one duly authorized to prescribe remedies; a doctor of medicine. According to Webster, a Neuropathic Physician would be a medical doctor suffering with a nervous disease.

---

"Spend a few moments in getting firmly fixed in your mind the principles of Chiropractice, a system of adjustments which remove the cause of disease and does not treat the effect. Dr. D. D. Palmer, the founder of Chiropractice, describes it as the 'art of adjusting by hand all displacements, subluxations of the 300 articular joints, more especially those of the vertebral column, for the purpose of removing nerve impingements, which are the cause of deranged functions (disease). By so doing, normal transmission of nerve force is restored.' Pressure on nerves reduces supply of nerve force to various parts of the body. The Chiropractor locates this pressure, removes it, a **full supply of nerve force** reaches the **starved** and so-called diseased part of the body, normal conditions again exist, and permanent relief follows. Simple?—because it's Nature's own way. Without a full nerve force we cannot have a free circulation, Nature's method of removing the refuse or wornout tissue of the body, **impure blood** follows with its long train of ailments."

The author of the above is the president of a Chiropractic college. Ignorance of the nomenclature (Chiropractic spelled with an "e") and a misunderstanding of the principles of Chiropractic occupy the same brain. How can he teach the principles of Chiropractic when he is unobservant of them? "Pressure on nerves" in a large share of diseases does not "reduce the supply of nerve force." but on the contrary augments it. The "diseased part of the body" is not "starved." "A full supply of nerve force." The cause of nearly all diseases is an over-supply of nerve force; therefore, we have fever. Allopathic "impure blood follows with its long train of ailments."

"Dr. W. O. Powell ease for all diseases."

Would it not be well to get "the principles of Chiropractic firmly fixed in your mind" before trying to explain them to others?

Dr. D. D. Palmer:

Your School Announcement received.

On the right of page 13 you mention "normal nerve vibration is about 200 a minute." Is nerve vibration in fever increased in the same ratio?

Why does death result from a temperature of 106 to 108 degrees?

Death does not always ensue when the bodily temperature rises to 106 or 108 degrees.

McNabb records a case of rheumatic fever in which the temperature was 111.4 degrees, as indicated by two thermometers. This high degree of temperature was maintained for some time after death. Teale reports a case in which, at different times, there were recorded temperatures from 110 to 120 degrees in the mouth, rectum and axilla. In the Adelaide Hospital in Dublin there was a case in which the temperature registered 120 to 130; one day it reached 130.8 degrees. Omerod mentions a nervous and hysteric woman of thirty-two, a sufferer with acute rheumatism, whose temperature rose to 115.8. She insisted on leaving the hospital when her temperature was 104 degrees. Philipson gives an account of a female servant of twenty-three who suffered from neurosis. On the evening of July 9th her temperature was 112; on the 16th it was 111; on the 18th, 112; on the 24th, 117; on the 28th, 117; on the 29th it was 115. The patient was discharged the following September. At a meeting of the Association of American Physicians in 1895, Jacobi of New York reported a case of hyperthermy reaching 148 degrees Fahrenheit.

As for the molecular vibration being normally 200 a minute, I have, on several occasions, verified this result on myself. By a little practice I counted every other vibration and doubled the amount. As for the number of vibrations in fever, that is conjectural.

If bodily temperature may be increased from 97 to 148 in fever, it would not be exaggerating to say that normal nerve vibration may be raised in fever from 200 to 300 per minute.

Why does death result from high temperature?

Because extreme vibrations destroy all metabolic action; high temperature, necrosis, liquifies tissue, rendering it unsuitable for vibrations. When tissue becomes too soft for circulation, innervation or respiration, one of the three vital functions ceases to be performed.

---

Physicians and osteopaths aim to correct the errors of metabolism—the group of phenomena whereby organic beings transform food stuffs into tissue and the production of kinetic energy.

## "SEROUS CIRCULATION."

Serous is a word always used as an adjective. It means watery, like serum, as the serous fluids; of or pertaining to serum. The serous fluids are the thin, watery fluids in the cavities of the body, more especially, those which are lined by serous membranes. The serous glands secrete a clear, watery secretion. Membranes comprise three orders, mucous, fibrous and serous. The serous membranes are the arachnoid, pleura, peritoneum and tunica vaginalis. They facilitate the motion upon each other, of the organs they envelop. Serous cavities are lymph spaces lined by serous membranes. Serous inflammation is an inflammation of the serous membranes attended with exudation of serum. Serous cysts are pouches or sacs filled with liquid.

Anatomists and physiologists are not acquainted with a "serous circulation." I presume that the author of the above headline meant to say that serum had a circulation. If so, he made a serious mistake in that he did not say what he intended to, and if he had expressed himself as he had desired, it would have yet been a grievous mistake, for serum does not circulate, does not make a circuit. Serum is transudated, passed thru membranes and other tissue, never to return—does not make a circuit.

"Liquid food (serum) is also absorbed but by a distinctly separate and complete serous circulation. This is as thoro, as to starting and ending, as the arterial or venous circulations."

Food is any article of diet which, when taken into the body, serves to nourish and build up the tissues. Liquid or solid food is known as ingesta as soon as it is introduced into the body. Ingesta includes that which is taken into the body, and egesta that which is thrown off from the body by the various excretory channels. Consequently, liquid food and serum are not one and the same liquid.

Physiological absorption is external when it takes place thru the external surface of the body. It also occurs thru the mucous membranes of the digestive and respiratory passages; hence it is known under the three forms of cutaneous, intestinal and respiratory absorption. Internal absorption is organic—deposition and decomposition, the intake and output. Transudation and circulation do not absorb "liquid food" or "serum." Absorption of fluids or other substances is performed by the skin, mucous surfaces and absorbent vessels. The serum has a "starting and an ending," but does not circulate as does the fluid that circulates thru the heart, arteries and veins, supplying nutritive material to all parts of the body.

"Closely investing every organ and thoroly entering every tissue in its serous membrane."

In biology, any part of the body having a special function is an organ. For example, the eyes are the organs of sight, the teeth are organs whose functions are to seize, cut, tear and triturate alimentary substances to change food into ingesta; therefore, serous membranes do not invest, envelop or cover every organ, nor enter every tissue.

"No physiology or anatomy gives these new thots."

I venture to say that he will not again give public expression, either vocal or written to these and other similar indeterminate, ambiguous "new thots."

"The small intestine is the true distributor from inside outward, and it is from this point that water is converted into serum. It is known as serum after having seeped, by osmosis, thru the walls of the small intestines into serous tissue. From here it completes a circle by way of all organs, and returning makes its completion at the kidneys."

The first serous glands to be met with by the food, as it enters the mouth, are those of the upper and back portion of the tongue. Anatomists find serous glands, not only in the small intestine, but also, in the large intestine, bladder, appendix, stomach, spleen, lungs, gall bladder, rectum, fallopian tubes and uterus. All of these secrete a thin, watery secretion known as serum.

"The specific function of these organs has never been solved up to this date."

Functions are discovered, not solved. We solve a doubt or problem.

"Chiropractic is the first science that dared to fearlessly pronounce subluxation to be the cause of all disease. The P. S. C. now takes another measure ahead and proves there is a serous circulation."

I was the first to announce that all diseases were the result of subluxated joints; about 95 per cent because of displacements of vertebrae, and the other 5 per cent from displacements of other joints, as corns and bunions from displaced toe-joints. I made this announcement before I developed the science which I named Chiropractic. It was not the science that "dared to fearlessly pronounce subluxation to be the cause of all disease." Imagine, if you can, a science being fearless, pronouncing, declaring, affirming, speaking out distinctly, being daring —a science personified.

I am sorry to learn that the discoverer of the "serous circulation" myth, blames that fad on the P. S. C.

"The P. S. C. now takes another measure ahead." The

measurer does not state whether he. took dry measure, wet measure, linear measure, or a printer's measure. I presume, he refers to wet measure, as he is measuring serum.

---

Dr. D. D. Palmer:

Since your call I am more interested in Chiropractic than ever.

I have taken an osteopathic course and one of Chiropractic of four and a half months. I would like to attend your school in Portland. I would consider it an honor and of great value to have a diploma with your name and photo on it.

Do you give credit to a student for time served in other schools? Yours for health, ——— ———

It is always a pleasure for me to meet any of the "Kiro Kids."

When I have passed to the Beyond, those who are fortunate in having a diploma, with a photo of the Fountain Head signed by the founder of the science and art, will appreciate it as a reward of merit.

The D. D. Palmer College does not allow credit for time served in any school of medicine, osteopathy or Chiropractic. With some, time is all that is served and the only proof of attendance. They may have absorbed some ideas which will have to be eradicated; therefore, it is no standard for us to go by. The benefits and disadvantages attained in other schools, as well as our own, will vary with each individual.

This doctor was under an instructor who had no use for the sympathetic nervous system, the cranial nerves or the communicating and accessory nerves. The "sympathetic nervous system is based upon superstition and while in vogue now, will not be in 50 years. It is unknown to the P. S. C. and is replaced with a direct brain cell to cell nerve connection." "We have said right along that the basis of the sympathetic nervous system was wrong because we are taught that man has 129 ganglions which are equivalent to 129 brains." "When I saw there was no use for a sympathetic nervous system, I threw it out, and then just had to put something better in its place, so I discovered Direct Mental Impulse." "Since D. D. Palmer ceased to be the editor of The Chiropractor, its pages and its clinics do not make use of the sympathetic nervous system, the cranial nerves, nor the accessory or communicating or recurrent nerves."

A case of hemiplegia will illustrate the difference between the "direct mental impulse" theory discovered by B. J. Palmer, and so taught to his students, and that of the nervous system found in man by all anatomists. To reach each portion of the body affected by hemiplegia by the "direct method" would require the adjusting of a half-dozen vertebrae, as given by the "combination of functions" methods. This form of paralysis is the result of one impingement and not of a "combination of functions." Considering the ganglionic chain of the sympathetic nervous system, the impingement is only on one nerve, one bundle of nerve-fibers which are distributed by the sympathetic ganglia. These ganglia are relays in the pathways for the transmission of impulses from the region in which they arise to the tissues in which they are distributed. Communication between the central nervous system and the sympathetic is established thru both efferent and afferent fibers. All the spinal nerves are joined by gray rami communicantes from the sympathetic trunk. Corresponding communications exist between the cranial nerves and the sympathetic, but these occur further towards the periphery and in not so regular a manner as the communications between the spinal nerves and the sympathetic system. Thru this ganglionic distributing agency the fibers of one nerve reach the whole half of the body. This impingement will be found at center-place. In the "direct system" the half-dozen or more places adjusted. none of which are displaced, will cause displacements, if moved, and impingement upon nerves, and affections in the portion where they end.

The cervical portion of the vertebral column sends out three pairs of nerves which supply the posterior portion of the cuticle of the neck and scalp. A student of the "direct system" tried to adjust the cervical to relieve paralysis of the face, one portion paralyzed in hemiplegia. He displaced a cervical vertebra, thereby impinging nerves which ramify the upper portion of the neck and the lower part of the scalp. This displacement caused an inflammation of the twig ends of the nerves which end in the cuticle, creating boils. The adjuster should have learned that hemiplegia is caused by an impingement at C. P. But he was not to blame for doing as he was taught.

By what deduction do I infer the above? From the fact that the patient in question had hemiplegia for three years and no boils; that immediately after the adjusting (?), the displacing of a cervical by one who had been taught the "direct impulse" system, the boils appeared; that anatomies describe nerves leading from the cervical to those portions where the boils appeared; that boils are caused by an inflamed condition of the peripheral ends of these nerve fibers.

---

A man is measured by his mind.

## OSTEOPATHY.

The Journal of Osteopathy, September number, is before me. I find the following items worthy of notice:

Elbert Hubbard says of Dr. A. T. Still: "At Kirksville I met the father and founder of Osteopathy. His name is Dr. Andrew Taylor Still. Dr. Still lives in a forest, but the world has made a path to his door. He is eighty years old, but looks sixty. He is tall, lanky, homely, angular and chews infinite tobacco.

"He was burning brush on his farm when I found him. His trousers were tucked in his boots, he wore a blue flannel shirt and his big brown hands were the hands of Esau. When a boy called him to come to the college to give a lecture he went just as he was without one plea."

A. T. Still is the kind of a man I like to rub up against.

The following is quite different from the older definitions of Osteopathy; it talks like Chiropractic:

"Osteopathy is nominally the science of the bones. Diseases come from mal-adjustment—a pressure on nerve substance by bone substance. Through manipulation a right adjustment is brought about, nerves act normally, circulation is equalized, the secretions flow, elimination follows—the man is well!"

"Neurology plays a big part in all diseases, and this is fully recognized."

Neurology—anatomy, physiology and pathology of the nervous system is all there is to it—bones, nerves and functions

"It seems impossible to hold our people to the Osteopath text; they insist on chasing off after strange gods."

It is true—they are not satisfied with Osteopathy as promulgated by the founder. Surgery, medicine and Chiropractic now constitute a large share of their practice. Many Chiropractors mix what they know of Chiropractic with other systems.

W. R. Archer makes some sensible remarks in regard to mixing medicine with Osteopathy:

"Dear Editor: It is regrettable to observe the tendency on the part of recognized Osteopathic colleges to desire a medical course and to confer the degree of M. D. on their graduates. The Massachusetts College of Osteopathy having already, we understand, put the plan into operation. The question arises, and it is a serious one, what effect will such mixing have upon the future welfare of Osteopathy? What better or stronger evidence does the medical profession want than this to prove to the world that Osteopathy alone is insufficient and of necessity has to turn to medicine for that which it lacks.

"Its success and reputation was never built upon that brand

of osteopathy which is given to the patient with a spoon and needs a medical license to protect it. And we stand aghast at the specter, and more so, if possible, at the reality of a recognized American college of Osteopathy doling out Osteopathy smothered in a tunic of medical theory or as an appendix to the very thing which its founder practiced for twenty years and discarded over thirty long years ago. Now we see it going forth in the wake of its fame as the protege of medicine—a lamb under the tender and protecting care of the lion."

The above remarks are fully as applicable to Chiropractor-mixers.

"In regard to anti-toxins, I have seen remarkable results from its use. I have used it in a large number of cases and would consider myself guilty of bad practice if I did not use it early with threatened exhaustion, laryngeal obstruction or any complication. I do not believe it necessary in every case of diphtheria and have treated many cases without it. But when time is an element, anti-toxin is more speedy than is natural recovery. Anti-toxin is not medication and is strictly Osteopathic in principle, founded as it is on the fact that the body must elaborate its own remedies."

Medication is the treatment of disease by medicines. Medicine is any substance given for the cure of disease. Anti-toxin is poisoned serum which is used as an antidote to prevent or counteract another poison; therefore, it is a medicine.

"That the body elaborates its own remedies" antidotes to counteraction of poisons is Osteopathic; therefore, to give suitable poisons to aid the chemical laboratory to combat disease is Osteopathic, but diametrically opposite to the principles of Chiropractic.

On the following page we find an Osteopath's opinion who has absorbed somewhat of Chiropractic. He says: "Why substitute or even mix a dangerous and unnatural theory with a safe and natural fact? Whatever value fresh serum may have, it deteriorates rapidly and becomes a dangerous poison, when exposed to light and heat of ordinary degree for only ten minutes, says the Medical Handbook, though it is labeled good for six months. All the serums are foreign substances and in the blood stream unnatural and very often set in motion destructive processes, which no physician can stop. On the other hand, the integrity of the nervous system means the normal functioning of the various organs of the body, which is health."

Another Osteopath says: "He believes the serum treatment the greatest advance made in medicine in the last 25 years."

There are medical, lesional and blood-poisoning Osteopaths.

The following is allopathic material used in building Osteopathy: "Smallpox is renovating, while vaccination is contaminating."

Don't that jar your mother's preserves? Smallpox a zymotic, filth disease renovating? No person is improved by being poisoned by either smallpox or vaccination.

The following is given on page 667 as Osteopathic treatment for typhoid fever: "Treatment—General treatment on spinal centers to assist elimination and to build up. Used some laxatives to control bowels. Special attention to cardiac and pulmonary centers. Controlled fevers by hydrotherapy exclusively. Fever diet with rectal feeding several days. Being some distance from the electric light wires, had a six H. P. gasoline engine and dynamo installed and used a 500 c. p. therapeutic lamp half an hour morning and evening. This, together with spinal treatment, seemed to stimulate greatly. The weak, thready pulse would become strong and full and would continue so for some eight to ten hours or nearly to the subsequent treatment. This, with the assistance of an efficient nurse, brought the case to a successful conclusion. Patient is now convalescing under observation. Much care is being given to the diet. We are in hopes that the pulmonary pathology will subside when the patient is able to ride to town to take treatment to assist the pulmonary circulation and be put under the rays of the Leucodescent Lamp again. No bacteriological or Midal test was made in this case."

A dynamo, run by a six-horse-power gasoline engine, to furnish Leucodescent Lamp rays of 500 candlepower, laxatives, hydrotherapy and spinal treatment on the side, is a powerful combination for an Osteopath. This simon pure Osteopathy looks as much like Chiropractic as a turnip looks like a rose.

The following items appear in the column of "business opportunities":

"For Sale or Lease—A well-established practice in a Missouri town of three thousand. Must change climate a while on account of health."

Why not change Osteopathy for Chiropractic "a while on account of health"?

"For Sale—My practice, running four hundred a month, in a rich, prosperous valley, and a most delightful climate, in California. Man and wife, or two men could take in two other towns. No competition. Schools and all churches except 'nigger' church. Reason is, 'I am going back to Dixie.' "

Going back to Dixie where there are "nigger churches."

"Excellent Opening—Good opening for a good, clean Osteopath in promising young city of more than five thousand people. No foreign or colored population, and small percentage of poor population."

Sequela—Clean Osteopaths do not want colored or poor population.

---

Do not append too many appendages to your name. It does not show good taste. Dr. John Smith, D. C. and John Smith, D. C. Chiropractor. This doubling up looks egotistical.

After John Smith has been in practice, or out of practice, a few years, he will write his name just plain John Smith.

Man is a physical and spiritual epitome of the universe. The spiritual is the cause of action. Action is life. The physical is that through which we see effects, changes. The spiritual always did exist and always will. It is eternal, it is changeless. The physical is transient, undergoing canstant change. The Spiritual is positive, the physical negative. The spiritual·acts upon and through the physical.

Man in his physical nature embodies the elements of the material universe. The spiritual controls the individualized portion we designate as an individual. The spirit manifests itself through the physical as a conscious intelligence. In the physical, man is of the earth, earthy. The spiritual is an individualized portion of Universal Intelligence—God—just as the material man is a portion of the material universe.

Through the five or more senses we take cognizance of, and become acquainted with, the physical world, its facts, laws and forces. Through the spiritual, by communication, we may receive intelligence from other spirits in or out of bodies.

This linking together of the spiritual and physical, makes it our duty to so keep the corporeal frame in proper alignment that the spirit may manifest itself in a natural manner. It is not only our inalienable right, but our moral duty, to become acquainted with the osseous and nervous makeup, that we may intelligently adjust any displaced portion of the skeletal frame, so that Innate (that portion of Universal Intelligence usually known as spirit) may manifest itself through, and take in a correct knowledge of, the material world.

---

Knowledge of a single fact does not make a science. To make an adjustment, as I did in my first case of Harvey Lillard 15 years ago, did not constitute a science. To know that a certain dorsal vertebrae wrenched from its normal position, was the cause of deafness; that the racking of it back into its former place would restore hearing; to know those two facts did not constitute a science; neither did it create the art of adjusting. But, so far, it was specific knowledge and specific adjustment. It was the beginning of a science, not a new science, for the principles existed as far back as there were vertebrae. The basic principle of Chiropractic and adjusting vertebrae for the relief of the disease has been practiced over 2,000 years.

---

## COMMUNICATING NERVES.

The connecting nerves between the central nervous system, the spinal, sympathetic and cranial nerves are communicants.

Nerves in their course subdivide into branches; these frequently communicate with branches of a neighboring nerve. They do not inosculate as do blood vessels; they may decussate, form plexuses, but each primitive nerve, or nerve-fiber runs a distinct course from the brain to its termination. The afferent, or sensory nerves, carry impressions to the brain; the efferent, or motor, convey sensations outward. They may, as communicating nerve-fibers, pass into the sheath of an adjacent nerve, become intermixed with its filaments, and again pass on, to become blended with other nerve-fibres in some adjoining bundle of filaments named funiculus.

The spinal nerves have their superficial origin in the spinal cord, and are transmitted through the intervertebral grooves and foramina.

The first spinal nerve, the sub-occipital, has its apparent origin in the oblongata, emerging from the neural canal between the occipital bone and the atlas. The vertebral nerves have their real origin in the substance of the brain, as in fact do all nerves.

The sympathetic system, also called the trisplanchnic, has its superficial, or apparent origin in the ganglionic cords, two chains of ganglia, which pass in front of the transverse processes and continue downward to the coccyx. These gangliated chains are accessories to the spinal cord, and are permanently connected with the spinal nerves. Therefore the trunks of these branches originate in the brain, descend as a part of the spinal cord, pass out through the intervertebral foramina to the ganglionic chains and from thence to the viscera, glands, heart, and blood vessels. In the ganglionic cords the spinal nerves rearrange themselves for the transmission of Innate impulses. This system is not independent, for it receives its fibers from the cerebro-spinal and the cervical. The gangliated cord are connected superiorly with the upper cranial nerves by branches which enter the cranium. Through this and the cranial system Innate Intelligence presides over the involuntary functions by directing its innervating force. The visceral branches of the third and fourth sacral nerves do not join the gangliated cord.

Figure 8 on page 168 shows fifteen of the connecting

nerve branches from the vertebrae to the chain of ganglia, on the right of the spine, eight of the cervical and seven of the dorsal. On the right of the gangliar chain is shown the sympathetic nerves as they pass off and proceed to the vital portions. It will be seen that there are many communicating nerve branches which connect the sympathetic with the spinal system. Communicating nerves are those which furnish other nerves with motor or sense nerves.

On other pages we have shown that spinal nerves are liable to be pressed against by the edges of the displaced articular processes. The branches of the sympathetic pass out through the spinal foramina as do the spinal nerves, therefore, the twenty-four pairs of ganglionic nerves are liable to the same pressure by sub-luxated vertebrae as are the thirty pairs of spinal nerves, and are as readily released by the hands of the Chiropractor.

The twelve pairs of cranial nerves have their origin in the brain, pass to their appointed places through foramina in the front and base of the skull; they do not occupy a part of the spinal cord, as do the spinal and sympathetic nerves. For this reason they are not thought to be subject to pressure by subluxated vertebrae, as are spinal and gangliated nerves.

We have seen how the spinal and sympathetic are connected in the gangliated chains by communicating nerves. May there not be similar communicating branches connecting them and the cranial?

The upper portion of figure 8 shows connecting branches from the ganglia to the third, fourth, fifth and sixth cranial nerves. These have their apparent origin in the ganglia. From there we trace them back to the spine, through the foramina into the spinal cord and from thence to the brain.

The third pair of cranial nerves are motores oculorum, nerves of motion, eye movers. They supply five of the seven orbital muscles, the other two being from the fourth and fifth cranial nerves.

The fourth pair are the smallest of the cranial nerves, the next in size are the sixth. They receive some communicating filaments from the cavernous plexus of the sympathetic.

While we differ in our osseous make-up, so much so that no vertebra of one spine will fit in any other, there is a great difference in our nervous construction. The ramifying, the blending and communicating nerves are not always the same, in fact, in some persons there are some nerves that are only rudimentary or missing. For further information on this subject see article on bones and nerves. We also find that the conducting qualities of nerve impulses is not always the same.

Fifth. The trifacial nerve sends branches to the teeth. While it does not pass down the spinal cord to the cervical vertebrae, there is a branch composed of filaments from the carotid plexus of the sympathetic which communicates with this pair of nerves, as has been proven by Chiropractors being able to relieve toothache instantly by adjusting the fourth cervical. A lesion in the cervical impinges a nerve which joins the superior and inferior maxilary, causing not only pain and decay in the teeth, but gumboils. When filling teeth, the nerves should not be destroyed, for they are the life thereof. Alveolar pyorrhea is a suppurative inflammation of the root membranes, and also of the connective tissue of the gums beneath the mucous membrane, the communicating nerves of which originate in the lower portion of the dorsal region. This disease can be as surely relieved as toothache, but it will take more time.

The trifacial nerve is often the seat of neuralgia. When intense it is called tic douloureux. Surgeons sometimes divide one or more of the three divisions, removing a portion of the nerve. The inflammation and distress cannot go farther than the excised portion, where pus is formed by reason of the excessive heat drying the serum. Unless special precaution is taken, Innate will repair the damage done by the surgeon, by causing a growth of nerve to fill the gap, and the pain is then resumed. If all the branches of the fifth are involved the sensory root is divided, or the Gasserian ganglion where the three branches have their superficial origin is removed. Why does the surgeon resort to neurectomy? Because he does not comprehend the cause, or knowing is not able to adjust it.

Chiropractors make use of the fact that the carotid plexus has its apparent origin in the superior cervical ganglion, that the fifth nerve is a branch of this complex network of nervous filaments, that the third cervical nerve which emerges between the third and fourth cervical vertebrae sends a branch to the superior cervical ganglion. Thus we trace one or more of the communicating nerves through the foramina to the spinal cord and to the brain. By releasing the pressure on the third cervical we relieve facial neuralgia.

The sixth or abducent nerve, is purely motor in its function, it supplies the external rectus muscle of the eye ball. It receives filaments from the carotid plexus of the sympathetic and communicates with the ophthalmic division of the fifth. It controls the external rectus muscle. Paralysis of this nerve causes convergent squint, owing to some of the sympathetic fibres going to the radiating muscles of the iris and passing along with this nerve. These abnormal conditions can be corrected by releasing the impinged branch of the sixth nerve.

The seventh, or facial nerve (not trifacial), has its communicating branch from the sympathetic by way of the geniculate ganglion, also a branch from the cervicofacial division, by way of the great auricular nerve, which springs from the second and third cervical nerves. The sympathetic, you will remember, is connected with the spinal nerves by the ganglia of the ganglionic cord.

The facial nerves consist of a pair, one on each side of the face. They are nerves of motion, and control the thirty pairs and one single muscle of the face.

This nerve is more frequently paralyzed than any of the cranial nerves. Surgical anatomy gives several may-be causes. Usually one-half of the face is affected, the forehead is smooth, the patient is unable to frown, the eyelids cannot be closed, the lower lid droops, causing the eye to look larger than its mate, the tears may escape down the cheek which is smooth and lacks expression, the nostril on the affected side cannot be dilated, the mouth is drawn to the sound side; there is inability to whistle, the food collects between the cheek and gum. All this because of the cervical communicating nerve being pressed upon by the displaced cervical vertebra.

The eighth or auditory nerve, is the nerve of the sense of hearing. It is soft in texture and destitute of a sheath, making it liable to injury. The superficial origin of this nerve is in doubt; while it is classed among the cranial nerves, it does not necessitate that its superficial or apparent origin is in the brain. Some consider it a branch of the fifth, others the seventh, while some think it a sympathetic nerve. While its origin and connections are in doubt, it remains a fact that by two adjustments, fifteen years ago, replacing a dorsal vertebra, I relieved Harvey Lillard of deafness. That established beyond a doubt that there was a connection between the dorsal vertebrae and the auditory nerve, more especially as he had felt a vertebra give way at the time he became deaf. I have relieved other cases of deafness by adjusting cervical vertebrae. What I wish to establish in this article is that all the nerves of the body, originate in the brain, pass down as a part of the spinal cord and emerge through some one of the foramina.

The ninth, or glosso-pharyngeal, is a nerve of taste sensation. It has branches of communication with the pneumogastric, facial and upper cervical ganglion of the sympathetic.

The mucous membrane of the pharnyx, fauces and tonsil are permeated by the filaments of the ninth nerve. Pressure on its communicating branches as they pass through the foramina cause over-action, an irritation, an inflammation in that portion just described, the nature of the disease depending up the age as well as other conditions of the patient and thon's surroundings. These parts become swollen, preternaturally hot, the mucous dries, producing an exudation named catarrh. Why not release the nerves from pressure and restore normal functions?

The tenth, or pneumogastric, supplies the organs of voice and respiration with motor and sensory fibres; the pharnyx, esophagus, stomach and heart with motor influence. It passes down the neck, through the chest and diaphragm and into the abdomen. In passing through the jugular foramen, it is accompanied with the spinal accessory. The vagus nerve is connected with ninth, eleventh and twelfth nerves, with the sympathetic, and the loop between the first and second cervical nerves.

The second cranial nerve, the optic, supplies the retina of the eye; it is the nerve of vision. It receives a communicating branch from the cavernous plexus for which it is indebted to the superior cervical ganglion. The Gasserian ganglion receives filaments from the cartoid plexus of the sympathetic and forwards a sensory branch to the eye balls. The optic nerve is considered a prolongation of the brain substance rather than an ordinary cerebro-spinal nerve, and the retina as an expansion of that prolongation. Gray tells us that "in ancestral vertebrates the general cutaneous sensor system was also capable of light perception. With the recession of the neural tube from the surface and in company with the morphological differentiation of the head-end, a light perceiving pair of organs arose as a special development. The distal end of the optic brain-vessicle becomes the retina, in structure like the brain wall, whose cell axones carry afferent impulses to the brain."

The optic nerve is peculiarly liable to become the seat of neuritis or undergo atrophy. Disease is the result of either too much or not enough impulsive force. If too much we have inflammatory conditions; if a lack of nerve force, nerve impulse, we have not enough of life force which results in the wasting away of that portion—atrophy. A light pressure on nerves serves to create an irritated condition; a heavy pressure decreases life force, producing paralysis. The anatomist and the investigator of Chiropractic would ask, where can bone pressure be brought to bear on the optic nerve? We have just stated that the optic nerve receives a communicating branch from the cavernous plexus. We trace it through that plexus to the superior cervical ganglion; from thence to the spinal nerves and into the spinal canal, passing through the intervertebral foramen. In the same manner we trace a sensory branch from the optic nerve to the Gasserian ganglion, from there to the carotid plexus and through the superior cervical ganglion to the spinal cord. Thus we trace branches of the cranial nerves as well as the sympathetic to the spinal cord. As all these branches have to pass through openings made by notches or grooves, they are liable to be pressed upon by displacements of the articular processes, striking against, making pressure upon the nerve they come in contact.

Diseases of the eye ball, such as exophthalmia (protrusion of the eye ball), inflammation and cataract, are readily relieved by adjusting the dorsal vertebra. The only possible explanation is that there are communicating nerves which go to the optic nerve from the spinal cord, that they are impinged upon, pressed against by the displacement of the articular processes, and that adjusting the vertebra restores the processes to their normal position.

The first pair of nerves are the olfactory, the nerves of the sense of smell. They are composed of forty or more filamentous bundles, which do not form one nerve trunk, but pass as filaments and are distributed to the mucous membrane of the upper part of the two passages of the nose, where they form plexuses with elongated meshes, making a fine net work of communicating nerves. The ophthalmic branch of the Gasserian ganglion sends a branch to the nasal.

The olfactory nerve is one of sense—the faculty by which certain qualities are perceived through the instrumentality of this nerve. Thus we sense odors, and in a measure our taste is qualified thereby.

In order to send a motor impulse to the olfactory nerve, we select a motor afferent nerve on the line over which we wish to communicate a movement. This has its motor root in the brain; the impulse is passed down the spinal cord, the elongation of the brain. It emerges through a vertebral foramen, proceeds to the upper cervical ganglion, leaves there and finds its way through the carotid plexus on the line of the trifacial nerve until it arrives at the Gasserian ganglion. Here it immediately takes the ophthalmic division, then selects the frontal nerve and proceeds on the infratrochlear branch for the nasal, where it delivers its message on time and in good shape, providing it has not been tampered with as it passed through the narrows, where there is a liability of impingement by pressure from displaced articular processes. On this line there was only one place (barring wounds) where this intelligence was liable to be interfered with, viz., the intervertebral exit.

Ninety-five per cent of all displacements which disarrange the transmission of motion and sensation will be found to exist contiguous to the exit of nerves from the spinal canal. Herein is the lock to which Chiropractic has at last furnished the key. This science has found the cause of disease and by hand adjusting is able to replace articulations to their normal position, thereby freeing any tension on nerves caused by bone pressure.

## JOY M. LOBEN, PH. C.

In the August number of The Chiropractor is an able article by Dr. Loben. It contains much that is Chiropractic and it is well expressed; but, there is one paragraph which is not up to date. The doctor will pardon the Fountain Head, the Discoverer, Developer and Founder of the science of Chiropractic for adjusting this paragraph, for the Fountain Head is now the Adjuster of Chiropractic literature. I claim the credit of the last mentioned, as well as of the former four—these five make me a full Chiropractic hand, every finger well rounded out.

The paragraph alluded to, on page 34, reads thus: "The only way in which any agency outside of man can interfere with the transmission of currents through a nerve is by cutting, by crushing, or constricting it in such a way as to break the continuity of its molecules and render it unable to transmit vibration. Only one place can be found along the path of a nerve from the brain to a cell in the body, at which such a pressure may exist. That place is at the exit of the nerve from the spinal column, for it is there and there alone that the soft nerve passes between two hard substances capable of producing a constriction."

This section is found under the headline, "The Completeness of Chiropractic Philosophy." The writer of this article is not complete in his Chiropractic education, although he appends to his name the degree of Ph. C. — Philosophical Doctor. Dr. Loben has attempted to make use of the molecular vibration theory lately put forth by the Founder of the science. He has not fully grasped the transference of impulses by molecular vibration.

He says in the first line of the second paragraph on page 30: "Chiropractic Philosophy is structurally complete." The text which Dr. Loben has furnished is not correct in its Chiropractic philosophy. It contains six errors. I am pleased to see that he has accepted molecular vibration as the kinetic energy, means used by Innate to transmit its impulses, to arouse energy, to functionate. It will take some thinking for Dr. Loben or any one else to fully comprehend and apply molecular vibration to the transmitting of impulses. If I rightly judge the doctor, he is of the right make-up to do the thinking.

From his first statement, in the above quoted paragraph, one might infer that there were some agent inside of man, "the individualized intelligence, or entity called Ego" that might interfere with the transmission of currents, as he refers to "any agency **outside** of man." Innate, the personified part of Universal Intelligence, cannot and would not if it could, interfere with or derange its own current of thoughts, its impulses. Innate being a personified portion of Universal Intelligence, the All Wise, is perfect in its intelligence, faultless in each and every impulse, its energy and function. But, from various causes (unknown before I brought them forth), these impulses are interfered with and deranged.

It will be observed that I have used the word agent, for the reason that agency is the state of being in action; while an agent is one who or that which has the power to act. An agent has the agency. In strict philosophical usage, the prime **mover** or **doer** of an act is the **agent.**

All agencies which derange normal action, increases or decreases functions, are from without—could not be from Innate.

Function is any specific power of action which belongs to an agent. The operator is behind the energy which is the force of action. This definition covers vegetative and cumulative functions. The action, itself, is a function performed. The process of digestion, the changing of food, so that it can be assimilated; assimilation, the alteration of digested food into fluids and tissue; absorption, promoting growth from nutriment, replenishing waste material; excretion, the method of getting rid of waste material, these are vegetative functions. Innervation furnishes vital force to energy.

Fermentation, decomposition and teratism are vegetative functions performed either in too great or too little degree.

Teratology is the science of abnormal growths—vegetative functions abnormally performed. Physiology treats of functions performed normally. Pathology of functions performed in an unusual manner. The performance of functions in a satisfactory manner is health.

All agents which cause increase or decrease of functionating (disease) are from without—could not be from Innate within.

Function is any specific power of action, that belongs to, or is caused by an agent. The operator is behind the power, vitality, that which accomplishes vegetative function. Vitality and intellectuality run the vegetative and cumulative functions. **As the vegetative function may produce teratism, so the cumulative may accumulate intellectual monstrous conceptions.** The transmission of energy from Innate to the physical and mental, if not interfered with by an outside agent will result in vegetative and cumulative functions being performed in a normal manner.

"Render it (the nerve) unable to transmit vibration." The **most** of **diseases are because of too much vibration,** creating **too much action.** For further explanation see other articles on molecular vibration; too much or not enough functionating.

Dr. Loben states that the only ways in which molecular vibration can be interfered with, is bẏ "cutting, crushing or constricting." This ignores poisons and impingements, the causes of the larger share of diseases. Some poisons irritate, excite molecular action, wave vibration, in excess—more than normal. Others are sedative, producing sedation, an under amount of molecular vibration, a reduction of vital power. A poison, therefore, is a substance which, when introduced into the body, augments or lessens the functionating of one or more of its organs. Impingement on nerves—pressure brought to bear against tubular cords, filled with fibers, the functions of which are to convey impulses and sensations to and from the brain—excites or retards molecular action, wave vibration. Any condition which will "break a continuity of its molecules and render it unable to transmit vibration." Whenever the connection is broken between the atomic particles of nerve-fibers, they are unable to transmit impulses by the aid of vibration—no vibration, no function—no function, no disease—no action, no life. This first sentence of Dr. Loban's is not expressed Chiropractically.

"Only one place can be found along the path of a nerve from the brain to a cell in the body, at which a pressure may exist." The developer of Chiropractic has discovered that any displaced bone may press against, impinge upon, a sensitive nerve, thereby exciting or depleting its conveying capacity. This pressure does not "break the continuity of its molecules and render it unable to transmit vibration" or impulses; it only modifies the transmitting force.

"That place (of pressure) is at the exit of the nerve from the spinal column, for it is there and there alone that the soft nerve passes between two hard substances capable of producing a constriction." Compression between two hard substances will not constrict, will not produce a constriction. Tubes or ducts can only be constricted; solid cylinders cannot be drawn together, made smaller. It is the channel, or opening, which may be closed by a ring-like pressure, as of a ligature, or some change in its walls by inflammation or cicatrix. Pray tell me, where do the first and second cervical nerves become "constricted" because of pressure between two hard substances or those nerves which produce corns and bunions because of inflammation.

The Developer and Adjuster of Chiropractic would correct the discussed paragraph as follows:

The only agents which can modify the transmission of impulses, are cutting, crushing, impingement, auto-suggestion and poisons. About cutting and crushing there is no chance for argument; but, how and where nerves may be affected by impingement, suggestion and poison is a much discussed question among Chiropractors. Impulses are transmitted by molecular vibration. Nerves may be severed or crushed anywhere. Impinged wherever there is a displaced bone, constricted, never.

---

Dr. Ross declared at the session of the eleventh annual conference of the American Hospital Association, October 2, at Washington, D. C., that 15 years ago the annual cost of medicines for each patient in the Massachusetts general hospital was about $2.90, while last year it was only 91 cents.

"It is difficult to predict what the future of medicine in hospitals is going to be," said Dr. Ross. "Undoubtedly, drugs will continue to be used, but other agencies or some agency still unknown to us will have a place."

---

"Do you want first or second-hand goods?"

If you want first-hand goods, you go to the first-hand man. If you desire Chiropractic first handed, you go to The Fountain Head, from which originated the first principle, not to any of those who were his pupils, who learned the principles from him. His graduates are not the first-hand man; to receive it from any other than the originator, The Fountain Head, is to get it second handed.

I, being the originator of Chiropractic, never had the degree of D. C. conferred on me. I was the first to put the goods on the market. All who have received the degree from me can not do otherwise than pass it on as second handed. Sand paper, paint or varnish will not make second-hand goods other than second handed.

Whenever any person states that he has Chiropractic first handed; that he is The Fountain Head; just ask to see his diploma. Enquire of whom he received his education; who conferred the degree of D. C. on him; who gave him his diploma. There never was but one Fountain Head of Chiropractic; all others are false, self-appropriated, for self-aggrandizement.

My students receive instruction first handed, direct from the Fountain Head; not one of them can ever step in his boots, or wear his hat.

Sheep's clothing will not change the nature of the wolf, neither will second-hand goods become first handed because of their being placed in a fountain. Water will not wash out deception, fraud and chicanery. Such trickery will not satisfy the public or the avariciousness of one who is "waiting just like a hungry wolf for a dinner."

## THE SKELETON.

The term skeleton is from the Greek skeletos, meaning dried. In its original sense it was applied to the parts which remained after the softer tissue of the body had been removed by disintegration or heat. It therefore, included the bones, cartilages and ligaments which bind the different parts together. The human skeleton consists of bones and cartilages.

A natural skeleton is a dried body; one prepared and held together by human skill and labor is artificial.

Therefore, a skeleton is an aggregation of the hard parts which give support, position and shape to the body. It also affords protection to many of the delicate organs which are lodged within its cavities. When each bone of the framework is normally articulated, occupying their normal position, there can be no displacement of the soft tissue; such a condition, in life, results in health. By the articulation of its several parts, its segments are used as levers which constitute the passive portion of the locomotory system.

A skeleton exists in almost all animals, altho not always formed in the same manner. In some, as the crustacea and testacea, it is wholly or partially external — exoskeleton or dermoskeleton. In others, as birds, mammals, etc., it is internal —endoskeleton or neuroskeleton. Some animals possess more or less of both the exoskeleton and the endoskeleton. The former is the outside skeleton—the hardened parts on the outside; such as shells, armor plates, scales, nails, hair, horns, teeth and feathers. The latter consists of the internal framework of bones and cartilage.

The number of bones in the human skeleton varies according to age. Owing to the process of fusion during growth, the number in the adult is less than in the child.

The axial skeleton is composed of the skull, sternum, vertebral column and the ribs. The appendicular skeleton includes the upper and lower limbs.

Including the ossicula auditus, there are 206 bones in an adult human body. Of those occurring in pairs, there are 172; of single bones there are 34.

Bones are divided into four classes according to their shape: long, short, flat and irregular. The limbs contain all the long bones except the clavicles. All the short bones are found in the limbs including the patellae.

There are 18 bones which have no muscles; 14 have one; 8 have two; 5 have three; 4 have five; the hyoid has eleven pairs; each hip bone has thirty-six.

All the bones of the body are articulated with each other, except the hyoid and the bones of the ears.

Strange but true, the position of bones determines the conditions known as health and disease. By their displacement, nerves are impinged upon. Pressure on nerves causes irritation, diametrical enlargement and longitudinal contraction. Change in the quality of nerve tissue modifies its capacity to carry impulses. The result is an increased or diminished amount of functionating which we name disease.

---

Chiropractic is not a science because it "stands in public favor," nor because of its marvelous results."

Chiropractic is a science because it comprises a knowledge of facts concerning health and disease. This knowledge reduced to law and embodied in a system makes it a science. Knowledge of a single fact or of many facts of several systems do not make a science. Knowledge of many facts concerning one subject, correlated in a system, creates a science.

---

An eigh-page Chiropractic booklet is before me. The author says of himself, "The Eminent Chiropractor. . . . He is a man of keen instinct, fine culture and excellent manners. . . . He alone knows the cause of your disease and just how to remove that cause. . . . Interview a man who knows something. . . . You could not do that which would be of more priceless value to you than to call on him at once. . . . Health is a pearl of great price." Of the school from which he graduated, he says: "The students of this school are pre-eminently the most successful of all Chiropractors."

Such remarks made in one's own literature by himself, shows the author to be an egotist. His neighbor practitioners look upon him as such. The printer took him to be a blow-hard. If a competitor should speak of himself in this manner, the writer of the above would look upon him as vain and conceited.

"The Eminent Chiropractor" before he opened an office. "A man of keen **instinct**.". Instinct is without reason, independent of instruction, works without a distinct object; what is accomplished is done without intelligence. Instinct performs its work blindly, ignorantly, without comprehension or knowledge. Others may know the cause of disease and be able to remove it, without a "**keen instinct.**" His "**keen instinct**" may be of "priceless value" to him, and not to his callers.

This kind of advertising not only brings reproach upon the author, but also reflects upon all others of his profession.

The above self-praise is copyrighted, 1908.

## A BACK-NUMBER.

A school announcement states: "Both your time and money are worse than wasted in attending a back-number Chiropractic School." We would add: "Go to The Fountain Head for a Chiropractic education."

Chiropractic as a science is being developed forward, not backward. To eliminate the sympathetic nervous system, is a step backward. Innate makes use of these nerves to run the vital functions. The apparent origin of the sympathetic nerves are in the ganglionic nerve trunks. From there we trace them by their rami communicantes back to their exit thru the spinal foramina where they exist as a part of the thirty pairs of spinal nerves. The trunks from the spinal cord contain three varieties of fibers. Those which go to the periphery, and do not pass into the ganglionic trunks; those which go into the sympathetic trunks, emerge therefrom, and go to and associate with the cranial nerves as accessory, and those which enter the ganglionic chains, rearrange, pass out and run the vital functions under the management of Innate. The cerebro-spinal nerves carry all the sympathetic fibers and the communicating accessory fibers of the cranial nerves.

This same school states in its literature that "The Innate brain is larger" than the Educated. Oh, no, the cerebellum is much the smaller of the two, being only ten per cent of the whole encephalon.

This "back-number" school states that the brain-cord represents the entire nervous system. "That the twelve pairs of cranial nerves are branches or divisions from the original 31 pair as they divorce." He should have said, as they divide.

The brain-cord does not contain or represent the entire nervous system. It does not take in the cranial nerves. It however sends communicating branches to join the cranial nerves; these are the sensitive communicantes which are traced by Chiropractors. Therefore, the twelve pairs of cranial nerves are not branches, divisions, or a part of the thirty-one pairs of spinal nerves.

Another statement is that "it is impossible to have a sympathetic nervous system." It would be impossible to live without a sympathetic nervous system, for all the vital functions depend upon it for their innervation. They are the only channels thru which Innate can run the vital functions. The sympathetic system is anatomically and functionally dependent upon the cerebro-spinal system.

Again this literature states that "the only place where pressure can be placed upon nerves is where they are entirely surrounded by osseous structure." Nerves are not pressed upon or against where they are entirely surrounded by an osseous structure. They are never pinched or squeezed in the spinal grooves of the atlas or any foramina, nor between any of the three hundred articular joints. They are **impinged upon, pressed against,** because of bones being displaced; these **projections** cause tension, irritation, contraction and enlargement.

Still another statement is that "we do not need a sympathetic nervous system to explain functions." We do most emphatically need a sympathetic nervous system to perform as well as explain vital functions. The vital functions depend upon the sympathetic nervous system for their innervating force; they and they alone, run all the organs of the body upon which life depends. The sympathetic system is that portion of the nervous system which is especially concerned in the distribution of impulses to the glandular tissues to the viscera in the four cavities, and to the vaso-motor fibers of the blood vessels.

The spinal nerves have two roots, the sensory or dorsal and the ventral or motor. The sensory is the larger of the two; it contains more filaments, therefore, needs more innervation. Each of these two roots is composed of many fibers which leave the spinal cord as such and immediately pass into sheaths which are then known as a trunk. These are enclosed in one sheath and go through the foramen as one nerve. Just as it emerges from the foramen it divides into four branches. One turns back and supplies innervation to the bones, joints, skin and muscles, and some fibers, the cephalic and cranial afferent, form cerebellar connections and convey impulses to both brains. The impinging of these brain filaments would cause an increase or a decrease of brain functions; thus we have brain fever and softening or hardening of the brain substance. The remaining one of the four branches, the ramus communicants, goes to the ganglionic chain and becomes a part of the sympathetic system. Each spinal nerve has one, two or three nerve branches which go to and and enter one ganglion, or one nerve may branch and pass into two ganglia. It will be readily observed that when tracing sensitive nerves, we press upon those which go to bones, joints, skin, muscles, brain or some one of the sympathetic or a branch of the cranial nerves. If it were not that these fool notions are being passed off as Chiropractic, we would not waste our time and space in this journal to refute them.

This same Chiropractor states: "If the fundamental principle of Chiropractic (pressure upon nerves as they pass through intervertebral foramina, caused by a vertebral subluxation) **is the cause** of all disease, then Chiropractors have nothing in common to do with the supposed to be, sympathetic nervous system. It exists in the ganglionic, external to the foramina, therefore, is **not** subject to pressure."

The Chiropractor who asserts that nerves are pressed upon as they pass through intervertebral foramina, is a "back-number." How are the first and second pairs of cervical nerves impinged? They do not pass through intervertebral foramina formed by two notches. Impinged nerves, which cause corns and bunions, do not pass through foramina surrounded by osseous tissue, nor between the articular surfaces of joints. Nerves are not pinched in the foramina of the sacrum, nor in the sacro-iliac articulations. They are, however, pressed against, impinged upon by the displacement of those joints. When the projecting articular processes are replaced, the pressure is removed.

The following certainly shows the ear marks of a back-number: "If the twelve cranial nerves originate within the brain and go direct to their organs without passing outward through the skull, there ought never to be a disease of these functions because they cannot be subject to pressure unless due to fracture or concussion of the skull.

The twelve pairs of cranial nerves have their origin in the brain and pass out of the skull through foramina; otherwise they could not perform their functions. They do not make their exit through the foramen magnum as a part of the spinal cord. They are reinforced by communicating nerves from the spinal and sympathetic systems. These nerves of communication originate in the brain, as do all nerves. They descend in and are a part of the spinal cord, pass out through the spinal foramina, and are liable to be pressed against by the displaced articular processes which have been wrenched to the left or right of their normal allotted space of movement. Their sharp edges impinge upon the nerves which they come in contact. Herein lies the explanation of the reason why we move the vertebrae from the side impinged upon in the dorsal and from the opposite side in the cervical and lumbar.

"Go direct to the organ." Only three of the twelve pairs of cranial nerves have organs to go to—the olfactory, optic and auditory, and these organs are not in the cranial cavity, necessitating the exit of the cranial nerves passing outward to reach them.

Chiropractors may trace some of the cranial nerves as they ramify the external of the skull, also their communicating accessories from the spinal and sympathetic which reinforce the cranial nerves.

"A disease of these functions." Functions cannot be diseased any more than "they can be subject to pressure." If, as the author asserts, the cranial nerves do not pass out of the skull to reach their organs, how would a fracture of the skull pinch a nerve? "Concussion of the skull." A violent jar or shock will not displace a bone so that its projection will press against nerves. In this last quoted paragraph of four lines are four anatomical and two pathological mistakes. Better go to the Fountain Head for a Chiropractic education, rather than to a back-number who claims to teach Chiropractic.

---

From page 26 of the July number of The Chiropractor I quote:

"D. D. Palmer is the acknowledged head, originator, discoverer and developer of the unique system of adjusting vertebrae by hand, using the processes as handles. There were in years past those who aspired to get that honor, but to-day I have acknowledgments from them that they did not discover the principles and movements named Chiropractic." Aspirants for those honors still exist.

---

I have a card 3 by 4 inches, containing 27 lines. The word functions is used 4 times; diseases 5 times; control 8 times and nerves 12 times. This repetition becomes monotonous.

"Mental impulses control all functions of the body." "Impulses are transmitted through the nerves." "All functions of the body are through the nerves."

Why not say, functions are mental impulses expressed thru nerves?

"All diseases are in and through nerves."

What? All diseases are in nerves? All diseases are through nerves? What about bones, joints, muscles, ligaments, blood vessels, membranes, glands and organs? May they not be diseased in their structure? Are not disturbed functions and displaced organs considered as disease?

"Blood is only a servant for the nerves."

According to Webster and March's Thesaurus, servant is always applied to **a person who serves**; therefore, it is improper to apply the term to any tissue. To make blood a servant of the nerves would be to make blood the employee and the nerves the employer; the nerves would be the master or mistress of the male or female blood.

The last two lines read: "Disease is Nature's way of telling something is wrong. A Chiropractor adjusts this wrong."

These two sentences tell us that a Chiropractor adjusts "Nature's way of telling something." Why not adjust displaced bones?

## DIABETES.

Diabetes is known by a superabundant discharge of urine, either with or without sugar; the urine is either limpid or saturated with sugar to the amount of four pounds or less in twenty-four hours. Constipation, loss of flesh and strength and a voracious appetite are manifest. The enormous quantity of urine passed thru the kidneys, robs the alimentary canal of its accustomed moisture.

Dorland says: "Diabetes mellitus, a disease marked by the passage of an excessive amount of urine containing an excess of sugar; glycosuria. It is attended by thirst, enormous appetite, emaciation, and loss of strength; it may occur in a temporarly form after the use of certain foods, with certain nervous diseases, and with congestion of the liver; but the disease is usually chronic and fatal, although in elderly people it may continue for some years."

Gould states: "**Diabetes mellitus,** glycosuria, **a disease of the metabolic functions** of the system, without gross or clearly defined anatomic lesions."

Pathologists are lost when they attempt to locate the cause of diabetes. The kidneys show no degeneration except what might be expected by the continued drainage of glycosuria. In diabetes we not only find that functions are performed in too great a degree as indicated by the amount of urine, but also, that the enormous quantity s either too limpid, being free from the ordinary solid constituents or is loaded with sugar. Where the kidneys are inflamed we find more or less albumin, blood, pus, fat, chyle, tube-casts and **diacetic-acid.** The latter is supposed by some physicians to be the cause of nephritis. In diabetes these are lacking. Normal urine contains no sugar, albumin, blood, pus, fat, chyle, tube-casts or acid.

Dunglison says, "There is no specific remedy for diabetes." The nerves which innervate the pancreas, those thru which it receives its impulses, which direct its functions, are derived from the hepatic, splenic and superior mesenteric plexuses, to which the pneumogastric and splanchnic nerves also send branches.

There are several tests for determining the amount of sugar in the urine. To know that the patient passes from ten to forty pints of urine in twenty-four hours, containing one to four pounds of sugar is of no value to the patient or the practitioner unless the latter is able to locate the cause and correct the same.

Gould says: "The etiology of diabetes is obscure. The causes are not well understood."

Delafield affirms: "The conditions leading to pancreatic hemorrhagia pancreatitis are not fully clear."

The pancreatic arteries are small and very numerous.

Stengel states: "The nature of the metabolic disturbances that lead to this inability to dispose of carbohydrates is still very obscure. The essential fact, is the inability of the body to consume carbohydrates for the production of energy. As long as excess of proteid and fatty food is taken and consumed, no disturbance of the general metabolism results; but when digestion fails or the diet is poorly regulated, destruction of the proteids of the body with increased excretion of urea occurs. Emaciation may be prevented for a time by increased consumption of proteid food, but eventually occurs."

Landois states as a fact: "After total extirpation of the pancreas, the digestion of albumin, fat and starches is impaired."

McFarland's query is: "What becomes of the sugar under normal conditions is a problem of great importance, concerning which we are still somewhat in the dark. The nature of this probable secretion is unknown to us, as is also the seat of its elaboration. That it may be owing to the absence of a ferment. The nature of the ferment, however is unknown.

McFarland states: "The removal of the pancreas invariably leads to glycosuria. The kidneys are frequently the seat of an acute parenchymatous degeneration that is probably caused by the persistent glycosuria."

Stengel says: "Disease of the pancreas is the probable cause in many cases, and may possibly play a part in all cases, though demonstrable lesions of the pancreas are not present in all.

"The nature of the metabolic disturbances that lead to this inability to dispose of carbohydrates is still very obscure.

"Total extirpation of the pancreas in the lower animals causes diabetes."

Another writer adds his opinion to this obscure metabolism. He says. "Up to the present time, we are in ignorance as to what part of the body is at fault in diabetes. As to what should cause this affection, we can as yet only speculate."

Kirk says: "Diabetes as it occurs in man may be due to disordered metabolism of the liver, to disease of the pancreas and to other not fully understood causes."

The pancreas is a compound racemose gland, resembling a bunch of grapes on a stalk. It is from six to eight inches in length and lies transversely across the posterior wall of the abdomen. In animals it is known as sweetbread. It is the abdominal salivary gland of the Germans. It secretes a limpid, colorless fluid that digests proteids, fats and carbohydrates. The secretion is conveyed to the duodenum by the pancreatic duct.

The most important carbohydrates are the sugars and starch groups, the saccharoses, glucoses and amyloses. They are constituents of almost all animal tissue known as fats.

Two hundred and fifty-six parts of glucose are equivalent to one hundred parts of fat. Carbohydrates are converted into sugar by the digestive process. A pure fat diet supports this proposition.

The pancreas furnishes a thick, transparent, colorless, odorless fluid, of a salty taste and strongly alkaline, which exerts an energetic characteristic physiological action upon digestion.

Kirk affirms that "pancreatic juice is the most powerful and important of all the digestive juices. The action of pancreatic juice on fats is a double one; it forms an emulsion and it decomposes the fats into fatty acids and glycerin by means of its fat-splitting ferment steapsin. The pancreatic juice does not act alone on the food in the intestines; it is assisted with the bile of the liver. The bile has little or no digestive action by itself, but combined with pancreatic juice it assists the latter in all its actions. This is true for the digestion of starch and of proteid, but most markedly so for the digestion of fat. Complete removal of the pancreas in animals, and diseases of the pancreas in man, produce a condition of diabetes, in addition to the loss of pancreatic action in the intestines. The disease as it occurs in man may be due to disordered metabolism of the liver, to disease of the pancreas and to other not fully understood causes."

Kirk continues: "How the pancreas acts other than in producing the pancreatic juice is not known. It must have other functions relating to the general metabolic phenomena of the body, which are disturbed by removal or disease of the gland. This is an illustration of a universal truth—viz., that each part of the body does not merely do its own special work, but is concerned in the great cycle of changes which is called general metabolism. Interference with any organ upsets not only its specific function, but causes disturbances through the body generally."

Kirk expresses, tho not clearly, a law of pathological physiology namely. that any one organ being inflamed, cannot suffer alone. It must, of necessity, transmit more or less of its surplus heated condition to those nearby. The pancreas may be the recipient of an undue amount of heat. As a result the liver becomes irritated, excited, performing its functions in too great a degree. One has received its inflammation from nerves being impinged upon or excited by poisons; its neighbor partakes, somewhat, of the same heat which also disturbs its functions.

Stengel states that "Total extirpation of the pancreas in the lower animals causes diabetes. The nature of the metabolic disturbances that lead to this inability to dispose of carbohydrates is still very obscure."

McFarland helps to clear up this mystery by saying: "Diabetes is a disease characterized by an erroneous treatment of carbohydrate foods, which, although properly digested and absorbed, are not utilized for the generation of force by combustion, or stored up in the form of fats and glucogen, but are immediately eliminated by the kidneys in the form of sugar. The removal of the pancreas invariably leads to glycosuria. The presence of sugar is the essential feature of diabetes. The kidneys are frequently the seat of an acute parenchymatous degeneration that is probably caused by the persistent glycosuria. Diseased kidneys have been thought by many to be the source of diabetes, but the improbability of this is shown by the fact that the glycosuria—the only symptom calling attention to the kidneys at all—is only a natural consequence of the hyperglycemia for which the kidneys cannot possibly be responsible."

Landois affirms that "after total extirpation of the pancreas, the digestion of albumen, fat and starches is impaired." Fat necrosis is usually associated with lesions of the pancreas—hemorrhagic infiltration, necrosis, gangrene and acute and chronic inflammatory processes. The lesion has been shown to be due to some substance in the pancreatic secretion, which splits the fat molecule into fatty acids (which may crystalize), and soluble substances; calcification is of later occurrence.

Brubaker states: "Removal of the pancreas from the body of a dog or other animal is at once followed by a rise in the percentage of sugar in the blood and its elimination by the kidneys."

Curtis says: "In a series of experiments made by Zambosi upon dogs, the nerves of the pancreas were not only cut, but the ends were tied 'in order to compare the behavior of the isolated segments with that of the central portion.' In no instance, however, was there any appearance of sugar in the urine."

The removal of the pancreas does not explain the change of function that takes place, when the heat is above or below normal. Pathologically, the change of functions is due to change of animal heat.

The pancreas secretes a juice which resembles saliva; its function is to convert starch into dextrine and glucose.

McFarland asserts that "Atrophy of the pancreas is not infrequent and is of regular occurrence in old age. It also follows local disturbances of the circulation, marasmus, diabetes, and cachexia. The organ becomes reduced in size, flaccid, and is often dark brown in color."

The atrophic pancreas of diabetes is said by Hansemann to differ from simple atrophy in that it consists of an interstitial inflammation associated with granular kidney.

Gregory loses sight of the fact that diabetes mellitus is not a disease of the kidneys, no more than diarrhea is a disease of and caused by abnormal functionating of the rectum. He says: "There is no doubt in the mind of the author that when we know more of the nerve supply and of the function that is controlled by the different nerve trunks or fibers, we will know more concerning the cause and existence of different diseases in any certain organ.

"For example, in the kidneys we have deranged function, and as a result we may have diabetes insipidus, or we may have albuminuria. Now, in either case, we have abnormal function, which is the result of the derangement of the nerve supply. To my mind, it is evidently a fact that the difference in the pathological lesions and abnormal functions of the kidneys are due to mechanical interference with some of the different nerve fibers that supply the kidneys, or to a derangement of the nutrition of some of the different portions of the central nerve cells in the spinal cord, or brain, supplying nerve filaments to the kidneys. The question is, What nerve or nerves cause one disease, and which causes the other?"

There is no doubt in my mind that, when we know more in regard to the effect that certain degrees of temperature have on metabolism, we will then know more in regard to the cause of and continued existence of different diseases of certain organs.

In diabetes mellitus there is no deranged functions of the kidneys. The kidneys merely take in and pass off what is given to them. There are no pathological lesions of the kidneys. The question is not "What nerve or nerves cause one disease, and which causes the other," but, what condition causes an increase or decrease in certain functions. **In disease there are no new functions added.**

Carver tells us: "**Diabetes,** so-called, **is** always **the termination** of chronic abnormality. It always follows a long period of chronic inflammation of the kidney. This inflammation, however, is of a character that the therapeutist is not acquainted with, and has no method of detecting. It is, however, of sufficient gravity to greatly **lessen depuration,** seriously affecting tissues generally, and to result in great change and debility of the tissues of the kidney. In this disease, "**The termination of chronic abnormality**" may last for many years. That would be a long termination, a lengthy end, a protracted finish, a far-reaching final. Diabetes never follows, nor accompanies "chronic inflammation of the kidney." Carver tells us that the therapeutist, the physician, has no means of detecting or knowing an inflammatory condition of the kidney in diabetes. Surprising, indeed, that in Bright's disease, there is no difficulty to determine on the operating table, in the recent state or post mortem, the morbid condition known as inflammation, but in this particular disease, "this inflammation is of a character that the therapeutist is not acquainted with." What is more surprising to me is, **how did Carver discover this chronic inflammatory** abnormality. "**Lessen depuration.**" Depuration is one of the cardinal principles of an obsolete doctrine of the nature of diseases which attributed all morbid phenomena to the disordered condition of the fluids, or humors of the body. That is known as humoral pathology. Friend Carver believes in humoralism; that is quite humoralistic when a Chiropractor tries to mix it with the science and philosophy of Chiropractic. The grandfathers of Allopathy believed in a process of depuration by which the animal economy is purified, either by the agency of some eruptive disease or some spontaneous evacuation, or by the assistance of some depurative medicine. Now, Friend Carver, why not be a full-fledged Chiropractor?

Ayers says: "No definite or characteristic lesions have been noted, though some degree of enlargement of the kidneys, together with sacculation, due to pressure backward upon the renal structure by the enormous quantities of urine in the bladder and ureters, has been observed. The ureters and pelves of the kidneys may be dilated, and the bladder, owing to constant over-distention, may be hypertrophied.

Delafield states: "Extirpation of the pancreas in man or dogs may lead to diabetes. While diabetes may occur without demonstrable lesions of the pancreas, it is fair to assume that functional lesions of grave importance may nevertheless be present. Under the influence of the doctrine of internal secretions it is now commonly assumed that the pancreas, in addition to its intestinal secretion, furnishes other substances to the body which are essential in the metabolic changes to which the carbohydrates and proteids must be subjected in securing normal nutrition. Interference with this internal secretion of the pancreas is thus assumed to be accountable for the faulty metabolism."

Stengel says that "pancreatitis may be acute or chronic. The acute variety presents itself in different forms, the most frequent being the hemorrhagic and the suppurative or necrotic. Chronic pancreatitis is analogous to chronic hepatitis and leads to similar induration or cirrhosis. Among the more or less characteristic symptoms of pancreatic disease are fatty diarrhea, imperfect digestion of proteids, rapid emaciation, lipemia and lipuria. All of these result from the cessation of pancreatic secretion and consequent disturbances of digestion and absorption of food. None of them is pathognomonic. A more important symptom is glycosuria and the role of pancreatic disease in the pathology of diabetes is a leading one. Atrophy, cirrhosis, carcinoma and other lesions of the organ may be found in diabetes. Whatever the nature of the disease, the results seem to be a disturbance of an internal secretion having importance in the consumption of sugar. When this secretion stops or diminishes glycosuria or diabetes results."

The pancreas secretes a fluid known as pancreatic juice which passes into the pancreatic duct at nearly the extreme left end of the gland and empties into the lower and inner part of the second portion of the duodenum with the bile which is conveyed by the bile duct.

The pancreatic juice has within it four drolytic ferments or enzymes, which make the juice of the pancreas an important digestive fluid. The secreted and excreted fluid of the pancreas is a "sugar-splitting ferment." If a solution of sugar is digested with an aqueous or glycerin extract of pancreas, the amount of sugar is diminished.

Pathologic physiology shows that from a lack of pancreatic juice, whether from the absence of the organ or its diminished functionating, proteids, fats and carbohydrate foods are changed into a limpid or sugared fluid.

The pancreas is primarily inflamed; its adjoining organs are somewhat overheated, secondarily, by contact.

Normal heat, normal tissue, and normal functionating are intimately connected and vice versa. The nerves which innervate the pancreas will be found emanating from the dorsal vertebrae.

---

Science is knowledge reduced to law and embodied into a system.

---

"Health is regained when these non-active nerves are compelled to again perform their work and carry new life to the affected parts."

Life could not exist with nerves non-active. Nerves are not compelled by physical or moral force to perform their work. Nerves do not carry **new life** to the affected part. Nerves transmit impulses; when impulses are carried in a greater or less degree than normal, such deviation is disease. The normal transmission of impulses, with functions performed in a normal manner, is health.

"I found in this case (diphtheria), as I have always, a displaced dorsal vertebra, and emanating from the occluded foramen, a sensitive nerve, which covered the membrane of the throat with its branches. These nerves were inflamed, expressed too much heat at their twig ends, because of being pinched in the foramina.

"Poisons taken into the system in food and water that is polluted or by breathing noxious effluvia from decaying vegetable or animal matter, or by the outrageous practice of the M. D. who injects vaccine poison into a healthy person, affects nerves, which act on muscles sufficient to displace vertebrae and impinge nerves, causing derangements which we name disease."

The above was written by me. It shows that I knew that throat diseases have their origin in the dorsal vertebrae, and that nerves may be inflamed and express too much heat.

I have learned since that nerves are not "pinched in foramina," but, instead, are **impinged upon** by the pressure of displaced bones.

As shown by the above, I was the first to advocate that poisons affect nerves, that affected nerves contract and by their contraction draw bones out of alignment. I was the first to affirm that nerves are impinged upon, not pinched. "Dr. D. D. Palmer by chance stumbled onto the basic principles of Chiropractic." Columbus by chance (?) discovered America.

---

Your thots are of little value unless you intelligently use them.

---

Innate and Educated. Innate existed before Educated. The latter is dependent upon the former for existence. Each of these entities has a mind, each has an intellect, a consciousness; each thinks, considers, understands, reasons, feels, perceives and wills. The knowledge and attributes of Innate has been acquired thru the countless ages of time; while those of Educated is limited to this, our life time and acquired thru the nervous system; that of Innate is the sum total of all life experiences.

The attributes of the Innate mind are directed thru the sympathetic nervous system to the upbuilding of the physical body, the sum total of all the processes known as metabolism; while that of Educated is directed toward our environments.

Innate is not the mind, any more than the body is the mind. There is a spiritual mind and a physical mind. The former is everlasting, the latter exists during life. The mind of the spirit is augmented by the experiences of the physical mind.

## THE SCIENCE OF CHIROPRACTIC, VOL. 3.

Has 337 pages of eleven-point type and 476 cuts. There are four views of the vertebral column, anterior, posterior and two lateral. As these cuts are of a normal spinal column, one lateral view would have answered all purposes. There are nine views of the torso (might have doubled the number by inverting), whereas three would have been sufficient. There are 238 cuts of vertebrae. Standard works on anatomy which contain much more information, have one or two dozen. Many of these cuts are indistinct, therefore valueless. There are three "enlarged views" of lumbar vertebrae, which views are of normal size. Many of the paired vertebrae used to show subluxations, are separated so far from each other that they are an absurd failure. There is not one pair which would give a physician or layman an idea of what a sub-luxation consists. Although there are 125 cuts of adjustments which make a great spread, they are entirely unfit to illustrate the philosophy and principles of Chiropractic. There are 17 beautiful cuts on scientific nail driving, which serve only to confuse the investigator.

The author learned from the writer all he (the author) knows about sub-luxations; that the nerves of innervation of the stomach, throat, liver and spleen emerge from one side of the spinal column, not from both; scientific nerve tracing; the function of the splenic fluid; the T. M. movement and all else of value mentioned in this book. Then how child-like to say, "This is my dollie, I saw it first." But he did not learn of me that near the center of the spinal column (page 230), "The vertebrae are less tightly wedged, more free and less force need be utilized." He has a vague memory of reading that the **sacrum is inserted like a wedge** between the two innominate bones; until I read this book, I was not aware that any of the vertebrae were tightly wedged, some more than others. This very thought was his from its inception and couched in his own language. Another new thought from this author (see bottom of page 154) "vertebrae can boast," brag, talk big.

Page 33: "Atlas is the fifth cervical expansion, considering the four superior cranial vertebrae as its predecessors." The atlas is not an expansion of the vertebral column. The four cranial bones, occipital, two parietal and frontal, are considered by some anatomists as the upper expansion, as is the sacrum of the lower. The cranial bones are not the predecessors of the atlas, they did not precede it in any office or position. Page 9: "The aim throughout this book has been to explain sub-luxations and their adjustments around six words."

He tells us that "this book is based around six words." These six "words" must be magical. He has found the talisman by which I discovered the principles of Chiropractic. By those "six words" he is enabled to "base" a book "around" and get a clear conception of the basic principles of Chiropractic. One page 284 and 295 he refers to these words and the basis. "Have one common **basis** and hold to that in preference to manufacturing such a **jargonity** of words and movements that mystifies the student. The thinker will observe that the larger number of diseases studied are followed in this region by strong, massive exostosis and ankyloses. It can be observed that the names of the diseases could be listed for pages." Those thoughts are his couched in his language.

Four hundred illustrated "foolers" count in numbers, make a great spread and a big show on paper, but are not worth the ink that is wasted on them. This book "based around six words" will be far from "convincing the masses that it (Chiropractic) can be and is for the first time adjusted to a practical art and science." The adjusting has dislocated the science of Chiropractic from a knowledge of anatomy; it has made several kyphotic curves in the science of Chiropractic.

The most of the descriptive part of anatomy is copied from McClellan's Regional Anatomy, which is copyrighted, and for which no credit is given. But no one must copy his literature, although written by another, without hearing a childish whine. "Somebody lied." Page 10 of the preface of this much illustrated book—it was much easier to make pictures than to advance the science of Chiropractic—says: "In this work not only does the language in which ideas are couched belong to the author, but the very thoughts themselves were his from their inception. Upon him has evolved the labor of their development. Even the methods used in illustration (with the single exception of the position of the hands in adjusting) are the children of his own ingenuity."

Page 88 and 92. "The axis covers the same **field** as the atlas and only in rare instances has any **keen** differences been noticed." "Research has not located a trouble at this subluxation other than what has been mentioned under the similar head of atlas." Better to have said, "What we have said of the atlas can also be said of the axis; rare exceptions to the contrary." In an experience of 13 years I have found but very few instances where the axis has been racked from its moorings; on the contrary, the atlas and the third cervical are frequently tipped, changing their relative position to the occiput and axis. On account of the superior oblique lateral and inferior oblique posterior articulations of this axis, it is rare that a wrench is received so as to change its position.

## ARTERITIS.

Arteritis signifies inflammation of an artery. It is also known as endarteritis. This inflamed condition may be of the intima, the inner coat, or it may involve the entire wall of the three coats, it may be acute or chronic. If the hyperthermia is confined to the middle coat it is called mesarteritis and peri-arteritis if of the external coat.

This disease is characterized by fatty degeneration of the arterial tissue and later by lime-salt formations. The chronic state produces arteritis deformans. Arterie-sclerosis is the last stage, the hardening of the arterial walls. Arteritis obliterans is a gradual hypertrophy of the arterial tissue with contraction and occlusion of the arterial lumen, the transverse section, the diameter of the artery. This is followed by collapse or closure of the vessel cavity, usually of the smaller branches. When the veins are affected in like manner, it is known as angio-sclerosis. The small blood vessels which ramify the outer and middle coats, the vaso-vasorum, may be congested, the tissue oedematous, or the enclosing structure necrotic, owing to an excessive heat condition.

The inner coat, known as the intima, if implicated, loses its natural gloss, looks a dull-yellowish color, is swollen and may ulcerate.

Rupture of the artery may follow acute suppurative and necrotic inflammation of the blood vessels. The inflammatory process may form new tissue within the lumen, named thrombo-arteritis, inflammation from a thrombus, a blood clot formed during life. These vascular, degenerative conditions may affect single vessels or a certan vascular territory or the entire vascular system. The lumen may be partly or wholly closed by the thickened walls and prevent circulation in the affected artery or vein, a condition known as obliterating endarteritis. Fatty degeneration, atrophy, or calcification may occur in the muscle fiber, or the membranous covering. Similar conditions may affect the aorta. Blood vessels may be affected with fatty degeneration, thickening of the intima, calcification and erosion and hemorrhages may occur.

Arterio-sclerosis may be limited to the aorta, to single vessels, or to special vascular tracts of the brain or heart. As a result of arteritis, circulatory disturbances may arise either locally or general. Sclerosis of the arteries consists of a deposit, in the vascular coats, of a quantity of hard, gritty, earthy, saline material which tho commonly considered as osseous, presents none of the true character of bone, there being no trace of bone corpuscles. Microscopical examination shows them to consist of an irregular, chystalline, granular mass, composed mainly of animal matter, phosphate of lime and a small per cent of carbonate of lime. The affected coats change from fatty to calcareous matter.

As a rule, as individuals advance in life, there is a progressive increase of earthy matter in the coats of normal arteries. Here, as elsewhere, sclerosis is pathological physiology, normal increased to abnormal functionating. The ash of the arteries of a newly-born child yields .86 per cent of phosphate of lime; of an adult 1.25; of an old man 2.77; the ossified arteries of an aged man contained 4.01. These changes are physiological when the lime salt is ordinarily increased, pathological, when deposited in too great a degree. Ordinary senile transformations are, therefore, physiological. We find arteritis and arterial sclerosis accompanying many inflammatory diseases, changes which are the direct result of inflammatory action.

Arterio-sclerosis in the limbs shows an abnormal condition of the nerves ramifying that region, indicated by coldness of the feet, cramps and spasms of the muscles. In organs there is manifested a softening of tissue, fatty degeneration, and later calcareous deposits.

Arteritis, inflammation of the blood vessels, may lead to ulceration of the coats which form the blood vessel walls; spontaneous rupture; contracture or occlusion of the interior of the cavity and lastly, dilatation and aneurisms.

The earthly matter may be deposited in the form of plates, laminar calcification, or it may be arranged in a concentric manner around the muscular fibers, known as annular calcification, and, when spread over a considerable length of a blood vessel, it is termed tubular calcification. The annular deposit may transform a blood vessel into a brittle, calcareous pipe, known as the "pipe stem artery." Necrosis, with erosion of the arteries in common in pulmonary tuberculosis, allowing rupture and hemorrhage. The intima may contain fatty, greasy, droplets.

Arterio-sclerosis is a physiological process of old age; it is pathological when occurring in youth or adult life.

The morbid appearance of a blood vessel affected with arteritis is that of redness, a deep claret color, and accompanied with a loss of its physiological properties. The local symptoms of arteries are pain, tension, stiffness of the affected limb, with extreme tenderness. As the closure of the vessels are of a slow procedure, anastomosing circulation is made compensatory. There is a cord-like feeling along the inflamed vessel in which there may be observed a jerking and forcible pulsation. The pain below the part of the artery affected is severe; it may be superficial or deep. The surface pain is in the skin, which is exceedingly sensitive to the touch, so much so, that the patient cannot bear the finger to be laid upon it, the sensation produced being similar to that of neuralgia. The deep pain is of a burning and lancinating character, usually following the course of a vessel. The limb gradually loses its normal temperature, becoming cold and of a dark or livid color, and yet the inordinate sensibility continues. As gangrene supervenes, sensation is lacking. Gangrene or mortification may be of the dry or moist variety.

Local physiological atrophy of arteries follows obstruction by ligation. In cases of amputation, the arteries of the stump diminish in size corresponding with the needs of the tissues to be nourished.

The arteries, like nerves and muscles are supplied with tension. Arterial tension is ever present. The observance of arterial tension, whether recognized as such or not, is one of the most important acts of the physician, in fact, more so, than the study of the pulse rate, for, bear in mind, the elastic tension and the pulse rate are quite different conditions. Arterial tension is the resistence of the arterial walls to the pressure of the contained blood. Arterial tension is the strain on an artery at full pulse. Tension, in physiology, is the condition of an organ when under a strain. The variation of temperature modifies the tension of the vascular system as well as that of the nerves, muscles and organs. Arterial tension is abnormal when it is too high or too low. High tension, when increased by exercise, excitement or hypnotism, is a natural, physiological response. High tension is pathological when the increase is caused by trauma, poisons, or auto-suggestion as in hysteria. Hypertension is functional; it may be normal or abnormal, morbid or physiological. High tension compresses the vasovasorum—the blood vessels of the blood vessel wall—between the inner coats and the fibrous coat, because the latter has reached the point of fixation by distention.

Many pathologists consider high tension and a rapid pulse, as exhibited in febrile diseases, as physiological—an effort on the part of Nature to supply more blood to certain parts for a protective purpose, a poison destroyer; that the increase in tension and circulation is essential to preserve life. Others consider high tension and a rapid pulse deleterious, evil, a condition which ought to be checked or reduced, therefore, they attack it instead of furnishing the best medical aid. It is a serious question among the medical profession whether high tension, high temperature and a rapid pulse are physiological, tending toward health, or a necessary, unavoidable evil; whether vascular relaxant medicines are beneficial or detrimental. Cardiovascular tension presents a grave consideration for the cardiovascular tension presents a grave consideration for the medical man. Excessive heat softens the vascular walls, causing them to become fragile, and, at the same time creates tension and high pressure, threatening rupture and hemorrhage. In disease the pathologist has hypotension to consider as well as hypertension, but the former is much more rare. Several years ago, before B. J. passed my examination for his D. C. diploma, the Ph. C. was conferred, not earned. I had a patient who suffered from hypotension when in a recumbent posture, but as soon as he assumed, or tried to assume a sitting or standing position, hypertension and increased circulation would compel him to lie down. This case I dismissed quite well, with normal tension (tone), standing, sitting or lying. It does not appear as one of B. J.'s cures in his revised issue of volume one, because I did not make a record of it in print.

Hypotension indicates a lack of power and circulation. The medical man has no all-powerful vascular stimulants upon which to rely. This condition of hypotension is illustrated in the critical period of acute infections. When the tension is relieved, going below normal, the patient approaches a condition of collapse.

An author on pathology says, "The causes of arterio-sclerosis are numerous and varied." Another writer states, "The cause of arterial inflammation are extremely obscure." And yet another says, "While the conditions under which arteritis develops are not fully understood, fruitful research may be confidently expected." The medical fraternity have always been hopeful.

In regard to the treatment of the narrowing or occlusion of the arteries, pathologists have but little to say. "Little can be done to cure the disease."

Pathologists think arteritis is the result of infection, kidney diseases, tuberculosis, rheumatism, gout, Bright's disease, syphilis, alcohol in excess, trauma, lead poisoning, overwork, overfeeding, or that it is inherited or constitutional. Others ascribe the majority of cases to the result of injuries, or from lodgment within its tubular walls of some foreign body of an irritating or infectious nature. It has been associated with cardiac hypertrophy, valvular lesions, chronic diffuse, nephritis, tumors, diphtheria, scarlatina and pyaemia. It is frequently associated with or follows these inflammatory diseases.

Many minute nutrient blood vessels course in the external and middle coats of large or moderate sized arteries. They arise from the vessels to which they are distributed or originate in an adjacent vessel. These small arteries are called vasa vasorum. The blood is returned from the vessel walls by small veins, named venae vasorum.

Arteries are supplied with nerves, medullated and non-medullated. A network of nerve-fibers exist, in the media (middle coat) and surrounds the vessels; these are vasomotor, they supply the muscle fibers.

The vasa vasorum and venae vasorum are supplied by nervi (plural of nervus) vasorum.

Nerves are supplied with nervous filaments, named nervi nervorum, which are distributed to their sheaths.

Nerves and blood vessels, themselves, are supplied with nerves and blood vessels. The nerves are from the sympathetic.

Thus, we see that vascular tension may be disturbed by trauma, poison or auto-suggestion, and may be returned to normal tone, the same as the elongated, thread-like structures.

---

## ADJUSTING.

"You state, as a rule, adjust from the side affected in the cervical and dorsal regions, in the lumbar vice versa. Is that a fixed rule? Will that answer the purpose in all cases?"

This rule, like all others, has exceptions. It is the abnormals, the exceptions to the rule, the Chiropractor has to deal with.

"You state that a light impingement on a nerve causes excessive heat, as a consequence, too much functionating; that excessive pressure prevents the transmission of a normal amount of impulse, therefore, less energy and a lack of functionating is exhibited. Please explain."

That is just what we have been attempting to do from time to time in the Adjuster; this may be more apparent with the above question before us.

The central extremity of a divided motor nerve may unite with the peripheral extremity of another nerve and still functionate. Langley united the central extremity of the vagus with the peripheral extremity of the sympathetic and found, after union took place, that the vagus had acquired control of all structures supplied by the cervical sympathetic, transmitting thru the sympathetic the vagus impulses. A light pressure on a nerve causes tension; a tension by nerve-stretching acts as an irritant. An increased pressure or extension up to a certain degree, increases irritation and functionating. A still greater pressure or extension causes a diminution of irritability until paralysis ensues. The process of nerve tension caused by impingement, acts as an irritant, if the pressure be light; greater pressure causes a diminution of sensation or of voluntary movements.

An impingement, on a nerve or muscle causes tension. An atlas displaced to the right or left may cause tension on one or both of the sympathetic chains of ganglia which pass in front of the transverse processes. Upon one side by crowding, and upon the other by drawing against the impinged nerve or muscle. Either condition amounts to a strain or tension causing irritation, super-heat and increased functionating. If the impingement is severe, a lack of functionating will result.

The effects of irritation or insufficient functionating caused by a displaced atlas, may be transferred thru the carotid or cavernous plexus to the cranial nerves. Or because of meningeal tension the nerve rootlets may become irritated.

A large share of diseases begin with a slight chill and fever which increases as the days come and go. Why?

Why does the chill period, the cold stage, the rigor, the involuntary contraction of the voluntary muscles precede fever? Why, in some instances, does it accompany fever. Why, in others, a sensation of cold, when in fact, the thermometer shows supernormal temperature. Why not have fever without the initial symptoms of shivering with cold? Why?

Just wait a minute while I ask the Bohemians (?), for they know all about Chiropractic (?). It is nice to stand in (?) with the Bohemians (?). While others have paid me from $100 to $500 to learn this science and art, it cost me nothing except a few hours' study and an intrigue with the Bohemians.

Pressure on nerves causes them to be excited, irritated; the peripheral nerves of motion become contracted, causing the sensation of cold or chillness.

It is a well known fact in physiology that physiological or pathological irritation of nerves causes contraction of the muscles to which they are attached.

Nerves of normal tonicity transmit a normal quantity of heat. When a nerve becomes unduly excited, irritated, it enlarges, and contracts on all the muscles with which it is attached.

Abnormal tissue and abnormal functions are inseparable; these two pathological conditions depend upon each other's abnormality. Increased diameter produces more heat until a crisis is reached by nercrosis of tissue. When it softens it liberates pressure. This necrôssed tissue may be bone or nerve, or both.

Pressure may be so great as to prevent, in a measure or entirely, the transmission of impulses—molecular vibration.

---

Chiropractic is a science, not a building; it was created, not built. Its foundation is not that of principles. It is founded on anatomy—otseology, neurology and functions. It is not built out of principles as a mason would build a house out of brick. Chiropractic is a science—a knowledge of health and disease, reduced to law and embodied into a system.

## LUXATIONS ADJUSTED.

"It has long been proclaimed that D. D. Palmer was the discoverer of the fundamental crude principles, and that B. J. Palmer, D. C., Ph. C., was the developer of this sicence. It is up to you to disprove that if you can."

I gave that journal the name of "The Chiropractor." It has been proclaimed for 13 years that I was the discoverer and developer of Chiropractic. The March, 1906, number says: "Dr. D. D. Palmer, Discoverer and Developer of Chiropractic, Editor." The next number does not state who is editor. The June, 1906, number, states M. P. Brown, M. D., is editor. On page 20, of this the June number, are cuts of eleven persons above the following statement: "The above represents some of the P. S. C.'s earlier graduates. First row on left, above downward: Raymond, '01; Simon, '99; Baker, '96. Second row: Christianson, 1900; Dr. D. D. Palmer, Discoverer and Developer of Chiropractic; Brown, M. D., '99. Third row: Miss Murchison, '02; B. J. Palmer, D. C.; Sec. the P. S. C. Fourth row: Stouder, '01; Schooley, '02; Graham, '99." Baker, Christianson and Murchison were not graduates of Chiropractic. The date of B. J. Palmer's graduation is not given. By turning to the February, 1905, number, page 21, the date is given as 1902, six years ago, which is correct.

"The above represents some of the P. S. C.'s earlier graduates." "Dr. D. D. Palmer, Discoverer and Developer of Chiropractic." When did he graduate? If the symptoms hereafter mentioned continue to develop, it will not be surprising to learn that D. D. Palmer graduated under B. J. many years ago. I was proclaimed as the Developer of Chiropractic as late as June, 1906, in The Chiropractor, managed by B. J. Palmer. The Adjuster is trying to adjust luxations.

There is not a Chiropractic principle that I did not discover and develop, as shown by back numbers of The Chiropractor. We do not use the term sub-luxations, because many statements made in the Chiropractor are complete luxations. They are not accidental, they are spontaneous. They are caused by a lesion, which has lost its natural connection.

On pages 31 and 47 of the August and September number, 1906, two class groups are given. They state, "Dr. D. D. Palmer, Discoverer and Developer of Chiropractic." In the November number, 1906, is an article of 18 pages written by "D. D. Palmer, discoverer and developer of Chiropractic." On page 47 of the January issue of 1907, B. J. says, in referring to The Science of Chiropractic, "It is written by Dr. D. D. Palmer, the discoverer and developer of Chiropractic." On page 29 of the January, 1907, number, I find a reward of $1000 offered to "The party who will produce the man, show him up, bring him to the front, who taugh Chiropractic to Dr. D. D. Palmer." "$1000 will be paid to any living being who will furnish the one who taught Dr. D. D. Palmer the science of Chiropractic." "This reward is offered in order to dispose of this question." "Chiropractic has passed through the crisis; it is now considered a distinct science." "The pseudo-discoverers are not to be found, thus it will be with pseudo-Chiropractors." "Dr. Parker and Dr. Story are both graduates under D. D. Palmer, the only discoverer of Chiropractic. If you can prove it otherwise, $1000 will be paid to you."

If Chiropractic had become a distinct science in January, 1907, how did it happen that B. J. developed the science? It is a dream, an hallucination, an insane effort of a disordered brain.

As no one has laid claim to the $1000, why dispute the fact yourself that I am the discoverer and only developer of this science? Why look further for the man who taught it to me.?

In the February, 1907, number, I find a cut giving a picture of "Old Dad." Underneath is "Dr. D. D. Palmer, Discoverer and Developer of Chiropractic."

I observe that there are eight months of quietude, during the period of incubation. I have analyzed the symptoms, and am now tracing The Chiropractor in order to locate the luxation causing aberration and kleptomania. I find on page 15 of the July number, "Everything is tried but the right thing—adjusting the cause—which remained for D. D. Palmer to discover." In this same number is advertised, "The Science of Chiropractic, by Dr. D. D. Palmer, Discoverer and Developer." Up to this date every vertebra examined showed proper alignment; due respect was paid by the son to his father for his untiring research from the time B. J., the son, was seven years of age up to three years ago. If the symptoms of aberration and kleptomania continue to increase, some number of the Chiropractor is the near future will give the date of the father's graduation as later than that of his son.

I have found the luxation on page 59 of the August and September number, 1907. It shows symptoms of aberration, hallucination, mental wandering, divergence from the truth and a well-defined case of kleptomania. The reader may notice the mental derangement, the incoherent, disjointed expressions, that have little relation to the subject; the delusions of the patient, imagining himself to be the discoverer, developer and Founder of Chiropractic.

In part it reads thus: "Twelve years ago D. D. Palmer had certain youthful principles that he based Chiropractic research around. Its early years were simple yet accurate and homely. The present day philosophy and adjusting of vertebrae is practical yet so unmixed and pure that it is technically scientific.. The application, today, is equal. This is now laid down in 2x2 exactness, reasons given for all deductions and conclusions. The stupendous development of the past two years in this respect alone marks another era in accord with Chiropractic's early teachings.

"For years we adjusted with a basis, although practiced, undefined and unprinted or written.

"**This book is based around six words.** The aim has been simplicity in preference to a jargonity that has no semblance to anything. It is absolutely plain, unadorned, undesigning and its art portrayed in detail."

I would like The Chiropractor to give its readers those youthful principles. Please describe that basis you adjust **with.** Above all I would like to know what those six words are that the forthcoming book is based around. It may be that the jargonity has no semblance to anything—never mind—please try to describe it. The symptoms have not entirely subsided, for as we still pursue The Chiropractor we read, "Chiro was discovered by D. D. Palmer and developed into a science by B. J. Palmer, his son." "Each one is talked in the cylinders personally by the discoverer and author." "Dr. B. J. Palmer is The Fountain Head (the worker, thinker and student) and that at his place is where Chiropractic was founded and developed." "Its development has taken place there by the same family through the son."

It is to be hoped that this adjustment may bring him to his senses, relieve him from kleptomania and wandering from the paths of truth and moral rectitude.

Chiropractors do not use drugs, water, heat or electricity in adjusting the cause of diseases. They do not rub, or manipulate; they adjust the bony framework, similarly as a jeweler does a watch.

---

"Ninety per cent of all disease is caused by '**Ligatights**' in the spine."

---

We possess two intelligences, Innate and Educated. Innate runs all the vital functions while we are asleep or awake. This intelligence which we are born with, knows how to run the functions of the body a hundred times better than the Educated. It remains for Educated Intelligence to be able to keep, fix, adjust the skeletal frame so that Innate can use it is a means of communication in such a manner as desired.

## SYMPTOMATOLOGY, SEMIOLOGY.

Is the science of determining the character and prognosis of disease by subjective and objective signs.

Science consists of ascertained facts in regard to the knowledge of principles and causes.

A compilation of recognized symptoms which denote the character and progress of disease would be the science of symptoms.

Determining the character of disease, also the decision arrived at, is diagnosis.

Prognosis, is the act of foretelling the course and termination of disease.

Diagnosis and prognosis are made by subjective and objective signs. The subjective signs are those noticed by the patient; those observed by the attendant are objective.

I have discovered and verified certain principles which determine conditions named health and disease; these constitute a science.

The science of Chiropractic is founded on quite different lines from that of medicine or any system of therapeutics.

The Chiropractor determines the nature of disease in a manner quite different from that of other methods. Disease, viewed from the standpoint of Chiropractic is of an entirely different nature from that accorded to it by any system of Therapeutics.

The physicians diagnosis and prognosis are made for the purpose of determining, beforehand, the progress and outcome of disease, as they expect diseases to have their usual run. Therefore, they desire to classify, not for the purpose of cutting short the duration of disease, but that they may know in advance, how long they can hold their job. A Chiropractor's analysis is made for the purpose of locating the cause of trouble, so that he can adjust the displaced portion of the bony framework, which, by its impingement on nerves and muscles, is creating disease. While the physician and the Chiropractor both use the subjective and objective signs, it is for quite a different purpose; the former for future need the latter for present benefit.

---

Facial hemiatrophy is akin to wry-neck; a progressive wasting of the bones, muscles and subcutaneous tissue of the lateral half of the face and head. It begins in early life, often at birth. It is due to a sub-luxated cervical vertebra. The affection becomes stationary at maturity. The medical profession agree that this disease is a nervous disorder and incurable. A Chiropractor should be able to replace the displaced bone, relieve the impingement and correct the deformity.

Kalispel, Mont., September 27, 1909.

D. D. Palmer, the Fountain Head of Chiropractic.

Dear Old Preceptor:—If I had known a month ago that you were in Portland, I certainly would have called on you.

As your sincere friend, I hope you are meeting with the success you so richly deserve. I was aware that there was something wrong, which should have been adjusted. Until now I did not know that others were trying to rob you of the honor and glory justly due you. Being one of your earliest graduates, I ought to know to whom that honor belongs. You and no other taught me the science of Chiropractic and the art of adjusting. I have every reason to believe that I received my knowledge of Chiropractic from D. D. Palmer, the fountain head of that science, of which I am proud. I prize the diploma I received from you, signed by yourself and no other, much more than any I have.

I am at the end of my outing, feel fine, feel as young as I did ten years ago.

Chiropractic has made a great advancement as shown by The Adjuster. It has a great future, if a few would-be leaders and dictators do not retard its growth or lead it astray. I was sorry to learn that you had been robbed financially and an attempt made to steal from you the honor of being the discoverer and developer of the grandest science on earth.

Dr. D. D., you will always find me standing by you as the fountain head of Chiropractic. I ought to know who is entitled to that credit. It is certainly not the little unruly kid that was in knickerbockers when you taught me the principles of the science of Chiropractic.

I remain as ever, yours very truly,

WM. A. SEELEY, D. C.

Spencer, Iowa.

---

Here's a problem. If one person who is exposed to smallpox contracts it, thereby proving it to be contagious, does not the fact that those who do not take it, disprove the contagion theory?

---

Stengel gives the relation of the mosquito to malaria, thus: "It has been positively demonstrated that when certain mosquitoes are allowed to feed upon malarial patients and later upon normal individuals, the latter acquire the disease." Where does the first mosquito get his first bite of poison to start malaria?

## GANGLIA.

The number of ganglia found in the ganglionic chains varies in different subjects. While the variation of the spinal nerves seldom deviate more than one pair more or less, the ganglia which receive the sympathetic fibers do not correspond in numbers, neither are they always the same in different subjects. Usually there are twelve ganglia in the thoracic region of the vertebral cord. This number is often reduced to ten or eleven by fusion. When there are only ten or eleven, the lower ganglia occupy the spaces between the heads of the ribs. The cervical portion of the vertebral cord usually has three ganglia, the superior, middle and inferior. The center ganglion is sometimes absent. The superior is supposed to be two or more fused in one. The lumbar portion of the sympathetic trunk generally contains four ganglia; this number may be decreased to three or increased to eight. Occasionally they are so fused as to form one continuous ganglion. The variation in size and number is more marked in the sacral portion of the trunk than in the cervical, thoracic or lumbar.

The sympathetic nervous system is connected with the alimentary canal, the vascular system and the glandular organs of vertebrates, by ganglia, plexuses and nerve cords. The sympathetic furnishes life force, functional activity through nerves which extend from and have their apparent origin in the ganglia of the two axial chains, similar to the way in which the spinal cord furnishes spinal nerves.

One spinal nerve may be connected with two ganglia, or two spinal nerves may innervate the sympathetic system by sending their fibers to one ganglion. The ganglia of the trunks throughout give off associate branches to the ganglia of the prevertebral plexuses and also several branches to the nearby viscera and blood-vessels.

To consider that any nerve or nerves are sympathetic with another, or that they may cause morbid phenomena to supervene without any direct morbific cause, acting directly because of reaction on another organ, primarily affected, is not Chiropractic, is not scientific, is not specific. While we may use the name sympathetic, accepted by common consent, we do not mean that, thru sympathy one disease causes another, that one organ or a portion of the body is in sympathy with another. These remarks are applicable to reflex action.

The two chains of ganglia which hold a similar relation to the splanchnic system of nerves, as does the spinal cord to the somatic nerves, run parallel to the spinal cord from the brain to the coccyx. They are connected with and derive their functions from the spinal nerves; in fact, the nerves of the sympathetic system, while having their apparent origin in the ganglia of the cord, originate in the brain, pass down the spinal cord, go out through the foramina of the spine, and are enclosed in the same perineurium. A bundle of nerve fibers containing spinal, ganglionic or communicating nerves to the cranial, are subject to the same liability of impingement of one or more fibers, regardless of their destination. These spinal nerves divide into branches, become accessory to certain nerves to which they communicate some one of their functions. Bear in mind that nerves do not anastomose; they pursue an uninterrupted course from the brain to the periphery, provided that they are not interfered with by pressure.

The twelve pairs of cranial nerves receive communicating fibers from the spinal and sympathetic systems with which they unite. These connecting branches of communication account for and explain the difference found in books on anatomy, which are compiled from dissections on the cadaver when nerves are lax, and the tracing of sensitive, rigid, tense, inflamed nerves in the living subject by Chiropractors.

While the cranial nerves apparently go direct to the organs of sense, muscles and membranes, passing through foramina in the skull, the spinal and sympathetic nerves assist in their makeup. Therefore, the cranial nerves receive more or less of their functional impulse by way of the spinal cord. This being the case, the functions of the splanchnic, spinal and cranial nerves are liable to be interfered with by pressure. By freeing the communicating branches which go to and assist in the makeup of the cranial, sympathetic and recurrent nerves, we do by them, as though they were named spinal nerves which in fact they are.

---

Brown's memory is so short that it only reaches to his knees, he therefore never pays for his boots.

---

Contradictory statements: "U. C. A.—Thousand years hence, aged sires, with heads of white, telling the children of this boy, who not only found the cause of disease, but told the world how to remove it." If a thousand years hence sires care as little for truth as the writer of the above, they will state that Daniel D. Palmer, Jr., a grandson of D. D. Palmer, is the man "who found the cause of disease." The above makes a strange contrast with the following statement made by the Portland, Oregon, convention, which were not aware that the honor of discovering "the cause of disease" had been stolen from its rightful owner. "That we recognize Dr. D. D. Palmer as the discoverer of the science of Chiropractic."

## TREE VS. MAN.

On page 78 of No. 4 Announcement is a cut of a tree trunk with branches and fruit. Pliers are represented as pinching a limb—result—immature fruit, because of a lack of function—a portion being "shut off." In order to show the likeness, there is also a cut of a spinal cord, branches of which proceed to the vital organs, heart, stomach and kidneys. Pliers are shown as pinching the nerve going to the stomach. To use the words of the writer (third line from bottom of page), "The organs of the body are at the **perpetual endings of the spinal nerves.**" He says, "The trunk corresponds to the spinal cord, the branches to the nerves, and the fruit to the organs of the human body."

"Perpetual" should be peripheral, an overlooked mistake of the printer.

To put that page in the hands of an anatomist, or one who knows anything of morbid physiology, would be to belittle the author and the science which he claims to represent. For me to allow it to go unnoticed would be to sanction its teachings, as he was a student of mine. I conferred the degree of D. C. on him and gave him a diploma, which is equal to saying I endorse the principles of Chiropractic as set forth. I assure the reader I never taught the author of that page that all diseases were because of functions being "shut off." On the contrary, I tried to teach him that diseases were results from too much or not enough functionating, that all diseases are because of (in their onset) an overproduction of heat—too much functionating—known to physicians as fever.

These cuts and their explanation are misleading; they are not Chiropractic. The nerve is represented as being pinched between the jaws of pliers. Nerves are never pinched between two hard substances—they are impinged upon by pressure, pressed against by protruding bones. Spinal nerves do not go to and end in the vital organs, as there represented.

"The organs of the body are **(not)** at the peripheral endings of the **spinal nerves.**" The sympathetic nerves, not the spinal, reach the vital organs.

The reader may think these principles are not taught at the P. S. C. Please turn to the inside cover of The Chiropractor and find, "Health is restored by **completing** the mental and physical circuit; **restoring** the currents. . . . to **replace** the **full quota** of positive . . . **permitting** the **reconveyance** of the intelligent immateriality. . . . to **re-establish** equilibrium . . . for the purpose of all normal . . . currents through **nerves** that **were formerly not permitted** to be **transmitted** through impingement, but have **now assumed their normal size** and **capacity** for conduction."

I have in many places in the Chiropractor and Adjuster stated that disease is the result of too much or not enough functionating. In all pathological derangements there is exhibited a surplus of heat as a prime factor—heat and the performance of functions are increased primarily. After the crisis, functions may be performed with less frequency and energy; may fall below normal, but even this condition is not because the function is "shut off," but because of softening of nerve tissue. Free the nerve from impingement and Innate will restore function to normal activity.

Neuritis precedes degeneration of nerves. Local heat may be so intense as to cause the complete disappearance of nerve-fibers. Nerves suffer as much or more than other tissue. Inflammation follows nerve impingement. Excessive heat continues until the nerve tissue becomes softened even to necrosis. This condition and change is manifested more at the point of pressure than elsewhere, leaving a depressed condition, injuring the fibers at that point, causing sequela affections.

We find an undue amount of heat and too much functionating present at the onset of every disease.

---

How some are prone to distort the truth is shown in a booklet of 26 pages—numbered 32, which the author says he wrote in an afternoon. As I looked it over I wished for a typewriter that would help me to make copy that fast.

He states: " D. D. Palmer made the discovery of Chiropractic accidentally while examining a patient's back, and that he noticed a bump"; this gave him food for thought. "Somebody lied." For ten years I had been looking, thinking, asking myself and others the question, why does one person have a certain ailment and another remain well, although both may be eating the same food at the same table, sleeping in the same bed and working side by side? At last Harvey Lillard assisted me in answering my question. He told me that while he was in a cramped position he felt something give way in his back and from that time he was deaf. Upon examination I found a vertebra out of alignment, racked out of its normal position. I replaced it by two adjustments and restored his hearing.

The principles of Chiropractic as taught by me have been developed by 23 years of close study. The discovery of Chiropractic has been commensurate with its development; as discovered it was developed. This D. C. would have his readers believe that the discovery consisted of "accidentally finding a bump on a man's back."

## NERVES AND BONES.

Chiropractors are especially interested in nerves and bones. By the nervous system we become cognizant of our surroundings, because of impressions made upon their peripheral endings. It is through them that we regard the outer world. By the knowledge thus derived we are able to adapt ourselves to our environments, receive sensations and direct motions. By a knowledge of their ramifications and functions Chiropractors are enabled to reinstate tone by placing this system of nerves in a normal position and relation. All parts of the body are intelligently connected by the bodily functions acting as a unit through this nervous system. It is through the nerves that all functions and actions are conducted; they are the channels of communication through which life is manifested and maintained.

The central nervous system exercises control over its nerve endings in the periphery. The cerebro-spinal nerves, even to their twig ends, do not anastomose, run together as one; the sympathetic nerves frequently do. While the spinal nerves very often send back recurrent nerves to the membranes of the spinal cord, the sympathetic ganglia never return any fibers to the central system. The cerebro-spinal nerves are distributed to the sensory surface, the organs of special sense, the voluntary muscles and the projection system of nerve-fibre tracts in the brain, by means of which external objects are brought into consciousness. The sympathetic fibers go to the involuntary muscles of the viscera, blood vessels and the lymphatic system. The nervous system permeates every portion of the body. The nerves divide and sub-divide into smaller branches until the division results in individual nerve fibers, and then these bifurcate repeatedly before they terminate in their twig ends. So intimate and extensive are the nerves distributed throughout the body that if all the other tissues of the body were dissolved there would be left, in gossamer form and bodily shape, a phantom of the cadaver.

Of the lymphatic, adipose, alimentary, vascular, dermoid, glandular, muscular and nervous systems, the latter, anatomically and functionally is the most highly developed and definitely distributed. A knowledge of this fact is very important to the Chiropractor.

The bones are the framework of the body. We owe to them, in a great measure, our shape and vigor. By their arrangement the viscera are maintained in proper position, one which is neither lax nor tense. By their displacement nerves may become tense by being stretched; bones being the only hard substance which will not yield. On the contrary, they displace the soft tissue in proportion to their own displacement. Thus by bone displacement nerves are injured, weakened or animated more than normal; either of which conditions cause too much or not enough functionating, a condition we name disease. So, to a Chiropractor, life depends upon the ability of Innate Intelligence to send out and receive messages in a correct manner, as the lines of communication may be interrupted by impingement because of displacement of any one of the bones which form the skeletal frame. The first and second pair of spinal nerves pass out through grooves —lengthened foramina, so as to permit the rotary movements of the atlas.

With the evolution of man the nervous system and the skeletal bones have undergone remarkable changes. There are no two persons formed alike in their osseous and nervous makeup. There are no two bones exactly alike, no two articular surfaces, outside of those which belong to each other, that will accurately fit. The spinal cord of the adult extends downward to the second lumbar vertebra, but occasionally to only the last thoracic. We find an occasional increase or decrease in the number of vertebrae in a column; there is always a corresponding variation in the number of spinal nerves, which may make a similar difference in the sympathetic and cranial nerves. These variations make it impossible and inexpedient for Chiropractors to confine themselves to any set rules; but by understanding Chiropractic principles of the nervous system in health and disease, impinged, sensitive branches can be located and followed, although in no two persons do the same nerves ramify the same tissue.

There are forty-two pairs of cerebro-spinal nerves; thirty are attached to the spinal cord and twelve to the encephalon. The spinal nerves have two roots. The sensory is ganglionated and afferent, it needs the ganglion to sense the incoming messages The dorsal roots of the thirty spinal pairs of nerves have 653,627 root fibers, the ventral 233,700; the proportion being 3.2 to 1.

The area of distribution of the spinal nerves is very variable, some nerves usually found are absent in some subjects. While each nerve has its own prescribed course of sensation and motion, no one has a definite area of distribution.

The nervous system is the first in the embryo to assume form and function. The remainder of the bodily organism is formed through and by it.

In order that we may more fully comprehend the great difference in our nervous construction, we will cull from Gray and Morris a few of the exceptions to the general rule.

Besides the thirty pairs of spinal nerves are two rudimantary relics of a tailed, vertebrate ancestry. Sometimes below the usual spinal nerves there are one or two pairs of filaments which do not pass out of the vertebral canal. The sensory root of the coccygeal nerve is also quite frequently absent. The dorsal root of the sub-occipital nerve may be rudimentary or lacking. It occasionally gives a cutaneous branch to the skin of the upper part of the back of the neck and the lower part of the scalp. Occasionally the ventral cutaneous of the first thoracic nerve is wanting. The first intercostal nerve, as a rule, gives off no lateral cutaneous branch, but, sometimes, a small filament communicates from it with the intercosto-bracial. Occasionally the lateral branch of the last thoracic nerve is absent and its place is taken by the iliac branch of the ilio-hypogastric. In such cases, the communicating nerve from the last thoracic to the first lumbar nerve is larger than usual. The first intercostal nerve frequently receives a connecting twig from the second thoracic nerve. The last thoracic is frequently connected with the first lumbar nerve by a slender branch. The ilio-inguinal nerve arises principally from the first lumbar nerve, but it frequently contains fibers of the last thoracic nerve. Sometimes the ilio-inguinal nerve is very small, and ends by joining the ilio-hypogastric. In such cases a branch from the ilio-hypogastric takes the place of the ilio-inguinal, or the latter nerve occasionally communicates with a branch of the long saphenous nerve. The accessory obturator nerve arises from the third or fourth or from the third and fourth lumbar nerves. It is not always present, sometimes it is very small, and becomes lost in the capsule of the hip-joint. It is present in about ten per cent of the cases examined. The anterior branch of the obturator nerve occasionally has a communicating branch to the internal cutaneous and sphenous nerves. When this branch is small, its place is supplied by the internal cutaneous nerve. A cutaneous branch is frequently given off from the muscular nerve of the ventral division of the sacral nerves, though sometimes from the pudic. It is often closely associated with the obturator nerve to the level of the brim of the pelvis. The lumbo-sacral trunk is usually formed by the union of the smaller part of the fourth and the entire fifth lumbar nerves. Sometimes the larger part of the fourth nerve may help to form the trunk. It may receive fibers from the third lumbar nerve or be formed entirely from the fifth. The sacral plexus is usually composed of the ventral divisions of the second, third, fourth and fifth sacral nerves, and the coccyx receive fibres from the third lumbar nerve or is formed entirely from the pudendal plexus which has its origin in common with the nerves of the sacral plexus. The division of the great sciatic nerve may take place at any point between the sacral plexus and the lower third of the thigh. This, when apparently single, is really two nerves appearing as one. The lateral cutaneous branch of the common peroneal nerve occasionally exists as a separate branch. The ultimate distribution of the twigs connected with the sympathetic and the vagus is not known. The phrenic nerve usually receives a twig from the third and another from the fifth cervical nerve, a small communicating branch from the sympathetic, and, rarely, a branch from the vagus. The twig from the fifth cervical is frequently connected with the nerve to the subclavius. As a rule the right phrenic branch divides into two main terminal branches. The brachial plexus is usually joined by small communicating twigs from the fourth cervical and second thoracic nerves. The fifth and sixth nerves of this plexus often unite before branching and dispose of their posterior branches as a common trunk, and the eighth often receives its communication from the first thoracic nerve before giving off its posterior branch. The branches of this plexus are given either from the roots above the clavicle, or from the cords behind and below the clavicle. The long thoracic nerve usually arises, by the roots, from the fifth, sixth and seventh cervical nerves. The last is sometimes missing. The nerve to the subclavius is a small twig which arises from the fifth nerve or from the upper trunk of the plexus, but occasionally it receives additional fibers from the fourth and sixth nerves. It sometimes gives off a communicating branch to the phrenic. In rare cases the entire phrenic nerve may pass by the way of the nerve to the subelavius. The medial brachial cutaneous nerve sometimes contains fibers from the eighth cervical and first thoracic nerves, but usually fibers from the first thoracic alone. This nerve may be absent, its place being taken by the intercosto-braciai or by part of the posterior, brachial cutaneous branch of the radial, or, rarely, by a branch from the first intercostal nerve. The radial nerve is the largest branch of the bhachial plexus. It contains fibers from the sixth, seventh and eighth cervical nerves, and sometimes from the fifth cervical and first thoracic nerves. The median nerve contains fibers from the sixth, seventh and eighth cervical nerves and the first thoracic, and, sometimes, from the fifth cervical nerve. The first thoracic nerve frequently receives a communication from the second nerve; in some instances it gives off a lateral cutaneous branch. The intercosto-brachial may divide into a small anterior and a large posterior division, or the anterior division may be absent. When the latter nerve is lacking, the intercosto-brachial usually takes its place. The lumbo-sacral plexus, in about half of the cases, receives a branch from the twelfth thoracic nerve. The first three lumbar nerves and the greater part of the fourth enter into the formation of the lumbar plexus, the smaller part of it and the fifth nerve commonly uniting to form the lumbo-sacral cord. It is subject to considerable variation in the manner of its formation. The slighter degrees of variableness may consist only of changes in the size of the portions contributed by the different spinal nerves to a given peripheral nerve, and a smaller share from a more distal nerve, or vice versa. In the more noticeable deviation, the origin of a given peripheral nerve may vary in either direction to the extent of one spinal nerve. The extreme types of the plexuses are sometimes associated with abnormal condition of the vertebral column. The ilio-hypogastric nerve springs from the first lumbar nerve, after the latter has been joined by the communicating branch from the last thoracic nerve, as found in about fifty per cent of cases; it frequently communicates with the last thoracic and the ilio-inguinal nerve. The lateral cutaneous nerve frequently receives some fibers from the first lumbar. The nerve to the articularis genu, usually a terminal branch of the femoral, frequently arises from the nerve to the vastus intermedius. This nerve is represented by two or three branches which enter the upper part of the muscle. One of them very often sends a twig to the knee joint. The obturator nerve sometimes receives fibers from the first and third lumbar nerves. It divides into two branches, the anterior branch forming a communication with the accessory obturator nerve, if that nerve is present. The articular branch of the obturator nerve is not uncommonly missing. Occasionally the posterior branch of the obturator nerve also supplies a twig to the hip-joint. The middle cervical ganglion of the sympathetic ganglionic cord is sometimes entirely absent. The number of the sympathetic ganglia is not always the same; sometimes an accessory ganglion is found, or a normal one is divided.

The sacral plexus has its variations, similar to the lumbar. It has seven types of arrangements; this includes the sciatic nerve. The pudendal plexus, the external genital, varies greatly in its formation.

Thus we might give the variations in the cranial and sympathetic nerves. But enough has been given of the spinal nerves for the student to understand that no set rules can be made for tracing or adjusting, on account of irregularities. He can, however, learn to trace sensitive nerves to and from displaced articular surfaces, which chafe, rub, or press against the side of the sheath forming the filaments, as we move that portion of the body where the pressure against nerves cause them to become limpid, or swollen and tense, drawing vertebrae and other joints out of alignment.

While anatomists divide the nervous system into the cranial, spinal and sympathetic, it suits Chiropractors better to consider a certain portion under the care of educated and the balance as belonging to Innate, as these two intelligences care for their respective lines of communication.

A plexus is where two or more nerves communicate, come together, then branch off to their respective terminations. These branches are composed of filaments of the primary trunks which form it. The two series of ganglia receive their filaments from the spinal cord. A portion of the nerves which emerge from the spinal foramina go to and enter the two chains of sympathetic ganglia; they control the nerves of organic life which include the arterial, venous and the lymphatic circulation, respiration, nutrition and all the vital processes.

The efferent nerves transmit impulses from the brain to their peripheral endings which excite muscular contraction. and influence the vegetative functions.

Nerves are distributive and communicative. The former supply the internal organs and the coats of the blood vessels with life force. The latter become enrapport, change their filaments more or less with each other, reinforce the receiver with either motor or sensory nerves which it stands in need of, and the giver can spare, thereby economizing space by running sensory and motor fibers in the same sheath. Communicating nerves. rami communicantes, communicating branches. whether they be motory or sensory, are those which go to, and join, other nerves, entering their sheath and sharing in common, the same covering. But the functions of the different filaments do not become blended, for each fiber carries its own impulse from center to periphery or vice versa.

The above variations will, in a measure, explain why the principles of Chiropractic have to be learned as a practitioner would gain information concerning any other profession; why he should have a knowledge of anatomy, more especially of nerves and bones; why a "key" is both a fraud and a graft.

---

Every Chiropractor should be well versed in the principles of Chiropractic.

---

"If I cut off your head, you die. Did you die with an organic disease or a function?" Neither. Decapitation eliminated the three essential functions which are essential to life (not health in this instance), circulation, respiration and innervation.

## CHIROPRACTIC HISTORY.

The following is copied from the Second Edition of the Annual Announcement of The Palmer School of Chiropractic, Davenport, Iowa:

"Dr. D. D. Palmer occupies the enviable position of being the discoverer and developer of the **only system of adjustment,** fixing what is wrong."

"He was born of humble parentage, reared in an atmosphere of independence and self-reliance; he never failed to think and delve where others failed to penetrate into the mysteries of the cause of disease."

"Within him were combined the rare qualities of **genius** and the ability to do hard work. There were others who were similarly gifted, but **none possessed that peculiar quality needed to originate and develop such a system.** No sooner did he become fully convinced of the vast importance of this method, than his attention was turned to the problem of how it would be best to fit others, so that they, too, could do what he was doing. **Hard work,** time and **genius was the solution.** He set about his task with no thought but that of success."

"Today he is at the head of a well-organized school, teaching a science that will do more to bless humanity than all the methods of therapeutics that have been promulgated. He creates an enthusiasm in those which are around him; he inspires a spirit of ambition which have for ages enshrouded the hidden cause of disease."

"**No one can possess the same depth of knowledge of a science as the person who discovered and originated it; no one can possess the same peculiar ability to impart that knowledge to others.**"

"Those who know the value of getting their information first-handed will appreciate what it means to study the different branches of Chiropractic **under the founder and originator** of this unequaled science."

We copy the above with pleasure and gladly give it space. D. D. Palmer is the creator of the science and art of vertebral adjustment. This "master mind" who "originated" the science and developed the art of adjusting is now rounding out, finishing up his work. The Adjuster is giving to the world these advanced thoughts and finishing touches.

On page 153 is a picture of "Dad Chiro" as he may be seen daily, preparing copy for The Adjuster. The Underwood typewriter records his thoughts. Behind him stands his ever-willing wife, to whom the readers owe much, for all copy is submitted to her as soon as written. She assists in cutting out personalities, smoothing down the rough places.

A Chiropractor of Oskaloosa, Iowa, says: "A correct diagnosis made without asking a question. It's wonderful." It certainly is wonderful how little some Chiropractors know.

He says: "The spinal nerves are pinched at their exit of the intervertebral foramen." Get a move on you; read the Adjuster; be up to date on Chiropractic.

He uses the illustrations of the tree and spinal cord; showing limbs and nerves pinched.

To clinch the whole as being Chiropractic, he states, "Article by Dr. D. D. Palmer, Discoverer and Developer of Chiropractic."

---

Normal tissue produces normal functionating. Normal functionating creates normal tissue. The two conditions are inseparable. We cannot have abnormal tissue without abnormal functionating. Abnormal functionating produces abnormal tissue; they are concomitant.

---

Spirit, soul, mind and body—four different entities. The first three are imponderable; the last ponderable. The first three cannot be weighed on scales, the latter can be.

Spirit is God, the Eternal, the All Wise, the Universal Intelligence.

Soul is life directed by an intelligence. The intelligence is the mind directed by Innate or Spirit.

Vital functions constitute life. They create vegetative functions. Vital functions are an expression of the soul. The soul owes its existence to the spirit. The spirit can exist without the soul or body. The soul is dependent upon both spirit and body.

Mind is dual in its nature; it is intelligence expressed by individualized spirit. Spirit furnishes mental force to run the vital and intellectual functions. The vital functions cause vegetative growth. The accumulated intelligence is acquired by the intellectual functions.

The body is a physical structure of fixed shape. It is supported by a bony frame-work, having within it an assemblage of related organs, which in health, work in harmony. A body has a vascular, nervous, lymphatic, alimentary, dermoid, glandular, muscular and kinesodic system whether dead or alive.

Spirit, soul and mind are distinct from matter. Spirit can exist without matter. Mind depends upon individualized spirit—Innate—for its existence. Soul is that which unites the immaterial spirit with the physical body.

## NEUROLOGY—CHEMISTRY.

Neurology states: "As all heat (page 505) is due to molecular change or friction, or chemical changes, it is very reasonable to attribute the cause of fever to bi-chemical changes, causing increased molecular action."

While it is true that **heat is generated by** both **molecular and chemical change,** there is a vast difference between these two forces, which are in no way related to or responsible for each other.

**Molecular** action creates heat, the amount being determined by the quantity of **atomic friction. Chemical heat is induced by combination** of substances of varying qualities.

Molecular change creates heat by and thru the **force of gravitation** acting upon particles of matter without reference to their character. There is another form of force found in the realm of atoms, which is effective **between** the atoms of **chemically different bodies, namely, chemical affinity.**

**Mechanical action and chemical combination create heat, but by quite a different process.**

**Gravitation and affinity** are very different forces.

Molecular change of atoms is operated upon by **interaction of forces, while chemical change,** known as **chemism, is dependent upon elective attraction, affinity,** the tendency or ability of one substance to unite with another.

The force which unites the particles of any body is known as **gravitation**; that which **combines,** fuses, **two or more** bodies of different natures into one is called chemical affinity.

The molecular or anatomic friction creates heat by **vibration** of its particles. In a chemical process, when affinities are satisfied, heat is set free — generated by the **force of unition** because of their affinity.

**These two forces, gravitation and affinity,** are present in the human body and the chemical laboratory. The former is operated by an **intelligent vital force,** which I saw fit to name Innate—born with. The chemical is directed by the **educated mind of man.** One is governed by an **unerring intelligence**; the other is **laboratory experimentation.** These two branches of knowledge are known as **metabolism and chemism.** The laws of **gravitation and affinity** are present in both. **Innate Intelligence runs the former** and a **chemist, one given to** chemical investigation, one versed in chemistry, **the latter.**

**Adhesion** (molecular gravitation) and **chemism,** the force exerted between the atoms of elementary substances, whereby they unite to form chemical compounds, are quite different attractions.

A laboratory is the workroom of a chemist, a place devoted to experiments.

I think it will be readily seen, that **all changes in the body are molecular** and **those in the laboratory are chemical. Molecular action, therefore, is not caused by chemical or bi-chemical changes. Molecular and chemical changes are in no way related to or dependent upon each other.**

**It is not reasonable, logical or within the realm of facts, to state that chemical or bi-chemical changes cause increased molecular action, inflammation or fever.**

If an undue amount of heat is confined in one locality of the body, it is known as inflammation. If this elevation of temperature is generally diffused thruout the body it is termed fever.

In health, heat production and heat dissipation are evenly balanced. In fever, the body is in a large measure incapacitated for normal activity, anabolism is decreased and katabolism is increased. The pores of the protecting covering of the body are closed, preventing the escape of the superabundant heat. In health, if heat production is increased, so also is heat dissipation. Under normal conditions there can be no elevation of temperature, or an accumulation of heat.

Fever is an overproduction of heat retained in the body by the closing of the pores of the cuticle.

---

"Lack of current is the cause of disease."

A current is a body of fluid moving continuously in a certain direction. Thus, we have currents of water, air and electricity. In the body, we have the blood current. If the author of the above quotation was an osteopath, I would think, he referred to the blood current, as that is the only current in the body. The author being a Chiropractor certainly did not refer to blood. In disease, the blood current may be diminished or increased. I am inclined to think the author had in mind transmission of impulses; if so, impulses do not flow as a current. **An impulse is a thot impelled or driven onward with force.** Thots are things which are transmitted by vibration; in the body, by nerve vibration; externally, by ether vibration. The force of an impulse depends upon the amount of vibration; the speed of transmission determining the momentum of impulses.

---

Howe says: "Esquirol possessed the skeleton of a woman, in which the traces of more than two hundred fractures could be counted." She was all broken up.

## THE TONGUE.

The tongue and heart are the only organs which have a body, a base and an apex. The tongue is the only portion of the body that has a special sense, motion and ordinary sensation. It is capable of assuming a greater variety of shapes and motions than any other organ. During mastication it keeps the food between the opposing surfaces of the teeth. With the saliva it forms the particles of food into a bolus, transfers it backward and into the pharynx for deglution. Its varied movements are controlled by the longitudinal lingual, transverse lingual, geniohyoid, mylohyoid, genioglossus, hyoglossus. chondroglossus, styloglossus and plataoglossus muscles. Most of these are attached to the hyoid bone, so that by its elevation, depression, forward and backward movement, the muscles of the tongue are in a great measure controlled. It will be observed that the hyoid bone contributes largely to the use of the tongue.

The hyoid bone's functions are somewhat similar to a derrick. It has no immediate relation with the bones of the skeleton; it lies in the soft parts of the neck and possesses great mobility; it is slung from the styloid processes of the temporal bones by the stylo-hyoid ligaments. Inferiorly it is connected with the thyroid cartilage of the larynx by the thyro-hyoid ligaments and membranes. Posterior it is intimately associated with the epiglottis. The cartilage which joins the lesser cornua of the hyoid process in early embryonic life, eventually becomes converted into the stylo-hyoid ligament. It is not uncommon to find this ligament ossified in some part of its extent, and occasionally in its entirety, as shown by a specimen in my possession, in which this process is replaced by a styloid ossified ligament which articulates with the temporal and hyoid bones.

The muscles of the hyoid bone and the tongue are for the most part supplied with innervating nerves from the hypoglossal and the ansa cervicals (a loop which takes in the first, second and third cervical nerves). It will readily be seen and understood by those Chiropractors who have been students of the Adjuster, that paralysis of the tongue as noticed in speech and swallowing, might be looked for in one of the ansa cervicals; that the displacement of any one of the first cervicals might produce a large portion of the inflammatory and paralytic conditions. Inflammation of the tongue is known as glossitis.

To make a success of Chiropractic, we should know it as a science and the art of specific adjusting.

To be able to locate the cause of disease, we must become acquainted with the principles of Chiropractic; practice and knowledge, will give us skill in adjusting. We should know that all vital and mental functions are the result of impulses sent out by the Innate through 43 pair of nerves; 12 cranial, 8 cervical, 12 dorsal, 5 lumbar, 5 sacral and one cocygeal; that when functions are performed in a normal manner, as Innate desires, we have health; that each of the 86 cranial and spinal nerves contain fibers which ramify certain portions of the body; that conditions known as health and disease depends upon the condition of these nerves; that a pressure on a nerve deranges the impulses sent out through it by changing the shape and size of its tubes which contain functionating filaments; that all there is of disease is too much or not enough functionating. For example: diabetes is an over-action of the kidneys yet, not a disease of the kidneys, but of other organs. Bright's disease is under-action; each disease having its special symptoms. If we can place the innervating nerves of the kidneys in a normal condition, so that Innate can send out impulses without hindrance, functions will be performed in a normal manner—which is health.

The Indian said that a white man was like a loaf of bread not baked; that the negro was like a loaf of bread all burnt black, but the Indian was just right, just baked brown. Thus it is with disease and health; disease burnt black or insufficiently baked; health just baked brown.

Remember that we are building a science. Consequently the more knowledge we have of the principles upon which that science and its philosophy is founded, the more we shall know it as a science.

---

Toronto, Canada, March 12, 1909.

Dear D. D. Palmer:

I am glad The Adjuster is out for the purpose of bringing into proper relation portions of anatomy which have been displaced by others. I hope to God to see your task accomplished soon.

Stick to your announced principles and yours will be the recognized school. Keep it free from anything which savors of graft or quackery.

The people are waking up to modern methods; it will not be long until legislatures hum with Chiros.

The Adjuster shows which is which — where the genuine Chiropractic school is located. The founder of any system has to come out good and strong these days. Yours for pure Chiro.

T. M. WOODHOUSE, M. D.
52 Cecil Street.

## THE STEAM PIPE.

The sympathetic nervous system consists of nerves and nerve ganglia, connected in most vertebrates with the alimentary canal, the vascular system and the glandular organs and controls, in a greater or less degree, their activity. I think the axial part of the system and its principal ganglia and nerves are situated in the four cavities of the body; they form a chain of ganglia, on each side of the vertebral column which are connected with numerous other ganglia and nerve plexuses.

This part of the nervous system has been named sympathetic because it was supposed by all schools that this system conveys sympathy, sympathetic impulses, from one portion of the body to another; that there is a mutual relation between certain parts, more or less distant, whereby a morbid change in one has an effect upon the other.

Chiropractic has accepted the distribution of nerves and the names as known by anatomists, and explains this apparent sympathy, why two or more organs or parts may be affected at the same time or continuously from one and the same cause. From the nerve-trunk branches continue to pass off, some to one portion and some to another. This nerve-trunk filled with fibers may be impinged upon by a displaced bone. This hard, unyielding substance striking against one side of this sheath causes the carrying capacity, conducting power of the various filaments pressed against, to become greater or less according to the degree of pressure they severally receive. A slight change in the position of the bone pressing against this sensitive bundle of fibrilla, may change the impingement from one or more filaments to others. If so, there will be a corresponding change in the portion of the body affected. Whenever a bone strikes against a nerve trunk or a nerve branch the nerve is impinged upon. It is not squeezed, pinched, compressed or constricted. To cause the three former conditions, the nerve must be confined between two hard substances. A nerve cannot be constricted by the pressure of two bones, by the closing of two notches of an intervertebral foramen, or by that of two grooves. Neither of these conditions would constrict or bind a nerve in a circular direction, as would a ligature. To say that a membrane of tubular form where its cavity is filled with nerve filaments, or a pipe conveying steam or water, can be constricted by the pressure of two hard, opposing substances, betrays as much ignorance of the English language and a lack of judgment in making comparisons, as did the assertion of the man who said that a cloud burst and let out all of the water. He should have captured the empty cloud and hung it on the fountain which adorns his letter head. It is equally inconsistent to state that a pipe is not a steam pipe because it is not made of steam. It is called a steam pipe because it conveys steam. A water pipe is so named because it carries water. We would not for a moment think of denying the existence of those pipes because they were so named.

The **sympathetic** nervous system was so named because it was thought to convey sympathy, or impulses, from one nerve to another. The cranial nerves receive their name because they belonged, and were confined to, the cranium. The steam and water pipes exist and will continue to perform their offices. The cranial and sympathetic nerves will continue to direct vital functions despite the anathemas hurled against them and their excommunication; forcibly expressed, by their erasure from a wax model.

It is better that we, as Chiropractors, learn how and why there exists the seeming sympathy between certain portions of the body.

When we can illustrate by actual demonstration that by the replacing of one vertebra we remove the cause of two or more diseased portions of the body, that instead of being in sympathy with each other, the affected nerves arise from one nerve trunk, that because of a displaced bone certain nerves were impinged upon, and that by removing the impingement, we restore co-ordination in more than one affected part; we have demonstrated that tension and laxity are the causes of disease, and how to reduce tension and take up the slackness of fibrous tissue.

---

Speaking of paradoxes; did you ever notice how slow time flies in fly time?

---

A certain would-be developer eliminates the sympathetic nervous system runs the twelve cranial nerves from the cervical vertebrae, where they originate, to their organs (?), they have but three—ear, nose and eye—and from thence to the brain. To use his own language, "obliterating the 'sympathetic nervous system' knocks the props of 'reflex action,' which is supposed to be the movement that takes place within this starting from somewhere—and going to nowhere system." That such teaching should be palmed off as Chiropractic I consider shameful. We have elsewhere shown what and where the sympathetic nervous system is. We also endeavor to throw the same Chiropractic light of reason on "reflex action." "Remember, boys, greater movements, all realities of life are based around simple principles. To act big when you have nothing behind it is but to heap ridicule upon your empty craniums."

## DRUG IDIOSYNCRACIES.

In the absorption and assimilation of drugs, idiosyncracies are often noted. In fact, they are so common that we can almost say that no one drug acts in the same degree or manner upon different individuals. In some instances the untoward action assumes such a serious aspect as to render extreme caution necessary in the administration of the most inert substances. A medicine ordinarily so bland as cod-liver oil may give rise to disagreeable eruptions. Christian speaks of a boy ten years old who was said to have been killed by the ingestion of two ounces of Epsom salts without inducing purgation; yet this common purge is universally used without the slightest fear or caution. On the other hand, the extreme tolerance exhibited by certain individuals to certain drugs offers a new phase of this subject. There are well-authenticated cases on record in which death has been caused in children by the ingestion of a small fraction of a grain of opium. While exhibiting especial tolerance from peculiar disposition and long habit, Thomas De Quincey, the celebrated English litterateur, makes a statement in his "Confessions" that, with impunity, he took as much as 320 grains of opium a day and was accustomed at one period of his life to call every day for "a glass of laudanum negus, warm, and without sugar," to use his own expression, after the manner a toper would call for a "hot-scotch."

The individuality noted in the assimilation and the ingestion of drugs is functional as well as anatomic. Numerous cases have been seen by all physicians. The severe toxic symptoms from a whiff of cocain-spray, the acute distress from the tenth of a grain of morphin, the gastric crises and profuse uticarial eruptions following a single dose of quinin—all are proofs of it. The "personal equation" is one of the most important factors in therapeutics, reminding us of the old rule, "Treat the patient, not the disease."

The idiosyncracy may be either temporary or permanent, and there are many conditions that influence it. The time and place of administration; the degree of pathologic lesion in the subject; the difference in the physiologic capability of individual organs of similar nature in the same body; the degree of human vitality influencing absorption and resistance; the peculiar epochs of life; the element of habituation and the grade and strength of the drug influencing its virtue—all have an important bearing upon both the untoward action and tolerance of poisons.

I have taken the foregoing information from Gould and Pyle's Anomalies of Medicine.

In confirmation of the above statements, they give thirteen pages of the idiosyncracies of twenty-seven drugs, from which I cannot take room to quote but one, carbolic acid, which is known, also, by the name of phenol. This substance is procured from coal tar by fractional distillation. It has a very peculiar and characteristic odor, a burning taste, is poisonous and has preservative qualities. It is used in vomiting, intestinal fermentation and as an antiseptic.

Gould and Pyle state: "In recent years the medical profession has become well aware that in its application to wounds it is possible for carbolic acid or phenol to exercise exceedingly deleterious and even fatal consequences. In the earlier days of antisepsis, when operators and patients were exposed for some time to an atmosphere saturated with carbolic spray, toxic symptoms were occasionally noticed. Kohler mentions the death of a man suffering from scabies who had applied externally a solution containing about a half-ounce of phenol. Rose says gangrene of the finger appeared after the application of carbolized cotton to a wound thereon. In some cases phenol acts with a rapidity equal to any poison. Taylor speaks of a man who fell unconscious ten seconds after an ounce of phenol had been ingested and in three minutes was dead. There is recorded an account of a man of sixty-four who was killed by a solution containing slightly over a dram of phenol. A half ounce has frequently caused death; small quantities have been followed by distressing symptoms, such as intoxication (which Olshausen has noticed to follow irrigation of the uterus), delirium, singultus, nausea, rigors, cephalagia, tinnitus aurium and anasarca. Hind mentions recovery after the ingestion of nearly six ounces of crude phenol of 14 per cent strength."

I have made the above quotation, in order to illustrate its application Chiropractically.

A few years ago I was called to see a student who had taken carbolic acid with suicidal intent. An adjustment, in the presence of the clinic, of one vertebra—the 6th dorsal—gave instant relief. On the following day he repeated the dose and I the adjustment, which gave the same relief as the day before; but, on the next and third day I was out of the city. I arrived in time to find him in convulsions.

Dunglison's Dictionary gives "a strictly physiological classification of drugs, substances employed as medicines in the cure of disease."

Drugs are pathological in their action on the nervous system; they are given to produce a change in function. Any act of the nervous system which accomplishes vital phenomena is a function. Any substance which causes a change in function is pathological in its action. In our nervous makeup, no two of us are alike; therefore, the difference in the effects of ingesta on the nervous system. That which is considered food for one is an irritant, a poison, for another. Drugs not only change functions, but, also, the anatomical structure; they are disease producing in their action upon both function and tissue.

"Personal equation" is a factor in therapeutics which cannot be positively foretold, because of personal idiosyncracies in the nervous makeup of individuals, and also because of variations in the quality of the nervous system of the same individual at different periods. I would say, "Adjust the bony framework of the patient to normal, instead of treating the disease."

Poisons are those substances which destroy life or impair one or more functions of the body, no matter by what avenue they may be introduced. These pathological changes and results are made in a healthy body; not by traumatic injuries.

Pathologists divide poisons into two classes; irritants and neurotics; an irritant poison causes irritation, pain, heat and tension of the nervous system. Neurotics are those drugs which have special influence upon the nervous system. Either class modifies functions. All poisons act on the nervous system as an irritant or a lenitive. By their action they draw vertebrae out of alignment. Poisons may be antidotal—having a tendency to draw vertebrae in an opposite direction to that of another poison for which it is given to counteract. The Chiropractor, instead of using a counter-irritant or a lenitive drug, accomplishes the same purpose sooner and without danger by adjusting the displaced vertebra by hand.

The bony and cartilaginous structure of the body—the endoskeleton—holds the soft parts which the nervous system ramifies in position. The disarrangement of any portion of this skeletal frame, displaces the soft tissue attached, in which certain nerves are located. The adjusting of the bones, together with the soft tissue, rearranges the nervous system so that normal action is restored.

---

"Medical chemistry." Medical, pertaining to medicine. Medicine, any drug or remedy. Chemistry, the science which treats of the elements and atomic relations of matter and of the various compounds of the elements. These two words are incongruous, inharmonious in the above combination. They are incompatible one with the other. They do not conform or agree with each other. Their connection is not suitable or agreeable. Medical science and chemistry are entirely and distintly two separate and unconnected sciences.

## DATES MIXED.

"The Palmer School of Chiropractic was established 1885." On page 18, "The P. S. C. was founded in 1885; twenty-three years experience." Page 25, we are told, "The P. S. C. . . . twenty-three years' existence." Page 27, "The P. S. C. located in Davenport **since** 1885." Page 56, "The Palmer School has been in active service for nine years." Page 107, "The P. S. C., during thirteen years' existence."

The first Chiropractic adjustment was given in September, 1895; see the History of Chiropractic, Vol. I, No. 1, page 11.

The earliest graduates of Chiropractic were A. P. Davis, 1898; Wm. A. Seeley, 1898; O. G. Smith, 1899; Helen De Lendrecie, 1899; Mrs. J. C. Bowman, 1899; M. P. Brown, 1899; Dr. Simon, 1899; O. B. Jones, 1900; T. H. Storey, 1901; S. M. Langworthy, 1901; Allen Raymond, 1901; E. E. Sutton, 1901; H. R. Stouder, 1901; B. J. Palmer, 1902.

How do these dates correspond with "1885?" There is a discrepancy of 13 years, if we count one student and one teacher as constituting a school. Three years after the first adjustment, the first student—B. J. was a student seven years after the first adjustment was given in September, 1895. B. J. passed an examination at the age of 20. The family register in the Good Book says: "Bartlett Joshua Palmer, born Sept. 10, 1882."

Page 6, 16th line from bottom. Make the "additions, subtractions and corrections," and see the result.

Page 7 tells us that B. J. Palmer is the author of Vol. I. The introduction of Vol. I says, "The Palmer School was named after the **honored discoverer**, Dr. D. D. Palmer . . . It shall always bear to him the **palm and token of appreciation**, deep feeling and **reverence for the man who discovered the cause of disease.**"

"To this man (Dr. D. D. Palmer) student, scientist and philosopher the world owes much. . . . His teachings, works and collections are represented in the P. S. C. only."

"To my **honored and devoted father** should be credited the bulk of responsibility for the issuance of this work. . . . I should come to the rescue with another article, which would prove the necessity of making this statement public.

I am the writer, the author of nearly every line in Vol. I.

I am the author of nearly every line in Vol. I.

The teachings of D. D. Palmer are not represented in the P. S. C. today (1910).

---

Why are cats like skilled surgeons? Because they mew-tilate and annoy our patience.

## CHIROPRACTIC ACROSTIC.

Chiropractic! What is it for?
Health restorer! And something more;
Invalid in body or mind,
Relief given, soon you will find.

Osteopathy—not up-to-date.
Physic and drugs eliminate,
Remove the cause of the disease;
Affect—a cure and give you ease;

Common sense should replace displaced;
The cause with the effect efface;
Ignorance to knowledge give place;
Cease old style, it is a disgrace.

—John Burrows, age 76, Portland, Ore., Dec. 10, 1908.

The above bouquet was presented to D. D Palmer near the close of his lecture and read on Dec. 10th, 1908.

---

## LONGER LIVES AND BETTER HEALTH.

There is much interest being manifested in regard to sanitation and health. Human life has already been lengthened. Smallpox, diphtheria, the itch and other zymodic diseases which are of filth origin, depending upon poison generated by decomposition, are now less severe, fatal and less frequent.

The treatments of physicians are more intelligent and humane, there being quite a contrast between the present and 100 years ago.

Cities and country homes are more sanitary, less filthy, cleaner, therefore healthier. We often think that we were born too soon, but no dog can choose his day. We are here making this trip which will never be made again, so let us each do the best we can.

Now, that we have learned the cause of disease—displacements of some part of the skeletal frame superinduced by accidents and poisons, we should make much more rapid strides toward health and longevity.

---

Vital functions. Vegetative functions. Food converted into tissue growth.

Animal functions. Consumative functions. Intellectual spirit growth.

## NAPRAPATHY.

The "Journal of the Society of Modern Research, with special articles on Naprapathy and other sciences," is the biggest little magazine I have seen.

This Journal is made of one sheet of four pages; all told, including the cover, the size of one leaf of The Adjuster. It is "Entered as second-class matter." It is not copyrighted.

The "special articles on Naprapathy and other sciences," with the general news, is contained in 43 lines.

The first "special article" has five lines. Four of which read: "Ninety per cent of all chronic disease is caused by 'tightened' ligaments in the spine." "90 per cent of chronic diseases all arise from **tightened spinal ligaments.**"

The next article we quote entire, as it is a "most valuable paper, contributed to the society by Dr. Oakley Smith."

"To the Bohemians is due the credit of discovering the **secret** of easily and quickly overcoming these tightened ligaments. Thus it was that they were able to bring about such astounding cures. This wonderful principle and method of the Bohemians has been highly developed within the last decade. Diseases that are conundrums to the ordinary methods are solved successfully by recent new discoveries and developments."

We are not informed who kept the secret a secret; it certainly was not a woman. But, "**thus it was** that the "conundrums" were easily and quickly solved, and the highly tightened ligaments successfully overcome by the wonderful, astounding, highly developed discoveries of this secret.

The next article informs us, "It is the **simplicity** of this method that **makes it so powerfully effective.**"

In the next item we are told, Dr. Oakley Smith will contribute most valuable papers to the society; his position "gives a unique force to what he may have to say."

An important news item states: "Furthermore, Dr. Smith is planning on spending the latter part of June, July and August in Europe, doing valuable research work for the society and science. The influence of the work of this society is rapidly spreading to every corner of the United States." Dr. Smith intends spending the **latter part** of these **three months** in Europe. Where does he intend spending the **fore part of each month?** I think, at home. As the United States has only four corners, the N. W., N. E., S. W. and S. E., it will "easily and quickly" spread to every corner.

---

Symptoms to a Chiropractor are sign-boards pointing to the location of the lesion.

## PAINLESS ADJUSTING.

Adjusting is an art. It is the application of Chiropractic knowledge in replacing displaced vertebrae. There is a vast difference in the ease with which the vertebrae of different persons are adjusted. Some can relax during adjustment, others will brace against the adjuster. Displaced vertebrae may be ankylosed by true or false ankylosis. The ankylosed tissue may be of a bony, cartilaginous or ligamentous nature. The displacements may be recent or of long standing. They may have been slowly or suddenly drawn out of alignment either by poison or by an accident. The vertebra may have kept its normal shape or it may have become deformed. All of these conditions must be taken into consideration; also, that some patients are more sensitive than others. Some adjusters have the knack of adjusting and others have not; some have the know how, while others think that the more strength they exert the better will be the adjustment.

Dr. Alma C. Arnold is said to be able to adjust vertebrae without any pain whatever. One who witnessed them says: "Her adjustments would hardly waken a sleeping child." I am told that she starts at the sacrum in all cases no matter what affection or vertebra has been displaced. She separates the sacro-lumbar articulations, then replaces them. She then loosens the articulations between the 4th and 5th lumbar and resets them. She thus continues from the sacrum to the occiput. She is said, also, to adjust ribs, tarsal bones, etc., that are out of joint. It is said that Dr. Arnold uses a movement that is more of a pressure than that taught by me for adjusting. It is said "There is no thrust or perceptible pressure." It is also said that when she separates and replaces the vertebrae, that the patient can hear and feel the movement of the processes as they disarticulate, this being the case along the whole of the spine with each and every vertebrae. The separating and replacing of vertebrae causes no pain whatever. She is said to be an adept at replacing the ribs and tarsal bones.

If Dr. Arnold has learned to handle vertebrae as readily as a Chinese lundryman does the balls on his abacus, or counting rack, it would be no more wonderful nor strange than was the moving of vertebrae by me fourteen years ago.

The above description of Dr. Arnold's adjusting was formulated after corresponding with several D. C.'s who saw her give adjustments. I thought then and do now know, that she was misunderstood, as evidenced by her letter which lies before me. In this she states that the above exposition of her adjusting is the most intelligent, except one; that she does make perceptible "pressure of from one pound on an infant to 125 pounds on a strong back." She further states, "My skill is shown by the fact that I give no more pressure than is needed to move the vertebrae; I give pressure rather than thrust. I know that my thrust is not entirely painless except on nearly normal spines. Old chronic luxations, I must hurt to some degree, but my work is as near 'painless' as is possible to make an adjustment of spinal luxations."

Dr. Arnold and I agree, in that skill in adjusting is shown by the ability of the adjuster to move vertebrae with the least force or pressure possible. She gives "pressure rather than thrust." I give thrust rather than pressure; that is, I find that the quicker the same amount of force or pressure is given, the more effectual is the result. I desire to move vertebrae with as little force as possible. In order to do so, the thrust must be made quickly, avoiding the push or shove.

I fail to see any special feature in Dr. Arnold's adjusting, except that she starts at the sacrum. Many Chiropractors adjust the entire spine as does Dr. Arnold, except that they start at the atlas and work downward instead of upward.

---

A "Chiopractic Spinologist" card reads: "Chiropractic (c-h-i-r-o-p-r-a-c-t-i-c) is the latest and most practical discovery of the age in restoring all the normal functions of the body. Abnormal function is caused by impinged nerves as they pass from the spinal cord thru the foramina in the (vertebra). Hence, the lack of expression, producing abnormal condition (poor health).

"The genuine Chiropractor does not treat, heal, rub or manipulate, but adjusts by hand. Chiropractic is purely a mechanical art."

"I have had quite a number come to me to fix their corns, bunions and ingrowing toe-nails."

I presume the writer of the above turned these cripples away without benefit to them or himself. I have taken in quite a number of dollars and relieved many of these cripples instead of sending them to the toe-butchers. Bunions and corns can be relieved by adjusting the contiguous joints. For those on the plantar surface, adjust the displaced tarsal bones. For ingrowing toe-nails adjust the last lumbar. Only last evening, I relieved a bad case of ingrowing toe-nails by one adjustment. Why not? Remember, that displaced bones press against, impinge upon nerves. If the nerves of the toes are impinged upon the above diseases occur.

## TYPHOID FEVER.

Its onset is gradual and insidious. The patient experiences chilly sensations, shivering and pronounced chills. He suffers from headache, his mental faculties are obtuse, he is unable to concentrate his thots with the usual vigor, he feels prostrated and languid. He experiences lack of appetite, nausea and even vomiting. In the early stage there is a tendency to diarrhea which becomes pronounced as the disease advances. Usually there is backache and a slight cough.

The recognition of typhoid fever does not depend upon one or two special symptoms, but upon the grouping of several, some of which may be absent.

As the disease progresses, the patient becomes listless and stupid; he answers questions incoherently. A muttering delirium becomes constant. He makes feeble efforts to get out of bed. His ideas are disconnected.

There are exceptions to this rule. The patient may be active and boisterous. His delirium may take the shape of a delusion. He may be indifferent to physical comfort, and desire nothing, except to be let alone. Sight and hearing are commonly impaired.

The idiosyncracies found in typhoid cases, the characteristic peculiarities of variation in individuals in this and other diseases, are accounted for by the difference in the nervous structure: no two individuals sense poisons just alike.

Typhoid fever patients are unable to sleep. They may bleed at the nose. There is a tenderness in the right side and lower portion of the abdomen. The gums may become swollen and bleed readily upon pressure. Many cases show an eruption on the abdomen and chest consisting of a few scattered, red pimples. The spleen may become enlarged. There is fever, which increases each day until it reaches its maximum of 104 or 105 degrees. A degree of heat sufficient to soften the nerve tissue. It lowers each afternoon and raises during the fore part of the night. There is catarrhal inflammation. ulceration and necrosis of the intestinal mucous membrane. The abdomen becomes distended with gas, and a peristaltic movement may be felt by pressing over the right groin. The patient's mouth is dry and parched; altho he endeavors to moisten his lips with his tongue, he does not ask for water. Flies creep over his face without any visible annoyance.

Etiology:—Typhoid fever is most abundant in the autumn, because of decaying animal and vegetable matter. This poison enters the body by inhalation, food or drink. The lesions of typhoid fever suggest an intense affection, constitutional poisoning.

Pathological Anatomy:—Widespread changes may occur in the lesions of the intestines as a result of the toxin introduced. There may be focal necrosis in the spleen or liver, degenerative changes in the kidneys, muscles and nerves, and the various glandular organs may become inflamed.

---

Chiropractic is economy; it was so built by its discoverer and founder.

---

Is the science of Chiropractic specific?

If it is not specific, it is not a science.

Science is knowledge reduced to regular rules and embodied in a system.

Art refers to something to be done; science to something to be known.

To have a knowledge of the principles of Chiropractic is to know it as a science.

To know how, the ability to make use of that knowledge is an art.

If Chiropractic embodies science and art, it must be knowledge reduced to certain rules and formulated into a system.

---

Osteopaths in the November number of the Osteopath Journal recommend mercuric and copper lotions for barbers itch. Nitric acid for warts. Hot air for arthritis. Salt water and lemon juice for constipation. Bi-chloride dressing for a scratch. Leucodesent Therapeutic Lamp for a swelling on the arm. Hot fomentations seasoned with red pepper, mustard and ground horse-radish for rheumatism. One writer has faith in X-ray treatment. Another relies a great deal on hydrotherapy, cascara sagrada and worm seed. One writer says, if antitoxin is one of Nature's remedies, it is osteopathic. An honest osteopath states, if he would only give lesional treatments his practice would go down to nothing in a short time. The treatment recommended for stammering is: have the patient speak slowly, tap on the floor with the foot, keeping time with the speaking of each word. One offers a solution of "one pound of Epsom salts, three ounces of borax to one gallon of water," and adds, "This is as good as anything the skin grafters can offer."

While we as Chiropractors may think the Osteopaths are using many adjuncts which are not osteopathic, we have nothing to say, for, are we not also "skin grafters" with our adjuncts?

## CHIROPRACTOR'S REQUIREMENTS.

Each school of practice should require of their graduates an examination based upon their future needs. Different schools modify their examinations every few years No change—no improvement. The old school of medicine must have had quite a different examination 200 years ago from that which it has now. Fifty years ago a knowledge of bleeding was considered essential. An examination a century ago would not be a standard for the same school today. There is fully as much difference in the schools of this advancing age as there has been in the past and present in the medical. Therefore, it would not be just nor in accord with the spirit of our age to give the same examination to all schools.

By the dozen or more schools of medicine, it would be thot there could be little or no variation in the teaching of anatomy. But for some reason there has been a great change in this branch in favor of Chiropractic. Thirteen years ago when I made my discovery of subluxations of vertebrae, Gray, a standard author, said, under the head of surgical anatomy: "The ligaments which unite the component parts of the vertebrae together, are so strong, and these bones are so interlocked by the arrangement of their articulating processes, that dislocation is very uncommon, and indeed, unless accompanied by fracture, rarely occurs, except in the upper part of the neck. Dislocation of the occiput from the atlas has only been recorded in one or two cases; but dislocation of the atlas from the axis, with rupture of the transverse ligament, is much more common, it is the mode in which death is produced in many cases of execution by hanging. In the lower part of the neck—that is, below the third cervical vertebrae—dislocation unattended by fracture, occasionally takes place."

Gray refers to a complete dislocation; in that he is correct. But since the advent of Chiropractic, that statement, altho true, is misleading. In reading the above quotation, we must consider that Gray refers to a complete luxation; he does not know of or recognize such a condition as a partial dislocation of vertebrae, a subluxation. Authors of standard text books desire to make such changes as will keep them abreast of the times, up-to-date. Since the advent of Chiropractic there has been a radical change in opinions among medical men in regard to dislocations of vertebrae. For some reason Gray has put in place of the above the following: "The main joints of which the spine is composed, together with the very varied movements to which it is subjected, render it liable to **sprains**, which may complicate other injuries;" that is, this lesion may make other morbid changes.

That which is known to a physician as a **sprain,** to a Chiropractor is a partial dislocation, a sub-luxation of vertebrae. That which is recognized today as a **sprain,** because of an overlift, or an unexpected jolt, a sudden shock or jerk which **strains** the spine, even to slipping a vertebrae ever so little, closes just so much of the foramina next above the vertebrae strained from its normal position. The result is an impingement of the nerve which before was free. This slight pressure irritates, excites, inflames the nerve. It becomes swollen and enlarged, filling its confines more fully; the walls of the foramen bind and compress it so much, that, altho, the foramen remains of the same restricting size, the enlarged overheated nerve is cramped in its passage from the spinal canal. That which was only a sprain becomes a lesion causing altered functions—disease.

Future copies of anatomies will contain a section on sub-luxation and its results.

Chiropractors have need of some branches of study not taught in other schools which are the outgrowth of this science. Among these are the art of nerve tracing and adjusting, discovered and brot to their present perfection by me. Chiropractic orthopedy and principles of Chiropractic are also peculiar to this science. Affected sensory nerves are traced externally in the living subject, and displaced vertebrae are replaced by hand adjusting. A knowledge of these two branches are prerequisite to success; they should be studied and practiced under a competent teacher. They are unknown in medical schools, therefore, are not taught by them. To realize the difference between a scientific adjuster and one who only knows enough to give a hand-thrust, one should take a hand-thrust and afterward an adjustment from Dr. Fite. He has had special instruction from the developer of this art. There is just as much difference in adjusters as in other lines of work. Some cannot, or will not get the knack of doing it just right; they will be awkward as long as they live, always doing as much harm as good. Dr. Fite's teacher points to him with pride as one of the best adjusters with the best results of any he has ever taught.

Chiropractors should make a special study of anatomy, more particularly that of osteology, neurology and arthrology. Bones, nerves and joints are to a Chiropractor what medicine, chemistry and bacteriology are to a physician.

Orthopedy has become a part of Chiropractic but with the difference that when Chiropractorized, it has but little or no resemblance to Medical orthopedy. A physician would not recognize nor own it.

Chiropractic is founded upon the principle that, all functions are performed thru nerves; that health is a condition where the controlling intelligence is able to send mental impulses outward thru nérves; that disease is a condition caused by bone pressure on nerves. This impingement creates aberration of nerve impulse.

Physiology is the science of the vital phenomena of organisms and of their relation to chemical and physical laws.

Innate (the intelligence born with us) runs the vital functions of the body with perfect precision, at birth and during life, providing that its impulses are not interfered with. This being the case, the intelligent director **knows all** about the running of the vital economy; it only remains for us as Chiropractors, fixers, adjusters, to learn the condition of nerves which favor health and **vice versa.** There is no more harm for a Chiropractor to be versed in physiology than in that of medicine, providing he does not hinder or disturb Innate in the performance of a work of which it knows much more than we can ever know. Educated Intelligence should learn to make it possible for Innate to have free control of all the vital functions. When we, as Chiropractors, have adjusted all displaced bones of the skeletal frame, made it possible for Innate to perform all the functions in a natural manner, what more can we do? What more should we do? We might as well try to inform the tree how to run the functions of its roots, bark, leaves and sap. The tree could well reply by saying, "I know better how to run the functions of my existence than you. Make my environments suitable and I will look after my vital economy." We can not impart information to Innate on a subject of which we know but little and of which it knows all. Innate has always existed; it is a scion of Universal Intelligence. We can no more direct the vital functions of the animal economy than we can that of the plant. Christion Scientists have made their success by saying to Educated, "Mind your own business, let the All-Wise-Goodness care for that of which it knows vastly more than perverted man will ever know. Eat what you want then attend to your intellectual pursuits, leaving digestion to the All-Wise; the digestive organs will care for its business. By constantly thinking about your digestion, what and how you shall eat, wondering whether your meal will hurt you or not, you just embarrass, interrupt and retard digestion." Thus they reason correctly on vital functions and make remarkable cures "where there is nothing the matter." Have not physiologists done more harm than good to the management of vital economy by making suggestions that are not in accord with its laws?

Pathology is the science which treats of diseases, their nature, symptoms, causes, progress and prognosis.

Chiropractors study pathology; or rather they analyze the

objective, subjective and local symptoms to determine what nerves are interfered with and at what point in their course the interference exists. But the purpose for which this is done is quite different from that of other schools.

Chiropractors look upon disease as a misfortune rather than an enemy. They consider that it needs assistance rather than subjection; liberty rather than slavery. As to the nature of disease their opinion differs from that of all other schools. Their view is that the phenomena called disease are the result of functions performed not in accordance with the rules and laws described by Innate.

Symptoms were formerly synonomous with signs, certain symptoms were signs of a certain disease. Today symptoms are regarded by physicians as vital or functional phenomena. morbific functions. To this we agree. If the medical profession could now be shown that impinged nerves cause "morbid functions," and that they can be returned to normal by releasing impingements they would be coming our way."

As to the progress of disease, the various schools agree. A large share of diseases are self-limited (cannot be cut short of their ordinary run by any known method) in the hands of all schools except that of Chiropractic, which limits them to a few minutes, or an hour at most. The former treats the effects; the latter adjusts the cause, as unlike in results as in methods.

The Chiropractor's prognosis does not agree with that of the physician as might be expected. The various schools of medicine study the nature and probable results; they know by past experience that the most of diseases are self-limited, have their usual run, that no treatment known will cut short their duration. During the first week or two, they study the nature of the disease, judge from symptoms and watch its progress; from their notes they make their prognosis. Chiropractors are expected to cut short, to abort the disease before it has declared itself or made known what kind of fever; if they do not, they are not wanted. A Chiropractor is employed to relieve the patient of the disease; a doctor to care for and watch the progress of the disease.

Theraupeutists are concerned in discovering and applying remedies for diseases. Chiropractors do not treat diseases; they adjust causes instead. They do not use remedies of any school to treat effects; therefore, Chiropractors are not concerned about remedies.

Hygiene is a sanitary science; a system of principles and rigid rules designed for the preservation and promotion of health. As a rule, those who give the closest attention to the laws of right living have the poorest health. For example, look to the Chiropractors of Oklahoma City; Gorby, Gregory and

Palmer eat all they want, and whenever they have a desire, of anything that will tickle their palates. The Carver-Denny School have specimens of those who are abstemious in their diet, observe and teach certain fixed rules for the promotion of health; they hire a man for the express purpose of giving a series of lectures on right living. From 63 years of experience and observation, I would say, "Take thine ease, eat, drink, and be merry."

Materia medica treats of drugs, their preparation and respective doses; and the physiological phenomena produced by them in the human economy. As Chiropractors do not prescribe or use drugs, an education in this branch would be useless.

Toxicology. To round out and complete a practical education of a Chiropractor, he should be acquainted with the action of drugs on the functions of the human body, so that he may know what nerves are affected by their introduction and what vertebrae to adjust to counteract their effects.

Toxicomania is an insane desire for intoxicating liquors and poisonous drugs. Chiropractors are able to relieve these abnormal cravings by correcting vertebrae which by constant use of poisons are drawn out of alignment.

Of what use is chemistry, histology, bactheriology and pharmacy could be to a Chiropractor, I am unable to say.

Jurisprudence is the application of forensic knowledge to the solution of questions concerning the administration of justice. Any Chiropractor may be called to testify in courts of judicature. When so called they ought to know somewhat of those subjects which are liable to be connected with court cases.

Obstetrics is the art of midwifery. It has to do with pregnancy, childbirth and the puerperium. A Chiropractor should be able to care for any condition which may arise in the families under his care, the same as a physician; this we intend to make possible in a two year's course. Mothers and their babes are liable to be injured at child-birth. Many have their vertebrae displaced at this critical period, causing acute and chronic diseases. If the accoucheur is a Chiropractor, he can adjust such, thereby preventing disease.

Gynecology is that part of education which has to do with diseases peculiar to women. All ailments from female weakness to fibroid cancer can be traced to subluxations of vertebrae in the lumbar region.

Surgery relates to injuries of any part or organs, and the adjusting of these, be they fractures or displacements. The Chiropractor should look well to conservative surgery—the preservation of a part rather than its removal. In the education of Chiropractors, dissection has been neglected. In our course of the first year we will give the arrangement of the viscera, osteotomy and neurotomy.

Diagnosis is the act of recognizing disease, and from its symptoms deciding as to its character; what lesions have occurred and will occur, how long it will endure and what will be its probable outcome.

Chiropractors do not treat, cure, heal or diagnose disease. As a science it is unlike any other system; it will not mix with any other. Chiropractors do not treat, cure or heal effects named disease in the sense that a physician or an osteopath does. They enquire for the location of the symptoms, in order that they may determine what nerve or nerves are impinged upon producing the undesirable effects. Having analyzed the case, they adjust to relieve the confined nerves. They do not wait for special symptoms to develop in order that they may determine the disease so that they may decide on the proper treatment.

---

A subluxated vertebra does not **shut off** the transmission of power; does not disorganize functional or organic action.

A subluxated vertebra may press against a nerve or muscle, causing it to be irritated, more tense and contracted, thereby changing functional activity. Functions are not disorganized, broken us, thrown into disorder or destroyed. Functions are increased or decreased because of pressure.

---

P. H. May, writing about the art of adjusting vertebrae, says: "Disseminate his art."

To whom does the art of adjusting vertebrae belong? I adjusted vertebrae three years before I taught it to anyone. A. P. Davis was my second student, October 18, 1898. B. J. Palmer graduated four years later. During the next four years I taught it to many persons who are practicing Chiropractic today, and they have taught it to many others. While some of these are mean enough to state that I stole the art, there is only one mean enough to wait until 10 years after my discovery, then claim that he was the originator, the fountain head, of the art of adjusting vertebrae, and that his alleged discovery was made 10 years previous to the time I gave my first adjustment.

P. H. May further adds: "Now, may the man who gave to the world this great science live long and to a ripe old age and when his labors are ended and when his innate will be united with the great universal intelligence, the Ruler of mankind, and of áll things and the world at large will say unto him, 'Well done, my good and faithful servant.' "

Thanks, Mr. May, for your good wishes. I have 37 years yet to live. If I had had the benefit of Chiropractic from infancy, I would place my somatic death at 150.

## THE PER CENT QUESTION.

"As to the per cent question. Of course you are technically correct, but I think it is **proper to assume a percentage of things that are not** physically **divisible.** This is especially the case in instances where we judge of anything by its effects.

"Thus: one can say that 25 per cent of heat in a pipe is lost by radiation and that at least 95 per cent of this loss can be prevented by covering the pipe with a certain kind of nonconductor; whereas another inferior nonconductor will prevent only 80 per cent of the loss.

"By the same reasoning, I contend, that it is proper to say that an estimated per cent of **vital energy fails to reach a given organ on account of the restraining influence of a subluxation.**"

Technically and mathematically you are wrong. Your conclusion is erroneous because your premises are incorrect.

"Loosely" says Webster as "a part or proportion of a whole" you are correct.

**Percentage is a mathematical calculation, and as such, it is precise, accurate and exact. It is not mathematical to assume to do a thing, nor to per cent things which are not divisible into 100 equal parts.**

"One can say" or "assume" anything, even an impossibility, but neither you nor I can do an impossible act, **cannot divide heat or steam into 100 equal parts** so as to determine the gain or loss.

Heat cannot be weighed, measured by the yard or bushel, nor per-cented by the hundred. Temperature is indicated by sensation, the thermometer or pyrometer.

Heat energy is designated by units of power; 550 pounds per second being considered equal to one horsepower. Its pressure is known by an indicator.

Tone is measured by a tonometer, an instrument for measuring tension, or the degree of resistence to pressure, as in estimating the tension of the eyeball, blood pressure, etc. It is not weighed on a scale, nor measured by the gallon. Different terms, words, or expressions have precise, limited meaning in certain relations and uses; they may be peculiar to a science, art or profession. They cease to be technical when used for anything and everything at all times.

Mathematical percentage is exact regarding the gain or loss or the divisibility of qualities, operations or magnitude which have been divided into 100 equal parts.

Heat, steam, impulses or vital energy, cannot be per-cented, an exact amount cannot be noted as gain or loss.

It is not proper to say "that an estimated per cent of vital energy fails to reach a given organ on account of the restraining influence of a subluxation."

A subluxation does not restrain or liberate vital energy. Vital energy is expressed in functional activity. A subluxation may impinge against nerves, the transmitting channel may increase or decrease the momentum of impulses, not energy.

Vital energy is not transmitted thru the nervous system or any other; it is expressed in functional acts.

Nerve tension determines the velocity of the impulses transmitted. Vital energy is expressed at the peripheral nerve endings.

The momentum, the quantity of motion received thru vibration (the amount of vibration is determined by tension), determines the amount of energy.

A subluxation does not restrain. Vital energy is not transmitted over, thru or by the nervous system. Vital energy and impulses can not be per-cented.

---

The fly is blamed for carrying all kinds of germs. This is one of the medical scape-goats: one of their explanations intended to cover a lot of ignorance. Did you ever watch a fly clean his feet and body? The fly keeps himself cleaner than many of those who talk about him.

---

The ophthalmic nerve communicates with the cavernous plexus of the sympathetic and the trunks of the third, fourth and sixth cervical nerves. Cunningham states, on page 552, that there are other fiber connections of which we at present possess no precise information.

I demonstrated, in the early years of Chiropractic, that the eyeball receives accessory nerves from the center dorsal; that diseases of the eyeball were because these communicating nerves were impinged upon. Cataracts are among the diseases we relieve.

The optic nerve occupies a peculiar morphological position in the cranial series of nerves. The optic nerve stalk, with its optic cup—the sensitive lens—appears to be a projecting portion of the brain. It does not connect with the ectoderm, the peripheral cell membrane. An extended portion of the brain is expanded at its peripheral ending; this expansion is the retina. The special nerve directing the sense of sight is distributed to the eyeball.

Thus it will be seen that Chiropractors adjust the communicating nerves of the eyeball, as they leave the vertebral column, at which place they may be impinged.

## PTOSIS, OPHTHALMOPLEGIA, DIPLOPIA, LACHRYMATION, AND BILATERAL ATROPHY OF THE TONGUE.

Mrs. S—, age 45, had all of the above affections in the left eye and left lateral half of the tongue.

The onset, two years previously was marked by four days of violent headache. The eyelid drooped, covering the entire eye. The patient was unable to use the palpebral muscles, not even sufficiently to cause a tremor of the eyelid. Ophthalmoplegia was present in all the muscles of the eyeball. Diplopia, heteronymous views, double vision, seeing two objects instead of one, was present, because of the visual divergence of the two axes. Lacrymation, profuse secretion, an overflow of tears was constant. Trophoneurosis of the left lateral half of the tongue was also present. The five affections named, consisted of paralysis of the motor nerves.

By a close study of the following nerve ramifications, the reader may be enabled to see why I adjusted the third cervical vertebra **to increase nerve tension and relieve atony; to stiffen relaxed nerves; to take up the slack and create a degree of tension known as tone;. to cause the proper firmness of nerve tissue necessary to transmit impulses at a rate adapted to the momentum needed to create the normal force required by each organ for ordinary activity, that functions might be performed with the usual expenditure of energy.**

**Health and disease are conditions created by normal tone, too much or not enough tension.** We, as Chiropractors, should find the displaced portion of the neuroskelton which by its **displacement tightens or slackens the lines of thot transmission.**

The nervous system consists of the cerebro-spinal axis, the sympathetic system and the nerves and organs of special sense formed by modifications of the peripheral nerve endings.

The cerebro-spinal axis consists of an enlarged portion, the brain, or encephalon, and a prolongation known as the spinal cord.

The encephalon is enclosed by the skull and extends to the lower margin of the foramen magnum; it weighs about fifty ounces in the male and five less in the female. It consists of the cerebral hemispheres, cerebellum, midbrain, interbrain, pons and medulla.

The cerebral hemispheres occupy the lateral ventricles (cavities) of the brain bladder. The cerebellum weighs about five ounces; is about five inches wide, two inches long and two inches thick. The mid-brain connects the pons with the cerebrum. The inter-brain is connected with the mid-brain and the two hemispheres. The pons is three-quarters of an inch thick, one inch long and an inch and a quarter in width. The medulla is about an inch long, three-quarters of an inch wide and a half inch thick. It fuses with the spinal cord at the lower margin of the foramen magnum. The spinal cord is about eighteen inches long and weighs about one and a half ounces. It is lodged in the vertebral canal, from the upper margin of the atlas to the lower border of the body of the first vertebra.

The twelve pairs of cranial nerves arise from the brain, the oblongata or the cervical portion of the spinal cord. They are called cranial nerves because they make their exit thru some one of the foramina of the skull.

The sympathetic nervous system consists of ganglia, connected by nerve-cords; one vertical nerve-chain, on each side of the vertebral column, which extends from the skull to the coccyx. **Each gangliated cord has an ascending branch which passes thru the carotid canal and into the cranium where it forms plexuses and communicates with the cranial nerves,** particularly the fifth, and the Gasserian ganglion. Both cords unite in front of the coccyx.

The **nerves** are filamentous bands of nervous tissue that connect the various parts of the nervous system with each other and the different organs of the body. **They conduct nervous impulses to and from the brain**—not force or energy.

The organs of special sense are those of touch, taste, smell, hearing, and sight. The skin is the organ of touch. The tongue contains most of the organs of taste. The nose incloses the organs of the sense of smell. The ear is the organ of hearing. The eye the organ of sight or vision.

The skin, tongue and the mucous membrane in the concha of the nose, receive their sensations by touch. The eye and ear by vibration. The brain may receive impressions from a distance, far or near, by that transference, known as telepathy, thru mentiferous ether vibration. Our next great advancement will be the recognition and use of ether vibration. Advanced thots in this and other books are largely due to, and are now being recognized as, thot transference transmitted by ether vibration.

The reticular (net like meshes) formations in the pons and medulla are more abundant, than in the spinal cord; they form a considerable part of the medulla, but are less in the cord, being most plentiful in the cervical region.

The spinal nerves are so called because they originate in the spinal cord and are transmitted thru the intervertebral foramina on either side of the spinal column. There are thirty-one pairs of spinal nerves. Sometimes the thirty-first pair is lacking; however, there may be one or even two filamentous pairs which do not pass out of the spinal canal. Occasionally there is an increase or decrease in the number of vertebrae in the column; such variations always have a corresponding number of spinal nerves.

Each spinal nerve arises by two roots, an anterior or motor root and a posterior or sensory root, the latter possessing a nerve center known as a spinal ganglion. The posterior root of the first cervical nerve forms an exception to the rule. It is smaller than the anterior and has occasionally a ganglion which is often situated within the dura mater.

The roots of the spinal nerves coalesce just beyond the ganglion and form a trunk, which emerges through the intervertebral foramen. It gives off a recurrent branch to the dura mater of the spinal cord and brain. It communicates with the sympathetic and divides into an anterior and a posterior portion. The posterior primary divisions arise from the trunk formed by the union of the roots, in the intervertebral foramina, and are distributed to the muscles and integuments behind the spine. The anterior, primary divisions supply the parts of the body in front of the spine, including the limbs. These two divisions innervate the somatic portion of the body.

The roots of the cervical nerves increase in size from the first to the fifth and then remain the same in diameter to the eighth; the posterior roots are three times as large as the anterior.

The first pair of nerves pass between the occipital bone and the posterior arch of the atlas; the second pair between the posterior arch of the atlas and the laminae of the axis. Therefore, **it is an utter impossibility for the first and second pairs of spinal nerves to be pinched or squeezed, in these lengthy gaps, by the closing of these bones.** Even if they were flattened in their horizontal diameter and narrowed in their vertical thickness, a slight bending forward of the head or a nodding movement would release the compression. The eighth pair of spinal nerves pass between the last cervical and first dorsal vertebra.

The sympathetic ganglionic chains have three pairs of ganglia in the cervical, twelve in the dorsal, four in the lumbar, and the sacral has four or five pairs. Each of these ganglia is a distinct center, with branches for distribution and communication. Nerve-fibers are of two kinds. Those of distribution supply the involuntary muscles of the blood vessels, hollow viscera and the secreting cells in the glandular viscera. The communicating fibers connect the ganglia with each other and with the cerebro-spinal nerves.

In the neck there are three sympathetic ganglia, connecting and communicating with the cervical nerves. The sympathetic system communicates freely with the **cerebro-spinal nerves.**

From the superior, cervical ganglion an ascending branch enters the cranium thru the carotid canal, making connections with certain cranial nerves. This cranial branch is divided into an inner and outer division. The outer forms the carotid plexus which sends some filaments to the Gasserian ganglion.

Gerrish says: "The gross anatomy of the cervical sympathetic gives no idea of its true anatomical relations as revealed by physiological experiments and pathological phenomena. The physiological connections as at present understood may be summarized as follows:

"Pupillo-dilator fibers pass by white rami communicantes from the first, second and third thoracic nerves, **ascend in the sympathetic cord to the superior cervical ganglion to form arborizations round its cells. Thence gray fibers pass to the Gasserian ganglion and reach the eyeball by the ophthalmic division of the fifth and long ciliary nerves.**

"Motor fibers to the involuntary muscles of the orbit and eyelids from the fourth and fifth thoracic nerves follow a similar course.

"Vasomotor fibers to the head, secretory fibers to the submaxillary gland, and pilomotor fibers to the head and neck are derived from the upper thoracic nerves and reach their areas of distribution after similar interruption in the superior cervical ganglion."

**The carotid plexus of the sympathetic ganglionated chain furnishes filaments to the Gasserian ganglion.**

**The Gasserian or semilunar ganglion receives filaments from the cavernous plexus of the sympathetic vertebral ganglionated cords. Three large branches—the ophthalmic, the superior and inferior maxillary, spring from its border.**

The fifth pair of cranial nerves, known as the trigeminal, meaning "three double" or "three twins," are the largest of the cranial nerves. They are nerves of motion, sensation and taste; they ramify the skin of the face, the tongue and teeth.

The ophthalmic nerve is entirely a sensory nerve. Before its division it receives communicating filaments from the cavernous plexus of the sympathetic. It supplies the eyeball, the lachrymal gland, the mucous lining of the eye and nasal fossa and the integument of the eyebrow, forehead and nose.

Each division of the fifth pair of nerves **subdivides into three** branches. It resembles a spinal nerve in having two roots, a motor and a sensory, and in having a ganglion on its posterior root; also, in being a compound or mixed nerve transmitting motion, sensation and taste.

The ophthalmic is the smallest branch. It **divides into three** terminal branches, the frontal, lachrymal and naso-ciliary.

Before its division, it has communication with the cavernous plexus of the sympathetic. It is connected with the third, fourth and sixth nerves by communicating branches. The frontal nerve has **three branches,** the supra-orbital, frontal proper and supra-trochlear. The supra-orbital is the largest of the three; it sends twigs to the pericranium, the skin of the scalp, the upper eyelid, the frontal and parietal regions. The frontal is distributed to the skin of the forehead and upper eyelid. The supra-trochlear pierces the palpebral (eyelid) fascia and sends filaments to the upper eyelid.

The lacrymal nerve is the smallest of the three branches of the opthalmic division. It receives a small communicating branch from the zygomatic nerve (the orbital branch of the maxillary nerve). This communicating nerve gives branches to the lachrymal gland, the conjunctiva and the skin of the outer canthus of the eye. A small twig passes beyond the lachrymal gland and pierces the palpebral (eyelid) fascia and supplies filaments to the conjunctiva (the mucous membrane uniting the globe of the eye with the eyelid) and is then distributed to the outer canthus (corner or angle) of the eye.

The naso-ciliary nerve divides into two terminal branches, the infratrochlear and anterior ethmoid. The infratrochlear nerve divides into two branches, the superior and inferior palpebral. The superior branch helps to supply the eyelids. The inferior is distributed to the lachrymal sac, the conjunctiva and skin of the upper part of the upper eyelid, the caruncle and the skin of the upper part of the side of the nose.

The naso-ciliaris or nasal nerve is **divided into three branches** —to the orbit, nose and face areas. The nasal nerve supplies two long ciliary (hair-like) branches to the eyeball. The roots of these ciliary branches are three in number and kind, motor, sensory and sympathetic. The branches from the ciliary ganglion are twelve to fifteen short ciliary nerves which pass to the eyeball in two groups above and below the optic nerve. They supply the coats of the eyeball, including the iris and ciliary muscles. The circular fibers of the iris and the villiary muscle are innervated by the third nerve; the radial fibers of the iris by the sympathetic.

The branch of the nasal nerve to the ciliary ganglion is a slender filament one-quarter of an inch long. One or two long, ciliary nerves pierce the sclerotic near the optic nerve.

There are four small ganglia connected with the fifth nerve. Each of these has **three roots** derived from the motor, sensory and sympathetic.

The ciliary ganglion is about the size of a large pin head, being one-twelfth of an inch in its greatest diameter. It has three slender roots which come from the cavernous plexus of the sympathetic.

The short ciliary nerves pass along the upper and lower surfaces of the optic nerve, subdividing until twelve to eighten fine filaments reach the sclerotic and pierce it in a circle round the optic nerve. They supply nerves to the eyeball, motor nerves to the ciliary muscle and sphincter iridis, and sympathetic nerves to the dilator fibers of the iris.

The supra-orbital sends palpebral filaments to the upper eyelid.

The main branches of the trigeminal nerve have anastomoses, inosculation, intercommunication with neighboring nerves. There are, in the course of the ramifications of the nerve, several other small ganglia belonging to the sympathetic system.

The branches from the ganglia in the neck are distributed to structures in the head, neck and thorax; the motor fibers going to involuntary muscles. For example, the dilator muscles of the pupil.

The branches from the cervical sympathetic ganglia and cord are divisible into two sets; central communicating branches for other nerves and peripheral branches of distribution which, alone or along with other nerves, form plexuses accompanying and supplying vessels and viscera of the head, neck and thorax. Altho, this distinction is made, it is well to bear in mind that the branches of communication are as much nerves of distribution as the others. Of the communicating nerves, one passes from the fourth to the fifth cervical and several from the loop between the first and second cervical, to the hypoglossal, vagus and sympathetic and the superior cervical ganglion. The branch to the hypoglossal, usually consists of one filament from the second and one from the third cervical.

Nervi communicans, the communicating nerves, are those which form a line of communication between nerves or ganglia; they may convey either sensation or motion. Distributing nerve is the name given to the nerve whose trunk branches are arranged for distribution of impulses. All distributing nerves are motor. We have, also, the sensory nerves of concentration.

The performance of functions depends upon the amount of energy stored and used. Functional abnormalities and structural alterations constitute the signs, symptoms and lesions of disease, but they involve no functional activities which the normal body does not already possess. These activities may be diminished, increased or entirely absent. **Action is dependent upon force; force is equal to the momentum of impulse; momentum is increased or decreased according to nerve tension.**

Ophthalmoplegia, a paralytic condition of the eye-muscles, may be partial or complete. Either the internal or the external muscles may be involved, constituting ophthalmoplegia interna or externa, and when both are affected, total ophthalmoplegia. The lesions may be nuclear or peripheral. Pressure due to neoplasms, gummata, aneurisms, or basilar meningitis may produce it, or it may follow diphtheria.

I have attempted to give a brief description of a portion of the nervous system, so far as it refers to the five pathological conditions which head this article.

The nervous system has been and is still undergoing a transformation in its ramification, its parts and quality. The higher the type in the scale of intelligence the more complex is the arrangement of the nervous system. No two of us are formed alike outwardly or in our internal construction. Anatomists agree in the general description of the nervous system, but in details they differ as the subjects from which the descriptions are given vary. Some authors give one, others two or three rami communicans from the spinal trunk to the ganglion of the vertebral chain. Where there are two, the rule is for one to contain the gray (sympathetic fibers) and the other the medullated fibers (white ramus). Morris says: "The trunk or anterior primary division of every spinal nerve has at least one of these; most of the nerves have two, and sometimes there are three." Of this variation Morris says: "The meningeal or recurrent branch is very small and **variable,** and is seldom seen in ordinary dissections. It is given off from the nerve-trunk just before its anterior and posterior divisions are formed. It consists of a few peripheral branches of spinal ganglion-cells (sensory fibers) which leave the nerve-trunk and re-enter the vertebral canal for the innervation of the meninges, and which are joined by a twig from the gray ramus or directly from the nearest sympathetic ganglion (vasomotor nerves). There is considerable evidence, both physiological and anatomical, obtained chiefly from the animals, **which shows that at times** certain of the peripheral spinal ganglion or sensory fibers **may turn backwards** in the nerve-trunk and pass to the meninges within the ventral root **instead of contributing** to a recurrent branch. The occurrence of such fibers in the ventral root explains the physiological phenomenon known as 'recurrent sensibility.' Likewise, **sympathetic fibers entering the trunk through the gray ramus may pass** to the meninges by way of the ventral root, and **at times the recurrent branch is probably absent altogether,** its place being taken entirely by the meningeal fibers passing in the ventral root."

Thus it is seen that authors differ. The statements of one who most widely differs from all others follows:

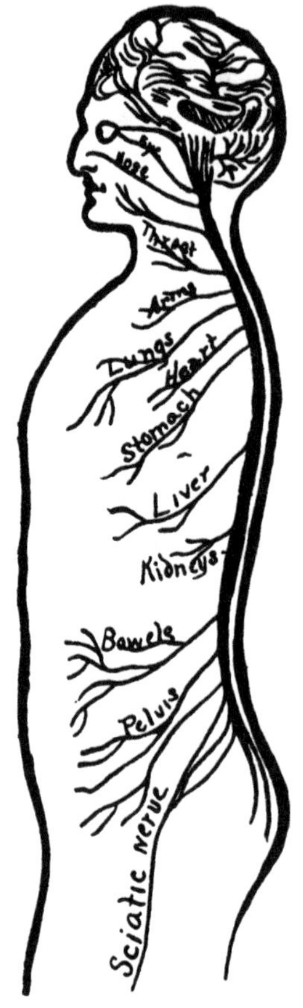


"B. J. Palmer, in one of his addresses to his class in Portland this summer, aptly quoted, '**that he who tears down must rebuild greater**,' and said 'when I saw there was **no use for a Sympathetic Nervous System, I threw it out,** and then just had to put something better in its place, so **I discovered Direct Mental Impulse.**' "

"Chiropractors have at all times denied the existence of the twelve cranial nerves as found in anatomies today. We have questioned their existence from the standpoint of what logic, nerve tracing and results have proven regardless of whether it seems reasonable to you or not."

I have never known any Chiropractic literature to deny the existence of the cranial or sympathetic systems of nerves, except that of the P. S. C., and that only since I ceased to be its president.

The adjoining cut obtained from one of the P. S. C. students "illustrates how the brain communicates with all the organs through the nerve system." "Every one of you know the history of Chiropractic. Chiro was discovered by Dr. D. D. Palmer and developed into a science by B. J. Palmer, his son."

---

"What is life? It evidently is something that can leave man in partial quantities or absolutely. It is life that is paralyzed in paralysis. Any intermediate stage between fullest life and death would be one of paralysis. A body without Innate is dead. A body with it is alive, but a stage between the two is paralysis."

The above lines remind me of Mrs. Brown whose husband was very sick. The doctor told her that he was half dead; so she hurried to the insurance office and asked for half of the life insurance; but she failed to convince the company that a partial quantity of life had left.

## "INNATE NERVOUS SYSTEM."

"I have often questioned the Sympathetic Nervous System. It seems that I have been grossly misunderstood. I do not wish to be understood as saying that we have no nerves, commonly known as sympathetic nerves, existing in the body. Those nerves are there; never have I questioned their existence.

"I wish to be clearly understood as saying that what has so many times been dissected as the Sympathetic Nervous System is there—I do not question that for an instant—it is there but its purpose and paths are different from those commonly ascribed to it in medical works.

"The Sympathetic Nervous System is a misnomer to express the real work that such a system does. I prefer the term **Innate Nervous System.**"

You "have often questioned the Sympathetic Nervous System." I hope your investigations have now given you decisive results.

You may "have been grossly misunderstood." Therefore. I will assist you in being comprehended aright.

You now state, "I do not wish to be understood as saying that we have no nerves, commonly known as sympathetic nerves." You should not have stated, "He graduated when we **did** teach the sympathetic system (nerve system)." That was when the discoverer and developer of Chiropractic was at the head of The P. S. C. You should not have stated "It is impossible to have a sympathetic nervous system." Hereafter, when you repeat "We do **not** need a sympathetic nervous system to explain functions," just leave out that one word "not." Hereafter you will not state "The Chiropractor has no spinal or sympathetic nerves to worry about." Such statements were misleading to your readers; they need adjusting. I feel that I have not spent my time in vain; but there are some persons who are so mentally put up that they will need continual adjusting. Your readers were not to blame for your being "grossly misunderstood."

"Those nerves are there." From the above quotations, your readers thought you "questioned their existence."

All right. "I do not wish to be understood as saying that we have no nerves, commonly known as sympathetic nerves, existing in the body. **They are there.**"

Are you now sure that you are awake; that it was all a dream? Look at that beautiful model. Do you see where you so ruthlessly tore from it that which represented The Sympathetic Nervous System? Be sure now that you are fully awake, and see things as they are. To be so "grossly misunderstood" was not to the advantage of Chiropractic.

"Right you are." We now understand you to say "That what has so many times been dissected as the Sympathetic Nervous System **is there**—I do not question that for an instant —it is there."

"**Chiropractors have at all times denied the existence of the** 12 cranial nerves as found in anatomies today. We have questioned their existence from the standpoint of what logic, nerve tracing and results have proven regardless of whether it seems reasonable to you or not." "Wake up. Wide awake." You are off again. I have never known any Chiropractic literature, except that of the P. S. C., to deny the existence of the cranial nerves. Nothing of that nature can be found in the writings of the Founder of Chiropractic. Nothing of that import ever came from The Fountain Head of Chiropractic. Rub your eyes. Wake up. Get out of that hypnotic condition. You have remained in that state so long some persons think you are in earnest. Now, wake up, get a move on you, tell your audience you were mistaken; that you have been under a hypnotic spell; that you now are awake and know the Sympathetic Nervous System and the "**12 Cranial Nerves** as found in anatomies today are there," that you do not question their existence for an instant. Look at those cranial nerves and see that there are 12 **pairs** instead of 12. When you get fully awake, you can then understand "the directions of their paths, their places of ingress and egress." Instead of "questioning the fact of fibers ending at ganglia and other fibers starting at ganglia," you will comprehend that ganglia are well defined collections of nerve cells and nerve fibers forming subsidiary nerve centers.

---

Function is any act necessary for accomplishing vital phenomena; the special action of a part.

Vital functions are those essential to life.

Vegetable functions are the results of vital functions; that which is accomplished.

Intellectual functions are those which pertain to our environments, our surroundings.

As the **vegetative** function is the culmination of the vital, the work performed, so comprehension bears the same relation to the consummative function of Innate that the vegetative does to the physical.

Physical growth and all that pertains thereto is vegetative. The advancement of the spiritual is the growth made by the intellectual.

Thus, we have four functions; the vital and vegetative of the physical, and the intellectual and consummative of the spiritual.

## DEATH.

Death is the cessation of life. It may be physiologic or pathologic. Molecular or cellular death is that of individual cells, which have ceased to perform their functions, the "wear and tear" of the system. This "tearing down and building up" is physiologic, pertaining to health. If the bodily heat becomes greater than normal, cell destruction is in mass, pathological, known as necrosis.

Life depends upon the performance of certain functions. When these cease to act, the whole organism discontinues to exist as a living, sentient being. Metabolism comprises those phenomena by which organic beings transform foodstuffs into tissue elements.

Metabolism consists of two separate and distinct functions. Katabolism, destructive metamorphosis, disassimilation, physiologic disintegration, and anabolism, constructive metabolism, activity and repair of functions. These two perform their operations of waste and repair, in health, by maintaining an equilibrium of forces. The same amount of material for the maintenance and growth of the organism is taken up and assimilated from the digested nourishment that is removed from the body thru the excretory organs in the form of waste material or end-products of retrogressive tissue-metamorphosis. The income must always balance the output. During the period of growth, a certain excess of formative activity corresponding to the increase must predominate. If in excess, a giant is produced; a deficiency makes a dwarf. In senility, the expenditure may be greater than the intake, to a reasonable amount; this loss in the aged is physiologic.

There are two forms of death recognized—molecular, the death of a part by the separation of minute particles, as occurs in ulceration and caries, and somatic, death of the organism as a whole.

Atrophy and hypertrophy may be physiologic or pathologic. The muscles in the athlete enlarge by exercise. When no longer in use their volume is a source of expense to the bodily economy; accordingly, they are permitted to waste. Remember that exercise excites, irritates nerves and muscles, causes them to contract lengthwise and expand crosswise. A lack of exertion allows them to be lax and physiological atrophy ensues. After the menopause, which is the physiologic cessation of menstruation, the uterus and ovaries, having no further function to perform, begin to atrophy. In the course of time they become quite small and relatively fibrous.

Extremes of temperature are destructive. Animal heat above 98 degrees destroys cell vitality because of necrosis. Temperature of the opposite extreme may cause gangrene by freezing.

Somatic death may be physiologic or pathologic. The former occurs at the close of a natural life-time, at an age recognized as normal to the species; such persons "die of old age." There comes a time when new matter is not taken in as fast as useless material is eliminated, and eventually actions cease to be performed; this is natural, physiological death. All the functions are essential to health; yet, only four are necessary to life—circulation, transudation, respiration and innervation.

**Bodily temperature above or below normal is pathologic.**

With the cessation of life metabolism ceases, and the temperature falls to that of the surrounding atmosphere. This change may occur in an hour or two or it may be delayed twelve or even twenty-four hours. In some cases, as death from tetanus, the temperature may continue to rise for a few hours after death.

When the muscle substance ceases to be controlled by intelligent life—ceases to act by or because of intelligence, it becomes rigid, a condition of rigor, it passes from a viscous to a solid state. The rigidity of the muscles after somatic death (not molecular) is known as rigor mortis—death stiffening of a cadaver. It may come on immediately or be delayed several hours. In from one to six days the muscles become lax and pliable.

---

A leaflet contains the following: "Are you tired of taking nauseous drugs, and medicines, and various treatments without getting results?" This might have been better said thus: Are you tired of treatments which do not give satisfactory results?

"Chiropractic, a treatment which treats the cause of disease and not the effect." Chiropractic is not a system of treatment; it is one of adjustment. Effects can only be treated, causes should be adjusted.

"Pressure on nerves reduces supply of nerve force." A light pressure irritates, excites the nerves to undue activity, causing too much heat—an increased temperature known as fever.

"A full supply of nerve force reaches the starved and so-called diseased part of the body." Most of diseases are because of an over action of functions, and not of a starved condition.

"Without a full nerve force, we cannot have a free circulation."

"Nature's method of removing the worn-out tissue of the body, impure blood follows with its long train of ailments." My boy, you are talking Osteopathy, not Chiropractic.

## THE SYMPATHETIC NERVOUS SYSTEM.

The great nervous mass which occupies the cavity of the cranium, is named the encephalon, or brain. From it extends twelve pairs of cranial nerves which leave the skull through openings at its front and base, not including the foramen magnum, and the prolongation extending downward, through the large oval aperture of the occipital bone and into the vertebral canal, where it is encased by twenty bony rings. The spinal extension is called the marrow or spinal cord. This stem-like division of the brain extends from the border of the foramen magnum to the first or second lumbar vertebrae. The remainder of the vertebral canal, which includes the sacral portion contains nerve filaments which protrude from the spinal cord. Above the foramen magnum, in the cranial cavity, the twelve pair of cranial nerves spring from the under side of the brain—their apparent origin. Their real origin is in the mass of the encephalon which is located in the brainpan, and consist of the fore-brain, mid-brain and hind-brain. These three are formed of the telencephalon, diencephalon, mesencephalon, rhombencephalon, metencephalon and myelencephalon. These six brains were originally developed from the primitive neutral tube; they are more prominent as individual brains in the early development of the encephalon. The real origin of the twelve pairs of cranial nerves is in these six primitive brains.

These cranial nerves are reinforced by spinal accessory filaments, which emerge by numerous bundles from the side of the spinal cord between the occipital and the seventh cervical. They ascend upward in the spinal canal through the occipital opening and join the cranial nerves. These accessory nerves do not emerge from the canal; therefore, so far as I know they convey their functions without danger of impingement, to be associated with the cranial nerves as communicantes.

As we return from the cranial cavity by way of the foramen magnum, which to all intents and purposes is a continuation of the vertebral canal, we find thirty pairs of openings, the intervertebral foramina, through which as many spinal nerve trunks pass outward. These contain the voluntary and involuntary, the Educated and Innate nerves, those which have to do with the animal and organic life. These have their apparent origin in the spinal cord arising from it by fibrous rootlets which form two roots, ventral and dorsal. They coalesce and compose the trunks of the spinal nerves, those which look after the welfare of our outward surroundings, and functionate the vital economy of our bodies. Immediately upon their exit they divide into four branches, one of which goes to and enters a ganglion of the gangliated chain, one of the two great sympathetic cords of ganglia and plexuses which become smaller as they go father from the base of supplies. These two chains of ganglia are occasionally connected by nerve trunks.

These sympathetic trunks of organic life pass in front of the vertebraterial foramina and lie close to and against the bodies of the dorsal vertebrae and the heads of the ribs, a ganglion occurring at the level of the head of each rib. On the lumbar vertebrae, they are more ventralward; on the sacrum they pass on the front of the sacral foramina. These two sympathetic gangliated cords are united in front of the coccyx.

Returning to the upper portion of the sympathetic cord, we find the superior cervical ganglion, fusiform, tapering from the center toward each end, one inch to one and a half inches long. It is often marked by one or more constrictions, appearing as though formed by the coalescence of four ganglia, corresponding to the four cervical nerve branches which enter it. The upper end of this ganglia barely enters the cranial cavity through the carotid canal (not the magnum foramen), sending upward the cavernous and carotid plexuses which are wholly within the cranial cavity from whence many communicating branches go to and form a complex relationship with the cranial nerves.

If we retrace our steps of investigation we will find that the branches of communication from the spinal cord carry, in their thirty pairs of trunk nerves, the filaments which go to and make up the sympathetic chains of ganglia where they are systematically arranged for distribution to the viscera and blood vessels. The solar plexus supplies most of the abdominal viscera with innervation; the cardiac plexus furnishes the heart with energy; the hypogastric plexus contributes the nervous influence to the pelvic organs; and yet they all owe their functional activity to filaments which originate in the six brains. These nerves of the sympathetic nervous system pass down the spinal cord and out through the foramina. The sympathetic ganglia receiving important branches which are distributed throughout the human economy in such matter and condition as is determinated by Innate and of necessity modified by the condition of its communicating fibers.

The cranial nerves are indebted for many of their accessories to this sympathetic nervous system. These communicantes can be traced from the cranial nerves to the sympathetic, then through some one of the ganglia and into the spinal cord, from thence to the encephalon.

We have been preparing the way, so we may intelligently

and successfully explain how and where nerves may be impinged upon. Perhaps some of those who have followed us closely are now able to do so.

---

Dr. D. D. Palmer, D. C.:—

The Adjuster received O. K. It seems to adjust many things, as well as teach how to adjust vertebrae.

I am writing to place my order for your text-book, hoping you have it already in the press at least and in a short time I shall receive it.

I remain yours very truly, ——— —————

We should know Chiropractic physiology so that we may discern the difference between it and Chiropractic pathologic physiology. For it is the latter we have to deal with. It is as much the Adjuster's business to adjust any and all idiosyncracies found in Chiropractic literature as it is to correct morbid physiology. If physiological functions and Chiropractic education were always correct, there would be no need for the Chiropractor nor the Chiropractor Adjuster. As long as luxations are found in vertebral columns or Chiropractic literature, there will be need for both.

I see you have added "D. C." to my name. That needs adjusting. Please tell me where the founders of Osteopathy and Chiropractic can obtain these degrees. All pseudo discoverers, developers and founders of Chiropractic have obtained that degree from me, the Fountain Head of the science.

"Pathology deals with the disturbance of functions and the alteration of structure in living beings, induced by unusual agencies and conditions."

In order to elucidate the above three lines. which may seem condensed, found in the center of the fourth paragraph, I will apply it to pleurisy. It is applicable to any disease.

The prominent **symptoms** of pleurisy are, pain in the thorax, followed by a chill—the sensation produced by the involuntary contraction of the cutaneous muscles—fever and a sharp sticking pain in the side.

**Symptoms** denote the presence of, as well as define disease; also the change in the patient's condition. As pleurisy advances, the patient coughs less, has less pain, lies upon the affected side, which heretofore he has not been able to do; he has less fever and his appetite may be improved. These symptoms are delusive, for we notice the breathing is more hurried, being confined to the unaffected side.

Ausculation by ear or percussion on the painful side will reveal less friction and a dullness, owing to serum or pus infiltration or both. These are **signs.** It is often difficult to draw the line of distinction between the signs of disease and symptoms.

The **functions** of breathing and blood circulation are accelerated; digestion and the serous circulation are impeded. Respiration is increased because one lung has to do the work of two. An undue amount of heat increases the number of red corpuscles in the blood and accelerates its action. Digestion and the serous circulation is retarded.

The pleura is a serous sac which envelopes the lung. The pleural cavity is a capillary space containing a little fluid which lubricates the opposed surfaces of the visceral and parietal membranes. Inflammation thickens and condenses the visceral covering of the lung; therefore, pus may result from the inflamed membrane, the passage of the serum may be withheld and an accumulation of serum or pus or both may fill the pleural cavity.

The **unusual conditions** referred to are those of inflammation and fever which produce abnormal metabolism.

Displacement of osseous tissue, whether by poison or traumatism are **unusual.**

"The development of diseases stopped."

Development in pathology means growth or increase. To merely stop development, growth or increase would not be "restoring health."

---

By one adjustment we can change the symptoms of pneumonia, typhoid fever and other acute diseases so that any physician would not recognize either as the same affection he had diagnosed five minutes before.

---

"A stream of water starting down a hill comes to an obstruction. By the time it gets here, you don't get the power it has here in case there is an obstruction."

A stream of water does not go down when starting. A stream of water would select a ravine, not a hill, to find its level. Dams are obstructions, used to obtain power.

This would-be illustration **does not illustrate pathological anatomy.** There is no similarity. One is animate, the other inanimate. One is a fluid searching its level, the other is impulses destined for expression. One is controlled by gravity, the other by molecular motion. One generates its power by attraction, the other by heat. One is visible, the other invisible. The former gains power by being obstructed, the latter will not pass an obstruction.

## OSTEOPATHY DEFINED.

Osteopathy is advancing towards Chiropractic. To progress they must take in the principles of Chiropractic. There is no other progressive road for them to follow. Chiropractors are losing nothing by their advancement; the world is being benefited.

Dr. A. T. Still, the founder of Osteopathy, says: "Natural flow of blood is health; and disease is the effect of local or general disturbance of blood—that to excite the nerves causes muscles to contract and compress venous flow of blood to the heart; and the bones could be used as levers to relieve pressure in nerves, veins and arteries."

Dr. A. P. Davis, a student of the first class in osteopathy under A. T. Still, the founder, and one of the first teachers of osteopathy, states in his masterly work on osteopathy, a book of 851 pages: "Diseases are recognized as only the result of the interruption of the onward flow of the fluids of the body, in their various rounds to build up and tear down the various tissues in itself, and that when these tissues are normally built up and the waste material properly eliminated, health is the inevitable result."

The reader will notice the advancement, from the above toward Chiropractic, in the following:

In the January number of the Journal of Osteopathy, on the inside of the front cover, we find: "A definition of osteopathy. A system of drugless healing by which a practitioner by a thorough knowledge of Anatomy and Physiology and by appropriate manipulation adjusts structure, so that nature can restore conditions of normal function to the body.—J. R. Davis."

W. Livingston Harold, D. O., is supposed to be authority. He defines osteopathy as follows:

"Osteopathy may be formally defined as the science which consists of such exact, exhaustive and verifiable knowledge of the structure and functions of the human mechanism, anatomical, physiological and psychological, including the chemistry and psycho-physics of its known elements, as has made discoverable certain organic laws and remedial resources within the body itself, by which nature under the scientific treatment peculiar to osteopathic practice, apart from all ordinary methods of extraneous, artificial, or medical stimulation, and in harmonious accord with its own mechanical principles, molecular activities and metabolic processes, may recover from misplacements, disorganization, derangements, and consequent disease and regain its normal equilibrium of form and function in health and strength."

W. L. Harold states that osteopathy is an "exact" science. J. R. Davis says "it is a system of drugless healing." Osteopaths, by their literature, give the public to understand that osteopathy is a drugless science. Their frequent use of drugs and surgery, and the teachings of their schools prove to the contrary. The parent school at Kirksville has a hospital where surgery is the last osteopathic manipulation.

Dr. F. Dudley Tait, of San Francisco, makes a public statement that I think is not far from the truth. "The osteopaths all over the country do practice medicine. They use drugs and the knife."

It is generally understood that osteopaths condemn the use of drugs and are opposed to their use. "Osteopathy is based on principles of adjustment, the harmonizing of the parts of the body, and the greatest argument against the use of drugs is that drugs are foreign to the body and **their injection produces a maladjustment** rather than harmony."

Dr. A. T. Still's book on osteopathy, pages 294 to 301, advises the use of glycerine in the ears to cure diptheria, croup, la grippe, scarlet fever, pneumonia, sore throat, tonsilitis and all diseases of the lungs, nose and throat. It has now advanced to a system of drugless healing—in definition only.

In acute poisoning, the usual medical antidotes are used—these are taught in all osteopathic schools the same as in the medical schools. In variola, they use carbolic acid or mercuric chloride solution to prevent pitting. Pumpkin seed infusion is used for tapeworm. In myxedema they resort to thyroid extract. In chronic cystitis, they wash out the bladder with solutions. In cholera infantum, hot injections and mustard plasters are used. "Osteopathy versus drug treatment"?

Osteopaths occasionally write prescriptions for drugs or give verbal orders for their use, notwithstanding their claim that they are opposed to the use of drugs as remedial agents.

It is stated that patients who were treated at the Philadelphia College of Osteopathy were advised to use certain medicaments at home, when osteopathic manipulations had failed to relieve. I have personally known them to advise the use of remedies that were not osteopathic, yet they state that they are opposed to the use of drugs because of their poisonous effects. Would we not be justified in believing that where diseases are treated by remedies other than osteopathic that "Osteopathy is a sort of gymnastic specialty"?

---

Nothing is as wholesome as a clear conscience. You may be able to get away from those whom you have wronged, but away from yourself, never.

## DISEASES OF THE SPLEEN.

The spleen is situated in the left hypochondrium, below the diaphragm, above the colon, between the stomach and the cartilages of the false ribs, above and anterior to the right kidney. It is about five inches in length and three in thickness. From one to twenty accessory spleens are found usually near it. But they may be a considerable distance from it; they have been found embedded in the head of the pancreas. Two spleens of equal size have been observed. One may be found on the right side of the body. These accessory spleens are of the same structure, and vary in size from a pea to that of a walnut.

The spleen is regarded by anatomists as a hematopoietic organ—one concerned in the process of blood making. It has no excretory duct, at least anatomists have failed to find one.

Removal of the spleen is not fatal. After its extirpation there is an overgrowth of the lymphatic glands to compensate for its absence.

Stengel states that the splenic functions remain in doubt. Dunglison says the exact functions of the spleen are unknown. Dutton affirms the office of the spleen is still involved in obscurity. Landois remarks that the spleen is a ductless gland whose activity is still, for the most part, shrouded in obscurity. Gould says its function is not certainly determined. How useless, then, have been the experiments of vivisection.

In malarial and typhoid fevers this gland is found to be enlarged; sometimes from two to three times its usual size, a condition usually the result of malarial poisoning and known as hypertrophy or in common language ague cake. It is subject to inflammation (splenitis), as are other glands and organs. Because of inflammation it may become necrotic, waxy, its texture degenerated. Abscesses are not uncommon near its surface and are usually multiple.

Splenomegaly is an enlargement of the spleen; this may be of the nature of a cyst or carcinoma or both. Delafield says, sarcoma and carcinoma may occur in the spleen by extension from some adjacent part, as the stomach. Enlarged spleens have weighed as high as twenty pounds.

A splenic cough may be recognized by being dry and unsatisfactory, no expectoration.

From my observations I have been led to believe that the spleen furnishes a fluid which passes into the stomach by physiologic organic absorption, osmosis and imbibition. This splenic fluid assists digestion; it is to the stomach what bile and pancreatic juice is to the intestines. During digestion the spleen is enlarged and more active; whereas the fluids from the pancreas and liver are poured into the duodenum a few hours later upon the arrival of food, thus showing their vital selective action. The stomach and duodenum attract these dissolving fluids when needed.

An extremely enlarged spleen was reduced in size by the writer in three weeks. Previous to adjusting, relieving the splenic nerves of innervation, the stools were few and scanty. While adjusting the dorsal vertebra there were twenty to thirty evacuations a day, all of which, except two or three, were apparently wholly of oil; the size of the spleen being reduced accordingly.

---

The cartilage which covers the articular surface of bones is called articular and is of the hyaline variety. It is firmly attached to the bone by its surface, while the other is smooth, polished and free, thus reducing friction to a minimum.

Hyaline is from a Greek word meaning glass. Hyaline cartilage was so named because the thin slices which cover the opposing surface of a joint are as hard and transparent as glass.

Hyaline cartilage is non-vascular and free from nerves. Lymph-paths permeate it, by which the interior is nourished. Cartilaginous fractures are repaired by straps and ferrules of bone. Permeation of cartilage with nerves causes ossification. Joints are well supplied with sensory nerves; but, neither the articular cartilage nor the articular surfaces have nerves.

---

On October 31, 1910, a policeman brot A. L. N., a young man, to me, in an automobile, thinking that he had his back broken. He had slipped on the post office steps, eight blocks distant. His screams on the street and in the hall attracted a crowd. We laid him on the adjusting table, his chest elevated on pillows. His twisting, deep breathing and his screaming, made the case difficult to adjust, as it was necessary to give him the thrust while slack, when the tension was off. One adjustment replaced the displaced vertebra, with a crashing sensation that could be felt and heard. In the meantime, the policeman had phoned for the ambulance. The man walked to the street without assistance. The first aid to the injured had been effectual, so there was no need of transportation to the hospital.

"Every cloud has a silvery lining." In the crowd were two Christian Scientists, who have an office directly opposite my rooms. Before adjusting I said to them: "This is the kind of a case you are looking for." They shook their heads and returned to their office, where they could think and pray for the poor man, while I adjusted the displaced vertebra.

## IMPERSPICUITY.

The object of language should be the expression of thot in the clearest and most attractive manner. Every writer or speaker will, of course, have a style of expression peculiar to himself, but there are some qualities essential to all good styles, namely, clearness, force and harmony.

Clear writing requires clear thinking. One cannot convey clearly to others what is vague and indistinct in his own mind. Every sentence should have one and only one, principal subject of thot. The sentence may be long and consist of many parts, but the parts should be so closely and skillfully combined as to give the impression of one symmetrical whole.

The following quotations are samples of indistinctness, inharmony and lack of understanding. I am sorry that they are put out as correct Chiropractic teaching.

"None but an experienced, specific, pure and unadulterated Chiropractor would have looked for the cause of these ankle and thigh affections in their spines, and only by the adjustment of such would he dismiss these cases well."

I can comprehend what constitutes an experienced Chiropractor. This experienced Chiropractor had had four months tuition in the school room and less than a month of practice when he wrote the above. A specific Chiropractor would be one specially indicated, as a sign or symptom, especially pointing out the proper course of treatment. A pure Chiropractor would be one free from mixture, in contradistinction from a mixed character or a mixture of ingredients. An unadulterated Chiropractor would be one who is free from admixture of inferior, impure, or of less valuable ingredients, for gain, deception or concealment. Some writers try to say too much. To have used the one defining adjective, experienced, would have been sufficient.

"It will be of interest to learn how the body is heated by mental impulses which creates combustion of chemicals arterially and seriously deposited, and not by blood, and therefore the blood acts as one of the attributes in preference to performing all the calorific duties thereof."

"B. J. was the first to discover and affirm that the heating of the body is by mental impulses, and not by blood."

There are two kinds of impulses; one is the sudden, spontaneous emotion of the mind, the motor, which goes from the center to the periphery; the other is the sensory influence acting upon it from the periphery. Neither of these create heat.

Webster's New International Dictionary, 1910, says of heat: "A form of energy variously manifested to sense, as especially in the effects of fire, the sun's rays, or friction. Heat was formerly supposed to be a subtle, imponderable fluid, to which was given the name caloric. It is now known to be a form of energy, probably the kinetic energy of confused oscillating motions of the particles of molecules of matter. Degrees of temperature represents intensities, not quantities, of heat, for when the same amount of heat is imparted to two bodies of equal mass but of different substances one is found to be hotter than the other; and we say that the specific heats of the two substances are different. The heat added to a body usually causes change of volume. It may go partly or wholly to producing change of state by fusion or vaporization of the body, or may cause chemical reactions. It may be transformed in part into other kinds of energy, producing the phenomena of light, electricity, etc. Radiation is not heat, but is the kinetic energy of vibration of the ether. It produces thermal effects when it meets bodies which absorb it, that is to say, bodies in which the regular undulatory motion of the ether is transformed into a confused motion of the confused particles."

"Mental impulses create combustion of chemicals."

A chemical is a substance obtained by a chemical process or used for producing a chemical effect. These processes are performed in a chemical laboratory. Therefore, the act of combustion, the burning of chemicals in the body "is not in it." Consequently, chemicals are never deposited in the body, either arterially or "serously." Webster is acquainted with the word serous used only as an adjective and the nouns, serousness and serosity; also, the Latin phrase, sero venientibus ossa — the bones (i. e., leavings) for those who come late; but, he does not know of such an adverb as "serously." Neither the serum nor arteries deposit chemicals. Chemicals are not burned in the body nor anywhere else.

"Hypertrophic rhinitis."

Rhinitis is an inflammation of the nasal mucous membrane. Hypertrophy is the morbid enlargement or overgrowth of an organ or part. Can you think of inflammation being an overgrowth?

"The mucous membrane is of serous origin, and is one of the transitional tissues of that character. We find serous circulation exceedingly complete in these tissues."

What? The mucous membrane originated from serum? That is the limit. Transition is a passing from one state or condition to another. We are told that the character of the mucous membrane is its change from serum to that of membrane. That exceeds the limit. The serum does not circulate, does not perform a circuit; it is transuded; the act is transudation, not circulation. Why say the "serous circulation is exceedingly complete"?

"The excessive heat proves the existence of stimulated, caloric, mental impulses ending in the membrane affected. Caloric chemicals are deposited in normal quantities but excessive mental impulses cause more than normal combustion."

"Stimulated, calorific, mental impulses."

An impulse is a sudden spontaneous emotion of the mind or the influence of sensation acting upon it; it may be mental or sensory. Mental impulses are motor. Calorific is heat producing. We are told that motor impulses are heat producing. Motor impulses are those which determine motion to nerves and muscles; they are not calorific. Excessive heat is the result of an increased agitation of the particles of matter. Excessive heat does not prove the existence of impulses, motor, sensation, mental, calorific or stimulated. Excessive heat is too much functionating, accompanied with inordinate molecular vibration.

"Calorific chemicals are deposited in" the body "in normal quantities."

Chemicals exist in the laboratory as substances which undergo alterations within certain limits of existence, as determined by temperature and pressure—two properties of chemical substances. Gould's Dictionary of Medicine gives 748 chemical tests. Dorland's Medical Dictionary 347. In chemistry a test is a characteristic reaction which distinguishes any one body from all others. In all these chemical tests, there is no mention of depositing any one of them in the human body—an impossibility, an incongruity. Chemists do not know of "calorific chemicals." The quantity of each chemical used is calculated on a certain per cent basis, not upon "normal quantities."

"Excessive mental impulses."

A mental impulse, one originating from Innate, the spirit, cannot be excessive or insufficient. The function may be performed in excess or insufficiently, owing to the force of transmission being increased or decreased. Heat is now known to be a form of energy generated by the oscillation of molecules, the more or less violent changing of the atoms of matter. Therefore, mental impulses do not cause normal or abnormal combustion—a process accompanied by the evolution of light and heat.

"Catarrh is universal in all states, and is one of the easiest and quickest effects to show Chiropractic results."

The author does not define "all states," whether he refers to conditions or the United States.

"Catarrh is universal." Were catarrh universal, each and every person would be affected by it.

Is it a fact that all persons have catarrh, that it is universal, usual, normal? I think not.

"Catarrh is one of the easiest and quickest effects."

Catarrh is not an easy or quick affection; its onset is insidious. Its effects may be easy or uneasy on the patient.

"The cause of disease is the inability of Innate to express her wonted mental functional abilities thru a certain organ by means of impulses that are carried by nerves and then placed into action to perform the functions of impulses. If hindrance occurs, disease is the result. The character of the disease depending upon what functions are being hindered and to what extent."

Please reread that sentence of 40 words without a punctuation, then assist me to analyze it. The cause of disease is the inability of Innate to express her abilities. What kind of abilities? Functional abilities, mental abilities, wonted abilities. Whose abilities? Her abilities. Who is her? Innate. The author says that the abilities should be expressed thru a certain organ. The abilities to be expressed by means of impulses. Innate was unable to express her abilities. Innate's inability to express her abilities are the cause of disease. Innate "wonted" to express her abilities by means of impulses. Impulses are carried by nerves. Impulses are placed into action. What for? To perform the functions of muscles. If muscles are hindered to perform their functions, disease is the result. Disease is characterized by what muscle function is being hindered and the extent of such hindrance. What do you think of that?

"Twelve years ago D. D. Palmer had certain youthful principles that he based Chiropractic research around. Its early years was simple, yet accurate and homely. The present-day philosophy of adjusting vertebrae is practical yet so unmixed and pure that it is technically scientific. The application today is equal. This is now laid down in 2x2 exactness, reasons given for all deductions and conclusions. The stupendous development of the past two years in this respect alone marks another era in accord with Chiropractic's early teachings.

"For years we adjusted with a basis altho practiced undefined and unprinted or written.

"This book is based around six words. The aim has been simplicity in preference to a jargonity that has no semblance to anything. It is absolutely plain, unadorned, undesigning and its art portrayed in detail."

---

He that cannot or will not reason is a fool.

## THE OPTIC NERVE.

A prominent teacher of Chiropractic states: "The optic nerve is presumed to pass directly through the eye to the brain without having exit from the skull."

Anatomists do not have to presume, and others should not, in regard to the path of the optic nerve. This nerve does not pass directly, or otherwise, **through the eye.**

The eye ball occupies the orbital cavity which is on the outside of the skull. Therefore, as the optic nerve has its origin in the brain, this nerve has to pass thru an opening in order to reach the eye.

The optic nerve and the ophthalmic artery pass outward, side by side, through the optic foramen which is at the apex, in the superior back part of the orbit. On entering the orbital space, it makes a curve down, out, inward and then forward to the globe of the eye.

The ophthalmic artery is a branch of the internal carotid, which, as we have just stated, with the optic nerve gains the orbital cavity through the optic canal, lying close to and on the temporal side of the optic nerve.

This nerve and artery have been examined and followed, their exit side by side has been noticed thousands of times. Every class should dissect this and other nerves before they receive their final examination.

It is the height of folly to state: "Optic nerve running from the outer margin of the eye to the fourth cervical." There are two communicating nerves which originate in the cervical region and pass to and in the cervical ganglion of the sympathetic nervous system. They reach the optic nerve, one by way of the cavernous plexus and the other through the semilunar, or Gasserian ganglion of the sympathetic nervous system, and they to the cervical ganglion. Following these communicating branches, we find their origin in the spinal cord, from thence to the encephalon.

Communication between the central nervous system and the sympathetic is established through both efferent and afferent fibres. In the region of the spinal cord both kinds of fibers pass from one system to the other by way of the rami-communicantes, delicate bundles of fibres connecting the near-by sympathetic trunk with their respective spinal nerves. Those fibers which transmit impulses from the central to the sympathetic system, are known as efferent, splanchnic fibers.

These two communicating nerves, for which the optic nerve is indebted to the cavernous plexus and Gasserian ganglion of the fifth cervical, are the ones which Chiropractors trace from their impingement at the exit from the spinal foramen.

or as we should say, from the cervical ganglion, which passes downward in front of the transverse process.

The spinal nerves, whether they be those which proceed to the ganglionic trunks becoming sympathetic, or those which do not enter as such, but remain as spinal nerves, cannot be reached by digital pressure until they have passed out beyond the distance marked by the chain of sympathetic ganglia in the cervical and the upper nine dorsal. Because of more space, they may be felt, when swollen, close in between the floating ribs, and against the bodies of the lumbar vertebrae.

---

Disease is functional derangement, or structural change, either in position or substance.

---

Blear eyes. Blepharitis. Conjunctivitis. Trachoma. Granular eyelids. Eyelids tumefied, inflamed and more or less painful.

Pyorrhea alveolaris. Suppurative inflammation of the root membranes of the teeth in connection with the tissue of the gums beneath the mucous membrane. The teeth become loose, the gums recede from the teeth. Hemorrhage is very liable to occur.

Individual teeth may be affected with alveolitis and cause gum boils.

The Chiropractor will find the above conditions traceable to k. p. The nerves which carry innervation to the kidneys, also, contain fibers which go to the eyelids, the teeth and gums.

Kidney diseases usually accompany affections of the teeth and eyelids.

---

Science is knowledge; ascertained facts; accumulated information of causes and principles systematized. I ascertained these truths, acquired instruction, heretofore unrecognized, regarding the performance of functions in health and disease. I systematized and correlated these principles, made them practical. By so doing I created, brought into existence, originated a science, which I named Chiropractic; therefore I am a scientist. I systematized the principles I discovered; I have reasoned from cause to effect; searched into the nature of physiologic and pathologic processes; investigated the phenomena embraced in health and disease; assigned rational causes for the existence of normal and abnormal functions; answered the question, "What is life;" and founded a science and philosophy upon the basic principle of tone. This knowledge I have given to the world; therefore I am a philosopher.

## FOUNTAIN HEAD.

I am the Fountain Head of Chiropractic; it originated with me; it was my ingenious brain which discovered its first principle; I was its source; I gave it birth; to me all Chiropractors trace their Chiropractic lineage.

Pseudos have drunk from the fountain of knowledge which flowed from this source; they have listened to the teachings of the discoverer and developer of the grandest and greatest science of this age. Would-be fountain heads have quenched their thirst at the debouchere for scientific knowledge, that which is specific, and then have contaminated it with streams of therapeutical ignorance. They parade themselves before the public with deceit, falsehood and self-egotism, proclaiming that they are the fountain heads, or that they have captured the fountain head school.

Webster says: "Fountain Head, primary source; original; first principle." There can be but one primary source of the first principle of Chiropractic. I am the originator of the fundamental principle that disease is a condition produced by sub-luxated vertebrae which impinge upon nerves as they pass from the occluded intervertebral foramina of the spine. To say that the building in which he conceived the principles of Chiropractic is the Fountain Head Edifice, or that the school he founded several years after the discovery, is the "Fountain Head School," or that Davenport, the city in which he first promulgated the science, is The Fountain Head City, or that a lad of thirteen years of age when I began to publish, for the first time in the world's history, that pressure on nerves is **the cause of disease,** was the primary source, the originator of the first principle which his father discovered, and, by years of close study, developed into a science, shows ignorance of the meaning of Fountain Head, or the innate desire of a rascal to rob his parental benefactor. This bare-faced falsehood reminds me of the obliging Turk who exhibited two skulls of St. Paul, one when he was a boy of thirteen and another when advanced in age.

The head that was, yet remains the primary source, the originator of the principle from which was developed the science of Chiropractic. Its owner lives, and is the author of this volume. Even death cannot rob him of being The Fountain Head of Chiropractic; it is a well-earned honor which neither he nor any other can bestow upon any one.

There can be but one "Fountain Head" of Chiropractic, one "primary source," one "original" who discovered the "first principle," and that one is myself.

I, and not another, discovered the first principle upon which I built the science of Chiropractic when I adjusted Harvey Lillard in September, 1895. We did not have a school until four years later. Where was The Fountain Head during that four years? Was I the primary source, the originator of the first principle, or was the school which came four years later? Can the Fountain Head of a stream be miles below its origin? Can the Fountain Head, the primary source, the origin of the first principle, be transferred from me to the building, or school, or city, or to a child?

During the first few years of Chiropractic's existence, when B. J. was a lad, sometimes we had a student, or students, but often we had none. Where was The Fountain Head when we were minus a school? No school, no Fountain Head; no school, no primary source; no school, no origin of first principle; no school, no originator. If the teachings of Chiropractic constitutes the Fountain Head, then there are as many Fountain Heads as there are schools; as many primary sources as there are teachers; as many originators of first principle as there are students. With such misconception born of absurdity, B. J. Palmer and others assume the ownership of the Fountain Head. Registering stolen property does not create ownership.

I am the Fountain Head of Chiropractic. I am the Discoverer, Developer and Founder of this, the grandest and greatest science the world has ever known.

On page 61, Vol. 2, of The Science of Chiropractic, date 1907, B. J. says of me: "His actions and thoughts are sharp, alert and ahead of the times. He holds an enviable and honored position because others are being taught to reach his intellectual level. His every thought was **Why?** Originality combined with strict discipline and stick-to-itiveness joined with principle and honor, has made him many enemies, the majority of which are, knowing him better, turning from enmity to respect and reverence. Many students have been placed on the royal road to wealth, and a very few have, for mercenary, avaricious green, tried to undermine his honor; these cowards have failed at every turn. One by one the increasing pressure of right has driven them into the line of truth and justice."

---

In that first adjustment given Harvey Lillard in September, 1895, was the principle from which I developed the science of Chiropractic. In that adjustment originated the art of replacing vertebrae. In the succeeding fifteen years, I have endeavored to develop from that demonstrated fact, such principles, together with the art of adjusting, as constitute the science of Chiropractic.

## KNOWLEDGE.

Knowledge is acquired by becoming intimate and conversant with facts; it is obtained by recognition and familiarity with our surroundings. Knowledge depends upon the scope of information. By actual skill we make practical that which we have learned. Knowledge is usually acquired by perception and reflection. However, we may perceive facts without reflection. Knowledge may be received thru intuition—an immediate knowing.

As our knowledge increases, nescience decreases, noumena becomes known. We desire to reach out and know the unknowable. In this volume I am endeavoring scientifically to replace belief with facts, nescience with science, error with truth. Heretofore, medical science has been swimming as a superficial film on the sea of infinite unknowableness. The sciences of geology, astronomy, psychology, biology, chemistry and last, but not least, Chiropractic, are shedding their rays of light on the heretofore unknowable. As Chiropractic becomes better known, methods based on superstition will grow upward out of traditional legendaries. Therefore, it is important that this newly discovered science should be dressed in proper garb and not be misrepresented by childish nonsense.

Great truths are not born suddenly; they come by degrees; they are the result of consecutive investigation rather than discursive reasoning.

What is life; of what does it consist; how does it adapt itself to its environments? What are the properties by which organs, or the organism as a whole, are maintained? Upon what does the performance of functions depend? What is metabolism and what relation does it bear toward vitality? These are questions of special interest. To reveal and disseminate the knowledge demanded by them is the object of this volume. To possess this knowledge will add much to our welfare and happiness in this world and also in that which is to come.

Life is evolutionary in its development. The mineral, vegetable and animal kingdoms are looking forward and upward, seeking a more refined and better method of expression. Growth, unfoldment is seen everywhere. Each individualized portion of matter is but an epitome of the universe, each growing and developing toward a higher sphere of action; intelligence expressing itself thru matter. The various methods of cure are intellectual advancement toward others.

Knowledge is power; it is eternal. Created entities, whether spirit or matter, are not lost. Changes there are, always have been and always will be, but existence will continue. The transference by death is but the stepping behind the curtain—just out of sight. Communication by thot and speech may continue.

In days gone by, knowledge was supposed to belong to gods; to become wise, was to bring condemnation, debasement, not elevation. Knowledge grows us out of superstition and the traditional cobwebs of antiquity. As we observe and learn to think, we advance intellectually; we coordinate self with our surroundings. Knowledge of the physical world and its phenomena is an index of successive classified pages of sense impressions; these enable us to find the information we desire.

The brain is not the ego; it does not retain consciousness of physical experiences. Knowledge is gained by intuition, or by perception and reflection. The brain is the center of the nervous system. By and thru the nervous system we obtain all reflective knowledge. Intuitive education is not obtained by experience or cogitation, nor thru the nervous system. Back of and behind all is a consciousness, the **I, myself**, which is greater than the body we see; an intelligence which controls all bodily functions, whether we are asleep or awake. All thots originate and emanate from the ego, myself. This fact is one of the fundamental principles of the philosophy of Chiropractic.

Science teaches us to know and art to do. Science is systematized knowledge. Art is knowledge made efficient by skill—the adaptation of intelligence in the physical world for the use of human needs.

Knowledge consists of all that is known, from whatever source derived or obtained or by whatever process the aggregate of facts, truths or principles acquired and retained. It includes all which has been learned respecting phenomena, causes, laws, principles or literature, whether by intuition or reason. Intuitive knowledge is not acquired thru teaching or the understanding; experience does not enter into its makeup. It is thot transference, a forerunner of the near future when mankind will become so sensitive that thots can be impressed upon the nervous system and language written or spoken will be obsolete.

Education refines mankind; to know all is to pardon those who do not fully agree with us. Experience develops understanding; we learn by actually living thru enjoyment or suffering. This sensation or feeling may be real or imaginary, personal or spiritual. By actually living thru events, real or fanciful, we gain knowledge. We are interested in getting all we can out of life, physically and mentally. How we may best accomplish this is the vital question.

## SOME EXPLANATIONS.

Dunglison says disease is the opposite state to that of health; any functional change or derangement.

Webster states that disease is a disturbance of the performance of the vital organs, or an alteration in some part of the body, or some of its organs.

Chiropractically expressed, functional derangement is disease; when functions are not deranged, but performed in a normal manner, we have health.

Disease, complaint, disorder, illness, indisposition, distemper, ailment, malady, sickness and affection are synonyms, that is, they mean the same thing.

Disease is the general term for any deviation from health; in a more limited sense it denotes some definite morbid condition. Disorder and affection are rather partial and limited; as, a nervous affection; a disorder of the digestive system. Sickness as generally used in the Bible, means every form of physical disorder. There is a tendency to restrict the words sick and sickness to nausea, or sickness of the stomach. Ill and illness are used in a general sense. We speak of a trifling illness, a slight indisposition, a serious or deadly disease, a slight or severe illness, a painful sickness. Complaint may be applied to any degree of health, slight or severe. Infirmity denotes a chronic or lingering disability, as blindness or lameness.

Antonyms, words of opposite meaning are: Health, robustness, soundness, strength, sturdiness and vigor.

Dunglison gives healing as curative. Medicine as the healing art.

Webster defines healing: Tending to cure; soothing; mollifying, as, the healing art, a healing salve.

Dunglison says of remedy; medicament; of medicament, remedy, medicine.

Medicine formerly meant any substance or remedy used in the treatment of disease. Of late, so many drugless methods are in use that there is a growing tendency and demand to restrict the word medicine to substances or drugs used as medicine.

Webster says of remedy: That which relieves or cures a disease; any medicine or application which puts an end to disease and restores health.

The special business of the medical practitioner, is to use drugs as medicine. That of a Chiropractor, to adjust displaced vertebrae, placing the articular processes in their natural position. Medical men are not supposed to know that vertebrae can be racked from their natural position; in fact, until of late, they had held such a thing to be an impossibility. A Chiropractor is not a drug user; he does not use remedies for disease.

Chiropractors and jewelers do not treat or cure, do not prescribe or apply medicine when they adjust, fix or repair vertebrae or watches. They do not use salve or other preparations to soothe or mollify abnormal functions, or when correcting an unreliable timekeeper.

Therapy and therapeutics are synonyms. Dunglison says of therapeutics: That part of medicine the object of which is the treatment of disease. A treatise on medical treatment.

Webster defines therapeutics as that part of medical science which treats of the discovery and application of remedies for disease.

Dunglison—Therapeutical: Relating to or pertaining to therapeutics.

Webster—Therapeutical: Of or pertaining to the healing art; concerned in discovering and applying remedies for diseases; curative.

Chiropractors are not concerned in discovering medical remedies for the curing or healing of disease. They repair, adjust, fix, replace displaced bones of the skeleton frame.

Dunglison says that a therapeutist is one specially trained in the treatment of disease.

Webster states that a therapeutist is one versed in therapeutics, or the discovery and application of remedies.

A Chiropractor is not a therapeutist, as he is not interested in discovering or applying remedies. To be versed in therapeutics would require one to be skilled in the use and application of remedies. Chiropractors do not use remedies.

Chiropractic principles are antipodal to therapeutics. They are neither related or pertain to therapeutics.

Chiropractors are not therapeutists. The Chiropractic science is not therapeutical. A Chiropractor repairs by adjusting, fixing, replacing; he does not use any therapeutical remedies. Chiropractic is nontherapeutical.

---

Some persons are too slow to catch cold.

---

Some Chiropractors waste much time using adjuncts. If this time was utilized in studying the principles of Chiropractic and their application, the profession would be advanced. Adjunct users should read and **study** Chiropractic literature; but, these are the ones who do not care to advance.

I would suggest that Chiropractors sign D. C. to their names when they have received that degree, as it designates what kind of a doctor they are.

"We do not treat effect. We adjust cause." And yet he says: "Chiropractic treatments free the circulation. Some of the diseases cured by Chiropractic treatment." "My treatment," is used three times in three short lines.

"Strange, but true, all the nerves of the body may be acted upon by the hands." I wish the doctor would show me how to act on the cranial nerves by hand.

"Chiropractic means hand practice." Not, if I know its Greek derivation.

I would prefer to use The Chiropractor instead of "the Chiropractic doctor."

"The two vertebrae being brought together create a window." The vertebrae are not brought together—they were created thus. A window is an opening in a building for the admission of light and air. The intervertebral notch is not a window. O. G. Smith calling it a window does not make it one.

"There is but **one place** where there can be any interference with the operation of this life power, **and that is in the spinal column, because** it is composed of bones and **boney** substance and the nerves extend through movable openings, while the rest of the body, through which the nerves pass, is composed of soft tissue, which is practically incapable of abnormal pressure upon nerves."

"Boney" is incorrectly spelled. Nerves may be impinged by the displacement of any one of the 200 bones, or by pressure of a hard substance. Bones are the only hard tissue of the body; when they project from their proper alignment, they press against sensitive nerves, deranging their carrying capacity. Elsewhere, The Adjuster describes the difference between pinching and impinging.

"Abnormal pressure on nerves." Any pressure is abnormal.

"If the cartilages between the vertebrae were abnormally thinned it will be readily seen that such a condition would allow the vertebrae to come closer together and make the openings between the vertebrae smaller; in fact, it would partially close these openings and the nerves laying within would be **impinged upon** and the nerve stimuli which should pass through would be **obstructed,** and the tissues, or organs, at the ends of these nerves would have **less than normal supply.**"

**Nerves pressed between two vertebrae are pinched. They are impinged upon when the pressure is brought to bear against one side.** Displaced bones usually excite nerves. Bones by impringement upon nerves, cause them to become irritated. Pressure on nerves causes local inflammation—general fever. A constant, heavy pressure on nerves will prevent normal vibrations which carry impulses. Blood vessels may have their channels obstructed. Nerves have no channels; their carrying capacity depends upon their ability to vibrate. Normal vibrations carry the normal amount in a natural manner. "Less than normal supply." The larger share of diseases are because of **more** than a normal amount of functionating.

"The **channels** through which the organs receive their power are the nerves, the place of emanation of this power is the brain. From whence the power comes. we do not know. If man is ever able to conceive and explain from whence this power comes and what it is, he will have solved the problem of the universe."

"The Chiropractor in making his diagnosis can, by examining the spinal column and noting the condition of the nerves and the position of the vertebrae, **accurately locate** the cause of ailments **and explain conditions and symptoms without asking a single question.**" He nor any other Chiropractor, cannot always locate the cause of ailments, or know the "symptoms without asking a single question." We make more or less mistakes in our analysis (diagnosis). Recent graduates are the ones who know the most—in their estimation. In proportion as we become acquainted with osteology, neurology, the principles of Chiropractic and a knowledge of functions, we shall make less mistakes. Failures made in diagnosis and locating causes, while I was in the author's adjusting room, showed me that the above statement is untrue and misleading. If we aim to tell the truth, we will lie often enough.

---

Better learn to adjust causes than to treat symptoms with drugs.

---

Seattle, Nov. 9, 1908.

The Seattle schools have sent home 717 children because they were not vaccinated. Their parents propose to fight for their right in the public schools—an education without being poisoned.

According to Dr. G. A. R. Steiner, there are 2008 children in the Seattle schools who are not vaccinated.

If vaccination is a sure protection against smallpox, why are the parents of vaccinated children not satisfied? Why demand that their neighbor's family should be vaccinated? Because they have no faith in its protection, fearing that their children who are immune (?) may catch it from those not vaccinated.

## SYMPTOMS.

"In all the vast lore of therapy appertaining to symptoms, there is nowhere to be found the expression of the faintest concept that a symptom properly applies or is related to anything but disease. In this connection Chiropractic teaches that a symptom is only an evidence of a condition, be that a condition of normality or abnormality. The symptoms of normal processes are fully as numerous and of as much value to the practitioner as those of abnormal processes. To determine that the individual has a certain disease, it is only necessary to observe all of the symptoms, both normal and abnormal. A Chiropractic diagnosis consists in an observance of all of the symptoms of the patient, those of normality as well as those of abnormality."

A symptom is a phase which occurs synchronously with a disease and serves to point out its nature, location and the changes taking place. Symptoms only exist during the period of disease. "In all the vast lore of therapy" or that of Chiropractic, symptom is not applied or related to any condition but disease. Symptoms always apply to functional disturbance or morbid tissue. Chiropractic teaches that a symptom is "an evidence of a condition named disease." Disease is studied by the symptoms exhibited. Normal processes and normal conditions do not exhibit symptoms—evidences of disease. Any perceptible change in an organ or function from that in health is a symptom; could not be otherwise than a symptom. The term symptoms of symptoms is used to denote the effects which are the result of certain symptoms and are not essentially or directly connected with the disease itself. The debility arising from dysentery is a symptom of symptoms. The word symptoms is never used in connection with normal functions or normal tissue.

"The Chiropractor, in making a diagnosis, first of all makes a very careful and thorough examination of the articulations of the skeletal frame to determine whether or not there are occlusions of nerves in the same."

To make a diagnosis is to distinguish one disease from another, by objective and subjective signs and symptoms. In making a diagnosis it should be the Chiropractor's business, first of all, to determine the nature of the disease by learning what functions are abnormally performed; what part of the body is affected. Then take into consideration the nerves which ramify the diseased portion in which they are likely to be impinged upon, and **lastly, not the first of all,** examine the locality where he has decided the luxation exists which by its displacement impinges upon those nerves. To examine "the (300) articulations of the skeletal frame first of all," would be to leave out the diagnosis.

The author of the above seems to think and would give his readers to understand that to make a diagnosis is to examine the articulations of the skeletal frame. It is safe to say that the author of Carver's Analysis, a teacher in a Chiropractic school, does not know what constitutes a diagnosis.

Most Chiropractors know but little or nothing of pathology or of the symptoms and signs of disease and normal or abnormal functions. They do not stop to make a diagnosis, but, straightway, first of all, make an examination of the vertebral column and adjust those they think out of alignment, regardless of the nature of the disease.

An examination of the "articulations of the skeltal frame" would be to inspect the 300 articulations. Why not make a diagnosis and determine therefrom which vertebra is displaced?

"The occlusions of nerves" has been noticed elsewhere; therefore I will only add that there are 76 articulations in the vertebral column; the uppermost five could not occlude foramina, for there are none to be occluded and the remainder outside (224) have no foramina to occlude. Why examine the 229 articulations which by their displacement could not possibly occlude foramina?

Any bone displaced may impinge upon nerves, but never squeeze or pinch them.

---

"Drugs have no place in this (Chiropractic) process."

Chiropractic is not a process. A process consists of a **series** of actions, motions or occurrences. Chiropractic is a science, not a process. Adjusting is an art.

---

Each and every Chiropractor who desires to achieve more than ordinary success should possess a thorough knowledge of osteology, neurology, functions and the principles of Chiropractic. If we desire to reach the intellectual class we must be educated in our profession. This should be the Chiropractor's stock in trade, his working capital.

We have the goods; you need them. If you can't do the best, then do the next best. If you cannot attend the D. D. Palmer School, thereby receiving Chiropractic direct from the originator, the Fountain Head, then take the Adjuster, study its pages, imbibe Chiropractic as developed by the founder. Be sure that your cumulative function accumulates these thots by physiological action. Remember, if you receive Chiropractic ideas pathologically, distorted, they are not physiologically Chiropractic.

## NERVE STRETCHING.

Landois gives us some valuable hints toward the philosophy of Chiropractic. He records: "Nerve-stretching is a mechanical procedure that has been employed for therapeutic purposes. If the exposed nerve is stretched, the tension acts as an irritant when it reaches a certain degree. After slight stretching the reflex irritability is at first increased; stronger stretching causes for a time diminution of irritability, as well as of reflex activity, and even temporary paralysis. The most extreme degree of stretching finally gives rise to permanent paralysis. It appears that the centripetal fibers (sciatic nerve) lose their conductivity earlier than the centrifugal fibers. In the process of stretching mechanical changes are induced in the nerve-tubes or in the end-organs that bring about alteration in irritability. The effect of the stretching may be propagated also to the central nervous system. Paralysis following forced stretching may undergo a marked degree of recovery. If, therefore, a nerve is in a state of excessive irritability, for example in a case of neuralgia, if this be due to inflammatory fixation or constriction of a nerve in its course, nerve-stretching may be useful partly by diminishing the irritability of the nerve, partly by breaking up the inflammatory adhesions. Nerve-stretching may be useful also in cases in which irritation of a centripetal nerve gives rise to reflex or epileptic convulsions by diminishing the peripheral irritability (in addition to the action described). In the case also of diseases of the spinal cord that have not yet advanced to a state of gross degeneration nerve-stretching is not to be neglected as a therapeutic agent.

"For physiological purposes R. Heidenhain's tetanomotor is employed to induce mechanical nerve stimulation. This consists of a vibrating ivory hammer attached to an extension of the Neef hammer of the induction-apparatus, which by a rapid succession of blows upon the underlying nerve develops a condition of tetanus lasting up to two minutes.

"Naturally, other mechanical stimuli of a similar nature will yield analogous results, such as contact with a vibrating tuning-fork, or with a sounding string, stroking with a bow-like apparatus, rythmic stretching of the nerve (longitudinal traction)."

Nerve tension, nerve stretching, acts as an irritant, causes too much functionating, too much action, a waste of energy. Extreme tension causes paralysis. Bones of the body framework give to nerves a proper and normal tension, known as tone. If they are displaced, they will cause either more tension or relaxation. If so, why not replace the displaced bone which is causing tension or relaxation?

A rapid succession of blows by a vibrating hammer increases tension and vibration. Vibration and tension coexist in nerve-tissue. Placing an exposed nerve against a vibrating tuning fork or a vibrating string of a musical instrument, will cause a similar vibration in the nerve, just as the contact of a telegraph wire will affect a telephone wire. Herein is an explanation for wireless telegraphy and thot transference. May this not account for the invalid feeling fetter or worse because of a neighbor's call?

---

It is said that Dr. McConnell, of Chicago, took dogs from the pound and wrenched their spines at certain points. A few weeks later the dogs were killed. The nerves near the strained vertebrae were examined with the naked eye and microscope; also the organs which those nerves supplied. In every instance the nerves and the organs innervated by them were found congested, inflamed and their functions disordered.

---

The O. G. Smith pounding tables used to make muscle; the Langworthy stretching machine; the throat punching; the no cranial nerves; the no sympathetic nerves and the no reflex action are not Chiropractic. They are antagonistic and detrimental to the philosophy of the science. The mission of The Adjuster will be to give Chiropractic up to date, throw down and out all rubbish that accumulated while I was "on a vacation."

---

"Ki-ro-prak-tic is the latest and most scientific method of removing the cause of 95 per cent of all acute and chronic diseases known, without Drugs, Medicine or Operation."

Why say "**most** scientific," when it is the only science which locates the cause of disease? Why not say Ki-ro-prak-tik is the only scientific method known which removes the cause of 95 per cent of all diseases without Drugs, Medicine or Operation?

---

Allopathy. That system of remedial treatment which seeks to cure diseases by producing a condition incompatible with the disease; opposed to homeopathy. "And poisons must, as Galen held, by counter-poisons be expelled."

Homeopathy. That system of medical treatment which seeks to cure a disease by administering medicine which would produce this same disease in a healthy condition; opposed to Allopathy. Similia similibus curantur. Like cures like.

## BIOLOGY.

Biology is the science of life; that branch of knowledge which treats of living matter as distinct from that which does not possess a living force.

It is divided into two main branches, morphology and physiology. Morphology deals with the origin, form, structure and distribution of living things. Physiology treats of the functions which create and continue a living existence, and the manner in which its individual parts perform their functions.

Anatomists study the structure of organs, their shape, size, the tissues of which they are composed and their relative position in the body.

Pathology treats of the modification of functions, changes in position and structure of parts. Pathological processes are but greater or less variations from those which are physiological. These deviations are regarded as morbid, since they pertain to abnormal functions or diseased structure. Disease is the result of the quickening or the retarding of impulses which excite, sway or modify the orderly transformation of energy. It is the amount of energy which transmits an impulse and gives it force; too much or not enough causes functions to be performed in too great or too little degree. It is the manifestation of perturbed functions or altered structure, or both; in fact, either cannot exist without the other. Pathology deals with the disturbances of functions and the alteration of structure in living beings which are induced by unusual agencies and conditions. The functional disturbances thus produced are embraced and known as symptoms of disease, or pathological physiology. The phenomena of pathological physiology are in no way opposed to those of normal physiology; they are their inevitable correlatives, when the living body is placed under sufficiently abnormal conditions. Pathological morphology is concerned with the structural alterations of the organism which result from abnormal conditions. It deals with the gross and microscopic alterations of structure; it embraces pathological anatomy and pathological histology. Alterations in structure are always associated with disturbance of function; both are dependent upon the inciting factors of disease. An intelligent study of morphology, of necessity includes normal anatomy and normal physiology, also pathological anatomy and physiology.

Physiology as defined by the medical profession includes the laws of chemistry and physics; that is, the same laws which regulate action of the mineral, organic world are believed to be operative in organic beings. Metabolism is supposed by the same fraternity to take place according to the laws of chemistry and physics. That is, food contains chemical substances which are acted upon in a chemical way by the various digestive juices in order to render them of service in building up the organism. Digestion is that to be a form of fermentation; when it is excessive or deficient there results a condition known as disease. McFarland states, "Until our knowledge of biology in its normal and abnormal relations is perfected, medicine cannot become an exact science."

Chiropractors consider that metabolism is dependent upon vital force, and not upon chemical action; that impulses sent out by Innate (Spirit) are normal, and would continue so to their nerve endings and functionate normally, if not interfered with by a change in the transmitting tissue.

The conductibility of impulses is modified by age. In general it may be said that the extremes of life show an increased disposition to disease. Certain diseases as mumps, diphtheria, croup, measles, chicken pox and pertussis affect children principally and occur only occasionally in adults. In advanced age we find diseases which are rare in infancy. Nerves become hardened and less sensitive as we advance in age; the glands, organs and cartilage become more fibrous and less elastic.

Functions are modified by traumatic injuries and various substances which, when taken inwardly or applied externally, impair the normal or special action of a part. Displacements of the osseous frame-work impinge upon nerves which direct the communication of impulses, and give an undue force to functional activity. Poisons just as surely act upon and cause contraction of nerves and muscles, drawing bones out of alignment. Local inflammations and fevers are due to traumatic injuries, inoculated virus or to poisons taken internally. An overheated condition, whether local or general, disturbs the functions of the body. All known diseases are the result of, and are accompanied by, deranged functions.

The body derives its nourishment from a circulating, nutritive fluid which is transuded thru the tissues by exosmosis and imbibition. When it is considered that the body contains in all its tissues about half its weight in water which is constantly being thrown off with the urine and feces, as well as by the skin and lungs; that, in the process of digestion and absorption, most substances must be dissolved in water; that water is a constituent of fluid-food, and, likewise, that numerous waste-products, especially in the urine, must leave the body in aqueous solution, the importance of a constant supply and continued renewal of water will be at once obvious. The transuded fluid, known as lymph, closely resembling the plasma in composition, but usually more watery, constantly passes thru the endothelial membranes, the capillaries, supplying such metabolic tissue elements as are not in immediate contact with the capillaries with moisture and nutriment. Provision is made for its removal from the tissues, after it has fulfilled its purpose, thru the lymphatic vessels which begin as mere clefts and gradually develop into larger vessels so as to provide a system of tissue drainage. I am now describing what is known by some Chiropractors as "the serous circulation" which, because it was a new thot to them, was considered a new discovery. All physiologists and anatomists know of, and have written extensively about, the "serous," the fluid transudation which pertains to all vegetable and animal life. There is a physiologic balance between the circulation and the amount of lymph, so that no more fluid exudes into a tissue than it needs. If the quantity of the fluid is increased the circulation is correspondingly accelerated. In diseased conditions this even balance is disturbed; either the transudate liquid is increased or the circulation is less active; the tissue becomes distended, saturated, macerated and tumefied, a condition known as edema or dropsy. Dropsy is not because of a surplus of the water drank as is often supposed.

Fatty infiltration is the accumulation and retention of fat. The physiologic functions of fat are, to protect the organs, maintain temperature and in time of need to become liquidized for nutritive purposes. Fat is a common physiologic phenomenon; it becomes pathologic only when it occurs in unusual tissues or in excessive amount. A physiologic function becomes pathologic when either excessively or deficiently active.

The science of Chiropractic has modified our views concerning life, death, health and disease. We no longer believe that disease is an entity, something foreign to the body, which may enter from without, and with which we have to grasp, struggle, fight and conquer, or submit and succumb to its ravages. Disease is a disturbed condition, not a thing of enmity. Disease is an abnormal performance of certain functions; the abnormal activity has its causes, as much so, as the windows which are bound and cease to be movable, or the transoms and doors which we are unable to close, because of the settling of some portion of the building. The morphological alterations of the body superinduced by displaced structure can be located and as surely corrected as can the sagging of the building. Disease is manifested by functional aberrations and structural alterations. These constitute the signs, symptoms and lesions of a departure from a state of health. Disease does not involve any new functional expression which the body does not already possess; it is only a change in the amount of energy and function performed. The body in disease does not develop any new form of energy; what it already possesses is diminished or increased, perverted or abolished. In health there is a constant physiological, invincible molecular change—the manifestations of energy. In disease this manifestation of energy is modified and the quality of structure is altered. The transmission of physiological impulses in normal amount is health; in a less or greater degree, disease. Physiological metabolism is health; pathologic metabolism is disease. The vital process known as metabolism, consists of osmosis, diffusion, elasticity, pressure and affinity. These are the energetical expressions of vital force.

---

## TAPE WORM.

This worm occupies the intestinal tract of man and the lower animals. It consists of a head, neck and a segmented body. The head is quite small, the neck long and slender; the body is flattened like a ribbon. The head is provided with four suckers and from ten to fifteen hooks. It varies in length from two to forty feet and consists of from two to a thousand joints. Each segment represents a complete organism. At maturity segments are discharged with the stool, its body ruptured and its eggs scattered. There is usually but one worm found in the same individual. Although the head is small and the neck slender, the segments of the body are half an inch in width. The number of eggs in a full-grown worm are estimated at from five to ten millions. It is parasitical, as it lives upon, and in, another animal.

The presence of this worm, in man, is supposed to cause indigestion. On the contrary, it is a scavenger living upon decaying food. If digestion were perfect, there would be no need of a scavenger; the food proposition would be reversed as the stomach would make food of its contents.

There are no signs by which a tape worm can be positively asserted, except the passing of its segments. There are many symptoms which are supposed to indicate the presence of a tape worm, among which are impairment of appetite and digestion, dizziness, diminishing of vision, itching of the nose and general emaciation.

It will be understood from the above dissertation that Chiropractically, to remove a tape worm, it is only necessary to improve digestion. The innervating nerve of the stomach will be found proceeding from the left side of the spine. Remove the impingement and allow the nerves to assume their normal tonicity.

## TYPHOID FEVER.

"The happy combination known as typhoid fever."

Some adjust in three places for this disease, therefore, the language of my text.

As there are quite different symptoms in three different cavities of the body, one vertebra is adjusted for each symptom.

Others, as well as myself, have relieved typhoid fever by one adjustment at center dorsal. If this disease can be relieved by the replacing of one vertebra—that is specific. That is what we as Chiropractors want to know.

I am well aware that three different portions of the body are affected. The symptoms in different cases being somewhat dissimilar.

There may be hemorrhage of the head, gums or bowels, because of softening of the tissue by too much heat. There is always present general, excessive heat. There is impairment of appetite, headache and diarrhea. The patient is stupid, somewhat delirious, sleeping but little, remaining in a semi-conscious condition. The teeth are covered with sordes, tongue dry and coated, abdomen inflamed and swollen with gas. The bowels may become ulcerated and perforated. There is inflammation of the meninges of the brain, lungs and bowels. There may be present suppurative lesions, such as osteitis, periostitis or osteomyelitis—inflammation of bones, their covering and their marrow. Meningitis, inflammation of the membranes of the brain or spinal cord may become prominent.

The predisposing cause is poison from some decaying animal or vegetable matter. Nerves sense this poison and as a consequence vertebrae are drawn out of alignment impinging upon the ganglionic chain of the sympathetic nervous system.

General, excessive heat points a Chiropractor to C. P. But how and why are such different portions affected? In order to explain, we will need to go over the distribution and the make-up of the sympathetic nervous system.

The trunks, or the gangliated cords of the vertical sympathetic nervous system, extend, on either side of the vertebral column, from the base of the brain to the coccyx. These chains are connected with the spinal nervous system by a series of branches springing from the spinal cord, which reaches from the occiput to the coccyx. These fibers go into the ganglia and their intervening nerve-cords and are distributed to the viscera by irregular branches. At its cephalic end, each sympathetic cord is continued in a plexiform manner into the cranial cavity, forming an intimate relationship with certain cranial nerves. At the lower extremity the two chains of ganglia are connected by the coccygeal ganglion. These two gangliated cords are also connected by intervening nerve trunks at various places.

The ganglia of these two important vertical chains are freely connected with the spinal nerves by what are called rami-communicantes. These branch from the spinal nerve trunks and pass into the various ganglia of the two sympathetic nerve chains of ganglia. They may be distributed directly from the ganglia reached or they may pass upward or downward and terminate in other ganglia from whence they are distributed to the viscera.

The sympathetic system serves to rearrange fibers derived from the cerebro-spinal system and distribute them to the viscera of the four great cavities of the body. In other words, it carries impulses from these fibers to the internal organs; the amount of functionating depending upon the extent to which the nerves leading to them are excited or depressed by impingements.

At C. P. we find a nervous center of distribution to all parts of the body. This discovery, as also were all other important developments, was made by me. The reader will please excuse the mentioning of this, for others claim to be the discoverers of 99 per cent of that which goes to make up the principles of Chiropractic. I would like for them to state any one principle of value which they have added to the science. As I have said, we find at C. P. a general, nervous center for all parts of the body. At this place we find the cause of hemiplegia and several other diseases which affect the body generally. Among these are typhoid fever. At the twelfth dorsal we find a Second Center Place.

Efferent splanchnic fibers transmit impulses from the central to the sympathetic system. We find hemiplegia has its cause in an impingement at C. P., because at this location there is a nervous center which controls the functions of half of the body; which half, depends upon which ganglionic chain is impinged upon. Where the face is affected on one side and the rest of the body on the opposite side, or the lower limb on one side and the upper on the opposite side, there is a crossed nerve trunk affected, producing a condition known as crossed hemiplegia. Cross nerve trunks connect the two gangliated cords at various places. Pardon my digression from the subject. I have made it, that the reader may the better comprehend the relationship that the various symptoms of this disease in different portions of the body bear to each other.

These gangliated chains are supplied with fibers from higher or lower levels, passing upwards or downwards to terminate in other ganglia of the same cord or in these of the opposite side.

The most pronounced lesion is ulceration of the intestines. It is characterized by a peculiar enlargement and necrosis of the lymphatic tissue owing to excessive heat. Diarrhea from too much functional activity--because of the excited condition of the nervous tissue of the intestines—is a prominent symptom.

The sympathetic fibers given off from the cerebro-spinal system may end in the ganglion with which it is related, or it may course upwards or downwards in the commissural cord in order to reach a neighboring ganglion, or it may even pass beyond all the ganglia and end with the peripheral cells along with the fibers of distribution from other sympathetic ganglia.

To sum up our findings. An impingement at C. P. irritates, excites the fibers of the nerve with which the displaced bone comes in contact. The vibrations of nerves is increased from 200 a minute to many more, increasing their carrying capacity, or rather their speed, accordingly. Too much heat is transmitted. If 200 is normal, then all over this is abnormal, excessive. This increased heat is transmitted to all parts of the body. The bones become softened and their color changed from white to that of a reddish-yellow. The vascular system is softened, giving way, at certain places, causing hemorrhage. The soft tissue of the intestines becomes more softened, even to the extent of necrosis, and perforation ensues.

Excessive heat is the cause of all abnormal conditions, the combination of which is named typhoid fever; an impingement at C. P. caused by a sub-luxated vertebra is behind that. And, behind all, is poison introduced into the system which acts on the nervous system—nerves sense poison.

---

What is better than a promising young man? One that makes good.

---

A Chiropractor's newspaper ad. reads in part:

"I'm in business for your health. Stop submitting to medical violence and get my opinion on your case, no matter what is your difficulty."

---

"Your body is a machine shop filled with a number of perfectly constructed machines." "Your body machine."

A machine shop is a workshop containing machines, where machines are made, where castings are finally shaped and finished. A machine is a construction or contrivance of a mechanical nature, the work of human hands.

## HEMORRHAGE.

The readiest temporary method of arresting hemorrhage is by pressure at the bleeding point or upon the artery above it. Never be afraid of a bleeding point, when you can place your finger upon it. If you make pressure at the proper spot, very little force is required; it can be easily maintained until permanent control of the bleeding has been secured. The stoppage of circulation by pressure has given the blood at the bleeding point time to coagulate. When the pressure is slowly removed, if no blood escapes, the wound may be dressed, leaving the blood-clot in position.

---

No. 2 of Vol. 1 of "Catalog Edition" is before me. It contains 29 pages. On page 28 I find: "Now that you have read the catalogue through, the question is, what are you going to do?"

I read the first 28 pages, but did not find a catalogue, list or enumeration of anything until the last page, which contained a list of students of the Oakley Smith College of Naprapathy.

The first of Prof. Smith's lectures, page 25, is "on hemiplegia or paralysis of one-half of the body." Page 26: "From the first day to the last the student's attention is gained and held by a stream of facts which at once build up an immovable foundation for the science of Naprapathy, and undo the formerly time-honored but erroneous teachings of medicine relative to the cause and cure of disease."

Let us see how they "undo the formerly time-honored but erroneous teachings of medicine relative to the cause and cure of disease."

Page 21: "In case of paralysis on one side of the body it is the sympathetic nervous system that is originally injured. This injury leads to an injury of the blood vessels in the brain. As a result of this sympathetic force being shut off, the blood-vessels swell or burst. Thus it is that paralysis is caused . . . This example is merely an illustration of the vital necessity of knowing intimately the course and distribution of all of the nerves of the body and the detailed relation of the various portions of the body which are in direct contact with the nerves."

This is the kind of interesting knowledge that Dr. Smith gives you in his daily lectures on anatomy. Dr. Smith yet holds to "the time-honored erroneous teachings of medicine"—a clot of blood on the brain and the "sympathetic force being shut off" as the cause of hemiplegia. The reader will refer to the section upon hemiplegia; he will see the difference between Chiropractic and the above view.

## THE CHIROPRACTOR'S WORK.

The Chiropractors are a band
Of noble workers, true and grand;
They truly labor all day long,
Striving to make right of the wrong.

They've studied well the human frame,
And of each part they know the name.
They know just where the nerves extend,
And on this fact much doth depend.

These tiny nervous threads doth play,
A most important part, they say;
In the condition of our health,
Which is to man far more than wealth.

The vertebrae compose the spine,
From which these slender nerves do wind;
Quite often from their duty stray,
From various causes in life's way.

Now, when these little bones go wrong,
The nerves as they ramble along
Are impinged upon here and there,
Causing disease which needs repair.

It seems to me 'tis plain to see
That vibration changed must be,
When pressure on these nerves doth come,
Making these nervous threadlets numb.

If the blood from its fountain source,
Does not well run thruout its course,
The body needs must suffer much,
This fact we know without research.

Chiropractor's must first inspect,
Remove the cause, not treat effect,
Impingements they seek to relieve,
And then much benefit receive.

So, to the vertebrae they go,
Adjust the displaced, just so;
That they in their places may be,
So that they from disease be free.

When the cause has been removed,
Kind nature can then do us good;
Disease no longer is within,
And we a happy life begin.

We know that without health 'tis vain,
Much pleasure in this world to gain;
But, with all things, changed doth seem,
Into our lives great joy doth gleam.

May God bless Chiropractors true,
That they still greater work may do;
For well we know that from on high
Great blessings come to those who try.
—The Health Journal, St. Paul, Minn.

---

## OSTEOPATHY.

"The human family needs **Osteopathy.** It has become a necessity, because it **embraces the whole range of human ills.**"

"Such success followed these manipulations that it was found to be **all that was needed** to restore harmony throughout the body, thereby obviating the necessity of drugs, they no **longer being necessary in the cure of disease**; and **these manipulations were found adequate and adaptable in every condition called disease.**

"Osteopathy is based upon a thorough knowledge of anatomy and physiology, which enables the skilled operator to correct any deviation of bony, muscular, ligamentous, arterial, venous or nerve structure found anywhere in the body causing inharmony and thereby restoring it to a normal condition.

"The following studies are taught by personal demonstrations: Hygiene, Dietetics, Hydropathy, Principles and Practice of Osteopathy, Naturopathy, Neuropathy, Chiropractic, Massage, Electro-Therapeutics, in fact **all systems** and methods of Drugless Healing."

Among all other systems and methods are, Ophthalmology, Suggestive Therapeutics, Phrenology, Mental Science, Christian Science, Hydro-Therapeutics, Electro-Thermal, Swedish Movement Appliances, Physical Culture, sun, water, light and air baths.

If "Osteopathy . . . embraces the whole range of human ills" and "all that is needed to restore harmony throughout the body," other methods being "no longer necessary in the cure of disease," and Osteopathic "manipulations are found adequate and adaptable in every condition called disease," **why use "all other systems and methods"?**

## TONE AND FUNCTIONS.

What is the basic principle of Chiropractic, the elementary proposition from which all other Chiropractic principles have sprung? It is tone.

What is tone? Normal tension.

What is tension? It is the renitency, the elasticity of tissue in a healthy state.

What is renitence? It is the normal resisting pressure acting against an impulse by elastic force, known as tonicity.

What is tonicity? It is the state of healthy tension or partial, normal contraction of muscles, ligaments and nerves.

What is contraction? It is the shortening of living fibers, with consequent thickening, by the application of a stimulus; it may be traumatic, toxic, auto or nervous.

What is a stimulus? It is anything which rouses or excites the vital energies of an organ or part of the body to increased functional activity.

What is energy? It is the power to produce action, the ability to overcome resistance.

What is functional activity? It is the action of an organ, whether physiological or pathological.

From whence does this power originate? It is inherent and dependent upon the tension of the organ whose function is being performed.

What is physiologic action? The normal functionating of the body and organs.

What is pathological action? It is vital action expressed in a degree either greater or less than normal, resulting in abnormal functionating and morbid tissue.

What is morbid tissue? The tissue of a diseased organ. Morbid is used as a technical or scientific term in contradistinction to the term healthy.

What is disease? A condition consisting of a change in position, or structure of a part or an organ, also, a change in one or more of its functions. Abnormal functions and morbid tissue are coexistent.

What view does the medical men take of disease? "An abnormal condition, general or local, marked by more or less characteristic changes of structure and function, generally having a definite cause, and running a more or less typical course, so that it may be considered as a distinct entity; a vigorous effort of nature to throw off morbific matter, and thus to recover the patient."

What are the most prominent symptoms of disease? Increased or decreased respiration, temperature and pulse. The vital tripod, the tripod of life, consists of the heart, lungs and brain; so named because their united action is necessary to the maintenance of life.

Why are abnormal functions and morbid tissue contemporaneous? Because normal and abnormal tissue can only perform functions becoming their condition; their structure and function depending upon their tension.

Why are not the functions of respiration, pulsation and temperature equally affected in disease? Because the impingement, poison or auto-suggestion may not change the tension of the innervating nerves of each function to the same degree.

---

## STRIP OF GAUZE IN BODY.

Depositions are being taken at Albany in a case pending in Oklahoma growing out of the peculiar fact that a physician, in sewing up a woman's body after an operation, is alleged to have left a piece of gauze 11 by 33 inches in size inside her body. Alice M. Elliott, of Lebanon, is suing Dr. U. L. Russell, of Guthrie, Okla., for $20,000 damages for malpractice.

On June 14, Dr. Russell performed an operation on Mrs. Elliott at Guthrie, Okla. She survived the operation and soon afterword came to Oregon with her husband, S. H. Elliott, and located at Lebanon. During the year following the operation she experienced considerable pain at times in her abdomen, but her condition did not become serious until early in August, 1908. She suddenly became very ill and Drs. W. H. and J. C. Booth, of Lebanon, who were attending her, saw that an immediate operation was necessary to save her life. She was brought to St. Mary's Hospital in Albany and an operation was performed by Drs. R. C. Coffey, of Portland, W. H. Davis, of Albany, W. H. Booth and J. C. Booth, of Lebanon.

When the physicians opened up the woman's body they were surprised to find a piece of gauze which had gradually collected into a solid mass and completely filled an intestine for a distance of about three inches. The gauze had clogged the intestine completely for probably 24 hours before the operation and had not the operation been performed immediately, death would have resulted. After the gauze was removed, Mrs. Elliott at once got well.

---

"Dr. Carver first became acquainted with Chiropractic through an application of its principles to his own case which was believed by therapeutists to be fatal." I made that application thirteen years ago, relieving him of consumption.

## NEURITIS.

Inflammation of a nerve is called neuritis. A nerve is an elongated, cord-like structure made up of an aggregation of nerve-fibers having the property of transmitting nervous impulses. Nerves which possess a degree of heat above 98.6 degrees are said to be inflamed.

Nerves overheated are enlarged, hardened, contracted lengthwise and sensitive to the touch. Microscopically, they seem to be partially degenerated with fatty myelin-sheaths and swollen axis-cylinders. Owing to the number of nerve-fibers occupying a nerve covering, we may have multiple neuritis, for fibers often leave their original trunk and pass into and become a part of other nerves. Several nerves, usually diametrically situated on both sides of the body, may be simultaneously affected with inflammation. Neuritis may accompany alcoholic, arsenic, mercury or lead poisoning, or such diseases as diabetes, measles, small pox, diphtheria, pneumonia and typhoid fever. Beriberi is a form of multiple neuritis.

Neuritis of necessity is attended with fever. The temperature may reach 104 degrees, or it may be subnormal after the fever crisis. Sunstroke may show temperature as high as 112 degrees or as low as 92.3 degrees. This latter condition is one of exhaustion instead of fever, a condition of collapse.

Because of inflammation, nerves degenerate, become atrophied. All this is due to impingement. If a nerve be examined immediately after an injury (pressure), there will be found only deformity of the nerve-fibers, a dislocation of the myelin and fibrilation of the axis-cylinder, appearing as though crushed. In a few hours the cells in the myelin-sheath begin to exhibit degeneration. Later the axis-cylinder is swollen. These changes are not uniform throughout the nerve; some portions may remain normal and others may undergo fatty degeneration forming small globules.

Chiropractically, the pressure should be removed. After this the nerve will gradually assume its former shape and appearance, the axis-cylinder becoming more distinct and the sheath firmer, until normal consistence of tissue exists and ordinary functions are performed. This is one reason why long standing cases require a corresponding length of time to return degenerated tissue to its former condition.

Unpleasant sensations in amputated limbs remain until the injured nerve is returned to its normal shape by removing the pressure.

If the temperature of the body is raised by sunstroke to 140 degrees, death is the result; molecular decomposition of the tissues, necrosis, sets in. With long continued, elevated temperature, distinct, fatty degeneration of tissue occurs.

Orthopedy is derived from two Greek words, **orthos** straight and **pais** child. Its derivation and earlier use implied the art of removing deformities in children. Its meaning and use has been extended until it now applies to the treatment of deformties in persons of all ages, more especially those of a chronic and progressive nature.

Orthopedics comprise that part of surgery known as orthopedic surgery which includes the mechanical and operative treatment of long-continued and progressive deformities with a view of preventing further development or straightening of bones which have become crooked. In this the vertebral column is considered as a backbone.

In the line of hygeia, gymnastics may be used and considered as a part of general surgery; in that of prevention and cure it is therapeutical.

Orthopedy treats such cases as club feet, wry neck, bow legs and spinal curvatures. In the treatment of these deformities, mechanical apparatus and operations are of special importance. The orthopedist must be a physician, a mechanician and a surgeon. As in ophthalmic practice refraction forms the greater part of the work, so, also, in orthopedic surgery, the application of mechanical appliances for those parts which are deflected from the normal, demand the greatest attention.

Orthopedy and ophthalmolgy by the use of appliances aim to **force** the crooked straight.

Chiropractic orthopedy makes a special study of etiology, desiring to know the why of these abnormalities and then correct the cause of deformities, for example: Club feet are drawn into abnormal shape because of displaced lumbar vertebral impingements; the proper thing to do as a preventative and a restorer is to correct the displaced vertebra, release the tension, restore tone. Wry neck is caused by the displacement of a cervical vertebra and the proper thing to do, is to return the osseous frame, the keyboard tension, to its normal position, thereby relieving the tension from the thread-like structures of the nervous, muscular and tendinous tissues. Where bones are softened by hyperthermia—an excess of heat—replace the 12th dorsal vertebra, thereby, remove tension, cause lower vibration, so that tissue may have tone, normal elasticity.

The reader will see that there is no resemblance whatever between surgical orthopedy and chiropractic orthopedy. The former aims to overcome and subdue the recalcitrant, rebellious, aberrant member, while the Chiropractor assists by adjusting the cause of wrong-doing. The Orthopedic surgeon looks upon deformities as something to be forced, fought, while Chiropractors desire to relieve tension by removing pressure which cause abnormalities.

## FORWARD.

The science of Chiropractic makes another step forward, one in accord with, and demonstrated by, anatomy. This advance, like all others, with the one exception of the bifid table which should be credited to Dan Riesland or T. H. Story, has been made by me.

It has long been held by Chiropractors and of late by Osteopaths that functions were abnormal because of nerves **pinched** in foramina or between joints. Now watch these two methods patch their sails.

We adjust the toes for corns and bunions. There are no nerves between the articulations, therefore nerves cannot be pinched by the displacement of these joints. The first and second pair of spinal nerves do not pass through intervertebral foramina, between two notches, but through long grooves which cannot impinge upon nerves as they pass outward. Yet we have many diseases which are caused by displacements of the atlas, where there is no possibility of a nerve being pinched in the superior or inferior grooves of that vertebra. The above are facts which every investigator will admit. The theory of subluxations closing the two notches which form the foramina of the dorsal and lumbar vertebrae, thereby impinging upon the nerves which pass through their openings, does look plausable when applied to those vertebrae, but it will not hold good in any other joint. The business of the Chiropractor is to adjust any of the three hundred articular joints of the skelctal frame, but why do so if there are no nerves between the articular surfaces?

We, as Chiropractors, never attempt to explain to a prospective student or patient how a displacement of the atlas pinches nerves as they pass outward through its grooves. True, we relieve abnormal conditions used by displacements of that vertebra, but it is not by relieving a pinched nerve.

There may be pressure by an impingement. But this does not imply that nerves are pinched between two articular surfaces—there are none. If we will use the word impingement in the sense of pressure and remember that an impingement instead of squeezing or pinching a nerve only increases its tension by stretching, we will have an explanation which will explain; one which anatomists cannot gainsay. Remember that the only sensational tissue are nerves; they sense everything.

It is a well-known fact that heat will relieve pain by relaxing nerve tension; also that by assuming certain attitudes we relax instead of tensify the already stretched nerves.

Now for an explanation which will intelligently explain. Bones cannot be displaced except at joints. This displacement causes tension on nerves because of the displaced portion projecting against them. This pressure causes not only a tension, but an irritation depending upon the amount of pressure and the character of surface or edge which is brought to bear against it. The difference between a rounded surface and a sharp edge will be apparent when we compare the acute excruciating pain of neuralgia with that of rheumatic aches.

---

Disease is a lack of co-ordination between Innate, the source of power, and its expression.

This book contains many Chiropractic pointers which have never appeared in print. It will now be in order for the second-hand fountain head, discoverer, developer and founder, to lay claim to them before they are eleven years old. Chiropractic furniture is second-handed whether received honorably or stolen.

---

## "THE PHILOSOPHY OF CHIROPRACTIC."

I expected to find in this book of 558 pages bearing the above title, the causes, reasons and laws concerning the philosophy of the principles of the science of Chiropractic. The binder's title is "The Philosophy of Chiropractic." In the preface it reads "The present volume on Philosophy of Chiropractic." The running head on each page is "The Philosophy of Chiropractic."

There is a lengthy preface; an introductory at the last of the book instead of the first; nineteen pages copied from an old book I gave the author; 198 on insanity, paralysis, tuberculosis, small pox, kidney diseases, hernia, rheumatism and contagious diseases; 47 on poisons; 78 on power; 142 on cycles. The 217 pages should have been placed under pathology; the 47 under toxicology; 78 under dynamics; and the 142 under cyclocephalus.

I failed to find a line on causation, the science of causes and principles, the relation of cause and effect. The philosophy of the science of Chiropractic is wholly lacking. The author did not know it, or he purposely or ignorantly left it out. The title is deceptive, misleading, designed and calculated, knowingly or unknowingly, to sell a book for what it is not.

A complete index is as indispensable to a book as a pen is to a scribe. An index for a student is as necessary as the finger-post guide is to the traveler. There is no index to its contents; no pass-key to locate its individual subjects. It is like a ship without a rudder or a compass.

## SHALL WE ADVANCE?

Shall we believe that the long, long fight against medical ignorance is wrong, is not going to triumph, or that the world is not ready for the change?

Is the stone axe better than the rifle? The mattox preferable to the gang plow? The mule pack more convenient than the express car? The tallow dip more commodious than the electric light? Shall we exchange the wireless for the hill-top signal? Trade the throbbing engine of the ocean steamer for the wind-jammer? Abolish our weather signal stations for Ayer's Almanac? Vacate our palatial homes for barbarian huts? Shall we refuse to advance? Do we prefer fetish charms and dope to that of adjusting causes? Is it not singular, with but few exceptions, that Chiropractic students prefer a short course, one which will enable them to do the work as a mediocre, rather than as an accomplished workman? Is it possible that the science of Chiropractic has arrived before its time?

The discoverer and developer of the greatest of all sciences finds but few who are willing or capable of taking in Chiropractice as a science. They prefer to know it as a chance method instead of one which is scientific.

Dr. Jim Atkinson, of Davenport, Iowa, found the world unwilling to recognize these advanced ideas and accepted the situation. Fifty years later there appeared in the same city one who was enthused with the same ideas.

Looking over the past fourteen years of Chiropractic development, it is strange but true that, with few exceptions, those who are indebted the most for benefits received along this line are the founder's worst enemies. The question is often asked by the originator of Chiropractic: "Is it worth while to be an advanced, original thinker?"

A short time ago a Chiropractor who thinks he is a scientific adjuster, spent a pleasant evening with me. I was surprised to hear him state, that he was a subscriber to the Chiropractor, and the Adjuster, but had not looked into either for many months. He is one of those who knows all that is worth knowing. I gave him the information of laying the hands along side of or on the back in order to prevent bucking. At that time he knew nothing of it; now, says he has been using that method for five years. He is a minister; therefore, I should not doubt his word.

It is but natural for physicians and others who have taken a course in the different branches of medicine to think they can learn the principles of Chiropractic in less time than those who have never seen the inside of a medical college. There are schools which cater to the above idea, knowing that, as a rule, it takes longer to uneducate than to educate. I would prefer a clean piece of paper to transcribe my thots on than one which has been used.

---

The Adjuster will adjust displacements which impinge upon the principles of Chiropractic, thereby advancing its progress instead of retrograding it.

---

In Chiropractic we comprehend the relation that physiological and pathological functions bear toward health and disease. We ascertain that the former becomes the latter when performed either excessively or insufficiently. In Chiropractic etiology we find an explanation for monstrosities of volume, form, color, structure, disposition, defect and excess in number. Regional anatomy of the vertebral column should be a daily study; it is indispensable to the Chiropractor.

---

## CHIROPRACTIC.

Los Angeles, Saturday, June 22.—Miss Maude Warmington of 1348 Figueroa street, sneezed her back bone out of joint last Monday.

She disarticulated the lumbar vertebrae by the violence of her sneeze, and heard the joints pop out of position.

It was just a simple, every day sort of sneeze that did the damage, a sneeze that should have been mildly enjoyable, but it has kept Miss Warmington in a state of excessive pain for three days, and has made her very much afraid of indulging again in what has proved such an expensive luxury.

As the tiltillation of the sneeze reached its emphatic degree, Miss Warmington was convulsed for a moment by the effort, and as she ker-ker-ker-achewed, she heard a sharp snap about her person, and the next instant was overwhelmed with pain and realized that something serious had happened to her spinal column.

She became prostrated at once and could hardly summon help. Aid was sent for to the California Hospital, and a physician, after a hasty examination, saw the trouble, and by a painful but not serious process replaced the rebellious vertebrae. The young woman is now said to be all right, but was advised to avoid catching any more influenzas.

Medical men generally say that this is the first instance of a sneeze producing such a serious result. Dislocations of the vertebrae are not at all common in medical practice, occurring only occasionally from violent causes.

## NERVE CONTRACTION AND STRETCHING.

Gray tells us: "The nerves supplying the abdominal muscles and skin are derived from the lower intercostal nerves and are intimately connected with the sympathetic supplying the abdominal viscera through the lower thoracic ganglia from which the splanchnic nerves are derived. In consequence of this, in rupture of the abdominal viscera and in acute peritonitis the muscles of the belly-wall become firmly contracted, and thus as far as possible preserve the abdominal contents in a condition of rest."

Lippincott says: "Nerve-stretching is the surgical operation of cutting down upon a nerve and stretching the exposed part. It is practiced for the relief of various neuroses. Nerve-stretching of the sciatic nerve may also be performed by extreme and forcible flexion of the limb."

Landois says that nerve-stretching is a mechanical procedure that has been employed for therapeutic purposes. If the exposed nerve is stretched, the tension acts as an irritant when it reaches a certain degree. After a slight stretching the reflex irritability is at first increased; stronger stretching causes for a time diminution of irritability as well as of reflex activity, and even temporary paralysis. The most extreme degree of stretching finally gives rise to permanent paralysis.

Landois' statement agrees with one of the earliest principles of Chiropractic, viz., that a light impingement increases tension with an increase of functional activity; whereas, a heavy pressure causes a lack of tension and tonicity, a condition we name paralysis.

---

## IRRITABILITY AND CONTRACTILITY.

Excitability or irritability is the quality possessed by nerve tissue to respond to a stimulus. This may be physiological or pathological. Physiological, when animated by impulses in a normal degree. Pathological, when excited by any other than bodily stimuli or impulses in an immoderate degree.

When nerves are irritated, stimulated, a nervous impulse is passed along the nerve, presumably by molecular action.

The irritability of a nerve is manifested by the results which the impulse produces in the muscles to which it is attached. Stimulation of a sensory nerve produces a nervous impulse which is conveyed to the brain. This is known as sensation. If a motor nerve is stimulated the muscles to which it is attached are contracted.

Muscles and nerves are irritable, but muscles only are contracted.

A student asked his teacher: "How are cerebrospinal meningitis and brain fever caused by a sub-luxation?

To one who knows nothing but "brain nerves direct to peripheral endings," it was unanswerable. These two diseases consist of inflamed membranes which envelop the brain and spinal cord.

Now, my boy, I will try to help you out. Let us take for illustration a typical spinal nerve, a middle thoracic. As it emerges from the intervertebral foramen, it divides into four branches, as we have fully stated elsewhere. This spinal nerve trunk is divided into the posterior primary and the anterior primary divisions; the ramus communicans, by which it is connected with the sympathetic ganglionic chain of the sympathetic nervous system, and the smaller ramus meningeus, a recurrent nerve, which, after it has been reinforced by a branch from the sympathetic, turns centralwards and passes back through the same foramen from which it emerged as a part of the mixed spinal nerve. This nerve, composed of the recurrent branch and a branch from the sympathetic, innervates the membranes of the spinal cord and the brain; its pathway being in the spinal canal. The meninges of the brain and spinal cord are their enveloping membranes.

Let us recapitulate, so that we may better comprehend this meandering. The spinal nerve as it emerges from the spinal canal through the intervertebral foramen, is composed of fibres which immediately divide into four branches. Now, observe closely: One branch proceeds to and enters a ganglion of the ganglionic chain of the sympathetic nervous system which supplies the vital organs and the vascular system with energy. A branch of this sympathetic system returns to the spinal canal by way of the same intervertebral foramen from which it emerged as a part of the spinal nerve. Just before entering, it is joined by a branch, the ramus meningeus which branches from the spinal nerve near the one which supplies the sympathetic. This nerve, composed of the two mentioned, named recurrent, because it runs back towards its origin, re-enters the spinal canal for the purpose of carrying the nervous influence necessary for the maintenance of various functions of the membranes which envelop the spinal cord and the encephalon. What we have said of this nerve is also true of the other fifty-nine spinal nerves.

Now, you want to know where these nerves may be impinged, where their carrying capacity is often interfered with.

You will remember where and how the sympathetic ganglionic chains trail on either side of the vertebral column; that these distributing nerve chains **lie close to and against the**

**heads of the ribs and the bodies of the vertebrae**; that, at each junction of the rib with the two vertebral bodies are demi-facets separated by a horizontal crest corresponding to the demi-facets of the centra. Close to and against this junction of the rib and the vertebral bodies is a ganglion of the sympathetic ganglionic nerve chain. Now watch closely. You will remember what we said in reference to the axial center of vertebrae; how each revolves around a center, circumscribing a portion of an arc. When a vertebrae is racked from its normal position, it is forced to extend the arc allotted to its normal revolution. To displace a vertebrae, is to change its articular surfaces with its adjoining neighbor. Now, look close. Do you not see that this cannot be done without disturbing the costo-central articulation. You will remember that I have just told you that a ganglion hugs close to the junction of the rib and the vertebrae. A displaced bone, whether of the vertebrae, long or short bones, projecting from its normal position, impinges upon such nerve or nerves, ganglion or ganglia as it comes in contact with. Not only that; the nerve which has a resisting substance striking against it, becomes tense as is manifested by its size and tenderness upon pressure. A vertebrae cannot be sub-luxated without disarranging the articulating surfaces of its processes and ribs. A displacement causes the body of the vertebrae to project from the median vertebral line, and impinge upon the contiguous nerve or ganglion.

A displaced vertebrae at C. P. strikes against a ganglion of the ganglionic chain, causing tension. The nerve connecting the ganglia becomes stretched tightly, strained to stiffness and rigidity, as are other nerves which we trace by palpation. This tension may be far-reaching, affecting more or less the proximal chain, as in hemiplegia, where the lateral half of the body is affected, or inaleterate hemiplegia, where the face on the one side and the limbs on the opposite, or the upper limb on one side and the lower on the opposite is affected. In the first mentioned instance, the ganglionic chain on one side is affected in its entire length, consequently causing a defect in the whole of that side, over which the sympathetic nervous system presides. The crossed condition of the two latter is explained by the crossing of the commisural branches, which connect ganglia on opposite sides of the mid-line of the body—the transverse branches which connect the two ganglionic chains of the sympathetic nervous system.

The recurrent nerve, composed of the ramus meninges and a branch of the sympathetic, may become impinged upon as they are ready to enter the spinal canal, by an articular displacement of the head of the rib with the vertebrae. This recurrent nerve carries a normal amount, or an excess, or not enough of innervation and heat to the meninges of the brain and spinal cord. A displaced vertebrae at C. P. strikes against a ganglion of the ganglionic chain, causing a tension—the nerves connecting the ganglia become stretched tightly, strained to stiffness and rigidity, as other nerves are which we trace by palpation. If this returning nerve is irritated by impingement, becomes over excited, too active, its capacity is augmented, its functions are magnified. There is an over supply of heat, producing inflammation in the membraneous coverings of the brain and spinal cord, conditions known as brain fever (too much heat) and cerebro-spinal meningitis.

If the teacher of the P. S. C. is generous, he will allow me one per cent on the above development, containing as it does, advanced ideas on Chiropractic. That will make him two per cent out of the 100—unless, per chance, he finds that this is copied from some article which he wrote previous to his establishing Chiropractic, in 1885, before he was three years of age.

---

Out of deep sorrows come high powers to comfort and strengthen.

---

## SYMPATHETIC.

Dorland gives the word sympathetic two meanings: pertaining to, caused by, or exhibiting sympathy, and the sympathetic nerve, or system of nerves. He says of frigorific nerve, the sympathetic nerve stimulation of which lowers the temperature.

McClellan's Regional Anatomy is a book in two volumes, from which the "Student, Author, Lecturer and Teacher on any phase of Chiropractic Philosophy, Science or Art, Anywhere at any Time," saw fit to copy many pages contained in Vol. 3 of the Science of Chiropractic, without giving due credit, although it is copyrighted. The purloiner evidently failed to notice the following paragraph found on page 157 of Vol. 2: "The pelvic sympathetic nerves consist of a chain of four or five ganglia extending along each side of the sacrum. The ganglia are brought into relation with the sacral nerves by external branches. The lumbo-sacral chain of ganglia is the sympathetic nerve-cord which passes downward on the bodies of the lumbar and sacral vertebrae. These ganglia are all connected by whitish nerve cords extending from one to the other, and they receive filaments from the corresponding spinal nerves."

If the name sympathetic is a bug-a-boo, why not use trisplanchnic, as Dorland says it is a general name for the sympathetic system?

## CORNS.

Dunglison says of corns: "Small, hard, corneous tumors forming upon the foot, generally the toes; commonly produced by the friction of ill-fitting shoes. The deeper portion, its base, is of conical shape, buried in the integuments, occasionally as far as the tendons and periosteum. Corns can be destroyed by the knife or caustic, or by paring them down and pulling them out by the roots. In that way of palliation they must be constantly pared; and to prevent pressure a thick plaster may be applied, with a central hole to receive the corn. Lunar caustic, rubbed over the surface, will generally diminish its irritability. A combination of salicylic acid, cannabis indica, and collodion has been found efficacious in removing the corn."

The above gives the generally accepted opinion in regard to corns. They may be cured or destroyed by the above treatment. It will be observed that the methods used are for the corn which is but an effect, therefore it can be treated.

Remember that effects can be treated; they cannot be adjusted. Causes may be adjusted, but they cannot be treated.

Chiropractors are the first to adjust the bones of the foot for the relief of corns; they do not treat effects, they adjust causes. The bones of the foot are displaced by the shoe cramping the toes, or they may be jammed against a chair leg while prowling around bare-footed in the dark, and in other ways too numerous to mention.

Soft corns are formed between the toes; be they hard or soft, they will be found contiguous to slightly displaced joints of the foot. Those on the sole are caused by the disarrangement of some one of the seven tarsal bones.

A graduate of a school where the "Dean of the Faculty stands at the head of the science of Chiropractic," told me that he was taught to adjust in the lumbar for corns and bunions, but so far he had not known of any being cured.

Chiropractors have learned that corns are the result of nerve impingement. A close examination of the joint adjacent to or next back of the corn, will show a slight displacement; the two articular surfaces will not lie in apposition. When these two surfaces are returned to their normal position and the nerve released from pressure, the painful sensation of the corn is gone.

I could give many cases where persons have been relieved of corns by returning the luxated joint to its normal position; but will only give one for illustration. Returning from Medford, a Choctaw Indian took a seat by me and removed his shoe, said that he had a corn from which he suffered greatly, that he had thought of having the toe amputated. I gave him an invitation to come to the clinic, which he did. He was the possessor of a very large corn on the small toe. I replaced the luxated joint. He felt of it, put on his shoe and said it was all right.

To my surprise, I have found dealers in shoes who knew years before I did, that corns were the result of nerve impingement.

Why use the knife or caustic? Why pull them out by the roots? Why not remove the cause instead of treating the effects? Why adjust in the lumbar for displacements in the joints of the foot?

---

The Chiropractor and The Adjuster have each their chosen field of information. The former gives the general news, the latter is endeavoring to look after the science, its development and the straightening of that which has become luxated, because of misunderstanding, or a desire to envelop that which I have developed. Reader, do you desire to aid in **developing** or **enveloping** this science?

---

## VACCINATION.

I want to thank Mrs. Little for her strong and truthful statements in the August Health-Culture under the title of "No Doubt About Vaccination." No, there is no doubt but that it is the biggest piece of quackery and criminal outrage ever foisted upon any civilized people. Medical ignorance is the greatest danger to humanity today. Medical tyranny by which criminal outrages are murdering our children all over this country by the enforcement of school blood-poisoning laws, is the foulest blot on our civilization.

It is the very height of absurdity to strive to "protect" any person from smallpox or any other malady by inoculating them with a filthy animal poison, and allowing the cause of such diseases to travel on! No one will ever pollute the blood of any member of my family unless he cares to walk over my dead body to perform such an operation. I am glad Mrs. Little is a genuine red-blood American. Every time I think of her, or see her name in print, my heart aches, for I know that she has laid away her only little son, who was foully murdered in this way by the medical profession. How any parent can tolerate this crime of blood poisoning upon their children, after reading the daily papers, is more than I can comprehent.—Harry B. Bradford in Health-Culture.

## THE KIDNEYS—THEIR DISEASES.

The kidneys are glandular organs which excrete urine. Each kidney is about four inches long, two inches wide and one inch thick. They are situated on the left and right side of the spine and in front of the floating ribs. Their nerves of innervation are derived from both halves of the spinal cord of the twelfth thoracic by way of the sympathetic and renal plexus, and accompanying the branches of the renal artery. The minute branches of the nerves form regular net-like plexuses on the walls of the fine arteries and kidney tubules. The kidneys are very vascular, being well supplied with blood vessels.

Remember: disease is too much or not enough functionating. The adult should pass three pints of urine in twenty-four hours. In Bright's disease the amount may be reduced to one-fifth; whereas in diabetes, instead of three pints, ten to forty may be excreted.

The kidneys, like all other organs, are liable to inflammation and a consequent modification of functionating. This condition, called nephritis, may be acute or chronic. It may accompany disease of other organs or one or both kidneys may be affected. The urine is diminished and contains albumen. Secretion and excretion are deranged and a portion of the fluid is withheld, inducing a condition known as dropsy. What urine is passed is of a deep color and deposits a sediment of serum-albumen, or a brick-red settling of escaped blood. The stool tract may attempt to carry off the accumulated liquid as a diarrhea.

If the kidneys have glandular functions other than those of filtration and excretion, or the pathological effect of uremia, such functions have not been satisfactorily explained.

Whether nephritis appears in company with other diseases, as a sequel, or independently, it will be observed that the patient, at the onset, experiences a chilly sensation which may be slight or amount to a pronounced chill, followed by fever. If one or both kidneys continue to be inflamed, the urine will be diminished or quite suppressed. Because of continued inflammation, the kidneys become degenerated. One or both may be enlarged, or softer than normal, the cortex becoming yellowish or of a light-gray color.

As to the cause of nephritis, pathologists disagree and are uncertain. McFarland says: "The true nature of nephritis is not known." Delafield states: "The nature of the excitants under these various conditions is most obscure." "The relationship between arterio-sclerosis and chronic kidney lesions is not clear. It should be remembered that in most cases the lesions of chronic diffuse nephritis are not independent, but are usually associated with those of other viscera. The significance of this association varies greatly. While the kidney lesions may be primary, they are very often secondary to other visceral abnormalities, or the whole series of lesions may be dependent upon a common known or unknown etiological factor. The nature of the excitants under these various conditions is most obscure; the exact mode of action of extrinsic or intrinsic poisons is almost wholly unknown. Stengel affirms that nephritis is due to poisons which reach the kidneys through the circulation, or micro-organisms may reach the kidneys through the circulation, their portals of entrance being entirely obscure."

Pressure on nerves, the fibres of which reach the kidneys causes them to be inflamed; the functionating power of the kidneys being increased or diminished in proportion to the degree of inpingement.

Those who have lumbago, pain in the back, may think they have kidney disease. Rheumatism in this region may exist with diseased kidneys, but not necessarily.

The inflammatory conditions known as nephritis or Bright's disease, cause degenerative conditions of the tissue. Deteriorated tissue cannot perform its functions in a normal manner. Whether the disease be acute or chronic, the kidneys larger or smaller than normal, the cortex white, red or mottled, too smooth or rough or a tendency to suppuration; no matter how these vary in extent, duration, intensity or relative preponderance, the cause of all is an excess of heat. Remember, that functions to be performed in a natural manner must have normal temperature.

---

## THE HOOKWORM.

Hookworm is the name of a disease caused by the uncinariasis, a worm about one-sixth of an inch long. Their natural habitat is in surface water or moist, sandy soil. They are supposed to be taken into the alimentary canal by drinking surface water or eating dirt adhering to vegetables. It is said, if not more than 100 of these worms occupy the intestinal tract, the symptoms are mild, but if this number is exceeded, the host becomes anemic, shiftless, lazy and good for nothing; death of the patient may be looked for in a few months.

The medical men look upon the hookworm as a "foe which they have to fight, combat, stamp out, wage a war of extermination" in order to "drive out the invader."

John D. Rockefeller has donated a million to furnish war material, soldiers and ammunition. How they propose to exterminate the hookworm from the surface water and moist soil, I am unable to say.

## DISEASES OF THE BRAIN.

All diseases of the brain are because of too much or not enough functionating—too great or too little heat. The larger part of the affections of the encephalon and its membranes are due to inflammation.

Hemorrhages of the brain may be minute or great, depending upon whether the escaped blood is from arteries or veins The rupture may be in the cerebrum, cerebellum or the pons. This rhexis is because of the softening, not of congestion.

Hydrocephalus—water on the brain, may occupy the space surrounding the covering or in its ventricles. It may be present at birth (prenatal) or acquired (postnatal). The fluid expands the sutures and fills in the gaps with Wormian bones. If this enlargement exists at birth, it interferes with delivery. Such children are usually short-lived. If they continue to exist, the head becomes enormous in size, because of the gradual pressure of the accumulated fluid. The appearance of cephalic infants is quite characteristic. The face appears small when compared with the large, globular head; the forehead high and bulging; and the facial expression is that of an aged person. Pathological works attribute the cause to a variety of lesions, then frankly admit the etiology is unknown.

Mollities and sclerosis of the brain substance—softening and hardening — represent opposite conditions of the effects of abnormal heat. Mollities is due to an over-amount of heat which produces liquidizing degeneration. Sclerosis is the result of a lack of normal heat—a condition which allows previously inflamed tissue to become hardened.

Hydrocephalus is a form of dropsy, an accumulation of water which should have been secreted and excreted by the kidneys. The recumbent position of infancy, in connection with the separation of the cranial bones, readily accounts for the location of the accumulated fluid. A careful examination will disclose a lack of kidney functionating owing to innervation, the nerves being impinged upon by displaced vertebrae. The tissue of the nervous system is so peculiarly delicate and sensitive that the least pressure by impingement interferes with the transmission of impulses and changes the amount of functionating.

Tumors are frequently found within the cranium, glioma being the most frequent and always found in the nervous tissue. Sarcoma is the next in frequency. The cause of tumors, here and elsewhere, is because of too much functionating, over nutrition, resulting in overgrowth.

Brain fever—meningitis, is an inflammation of the meninges or membranes which enclose the brain and spinal cord.

Our chief concern is in knowing where the primary lesion exists, how it creates abnormal conditions within the cranium, and, above all, how we may relieve the lesion so as to eliminate the effects.

As we have noticed elsewhere in The Adjuster, spinal nerves, as they leave the intervertebral foramina, divide into four branches, one of these proceeding to the sympathetic ganglionic chain. A recurrent nerve returns, reinforced with a branch from the sympathetic, through the intervertebral foramina to invigorate the meninges of the brain and spinal cord. These fibers may turn backward in the nerve trunk and pass to the meninges within the ventral root instead of contributing to the recurrent branch. If these fibers in the nerve trunk or the recurrent branch are impinged upon, pressed against by a displaced vertebra or the head of a rib, it becomes inflamed, tense and rigid and transmits an abnormal amount of heat to the contents of the cranium. The result is a diseased condition of the brain or spinal cord.

---

It is as easy to smile as to frown, and it gets more favors.

---

## QUEER NOTIONS OF THE CHINESE.

One day, says Mrs. Headland, my husband brought home a physiological chart about the size of an ordinary man. It was covered with black spots and I asked him the reason for them.

"That is what I asked the dealer from whom I bought it," he replied, "and he told me that those spots indicate where the needle can be inserted in treatment by acupuncture without killing the patient."

When a Chinese is ill the doctor generally concludes that the only way to cure him is to stick a long needle into him and let out the pain or set up counter irritation. If the patient dies it is evident he stuck the needle into the wrong spot. And this chart has been made up from millions of experiments during the past 2000 or 3000 years from patients who have died or recovered.

This was practically illustrated in our own family not long after we got the chart. Our house boy one afternoon came down with cholera. We gave him some medicine, but as he did not recover at once he was taken away. As I passed through the gate house a few hours later I saw him through the half-open door lying upon the brick bed and a native physician prodding him under the tongue with a long needle. —April Circle.

## CHIROPRACTIC HYGIENE.

My text will be found in the 19th verse of the 12th chapter of St. Luke, a portion of which reads: "Take thine ease, eat, drink and be merry."

Webster says of hygiene: The science of the preservation of health; sanitary science; a system of principles or rules designed for the promotion of health.

Chiropractic hygiene is the science of the preservation and restoration of health by retaining and restoring normal functions.

Chiropractic has not formulated a system of certain, prescribed, fixed rules, because what is food for one is poison for another. Therefore, "Take thine ease, eat, drink and be merry," knowing that Chiropractic as a science will not only preserve, but restore, your health. Observe Chiropractic hygiene, "That it may be well with thee, and thou mayest live long on the land."

Go where you may, you will observe that the man, woman or child who "takes no thought for the morrow," the one who takes life easy, eats, drinks and is merry, is the one who enjoys the good things of life and lives long in the land.

Collectively and individually, those who enjoy life, live to eat and drink and have a good time, are the ones who do not follow any prescribed principles or set rules, who do not measure their food, nor time their eating. St. Mathews tells us to take no thought for your life, what ye shall eat, or what ye shall drink.

When the men or women who have lived to a ripe age are asked how and by what means they have attained such longevity and retained good health, the universal answer has been and no doubt will continue to be, "I have eaten and drank whatever I desired, have aimed to enjoy myself and get the best I could out of life."

Longevity is most frequently found in the middle and lower classes; not among those who have "a system of principles and rules designed for the promotion of health."

The oldest person I have seen was a colored woman who was 125 years of age; her husband was 100. She was excusable for not marrying one near her own age. This old couple knew nothing of hygienic rules and certain regulations for the promotion of health.

The natural term of life of an animal is five times the period of its development. Man is not fully matured, all the epiphyses united to their diaphyses, until the age of 25 to 30 years. Five times 25 gives us 125 years as the natural life time, providing that the same care and judgment is used as that of the lower animals.

Of the human family, three-fourths of those which reach the age of a century are women, only one-fourth being able to "husband out life's taper," after a century. One reason for this difference is the tendency of women to talk, gossip and prattle—they live as long as they can talk.

In Haute Garonne, France, a venerable dame lived to be 150 years of age; she died peacefully in a hamlet where she had lived all her life. She had all her mental faculties and could talk till the last. Her body became greatly attenuated and her skin was like parchment. She died a natural death.

The fundamental principles of nearly every branch of modern science has been the gradual metamorphosis of investigators who searched for the "philosopher's stone" and the "elixir of life." The philosophers of the middle ages spent many long, weary hours of study and research chasing after what proved to be a will-o'-the-wisp. Those of the twenty-first century will, no doubt, look back upon us in a similar manner.

Daily exercise short of fatigue, calmness of mind, moderate intellectual powers, a family life and a merry disposition are aids to longevity.

Thomas Parr, an English farmer's servant, was born in 1743. He died at the age of 152 years and nine months. He had lived under nine kings of England. At the necropsy, his internal organs were found to be in perfect state. His cartilages were not ossified, as is the case usually in the aged. No doubt, normal temperature was maintained, which produced the usual amount of red and white blood corpuscles of middle age.

Many aged persons attribute their long lives to an excessive use of stimulants; at least they did not observe the rules and regulations of hygiene as laid down by The Laws of Life. Mary McDonald, a negress, who died at the advanced age of 135 years, was an inveterate smoker. Thomas Wishart died in 1760 at 124 years. He had chewed tobacco 117 years. John de la Somet, of Virginia, died in 1766, aged 130. He was a great smoker; the use of tobacco seemed to agree with him. William Riddell lived 116 years; he carefully avoided water all his life, but had a thirst for brandy; he was not a hydropath nor a temperance crank. Dr. A. T. Still is past 80 years of age, but looks like a man of 60; he chews an "infinitive amount of tobacco."

Eat, drink and be merry, that your days may be long in the land.

I have cited the above cases to show that hygiene, the laws formulated by hygienists, have but little if anything to do with health, its preservation or restoration. On the contrary it may have much to do with debilitation. For example, a lawyer told me that some years ago he made up his mind that a certain article of food did not agree with him, so he cut it out. The disagreeableness continued, so he began to cut out, one after another, different articles of diet, until he was a debilitated, starved wretch. He at last concluded to eat one good square meal, concluding that he might as well die for a sheep as a lamb. The meal consisted of a plenty of everything which others were eating. That meal and every one since agreed with him. It is "not that which goeth into the mouth that defileth a man."

The miserable dyspeptics are those who prescribe and dictate to Innate, not how fast, but how slow they shall eat; the time required to partake of a meal; what it shall consist of and how it shall be masticated. If they could, they would, follow every bite of food with special directions thru the thirty feet of alimentary canal, directing the assimilation and the transformation of food-stuffs into living tissue. If they could, they would advise Innate how to perform destructive metamorphosis; dissimiliation; physiologic disintegration; the movement toward a catastate.

The facts are, Innate knows far better how to digest and assimilate the food than man will ever know. The man we know as John Brown only bothers and hinders digestion by mental dictation.

What we eat is a matter largely of education. It is not that which goeth into the mouth that defileth a man. There are those who prefer meat and cheese well on the way toward putrefaction. What is food for one is poison for another.

We sense all animate and inanimate nature thru the nervous system. We perceive by the five senses that which is tangible. By that transference we receive impressions from tangible and intangible sources. Ether is one of the rarefied elements which is supposed to fill all known space, even that which is occupied by solids and fluids. The transmission of heat, a form of energy known by the effects of fire, the sun's rays and friction, are functions of ether; thots are also carried by ethereal vibration. Thots are real, veritable things; they travel thru space by ethereal vibration. The variation in the sensibility of nerves is past our comprehension. There are no two of us who sense alike. We differ in the makeup of our tissue, and in our likes and dislikes.

Considering the great variation in the sensibility and quality of the nervous tissue in health, it is not surprising that the variation is increased in abnormal conditions. The former variations are physiological; the latter pathological. Remember, pathological physiology is the result of functions performed by an excess or a deficiency of force. The Educated should see that all parts of the osseous frame is in normal position, as tonicity of the nervous tissue depends upon the position of the frame-work which supports the soft tissue.

---

## SECONDARY LESIONS.

Under "Abnormalities of the brain;" bottom of page 273 of Carver's Analysis, the analyzer advises adjusting **nine different vertebrae** for the "occlusion" of **nine pairs of nerves**; and yet their "Eight college year," (two college years of five months each in one calendar year) states, "**Chiropractic** is a new **specific, direct** and efficient system." If adjusting nine different vertebrae for one disease is specific and direct, the adjusting of twice that number ought to be still more specific and direct.

Page 276. "Upon the arrival of the Chiropractor, he should at once begin adjusting to remove the occlusions at all brain and heart places. **Following this,** he should carefully examine the patient to ascertain whether there are other occlusions and their gravity, and should especially direct effort to the removal of any occlusions that cause interference with depuration or absorption. It will be found that motor reaction is intense, and that frequent adjusting will be necessary at least for a few hours; at the beginning as often as every fifteen minutes."

"Begin adjusting." A Chiropractor who is "specific, direct and efficient" should be able to quit in a moment after he begins, as one adjustment which takes but a moment is sufficient for each disease, if acute; and but one adjustment each day is needed if the case is chronic.

"Following this (adjusting) he should carefully examine the patient." I would place the examination first and then do the adjusting.

"To remove the occlusions at all brain and heart places" and "other occlusions" and "occlusions that cause interference with depuration and absorption." The author evidently considers the brain occlusion the first occlusion or lesion and all others secondary, as he says, on page 272, "It will at once be understood that any abnormality of the brain instantly results in an abnormality of the body, and that the abnormality of the body will be in direct ratio with the abnormality of the brain. If a local area only of the brain is affected, then that part of the body ramified by nerves, which have origin in the affected area of the brain, will be affected, and the gravity of the affection will be in ratio with the gravity of the abnormality of that local area of the brain."

## THE NERVOUS SYSTEM.

Life is action. Without it there is death. All actions of the human body represent functions performed. Animal actions are functions animated by an intellect. Vital functions are those essential to life; when normal they are physiological; when pathological or morbid they are lesional; diseased when the structure is changed from normal consistency; disordered when the organs are displaced, or their functions changed from normal. Vegetative functions relate to growth by nutrition, apart from the sensorial and animal functions.

An, heretofore, unrecognied force which I chose to name Innate, because it unites with the body at birth, performs functions, creates life and produces all action. There are three kinds of functions; vital, vegetative and intellectual. The two former are under the control of Innate; the latter is directed by Educated mind.

Vital functions are those essential to life, such as innervation, circulation, respiration, digestion and calorification.

The vegetative functions are those which pertain to the nutrition, growth or decrease of the body. They are supposed, by physiologists, to be performed by trophic nerves. They include metabolism, which may be either constructive (anabolic), or destructive (katabolic), micturition, defecation, assimilation, absorption, exhalation, secretion and excretion.

The intellectual functions are those which run the voluntary movements, those which are sensorial, or distinctively animal, such as the affections, reasoning, formation of ideas, perception, locomotion, voice and memory.

Nerves which carry impressions from the periphery to the center are sensory. Therefore, they are named afferent, esodic or contripetal. Those which convey the nervous influence from the nervous centers to the circumference are called efferent, exotic or centrifugal. They are motor and cause action. If these nerves are unobstructed, free to act in a normal manner, we have health. But if they are interfered with by their tubes being bent or occluded, their fibers compressed, we have either too much or not enough action, resulting in conditions we name disease. The beginnings and terminations of nerves are known as central and peripheral; the ganglionic center and the outside. The spinal and cranial nerves, those run by Educated, respond instantly to sensory or motor impressions; while those of the sympathetic, which control organic life, act more slowly, being affected only by Innate. The vegetative functions are the result of vital action.

Animal life, controlled by Educated, connects man and animals with their external surroundings. The Educated sows and reaps the grain, grinds it into flour from which bread is made. The Innate (born with) assimilates it by a process known as digestion, through the "nervous system known as the automatic functions." Each intellect has its individual work to perform. It is but fair to say that either knows but little of the other's labor. The time is coming, however, when these two conscious intelligences will converse freely on matters in which they are mutually interested. We are bordering now on that junction which will give us a better understanding of our diseases and our duality, the seen and unseen, the spiritual and the physical. For example, the Educated presumes that Innate needs a physic. The taste and smell is objectionable, but as Educated is the intelligence that looks after and governs the outside welfare of the body, he imposes upon Innate by compelling thon to swallow the objectionable dose which is recognized by Innate as a poison. If thon fails to get rid of the noxious stuff by vomiting he does the next best thing, namely, causes water to flow into the alimentary canal, below the stomach, from the surrounding tissues, and washes it out. In the near future, these two intelligences, instead of warring with each other, will mutually work for their undivided benefit.

All vital and mental actions depend upon the condition of the nervous system for their expression. Either intelligence can direct its impulses without aberration if the lines of communication are clear and unobstructed.

We have the ganglionic nervous system of the "automatic functions," a collection of nerves which heretofore have been supposed to work without any governing power. The science of Chiropractic has demonstrated the fallacy of this assumption. The Good Book tells us that man became a living soul when he had the breath of life breathed into his nostrils. The infant becomes an individualized, living being as soon as it breathes the breath of life and not before. When it receives a life directed by an intelligence, a living soul, that which runs the vital functions when we are asleep and awake; that which knows much better how to mend a fractured bone the first day of its life than the surgeon will ever know; that intellect which is known as Hahneman's Vital Force; New Thought's Divine Spark; Hudson's Subconscious Mind; the Allopath's Vis Medicatrix Naturae, the healing power of nature; D. D. Palmer's Innate Intelligence; I repeat, when it begets a living soul, it (the immaterial) will live throughout the eternity.

The voluntary nervous system includes the 31 pairs of spinal and the 12 pairs of cranial nerves which Educated, during life, learns to control.

The organic nervous system, the great sympathetic group which distributes its fibers to the organs of the cavities of the cranium, chest, abdomen and pelvis, is the sympathetic.

All vital and intellectual forces depend upon the condition of the nervous system for their expression. Either intelligence can direct its impulses without aberration if the lines of communication are clear and unobstructed by pressure.

Each nerve is a cord or bundle of fibers containing many filaments, each forming a distinct route of intercourse, running a distinct separate course to its destination. They do not inosculate. This may be fully appreciated by seeing a Chiropractor trace a sensitive, tensioned, overheated, enlarged nerve.

Impulses are thoughts passed between two parts of the body more or less distant from each other. The nervous system is the means of communication.

The sympathetic consists of ganglia, plexuses and nerves which are connected with the organs, vessels and viscera. They control the fluid circulation, nutrition, respiration, in fact all the vital and vegetative functions. These ganglia are situated in the cavities of the head and trunk, forming a double axis extending from the cranium to the coccyx on either side of the vertebral column. They may be traced upward, even into the cranial cavity, where they communicate with cranial nerves. It should be observed that it is not an independent system, for it is connected by branches of communication with the spinal cord. These gangliated cords extend parallel with each other until they reach the sacrum, where they converge and form a single ganglion called the coccygeal. They might well be named the right and left vertebral cords. Its nerve fibers are of two kinds, distributive and communicative. These gangliated cords of the sympathetic system situated on opposite sides of the vertebral column are intimately connected by cross trunks, or branches, named commissural.

The cranial and spinal nerves are voluntary; they are subservient under the control of Educated. The sympathetic nervous system is involuntary as far as Educated is concerned, yet, it is under the control of Innate to the extent that its pathways for impulses are free from inpingements. Educated and Innate have each their special systems of nerves, or fibers, to convey their mental, vital and vegetative functions.

The cranial and spinal nerves proceed from the cerebrospinal center—the cerebrum, cerebellum and spinal cord. The 12 pairs of cranial nerves have their apparent origin in the base of the brain, but their real source is in the substance of that mass of nerve tissue. They leave the skull through foramina at its front and base. The spinal nerves are rooted in the spinal cord and pass through openings formed by the junction of the intervertebral notches. The spine has 31 pairs of nerves, while the two series of ganglia lie along either side of the vertebral column, contain 25 ganglia—three cervical, twelve dorsal, four lumbar, five sacral and one coccygeal. Counting the cranial and spinal nerves and the vertebral ganglia, we have 68 pairs which are liable to be impinged upon by subluxated vertebrae. This pressure is made apparent when we take into consideration the communicating branches which connect the spinal with the sympathetic, and the accessory nerves of the cranial derived from the spinal and sympathetic. We, as Chiropractors, should know the ramification and communication of these nerves in order that we may put to right and relieve ailments caused by their impingements. The thirty-one pairs of spinal nerves contain fibers which go to and make up the sympathetic nervous system, therefore, when the spinal nerves are impinged upon these sympathetic fibers are liable to suffer, causing too much or too little functionating, displacement of viscera from lack of tonicity, and degeneration because of too much heat.

In the cervical region, the sympathetic trunks pass in front of the transverse processes. In the thoracic region they lie close to the sides of bodies of the vertebrae and on the heads of the ribs. In the lumbar region they are nearer the front of the bodies of the vertebrae. They pass on the ventral side of the openings of the sacral foramina.

The sympathetic nervous system in vertebrates is connected with the alimentary canal, the vascular system and the glandular organs. It furnishes life force, functional activity, through 24 pairs of nerves which extend from and have their apparent origin in the two axial chains of ganglia. Each of the 12 dorsal or intercostal nerves are connected with the adjoining ganglia of the sympathetic system.

To consider that any nerve or nerves are sympathetic with another, or that they cause morbid phenomena to supervene without any direct morbific cause acting directly on the reaction of another organ primarily affected, is not Chiropractic, is not specific, is not scientific. While we may use the name, accepted by common consent, we do not mean to say, that through sympathy one disease causes another, that one organ or a portion of the body is in sympathy with another.

---

"Remember the same bee that stings you can also give you honey." Not a drop of honey will a stingless bee gather. For many years I produced tons of honey, but not from stingless bees.

## DR. THOMPSON.

The following article, consisting of the comments made upon a contribution to Everybody's Magazine, by Dr. Thompson, were penned at the request of a former student of Chiropractic who was medically inclined:

I am impressed with the honesty of the writer and with his desire to advance "Medicine." He strikes a vein of truth when he says, "A new era seems about to dawn upon us, both as respects the **understanding** and the **management** of these disorders." He then refers to a "derangement of the working, rather than of the structure, of the nervous system." Considering the great advancement Chiropractic has made during the last thirteen years, his prophetic sight seems to sense the need of the science which has discovered the cause of disease. Chiropractic has not advanced medicine nor any of the systems which it includes. It has discovered and developed a system which is unlike any other, as it adjusts causes instead of treating effects.

"We are brought to believe, with Dr. Thompson, that Medicine today is in the position of Columbus when he landed upon a West Indian island—it is a small island, but it is on the edge of a great world." You say he is one of those whom I ought to look up to as authority, one whom you think I unwisely turn down. Dr. Thompson says that medical men after studying medicine 2000 years, know in comparison as little of disease as Columbus did of the great continent of America on the first day of his landing on Hayti, one of its small islands. Columbus thought he had encircled the world, that he had returned home and landed on one of the East India islands. He was no more mistaken than are physicians in their erroneous reckoning concerning bacteria, microbes and pathology. Past generations have corrected the erroneous notions of Columbus and have benefited by their correction. It now remains for Chiropractors to rectify the mistakes of the medical profession.

Columbus was not mentally hide-bound. He dared to think and act. He did not stick to the shores of Italy, but set forth to discover other regions. Medical practitioners should not remain bigoted, nor stupidly conservative, for, as Dr. Thompson wisely remarks, "There is no telling into what unexpected paths a single scientific discovery may lead. The scientific investigator may start with a single aim in view, but on his way stumble upon a great principle in life reaching far beyond his original object. Nor does it matter if he begins with something rather unattractive in itself, for science does not mind that aspect of a subject in the least." Does not Dr. Thompson portray the beginning of Chiropractic? Does he refer to "D.

D. Palmer's stumbling by chance onto the basic principle of Chiropractic'' as stated by "Uncle Howard''?

Dr. Thompson uses an illustration. "Though a locomotive be perfect in every detail yet not one of its wheels will turn if it has no coal.'' The doctor does not observe the intellectual fireman behind the material coal, no more than you do the intelligence which is directing the functions of the sympathetic nervous system. The locomotive may be perfect in every detail, have an abundance of coal and water, and **lack a fireman, an intelligence to run it.** Thus it is with our bodies. They may be perfect in every particular, and every piece in proper position, but without an **intelligence to direct their vital functions,** they are inanimate and like the engine on the track must have an intelligence to run them. The locomotive and the body are both inert without an intelligence to direct them.

Dr. Thompson tells us that "insanity is a disorder of the blood.'' "That insanity is not a disease of the brain, because no anatomical investigation, microscopic or otherwise, can show the least difference between either brain cell or fiber of a person who died insane and the brain of one killed in an accident. The same absence of brain changes is noticeable in a whole class of important chronic nervous diseases, such as migrane, neurasthenia, hysteria and epilepsy. None of these show at **post mortem** any characteristic changes from normal brains.'' Just listen to that. We have been taught by medical men that insanity had for its cause a lesion in the brain. This last statement is backed up by "**post mortem** examinations in which the vessels of the brain were found torpid or diluted—a vaso-motor paresis causing an imperfect cerebral circulation.'' Just think of this radical change.

It will be observed that Dr. Thompson follows the trend of the medical profession by accepting, as final, the results of an examination of nerves after death. Chiropractors depend on the findings of examinations made during life, thereby giving the patient, instead of the undertaker, the benefit of their discoveries. Thus the medical fraternity continue to change their pathology, each time apparently proving their diagnosis. It takes years of facts to disprove each false statement, then they let go of one delusion to grasp another, which in turn, is proven incorrect and discarded.

Can you not be as honest and make the same confession as did Dr. Thompson in the article referred to, and say with him that physicians know as little of diseases as did Columbus at day-break when he took possession of the unknown New World?

Dr. Thompson alludes to what is known as the sympathetic nervous system by saying "The third great nervous system in us, a nervous system whose very existence the public has hardly heard of, but which physicians already know to be more directly connected with the life of the body than are brain and spinal cord put together. Physicians do not often mention it, simply because they know so little for certain about it."

Morris states: **The sympathetic system is intimately associated with the cerebro-spinal**, and consequently with the central system.

Gerrish says: **The gangliated cords are connected superiorly with the upper cranial nerves by branches which enter the cranium.**

Cunningham affirms: The sympathetic nervous system is intimately connected with the cerebro-spinal nervous system, and has a common developmental origin; it consists of a pair of elongated gangliated cords extending from the base of the skull to the coccyx; connected by a series of branches to the spinal nervous system and gives off an irregular series of branches to the viscera; **at its cephalic end each sympathetic cord is continued in a plexiform manner into the cranial cavity, where it forms a complex relationship with certain cranial nerves.**

McClennan sets forth that the cervical portion of the sympathetic nerve, on each side consists of a continuous cord in which there are three ganglia. The superior is the largest of the three. It is opposite the second and third cervical vertebrae, and is about an inch and a quarter in length. **It receives four communicating branches from the four upper cervical nerves.** From the upper portion of the superior ganglion, the cord is continued into the carotid canal to form the carotid sympathetic plexus **inside of the cranial cavity where it communicates with some of the cranial nerves.**

Gray avers: The sympathetic nervous system consists of a series of ganglia connected together by a great gangliated cord, extending from the skull to the coccyx; one gangliated cord on each side of the middle line of the body, partly in front and partly on each side of the vertebral column. Each gangliated cord of the sympathetic **may be traced upward from the base of the skull into the cranial cavity** by an ascending branch, which passes through the carotid canal, forms a plexus in the cavernous sinus, and **communicates with certain cranial nerves.**

Dutton declares: The sympathetic nerves are those of organic life. The cerebro-spinal nerves are those of animal life. The former control the circulation of the blood, respiration, nutrition, calorification, absorption, secretion and all the various vital processes; they are the involuntary nerves, not directly under the control of the will. The latter includes the functions which connect man and animals with external surroundings, as understanding, sensation, locomotion and voice.

A would-be lecturer and teacher "**on any phase** of Chiropractic philosophical science or art, anywhere at any time," contradicts the above anatomists by particularizing that **it is impossible to have a sympathetic nervous system**; that **he has eliminated it, thrown it out, has no use for it; that there is no such a thing and that we do not need it to explain functions.**

---

## A SCHEME.

The cut on the opposite page represents a scheme to cut out the cranial and sympathetic nervous systems and envelop the science of Chiropractic; to exchange vital force for water, functions for gravitation, the nervous system for rubber hose, the skull for a water-bag and Innate for an egotist.

The fountain head from whom this envelopment originated, aims to demonstrate by this water device how the flow of mental impulses may be cut off, or shut off in part or in whole. He does not realize that mental impulses are not made of substance, are not liquid, are not composed of particles, do not flow, can not be shut off, or cut off. His device does not demonstrate how an excess of vital energy causes nearly all diseases.

If the author of this and other schemes would put in as much time and energy in developing the science, art and philosophy of Chiropractic as he does in enveloping them, he would advance instead of retard them.

---

Depuration and absorption, as well as all other functions, will be performed normally when the osseous, supporting framework of the soft tissue, is in its normal position. There will then be neither tension nor relaxation of nerve-tissue.

It is not necessary to adjust for each and every symptom, regarding each as a secondary occlusion or lesion. No matter how many symptoms are manifested by each disease, they all arise from one osseous displacement which causes an impingement upon a leash or bundle of nerve-fibres, each of which are longitudinally stretched, put on a tension, causing derangement of the organ or portion it innervates. For example, in spinal curvature adjust the 12th dorsal and not every vertebra found awry.

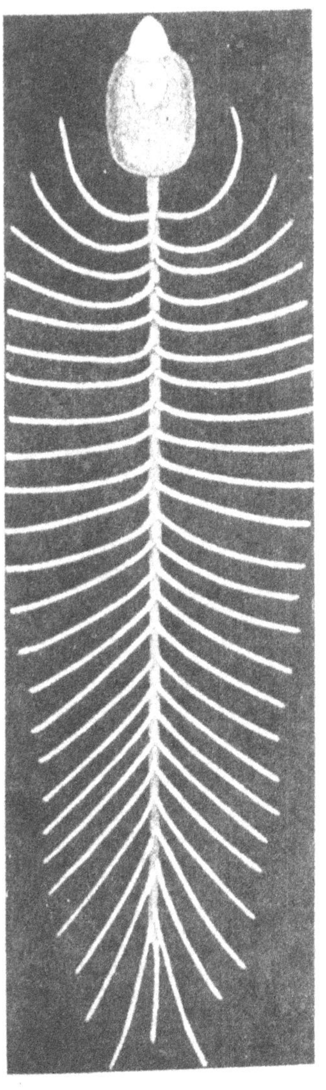

The "Therapeutical Idol Shatterer. Destroyer of superstitious ideas regarding creation, transmission and expression of life, in any form and replacer of impractical with practical studies, etc., etc.," states in **The Davenport Daily Times** of Nov. 12, 1910: "**No one, up to my knowledge and my time, ever dared to question the practicability of the sympathetic nervous system, and no one had the sand, daredevilism, as it might be called, to say it could not be, and proceed to prove that it was irrational. No one had the nerve, or perhaps the gall.**"

"B. J. Palmer, in one of his addresses (July, 1908) to his class in Portland this summer, aptly quoted, 'that he who tears down must rebuild greater,' and said, '**When I saw there was no use for a Sympathetic Nervous System, I threw it out, and then just had to put something better in its place, so I DISCOVERED Direct Mental Impulse.**"

This cut is used to illustrate the "Direct Mental Impulse" system, originated and devised by B. J. Palmer. It "illustrates how the brain communicates with all the organs through the nerve system."

He has the nerve, sand, gall and dare-devilism qualifications to place this piece of mechanism before an audience.

A child by nature's kindly law,
Is pleased with a baby's rattle,
And tickled with a tiny straw.

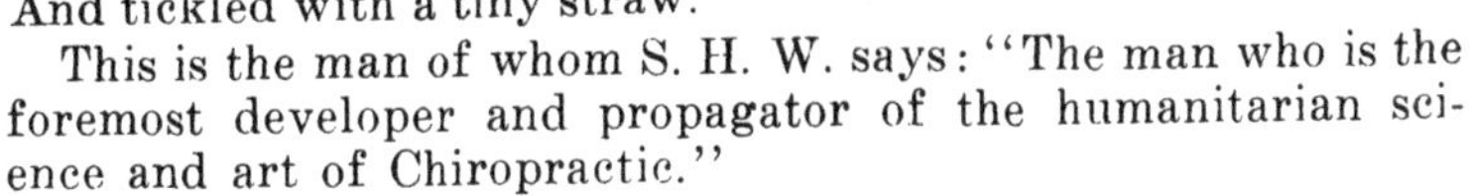

This is the man of whom S. H. W. says: "The man who is the foremost developer and propagator of the humanitarian science and art of Chiropractic."

---

A knowledge of the principles of Chiropractic, as developed by the founder, is necessary for the success of the Chiropractor.

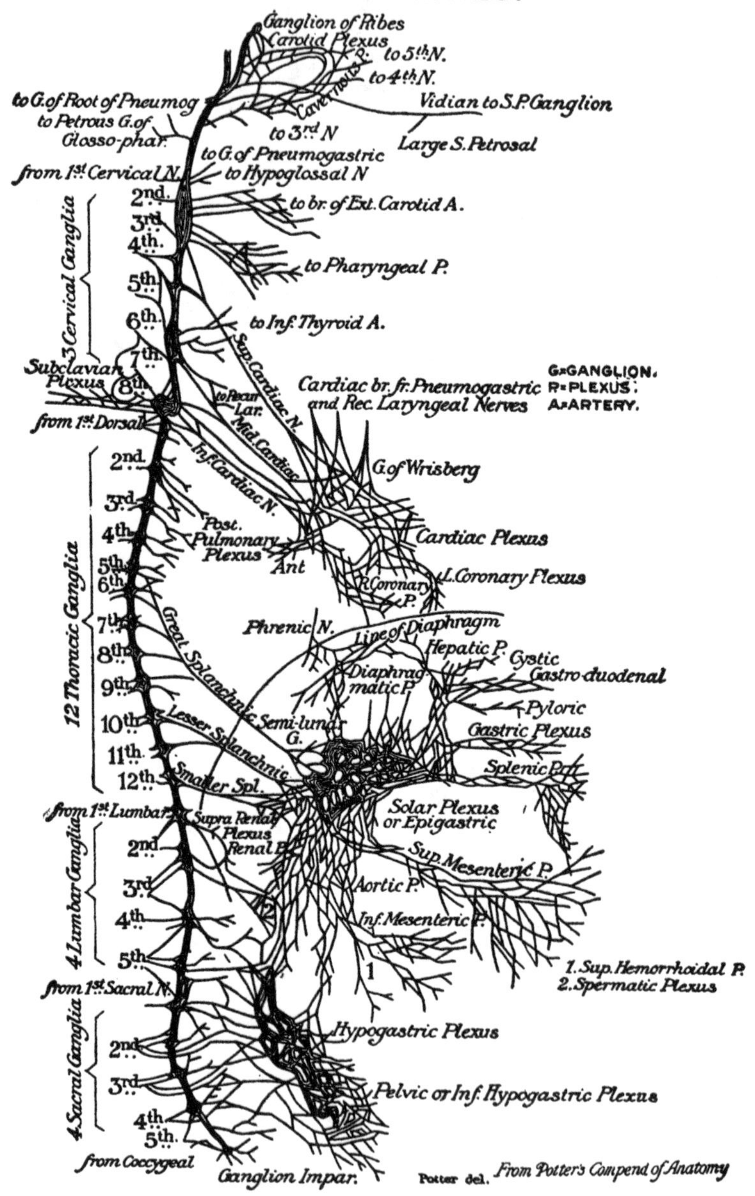


Taken from "Gould's Illustrated Dictionary," published by P. Blakiston Son & Co., Philadelphia.

## A LUXATION ADJUSTED.

The pseudo-developer of Chiropractic—the man who makes such changes in anatomy as seems best to suit his philosophy, that of no cranial or sympathetic nerves, says: "A superior sub-luxation of the atlas, determined by palpation of either or both transverses, would make compression between **that notch** and the occipital of frequent occurrence."

A sub-luxation consists of two or more bones, whose articular surfaces have **lost in part** their natural connection—one in which the articulating surfaces remain **in partial contact**—those which partly preserve their connection. If so, the atlas cannot be luxated or subluxated superiorly. To displace wholly or in part the superior or inferior articular surfaces of the atlas, it would have to be moved anteriorly or laterally from its adjoining articular surfaces. You cannot determine what does not exist. The atlas has no notch, either superiorly or inferiorly. The atlas has grooves through which the vertebral artery and sub-occipital nerves pass. The grooves correspond and take the place of notches of other vertebrae. Grooves are not notches.

---

"The sympathetic nervous system, in name and functions expresses no intelligence to a Chiropractor. The Chiropractor has no spinal or sympathetic nerves to worry about." The author of above only knows of "brain nerves," which expand from the brain, pass down the spinal cord and emerge through the foramina. That is the extent of his comprehension of the nervous system. The spinal, sympathetic and cranial nerves do not appeal to the Chiropractor who has not the intellect to comprehend the three divisions of the nervous system; therefore he bundles them into one, basing them around his talisman of six words. This is the man who is "the developer of this wonderful science and philosophy." He is "steadily developing the **theory** of Chiropractic" backward. "There is not in the length and breadth of the entire world any man or set of men that can tell you any more, or as much" which is misleading, degrading and which he calls developing, as can this pseudo fountain head.

He says that complete relaxation of the patient's back, arms and abdomen is desired, but does not inform us "how to get the patient to relax." Fellow students, I am going to tell you how you can keep your patient relaxed. Have the patient, while lying on the table, place thon's arms beside and parallel with the body, or the hands on the nates. Try it. I think you will be able to comprehend the direction and act accordingly without 500 cuts to show the great number of variations one might devise. This word **thon** was used by me years before the noted author, copyist and plagiarist got it. It will be found in the third edition of the Proofreaders' Stylebook, on page 30, where it is used as the third person singular.

"Notice how plum the line pierces all spinous processes." This is the first time I ever read of a "plumb line piercing spinous processes." I presume that the "author" meant to show that the distal ends of the spinous processes were in line. If so, that is one of his "foolers," as the spinous processes frequently fail to form a true mediam line. Some of them may incline either to the right or left of this line; the club ends may be unequally developed; the cervicals may have one or both prongs broken off. Therefore, they are not reliable guides for palpation or for vertebral deviations. He may have a befogged recollection that "the transverse processes of the cervical vertebrae are pierced by the vertebraterial foramen."

"Nerves can only be impinged in those parts of a cervical vertebrae where there are and can be pressure upon nerves by bone. The study of a cervical vertebrae usually shows that outside of the (intervertebral) foramina such is impossible." The developer of the Chiropractic science states that it is not possible to pinch or squeeze the first or second pair of spinal nerves by the closing of the atlas grooves and it is very doubtful that any nerves are pinched by the closing of any intervertebral foramina. I doubt very much that nerves are ever pinched, squeezed or compressed anywhere. Nerves cannot be **impinged** upon between any two bones, vertebrae or other joints.

What is valuable in Vol. 3 is either copied verbatim, or are the thoughts found in my writings previous to three years ago. That which is new and the very thoughts themselves of the "author" are not philosophical Chiropractic.

This book purports to give the inquirer information on subluxations, and how to adjust them; yet the author is shrewd enough to state that the essential features of Chiropractic cannot be taught by mail or in a book.

If the contents of this issue does not make plain the difference between humane feeling and a system of nerves then the unobserver has my sympathy.

---

Chiropractic "is for the first time, adjusted to a practical art and science." The seventeen illustrations of scientific nail driving is far from elucidating Chiropractic adjusting. A vertebra, racked from its normal position so that it is impinging upon a nerve, should be replaced by using the processes as levers, not driven like a nail. We have had far too much of that 'hammer and nail driving' already."

## SCARLET FEVER.

This disease is technically known as scarlatina. There are three varieties, named according to the degree of severity. Scarlatina simplex, scarlatina anginosa and scarlatina maligna. The specific virus of this disease enters the system by inhalation. It is a disease of childhood. Like most fevers it is generally ushered in by a pronounced chill. In some instances, however, it may be absent; there are no two cases precisely alike.

Lesions of the mucous membranes and glands similar to those of measles, but generally more intense, are present. There is usually intense fever, headache and general prostration, perhaps delirium. Soreness of the throat, pain upon swallowing and vomiting may be present. The glands of the neck may suppurate. Severe inflammation of the throat, middle ear, larynx, and trachea, with endocarditis and pericarditis are much more frequent than in measles. Diphtheria may be present as one of the complications. Focal necroses of various organs are observed in fatal cases.

Scarlet fever is one of the eruptive (exanthematous) fevers. The eruption appears as a rash of thickly set red spots. A peculiarity of scarlatina is its tendency to involve the kidneys, causing dropsical conditions.

---

Medical pathology states that bacteria excite the phenomenon known as inflammation; that inflammation is physiologic; that it frees the body of substances capable of producing disease; that it is a body cleanser; that it is "conservative in tendency, benign in disposition and evidently the result of a carefully adjusted protective mechanism."

I was the first person to deny the above proposition, for which I have the enmity of the medical profession and the hatred of many Chiropractors. I was the first to assert that inflammation, excessive heat, is the result of nerve irritation. That an increase of temperature means increased activity of body tissue, an exorbitant amount of functionating; that disease depends upon, and is never present without, a variation of heat from the normal. That nerves heat the body; that normal heat is health; that heat above or below normal is a sign of disease, creates diseased tissue, produces abnormal functions; that pressure on nerves cause an excess of heat named inflammation. To those who state that I stole the above fundamental ideas from the Bohemians or any one else, I have $500 to pay them for their time, if they will produce any such language used by Bohemians or any one else previous to my use of them.

**The Principles of Chiropractic** continue to be developed by the same mind which gave it birth—disease is the result of too much or not enough functionating — bone pressure on nerves cause impingements—pressure excites or depresses transmission. Its origin and all the principles upon which it is based, were included in the first adjustment.

Chiropractic came to the world as soon as it was ready to receive it. It came as an educator. The human intellect is outgrowing credulous superstition. There was a demand for this science, and a fit person who is destined to enlighten the world on that perplexing question—what is life—was prepared to present it. It did not come to antagonize other systems—they have served their time and purpose. This science is being appreciated: it is solving the problems of human life.

Therapeutic methods are absorbing the principles and movements of Chiropractic as fast as possible. The people demand that medicine and therapeutics shall move forward or step aside and allow this giant to pass.

Chiropractic is a proven fact—it is a science demonstrated by the art of adjusting. As we become acquainted with its principles, founded upon laws as old as the vertebra, we make less failures. The science can only be developed along the lines laid down by its founder.

The principles of Chiropractic should be known and utilized in the growth of the infant and continue as a safeguard throughout life.

The cumulative function determines the contents of the intellectual storehouse. The condition of the physical decides the qualifications of the mental. We take with us into the great beyond, when intelligent life ceases to unite spirit and body, just what we have mentally gathered, whether those thoughts are sane, or monstrous conceptions—are of reason, or the vagaries of a freakish mind.

This philosophy will make the junction between the physical and the spiritual comprehensive; it will advance mankind mentally, physically and spiritually.

---

How can Osteopathy be a "system of medicine" and "not a part of medicine?" Does Osteopathy embrace the whole system of medicine and not a part of it?

---

The bridge of life has many loose planks and others are greased. It does seem at times as though someone had greased the loose planks, thereby insuring our downfall. We are not always, to blame for our falling, but there is no benefit in remaining down; get up and go ahead.

## ILLINOIS SUPREME COURT TAKES COMMON-SENSE VIEW OF VACCINATION.

"This case is an attempt to have a writ of mandamus issued compelling a School Board to accept as a pupil a certain child that has not been vaccinated. This Court does not find that a healthy child is a danger, or a menace to pupils or teachers. Therefore, to deprive him of school privileges is to do him a wrong and an injustice. In the case at bar the child is not on trial. Of himself he could never be expected to go to a physician and ask to be vaccinated. All of his instincts are against the operation. This Court does not attempt to decide whether vaccination is a prophylactic against disease—we merely hold that it has not been shown that a healthy child is a menace or danger to his fellows. That the young shall be educated is very desirable; and the attempt to deprive certain children of the right of public school advantages is a very serious matter. The dangers arising from ignorance and idleness are quite as imminent as those arising from smallpox.

"To use the leverage of coercion or intimidation, with parental love as a fulcrum, and thus force parents to do certain things against their conscience, is neither ethical nor equitable. As a legal resort it is unjustifiable.

"Counsel has intimated that while the child may not at present be a danger to his school-fellows, yet the fact that he has not been vaccinated will in after years make a danger to society.

"**This is too anticipatory** for this Court to consider, but granting the argument, we do not see how the enforced illiteracy and ignorance of the child is going to limit the dangers of infection, if unhappily he shall at some future time contract smallpox. Let the writ of mandamus be issued."

**This is a hot dose for the medical trust vaccination grafters.**

---

I have just finished the reading of 558 pages on the "Philosophy of Chiropractic." My great surprise is, that so much was written without saying something.

---

The sympathetic nervous system is so named because it is supposed to convey sympathy, or sympathetic impulses from one portion of the body to another. The Chiropractor understands why two or more portions are affected at the same time. The impingement of a nerve-trunk may affect two or more fibers, or branches, which ramify different portions of the body.

## POISONING.

What can Chiropractors do for poisoning?

A few years ago I was called to the infirmary to attend one of the students who was suddenly ill with stomach and throat trouble. One adjustment at S. P. gave immediate relief. The next day I was called to the same man with the same ailment with the same result.

The following day was Sunday. I was absent from home until sundown. Upon my return I found him in convulsions. I then saw that he had taken poison. An examination of his room disclosed the fact that he had sought to take his life by corrosive sublimate.

November 7th, last, we had link veal sausage for dinner. I ate one, Mrs. Palmer one and a half. About five hours after, she became suddenly very ill. I saw that I had a case of ptomain poisoning. I could not leave her to call help. I gave her an adjustment with immediate benefit. She was relieved and went to sleep. During that day and the next, she felt as tho she had been sick. Ptomain poison is caused by decomposition without putrefaction. There are no characteristic postmortem lesions (molecular) except that of gastro-intestinal inflammation.

These are the only cases of accidental poisoning I can cite the reader to, where Chiropractic has been used with success. Without further experience I would advise the Chiropractor to adjust immediately and send for a physician. If the patient is relieved by the time the physician has arrived, well and good; if not, then you have complied with public educated demands. Until we have had more experience, I would not advise relying upon adjusting alone if a physician can be called.

Vaccine poisoning is readily relieved by adjustments, as experience has proven by a number of cases adjusted by the originator of Chiropractic.

---

The Chiropractor of August and September, 1908, page 43, says: "Dr. Palmer has several volumes on the basic principles of Chiropractic."

Basic pertains to the base, the foundation, the essential principle. Chiropractic has but one foundation, only one base, the essential principle, the fundamental truth upon which it was built. The basic principle of Chiropractic is not mentioned in those "several volumes." Strange that a man could write volumes on a subject of which he knew nothing.

I founded the science of Chiropractic upon the basic principle of tone. By reasoning upon the immutable laws of biology, which are based upon tone, the living principle of animal and vegetable life. Chiropractic philosophy explains the phenomena of biology, in health and disease. From that basic principle of tone many principles are derived.

A principle is the source or origin, that from which anything proceeds. It is the ultimate element, or cause, in Chiropractic, the primordial quality of tone.

Tone is the source or origin of all life, normal or abnormal, animal or vegetable. Tone is an elastic quality of tissue fiber upon which life depends. Tone is the element, the source of all life; its quality determines the character of life.

Upon the comprehension of tone I built the grandest science of this or any age. Tone is a law which can be comprehended; it is a principle upon which others are founded. It is an elementary proposition, a foundation principle which characterizes the Chiropractic science; it gives to it essential properties.

These "several volumes" do not contain the principle upon which the science is founded. Their author has not the faintest idea of what the basic principle of Chiropractic consists. Why write volumes upon that of which we have no conception? In all these volumes there is nothing on the basic principle, nor any principle concerning the science of Chiropractic; consequently, they contain nothing scientific, of the science, naught regarding it which is philosophical.

The "Therapeutical Idol Shatterer. Destroyer of superstitious ideas regarding creation, transmission and expression of life, in any form and replacer of impractical with practical studies, etc., etc.," states in **The Davenport Daily Times** of Nov. 12, 1910: "**No one, up to my knowledge and my time, ever dared to question the practicability of the sympathetic nervous system, and no one had the sand, daredevilism, as it might be called, to say it could not be, and proceed to prove that it was irrational. No one had the nerve, or perhaps the gall.**"

"B. J. Palmer, in one of his addresses (July, 1908) to his class in Portland this summer, aptly quoted, 'that he who tears down must rebuild greater,' and said, '**When I saw there was no use for a Sympathetic Nervous System, I threw it out, and then just had to put something better in its place, so I DISCOVERED Direct Mental Impulse.**' "

A cut of this "Direct Mental Impulse" system will be found on page 248. That cut "illustrates how the brain communicates with all the organs through the nerve system."

Nerve, sand, gall and dare-devilism are needed qualifications for a sciolist.

A child by nature's kindly law
Is pleased with a baby's rattle,
And tickled with a tiny straw.

Such hyperbole might be thot created to tickle the fancy and create laughter, just to kill time, were it not that many are cajoled into spending their time and parting with their money for such foolish nonsense, when they should be receiving something of value for their outlay.

---

## OPERATION A SUCCESS.

### Harrisburg Girl Suffering From Enlarged Tonsils—Doctors Remove Her Appendix.

New York, March 9.—A dispatch to The Herald from Harrisburg, Pa., says:—Eight-year-old Rosie Cohen and her brother Joseph, aged eleven years, were sent to the Harrisburg Hospital yesterday suffering from enlarged tonsils. The girl was given ether and by mistake was sent to the operating room with several other patients and operated on for appendicitis.

The surgeons say they found her appendix somewhat inflamed, and, therefore, were not aware that a mistake had been made until the parents called and found that the operation had been performed. The operation was "successful" and the child is resting easily.

**Strangely enough,** the doctors say she would have developed appendicitis before long and the operation would have been **necessary anyway.**—Toronto Globe, March 10, 1909.

---

"Dr. D. D. Palmer.

"Dear Sir: I am much interested in your explanation of why we adjust **from** the affected side in the dorsal region and towards the affected side in the lumbar. I think I know just what you mean; but, what you say in regard to the cervical and atlas, may get your readers mixed.

"In the January number of The Adjuster, you contrast the dorsal with the lumbar and cervical on pages 44 and 49. In the March number on page 5 you contrast the dorsal and cervical with the atlas and lumbar. On page 47 you contrast the dorsal, cervical and atlas with the lumbar.

"I think a short statement rectifying the error would be appreciated by your many readers.

"Your explanation of the difference between nerve 'pinching' and nerve 'impingement' is completely satisfactory. Sincerely yours, —— ———."

We take pleasure in answering questions from our subscribers, and above all, it is not only a pleasure, but a duty to correct mistakes as fast as they are known to us. We are not above making mistakes. You will understand that recent ideas need different descriptions and often a new nomenclature; in this way mistakes are liable to be made.

Page 44 should have read: "Herein is given the reason why we move the vertebra from the side impinged upon in the dorsal and the cervical, and from the opposite side in the lumbar." The same mistake was made on page 49, and was not noticed until The Adjuster was mailed. We take pleasure in adjusting our mistakes as well as those of others.

The statement in the March number is correct, but the adjusting of the atlas may need further explanation.

We adjust the atlas, cervical and dorsal from the affected side, that is, toward the shoulder of the opposite side but in the reverse direction in the lumbar.

We use the spinous processes as levers in the lumbar, dorsal and cervical, and the anterior ends of the posterior arch of the atlas when adjusting.

In the lumbar, the axis is between the distal end of the spinous process and the body of the vertebra, the proximal end of the spinous process. The distal end of the spinous process and the body form portions of a circle—the arcs in making a normal movement. A displacement consists in these arcs being extended more than normal. Adjustments should be made, so that the body of the lumbar is rotated, moved away from the vertical ganglionic chain of the sympathetic nervous system.

In the dorsal and cervical, the axial center is on the anterior of the bodies, therefore, to move the body of the vertebra away from the nerve which is being impinged by its displacement, we move the spinous process and body away from us and—away from the side affected.

The axial center of the atlas is on the anterior of the odontoid process. This movement changes the anterior arch away from you and the posterior arch relatively toward you.

---

Sight-seeing and adjusting literature is recreation for the editor of the Adjuster.

---

When the world demanded Chiropractic, "the man of the hour" was at hand. Two men were not needed. The man of the hour developed as he discovered. To discover was to develop.

---

Chiropractors state that all disease is the result of nerve impingement—a pressure because of a displaced bone. Medicine is not a mechanic; any amount of it cannot replace a bone that is displaced.

## DISEASES OF THE TOES.

The nails are thickened, hardened pieces of skin. They are subject to a number of diseased conditions, the result of functions performed abnormally. Hypertrophy of the nails is quite common. The toe nails may become quite rough, uneven, brittle, lusterless or elevated from the nail-bed. These conditions are liable to follow diseases of other portions of the body.

Ingrowing toe nails is a troublesome affection; pressure of the sharp edge of the nail may produce inflammation and ulceration.

One of the most painful toes I ever saw was occasioned by a corn which had formed under the nail. I relieved it by one adjustment of the first joint. Corns and bunions are because of luxated toe joints. Those on the plantar surface are because of luxated tarsal bones. These displaced bones impinge upon nerves which end just where we find the inflamed cuticle. Set joints for corns and bunions. For the other toe affections, look to the lower lumbar vertebra.

---

In the past, the Discoverer, Developer and Founder, the Fountain Head of Chiropractic, has been modest in stating what belongs to him. While he was diffident there were those who with bold effrontery stole from the Chiropractic line clothing that belonged to another. They have attempted to wear it, but it is unbecoming, does not look well and makes a laughing stock of the would-be owner. "Borrowed garments never fit." The Chiropractor Adjuster will aim to adjust these wrongs which are making a diseased condition in Chiropractic.

---

From a Chiropractic output we take the liberty of commenting: "The spinous processes must be exactly located and spaces discriminated. This is determined by placing the center finger on the posterior process and dropping the finger above into the space between, then compare the relative spaces."

The above palpation is very indeterminate and unreliable. Not only are the spinous processes often bent to the left or right, but diseased conditions, in which heat has been a factor, causes the supra-spinous ligament to become ossified more or less, uniting two or more processes, or partially filling in the gap between. The tips of the spinous processes differ in the normal. This variation is often increased by the addition of exostosis on the inferior or superior borders.

"Let arms be relaxed throughout, although remaining in position." In the Philosophy and Principles of Chiropractic Adjustment, published by this same school, we find 100 cuts of adjusting. In each the arms are represented as hanging downward; therefore, we presume that the author believes this to be the proper position. By laying the arms alongside the body as Jack Bones has done when taking his adjustments. as illustrated in nine cuts, the adjuster will find that the adjusted will have but little or no inclination to resist or buck against the adjuster. Now, this pseudo-fountain head will need to make another hundred cuts in order to show how he has developed the science of Chiropractic by changing the position of the hands and arms. By using the old cuts to show the old way, he can increase the number to two hundred, which will make a great spread, and draw lots of attention. Place the arms in proper position and you will not have to "wait until the patient is relaxed." This one idea, although not based around six words, is worth more to a Chiropractor than all that is new in Vol. 3 of the Science (?) of Chiropractic.

The man who had the brains to found the science of Chiropractic; who was able to dig from the mass of therapeutics the true cause of disease, and devise a method of adjusting racked vertebrae; who, as the Fountain Head, originated the principles of the grandest and greatest science of this age, which egotistical, kleptomaniac scavengers are devising every conceivable means to purloin with threats, trying to intimidate others from writing advanced articles on Chiropractic, while they are retrograding it into the ignorant past instead of developing; the originator of the science still lives, and is yet able to write articles for the advancement of the science to which he gave birth.

---

The All Wise Creative Intelligence is as expressed. The Creator is unfolding creation, developing it toward perfection.

---

The human race is divided into two classes—those who go ahead and do something, and those who destroy what the others have done.

---

Chiropractic is still being developed by its originator.

Readjust the skeletal frame; the recuperative powers inherent in the body will do the rest.

Art always relates to something to be done; science to something to be known.

A Chiropractor is one who has a knowledge of Chiropractic and is able to adjust vertebrae.

Chiropractors present to the world a system which is scientific and devoid of therapeutical experimentation.

Chiropractors use the long bones and the processes of vertebrae as levers to replace displaced vertebrae.

## MUMPS.

This is an inflammation of one of the glands which secrete saliva—the parotid, situated at the angle of the jaw, just below and in front of the ear. It rarely terminates in suppuration, or, upon recovery, in induration of the gland.

The disease frequently begins with a slight chill and a feeling of general indisposition; there is fever, altho not intense. The patient feels a tenderness at the angle of the jaw. which becomes quite painful during mastication. The parotid gland is also swollen, tender and red; the patient may be unable to take any solid food, the swallowing of liquids may be difficult. It is not unusual for the opposite side to become affected as the one improves, or both sides may be diseased simultaneously. The affection may not be confined to the parotid glands, but may involve the glands of the genital organs in the male and the mammae of the female. Orchitis—inflammation of the testicle, may be associated with mumps or venereal diseases.

---

A booklet on Naprapathy. We are pleased to see that the system is properly named; Naprapathy is not a misnomer.

For a time this method was confused with Chiropractic, inasmuch as the three originators took a Chiropractic course under the editor of this journal.

I am pleased to read therein: "Naprapathy should not be confounded with Chiropractic. There is no more similarity between Chiropractic and Naprapathy than there is between a wood sawyer and a carpenter." After reading this booklet. I fully agree with the writer.

"Naprapathy means to fix disease."

Chiropractors fix, put to right skeletal displacements.

Diseases, symptoms, effects cannot be "fixed." they can be treated. Causes can be fixed, adjusted, made right, placed permanently; but they cannot be treated.

Naprapathy treats and cures diseases.

Chiropractors adjust bones, relieve impingements on nerves

N. is "a system of healing."

C. is a system of adjusting; does not heal.

N. says, "Disease is brought on because of nerves and blood vessels being pinched."

C. holds that disease is because of nerve impingement.

N. affirms that "A disease is a coming together of several symptoms."

C. Disease is the result of functions performed in too great or too little degree.

N. "At least 90 per cent of disease has its deep-seated cause **in the spines.**"

C. At least 90 per cent of diseases are caused by impingements **outside of the spine,** near the foramina.

N. "A relaxed ligament is a result of mal-nourishment. Normal nourishment is the cure for a relaxed ligament."

C. A heavy impingement causes paresis directly of the nerve and indirectly of the muscles. Relief is given by removing the pressure.

N. "No tight ligaments; no disease."

C. No impingement upon nerves; no disease.

N. "Without a shortened ligament, disease cannot exist."

C. Without pressure on nerves, disease cannot exist.

N. "Ligamentous straps which were too tight."

C. Nerves which were contracted and enlarged.

N. "A slow pull on a ligament is of no avail; it must be acted upon by a short quick thrust."

C. A push is useless when replacing any joint; it requires a quick, energetic, decisive move.

N. "The short, quick thrust is delivered upon some bony process, so as to get the desired 'impact' upon the shortened ligament."

C. By using the long bones and processes of vertebrae as levers, adjustments are given, the movement being quick, so as to replace the bone to its normal position, relieving pressure from nerves.

---

No profession offers such an unlimited field of usefulness.

---

G. H. Patchen, M. D., of New York City, says: "I am always a seeker after truth. **It is the only authority I recognize.**"

---

Today a large number of Osteopaths have become believers in spinal lesions; they correct them in a manner similar to that made use of by Chiropractors, and by so doing, they have shortened the time of their treatments to one-fourth of that which was formerly required.

---

"Naturopathic physicians." A physician is one who practices medicine, a doctor of medicine. A Naturopath is one who uses natural remedies; he eschews medicine, he does not use drugs. These two words are opposite in their meaning, should not be used to express the same idea, because they are opposite, contradictory.

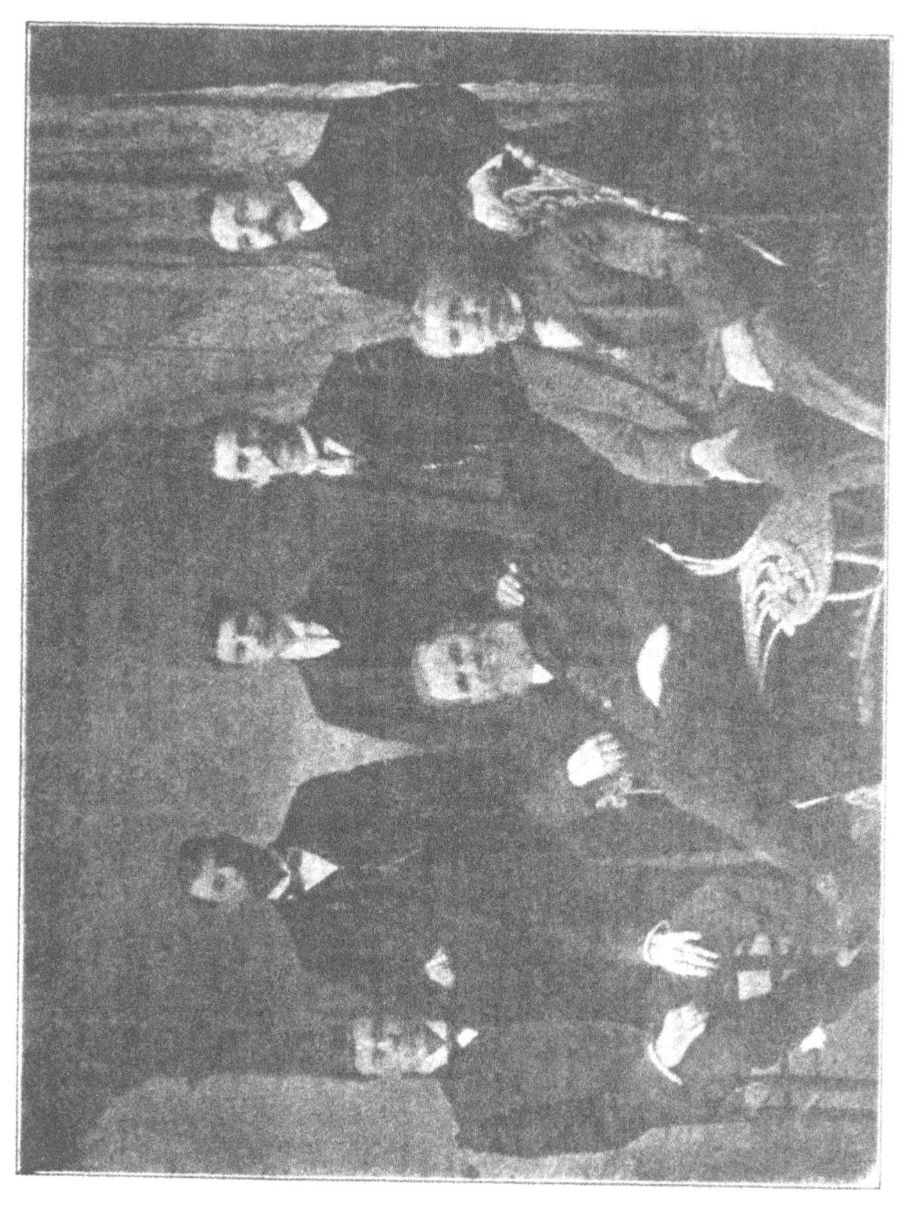

Cut of a photo taken at a reunion in Dec., 1902. Dates of their graduation: Smith, 1899; Jones, 1900; Sutton, 1901; Story, 1901; Langworth, 1901; B. J., 1902. B. J. was the 15th graduate up to 1903.

## THE MEDICAL PRACTICE ACT.

The doctors are wild with fear and alarm, they are trembling and quaking with rage.
They do not perceive, or understand that this is a progressive age;
With affected nerves, their pens dipped in gall, they seek to banish the fact,
That the tool they have used to gain their foul ends is the Medical Practice Act.

For years they have ruled the people, as slaves they bowed before them all;
Their arrogance is great; they forget that pride goeth before a fall;
These Allopaths would feign believe themselves safe, and as strong as the Czar,
And that naught could arise to cause them fear, or the ease of their lives to mar.

A sturdy young giant came out of the West, to battle for truth and right;
He befriends the weak, the maimed, the halt, and hurls proud defiance at might;
He fights with a will, and his enemies strong can never force him to yield;
This herculean giant has Chiropractic emblazoned on his shield.

The alarmed poisoners and butchers, much frightened, ran to their friends,
The monopolists, whom they hoped would help accomplish their foul ends.
"Oh, pass us a law; Oh, pass us a law; please pass us a law mighty quick
Which will fine and imprison all, save ourselves, who attempt to cure the sick.

"Make the law strong in every detail; protection is what you must give;
Protection, by forcing the sick of our land to pay us, so we may live."
Thus cried the doctors in the East and the West, and their pleas were not in vain;
In most of the States in this grand land of ours did they such protection gain.

Ohio, Nebraska and brave Illinois have bowed the menial's knee.
They stand for slavery, injustice and jargon, in this great land of the free;
In sickness and ailments you truly can't choose, if you obey the state's laws,
But must pay the fee to the Allopaths—it's all for the good of the cause.

The doctors worked hard to get their bills thru, and at a very late date,
Monopoly, by trickery, passed in the Hoosier and Badger States.
The devilish doctors now laugh and grin and chuckle in their ghoulish glee:
"Oh, we are the only, only ones, now, who can touch the sick for a fee.

"We can charge as we wish, and do what we like with poison and knife and saw,
And should we by chance kill a patient or two, it's in the name of the law;
The Chiropractors, altho they have brains, we have to acknowledge that fact,
If they practice, will be heavily fined by our Medical Practice Act."

## "ESTABLISHED 1885."

This head line of a letterhead adorns the top of a fountain in which is the head of B. J. The interpretation means just what is says on the basin below, "Chiropractic's fountain Head."

While he was making a date for the establishing of his fountain head, why did he not place it at his birth, Sept. 10, 1882; it would only be stretching an untruth three years more. As B. J. established Chiropractic when he was three years of age, why not have D. D., the Grand Son, also, establish a school as soon as he is three years old? The Grandfather had Chiropractic quite well established in 1900. With Chiropractic established in 1885, 1900 and 1909 it ought to be quite well and securely established.

---

Chiropractors and jewelers do not treat or cure, do not prescribe or apply remedies when they adjust, fix or repair displacements of bones or watches. They do not use salve or other preparations to soothe or mollify abnormal functionating in living organisms, or when correcting an unreliable timekeeper.

## BERNARD SHAW ON VIVISECTION.

(From the Portland Oregonian.)

"It is pretty certain that, if the great majority of sensible men were opposed to vivisection, the eminent George Bernard Shaw would favor it, but inasmuch as every scientist in the world of any repute and every ordinary citizen who cares a fig for the welfare of the human race, look to vivisection as our only salvation from numerous ills, Mr. Shaw violently condemns it. He has risen to a proud station among the members of the British Union for the Abolition of Vivisection. This was to be expected, for when Mr. Shaw made up his mind to join a society of fools, naturally nothing would satisfy him short of being the biggest fool of the lot. The ignorance and prejudice which he exhibited in a widely-published address to the union, not long ago, show that his eminence has been worthily won. An anti-vivisection speech, which did not contain at least a score of falsehoods, would be rather flat. If it treated physicians and men of science with anything like common fairness, the speaker would be hooted. Anti-vivisection thrives on a diet composed half of deliberate lying and half of mawkish conceit.

In the speech to which we have referred, Bernard Shaw says over and over again that vivisection has accomplished nothing for the good of mankind or the increase of knowledge. Statements of this sort display absence of conscience, which would be incredible in anybody but an animal worshipper, but it is notable that men and women who have devoted themselves to the religious cult of dogs, cats and monkeys lose every vestige of feeling for the woes of their own kind. No women are so utterly insensible to human suffering as those who have become the slaves of a pet dog. To see some of them grovel before their ugly little idols is enough to make a person ashamed of his species. The dog worshiper in general not only becomes dehumanized to an astonishing degree, but he even boasts of his mania as if it were something to take pride in. "I am a lover of dogs," he cries from the housetops. Did you ever hear one of these infatuated monsters proclaim his love for his fellow man? Or take a woman who has fallen a victim to the cat cult. Behold how she prostrates herself before her fetish. She consecrates every waking hour to its service, dreams of it by night and when she dies it is bounteously remembered in her will.

There are instances of besotted females who have left fortunes of $10,000 for the support of a pet cat! To a beloved and adored dog now and then $30,000 or $40,000 have been left by some dying idiot for luxurious maintenance. Only the other day there was a story in the papers of a poodle dog which had long enjoyed the income from a bequest of this sort. It finally died from a surfeit brought on by dining on a whole chicken, followed by a pound of candy. Meanwhile there were thousands of children in the same city who had not had a decent dinner in their lives. Such is the dire influence of dog and cat worship on the human intelligence and conscience, and yet the anti-vivisectionists boast of their addiction to the vice.

Everybody ought to read Mr. Shaw's speech, for it shows how inane a really able man may become when he devotes himself to a cause which is at the same time both silly and wicked. A good specimen of the dense ignorance he displays is to be found in this sentence: "I wish myself that the vivisectors could be induced to perform some really scientific experiments upon themselves." This implies, of course, that they never have done so, and doubtless Mr. Shaw would go on repeating his dull falsehood, even if somebody would tell him of the medical officers who inoculated themselves with the yellow fever at Havana; of the scientists who permitted poisonous insects to bite them on the Roman Campagna, and of the young experimenter who tried upon his own body the effect of cancer virus. Whatever may be said for or against the physicians and other men of science, they have never hesitated to put their theoris to the supreme test of a trial on their own persons. Their own courage in this particular far surpasses what is required of a soldier on the battlefield. It is easy for Mr. Bernard Shaw and the coterie of shrews and imbeciles who train with him to rail at physicians and assert that their experiments on living animals are a systematic cultivation of cruelty, but one may predict safely enough that in all the multiple of the anti-vivisectionists there is not a single individual who ever willingly made the smallest sacrifice of his own bodily comfort for the good of the human race. They are all of them completely satisfied when they have secured the comfort of their pet dogs and cats. They are the most selfish people in the whole world. Where will you find anybody else who is willing to doom thousands of human beings to death for the sake of gratifying his own vanity? That is precisely what the anti-vivisectionists would like to do.

The problems which now confront physicians cannot be solved without making experiments on living animals. We are compelled, therefore, to choose between inflicting some transitory pain on a few cats and monkeys and permitting such diseases as cancer to ravage mankind without a remedy.

The anti-vivisectionist prefers to spare the beasts and let human beings perish in hopeless misery. They have won so much support in Great Britain that they have substantially stopped the progress of medical research there. British physicians who wish to do scientific work have to go to the continent for an opportunity. If the animal worshipers can accomplish their purpose they will do the same thing in America. They openly avow their intention to close the Rockefeller and Buffalo research hospitals. They will put an end to medical experiment in every laboratory in the country if they can once get control of legislation. The time has passed when they ought to be treated leniently. They ought to be roundly denounced as enemies of the human race and every person who cares for the welfare of his own species should do his part to help thwart their wicked schemes."

---

The Sunday Oregonian of September 26th contained the above editorial on the question of vivisection—surgical operations upon living animals for the purpose of observing normal or morbid physiological processes. The Oregonian, instead of citing the reader to some knowledge gained by torturing helpless, dumb animals, uses slanderous epithets, such as fools, monsters, idiots, shrews, imbeciles, animal worshipers and besotted females. It says that the lovers of household pets were silly, wicked, fetish worshipers; that the eminent George Bernard Shaw, who has risen to the proud station among the members of the British Union for the Abolition of Vivisection, is the biggest fool; that he exhibits dense ignorance, prejudice, mawkish conceit and states falsehoods and deliberate lies in his speeches. Such vituperative argument is unbecoming.

Vivisection is supposed to be performed in the interest of pathologic physiology, with a hope of discovering the cause of abnormal metabolism, so that the surgeon may learn something regarding biology—the science of life. Thousands and thousands of helpless victims, unable to call down the vengeance of heaven upon their cruel tormentors, have been slowly tortured in the interests of science until a lingering death put an end to their misery. These deluded vivisectors imagine that, by observing, under the microscope, the behavior of the pathological conditions and processes induced by their cruel and unnecessary experiments, they will be able to discover the cause and nature of disease. But, with all of their efforts, these ardent enthusiasts have not disclosed the reason for functional derangement, or the cause of any disease.

McFarland truthfully and conscientiously states in his textbook on "Pathology for Practitioners and Students," "that a knowledge of pathology forms the only rational foundation upon which the art of medicine is perfected; medicine cannot become an exact science." The question arises, Is there any science in the practice of medicine and has vivisection advanced it along the lines of scientific investigation?

In a frank and honest manner McFarland states that the nature of assimilation of digested foods is still undetermined. The metabolic processes, while believed to be chemical, are as yet inexplicable. Traumatic fever remains unexplained. What becomes of the sugar (in diabetes) under normal conditions, is a problem of great importance concerning which we are still somewhat in the dark. The nature of this probable secretion (pancreatic juice) is unknown to us. The nature of ferment is unknown. It is not yet positively determined where urea is formed; it is a paradox. The relation of gout to uric acid is certain, though by no means clear. The origin of uric acid is obscure. The importance of bile salts, or rather, of the acid of which they are formed, is not known. The physiologic chemistry of gout is far from clear. The pathology of gout is bound up with questions. Curiously enough, the results of experiment and disease seem to differ. In the physiology of dwarfs there is probably some hidden error of nutrition or metabolism. The chemistry of the process of fatty metamorphosis is obscure. Experiments leave us in some doubt regarding the true nature of the process. The nature of the process of mucoid metamorphosis is obscure. The cause of colloid degeneration is not known. The mechanism of the formation of over-growths is not understood. The etiology of gigantism is obscure. Tumors arise without apparent cause. In truth, we are no nearer the correct solution of the etiology of tumors, so far as any accurate knowledge is concerned, than we were ten years ago. The cause of sarcoma is unknown. The cause of angioma is obscure. We have no positive knowledge of the nature of lymphomata. The etiology of carcinoma is very obscure.

The above extracts are gleaned from a pathological textbook which is intended to give physicians and students who "look to vivisection as our only salvation from numerous ills," more and better knowledge of pathological physiology.

Why not get wise and accept the truism of an illustrious medical grandfather of 1776, Baron von Swieten, counsellor and first physician to their Majesties, the Emperor and Empress of Germany; perpetual president of the College of Physicians in Vienna; member of the Royal Academy of Sciences and Surgery at Paris; H. Fellows of the Royal College of Physicians at Edinburgh. He said: "A pleurisy terminates either in a cure, in other diseases, or in death. This is a circumstance which a pleurisy has in common with all other diseases."

How long at the above rate of enlightenment before one will be able to tell us something in regard to metabolism? How many more thousands of helpless creatures will be made to suffer before we can be edified on biology, or told the origin and nature of any one disease? Pray tell us how much longer will you continue to callous your feelings before you will give up the bloody delusion of vivisection? How many more generations will come and go before you will be able to lesson the number of your self-limited diseases—those which run a definite course, notwithstanding your coveted ignorance gained by centuries of misdirected cruelty? McFarland says: "A knowledge of these specific actions of poisonous substances that form the foundation of therapeutics, and it is only a thorough knowledge of their pharmacology that gives medicine a firm scientific station."

The interest and energy shown by the medical fraternity is commendable; but the ignorance displayed is to be deplored. Vivisection and pharmacology have not and never will enlighten the world concerning pathological physiology.

If your windows fail to move freely and your doors to open easily, because your building has sagged, would you slash, cut and destroy others in order to learn the reason of their nonperformance of the acts which they were designed to do? Would you not rather make an effort to discover what part of the structure had become displaced, permitting the building to settle and thereby deranging some part of its architecture which in turn had been drawn out of alignment sufficiently to cause the difficulty with the doors and windows? You would not permit a would-be workman to butcher your doors and windows, but would employ a master-mechanic who would adjust displaced portions.

As it is with the building, so it is with our bodies. The skeleton forms the solid framework of the body. It supports the softer structures which are grouped around it, and affords protection to many delicate organs which are lodged within its cavities. By the articulation of its several parts, its segments are converted into levers which constitute the passive portions of the locomotory system. The various bones and cartilages are united by means of ligaments so arranged as to give the body definite shape and afford attachment to the muscles by which the various movements are accomplished.

Innumerable accidents make us liable to displace some portion of the bony framework, more especially the segments of the vertebral column. Poisons taken into the body by inhalation, food or drink, act in a noxious manner on the vital properties or the textures of an organ or the system at large, by and thru the nervous system, the nerves of which, being irritated, contract longitudinally and act on muscles which by their muscular attachment, draw bones out of alignment.

Bones displaced ever so little by accident or poisons, impinge upon sensitive nerves, the conveyors of impulses, thereby augmenting or decreasing functionating, which is disease. Why not relieve the pressure upon the nerves by replacing the portion of the skeletal framework? By this method all kinds of diseases are now being relieved.

This new system is founded upon the relationship of bones, nerves and muscles. If they are in their normal position we have normal functionating, which is health. This system has been discovered and developed without the shedding of blood or the taking of innocent lives.

The originator of this method stands ready to demonstrate these ideas by relieving typhoid or other fevers in a few minutes and that in the presence of physicians. Why not use as good judgment in adjusting displaced portions of the body as you would that of a building?

Why tell such improbable stories as that of the poodle dog dining on a whole chicken and sweetening its repast with a pound of candy?

Is there any harm in giving employment to the laborer in building tasty structures or caring for our horses, cattle, sheep, hogs, dogs, or cats? Supposing (in your mind) that a poodle dog ate a whole chicken and sweetened it with a pound of candy; the raising of the chicken and the making of the candy gave employment to labor wherewith to buy food for those less fortunate financially.

The officers who innoculated themselves with yellow fever, the scientists who permitted poisonous insects to bite them, and the young experimenter who tried to innoculate himself with vaccine or cancer virus, were bigger fools than the owner of the poodle dog who gave him a full stomach of chicken sweetened with candy.

The problems of metabolism and pathological physiology which have for centuries confronted physicians, cannot be solved by cruel experiments on helpless living animals. Humanity is awakening to the fact that there is no salvation from our numerous ills thru pharmacotherapy or vivisection.

---

"Your body is sick," is like having a bad taste in your mouth; where else would you have it?

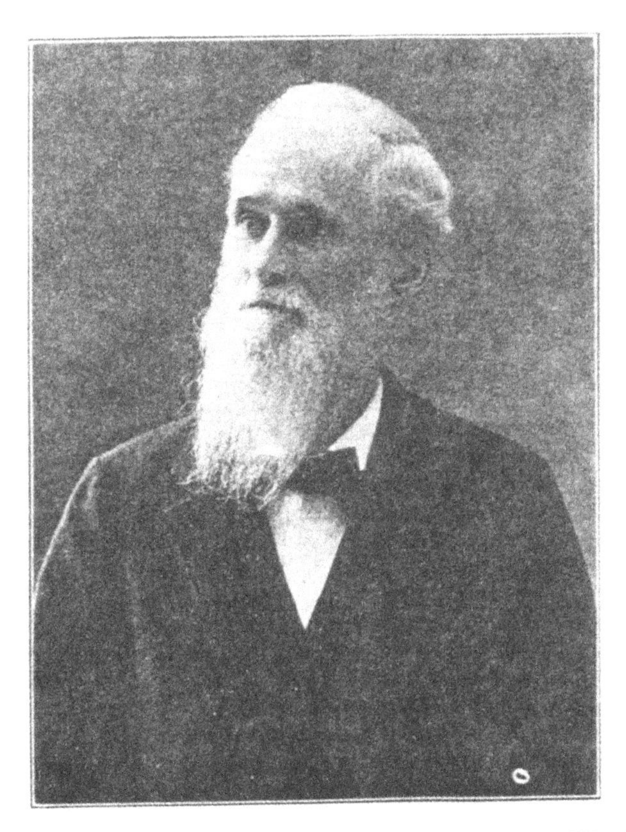

Rev. Samuel H. Weed, A. B., 1864, A. M. 1867 and B. D. 1867. Those degrees were earned and bestowed on him by the faculties. He was a member of Co. K., 133 Regt., Ind. Vol. Inf. His residence is at Monmouth, Ill.

Rev. Weed is a man not above manual or mental labor. During our early acquaintance he labored on the farm or in the garden, printing office, acted as Justice of the Peace and that of a Presbyterian minister.

"Mrs. Weed and daughter took Chiropractic adjustments in 1896," of me, "and were much benefitted, after which Mr. Weed also received adjustments "of me" for sciatica and was relieved. About this time he was asked "by me" to suggest a name for the science and art" which I had originated and was developing. To him I am indebted for the word Chiropractic. At the date mentioned B. J. was 14 years of age. Six years after, the "1896" he took a course in Chiropractic under me.

## AMBIGUITY.

"Chiropractic as taught by this college is supreme and foremost in rank and dignity. It is taught along the lines of the philosophical and physicological laws of nature.

"A golden opportunity awaits those who will take up this extraordinary profession, which is devoid of superiority or competition.

"A free clinic is maintained."

A college is a society of scholars, or friends of learning, incorporated for study, or instruction. This college consists of one man, who is the whole society, he fills all offices. He is the college, supreme and foremost in rank and dignity.

"Philosophical laws of nature."

Philosophy is the science that treats of the laws that govern facts or phenomena. Laws are not philosophical. Our reasoning upon them may be, or may not be philosophical.

"Physicological laws of nature."

The two words from which the above is compounded are heterogeneous, possessed of different characteristics, are dissimilar, are not in any way related to each other, or the subject (laws) referred to. Physico is used as a prefix, meaning natural; as, physico-philosophy, natural philosophy. Logical is the science or art of exact reasoning. The laws of nature—there are none other—are natural. Whether they appear logical or not depends upon our reasoning.

Extraordinary is the unusual, not customary, out of the ordinary; a word that is not applied to professions.

Devoid designates empty, vacant. Can you think of a profession being devoid, empty, vacant of competition and superiority. I presume that the doctor meant to have said, that the profession has no competition, nor a superior. He nor I will live to see the day when Chiropractic will not have competition, and as for its superiority, that depends upon who is the judge.

Clinics are held, not maintained.

---

Adversity is often a blessing. The man who has lost a leg never has corns on both feet.

---

Mr. McQuire (to hospital attendant)—Phwat did ye say the doctor's name was?

Attendant—Dr. Kilpatrick.

Mr. McQuire—Thot settles it. No doctor wid thot cognomen will git a chance to operate on me—not if I know it.

Attendant—Why not?

Mr. McQuire—Well, ye see, my name is Patrick.—Judge.

## GUARANTEES.

Many persons want a guarantee. Usually these callers think they are shrewd and capable of driving a sharp bargain; they want to gamble, bet on the other man's game, which is usually favorable to the man who is running the game.

If the practitioner cares to bother with these callers, he may show them the following forms of grafting.

"**Business Methods of Specialists,**" by J. D. Albright, M. D., 3228 Broadway street, Philadelphia, Pa., from whom I quote the following:

"The advertising specialists' guarantee is a unique document. Of which it may truthfully be said, it is 'fearfully and wonderfully made.' It is so skilfully constructed and so abounding in verbosity that the loopholes which it **always** contains are so neatly disguised that it fulfills its purpose as a decoy in a most satisfactory manner.

"In drawing up these guarantees, several plans are adopted, according to the circumstances under which they are made; that is, guarantees may be specific on a certain point in certain instances, while in others the point specified in one may be omitted in another, thus enabling the man who is willing to lend himself to this form of deception to write an **apparently** binding guarantee to suit any case, **even meeting the objections** of such as may be shrewd enough to detect certain discrepancies, and at the same time provide a safety clause or an omission for his benefit.

"The guarantee of advertising specialists are the subject of considerable inquiry from physicians who, like the patient, are not informed of their true nature, and, as it is rare that action for recovery is brought against the advertisers, and but little unfavorable criticism is heard against them, many of the regular profession are inclined to believe that the specialists are nearly in possession of wonderful secrets, and actually bring about the cures they so freely guarantee to effect. A careful reading of the various forms of guarantees which are here described will serve to classify the atmosphere to a considerable extent, and disseminate information that cannot be too widely known.

"Example 1. One of the simplest forms of guarantee is that in which the patient **is promised a cure** of whatever disease he may have, not only completely, but also permanently, at a certain fee per month, which shall include all medicines and services. Nothing is said of refunding money, **but the cure is guaranteed to be satisfactory to the patient.** In addition to making no reference to a penalty or providing for a refund, the important item of **Time is omitted.**

"**This practically binds the patient to continue the treatment for an indefinite period**, and when he refuses to pay the monthly installment, the treatment is discontinued. The doctor will plead his inability to effect a cure unless he is given every opportunity, and for as long a period as the disease will require, and assumes a grieved demeanor when the patient rebels at the expense. **As a matter of fact, the doctor is well pleased** with the amount he has received, and inasmuch as no further cash is to be expected, he is through with the patient.

"Among the more intelligent the absence of the time clause is frequently detected, and a more ingenious form of guarantee is employed, the doctor assuming, in such cases that the omission was an oversight and entirely unintentional.

"Example 2. A guarantee may be given to cure a certain disease, eradicating all traces of it from the system, within a specified time, for a certain fee per month, with a clause inserted that failing to perform his part of the contract, **the doctor will refund every cent paid him for services.** This looks good to the patient and acts as a clincher. It is especially gratifying to the doctor to book patients that seem to glory in being shrewd. They are meat and drink to him. The joker in this guarantee consists of this: As each month's payment is made, a receipt is given, usually on the back of the contract, '**For** medicines for the month of ———' and as time rolls by and the specified limit is reached, the patient, if dissatisfied, claims his money back. As pleasantly as possible the doctor informs his patient that he has been paid nothing for services, refers his victim to his receipts for medicine only, and appears to be sorry to say that there will be no refund.

"Example 3. Another form of guarantee is that in which a cure is guaranteed, regardless of the disease, completely and permanently, within a certain specified time for a certain fixed fee, with the following clause inserted. 'Should the cure not be entirely complete at the end of the above specified time, we reserve the right to furnish **all the medicines** required to effect a complete and satisfactory cure, without the additional charge,' or words to that effect.

"The doctor will argue that no one can definitely predict the exact date upon which all evidences of any disease will disappear, and while he has specified a period of time that is ordinarily sufficient to cure the condition, it is just possible that it may require additional time. As no further charge is to be made, there is usually no objection made to continuing the treatment for a supposedly short time in order to complete the cure (supposed to be almost effected), yet a careful reading of this clause does not warrant these assumptions.

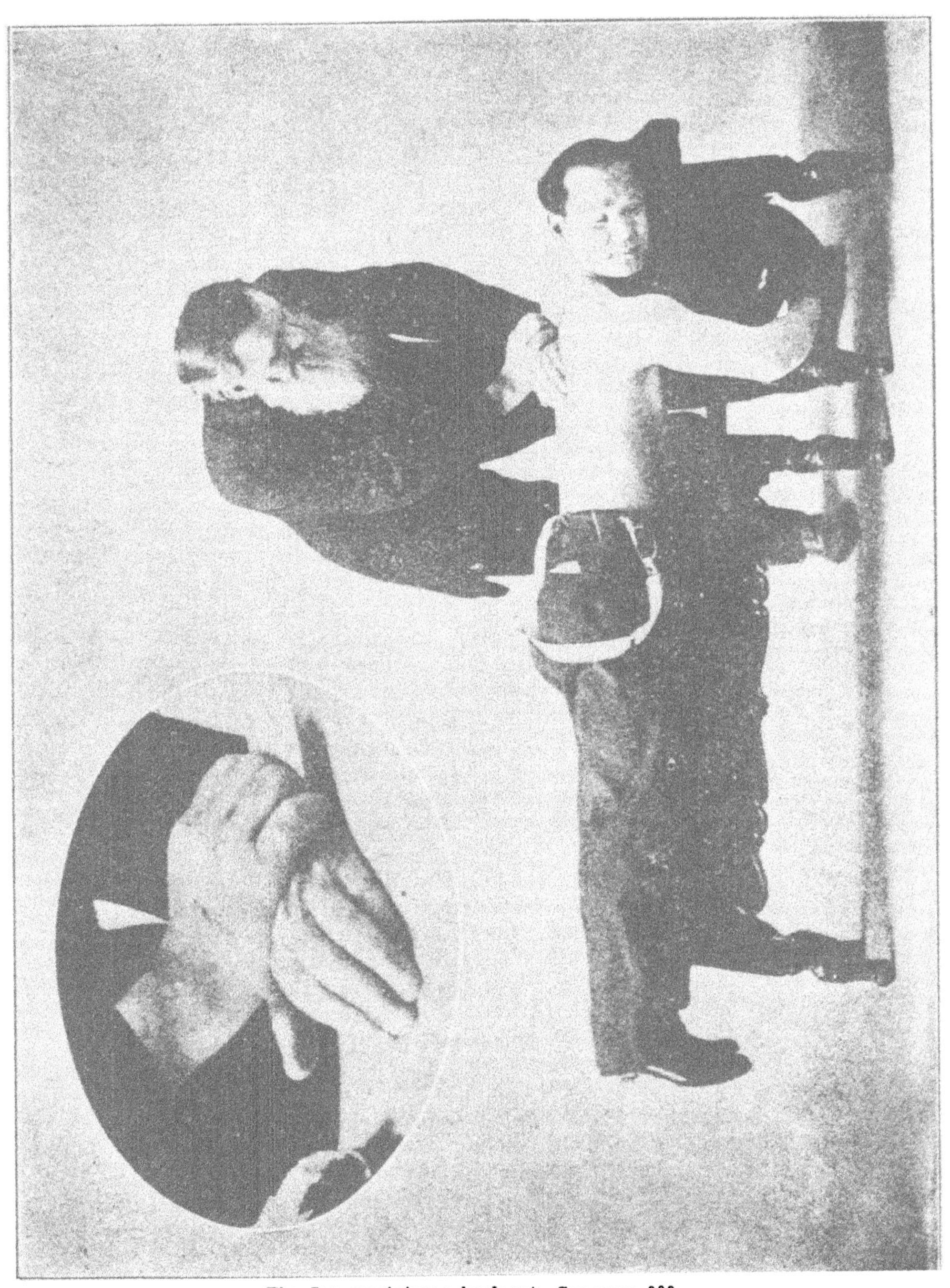

The Jap receiving a back-set—See page 908.

"When the patient has paid the fee agreed upon and taken the treatment during the required and specified period, if not satisfactorily cured, the free treatment is begun. This consists of one hundred pills or tablets, with instructions to take one at bedtime each night, with a request to report when they are all taken.

"If the patient does not suspect the trick at the time he receives his first hundred pills, he is due to awake when he receives the second hundred with similar directions, and if he refrains from certain pointed remarks at this time he will most probably have his say when he reports at the end of the second hundred days.

"When he finally appears, greatly dissatisfied, and possibly threatens the doctor with all manner of dire consequences, more pills are offered him in apparently the best of faith on the part of the doctor, who meanwhile continues to assure him of his best endeavors to complete the cure. Never does he recede from this point. He never admits any semblance of deception, but invariably masquerades in the disguise of a man much grieved at the ingratitude of the average patient toward a conscientious medical attendant. The patience of the ungrateful one finally deserts him, and he studiously avoids his one-time confidential medical adviser.

"Example 4. A guarantee for the cure of gonorrhea, 'lost manhood,' or some other secret disease **is usually made without a single legal flaw. The cure is guaranteed to be certain**; the time limit is specifically mentioned; the price of treatment is reduced to exact figures for the complete course of treatment.

"The doctor, knowing well the trend of human nature, protects himself against any legal action or unfavorable criticism by carefully and prominently mentioning the disease with which the patient is afflicted one or more times in the guarantee.

"Should treatment prove unsatisfactory after all the money agreed upon has been paid, an excuse is sought for to warrant further demands for cash. Very few men with gonorrhea follow directions to the letter in regard to alcoholics or sexual matters, and it is never difficult to secure an admission on the part of the patient that he has failed to follow strictly the advice or instructions given him in matters relating to diet, exercise, etc.

"Unless an additional financial consideration is forthcoming, the doctor politely dismisses his patient. The fact that, in order to secure any legal redress the guarantee with the secret diseases specified would necessarily become public property, is a sufficient assurance to the doctor that nothing of the sort will be attempted by the patient.

"In drawing up the guarantee, 'sexual weakness' is mentioned prominently in connection with catarrh, indigestion, kidney or bladder affections, or whatever the condition may suggest. As in the case of secret diseases, the reference to this delicate subject is sufficient to prevent any complaint on the part of the patient if he finds himself duped by the doctor.

"Example 5. This is a guarantee that is somewhat similar to example 3; yet is sufficiently different to warrant reference to it specifically.

"A guarantee may be drawn **which promises everything the patient might desire, everything the most exacting might demand,** for a certain fee within a specified time, and all money to be refunded in case of failure. It also contains the apparently reasonable clause that the patient will do his or her part toward effecting a cure by following directions faithfully, obey instructions and report for treatment regularly. This looks innocent indeed, and no one could possibly object to it, as the most skilled physician is powerless to cure unless he has the opportunity to treat his patient.

"As the time for making the last payment approaches, say from four to six weeks previous, the doctor begins to make demands upon his patient that subject him to great inconvenience. He will demand his presence in the office twice a day, and will perhaps pass sounds or dilate the rectum so frequently that considerable irritation will be produced; if the patient be a female he will use the speculum and apply local treatment for some imaginary disease in some portion of the genital tract; he will furnish medicines that will sicken the patient and order certain rules to be followed that will disgust and annoy the patient so much that continuation of the treatment is refused, or at least appointments will not be punctually kept, thus providing an escape from his agreement on the part of the doctor.

"Should the patient, however, endeavor to meet every requirement, the doctor will persist in his abominable tactics, and it requires no further illustration to convince the reader that a doctor thus disposed can make patients sick in considerable less time than he can make them well, and subject them to such a variety of indignities that the misnamed treatment is infinitely worse than the disease, and its continuation an absolute impossibility.

"Example 6. When dealing with persons who can well afford to pay a good fee, a favorite scheme of the advertising specialist is to accept a patient for treatment for a certain round sum, one-half of which is paid cash and the balance when the patient is satisfied that he is cured, even offering to permit six months to elapse after treatment is discontinued before payment, that the patient may determine the permanency of the cure.

"This is an alluring bait and often catches the biggest fish; businessmen who imagine they are shrewd; men who pride themselves on driving close bargains; persons who seek an advantage in their favor in business matters. This form of contract also appeals to those who are dishonest and accept the terms proposed with no intention of ever making a second payment, even though they should find themselves entirely cured. Such persons are reasonably certain that a cure is merely a matter of time and fully believe that the doctor must be convinced that he can cure them, otherwise he would not be willing to treat them on such reasonable terms. The biter is sometimes bit, and this is where it actually happens.

"Should the treatment prove curative the doctor will exhaust every legal means to collect the balance due, and as he is usually fortified by a contract, made in duplicate, which incidently refers to 'sexual weakness' or 'errors of youth,' he collects his fee in ninety per cent of cases, while those who escape payment are usually harassed and dunned more than any respectable person would care to endure.

"If the desired results are not obtained after due time the patient receives a placebo or some disagreeable medicine, given with the object of lengthening the intervals between visits, or provoking a loss of patince or even disgust. In this event the doctor never refers to the 'balance' of the fee. It is, of course, quite evident that 'half the fee' is all the doctor ever expected, and it was probably amply sufficient to repay him for the energy and skill he expended in his efforts to cure, at the same time taking a reasonable chance in effecting a cure and collecting the balance. In contracts of this sort, when the doctor displays such generosity in the matter of terms, no provision is made for the return of the fifty per cent of the fee paid in advance.

"Example 7. When promises are made to accept patients on this plan, some trick may confidently be sought for, and it will usually be located without much effort. The method most frequently employed is the taking of promissory notes from patients, payable when cured. The time for effecting a cure is estimated verbally, in conversation between doctor and patient, and serves as a guide in determining the date upon which first payment will be due.

"The doctor is always certain that the disease is curable, and continues the conversation in an optimistic manner until no doubt remains in the mind of the patient as to the eventual outcome of the treatment. However, as a matter of assurance,

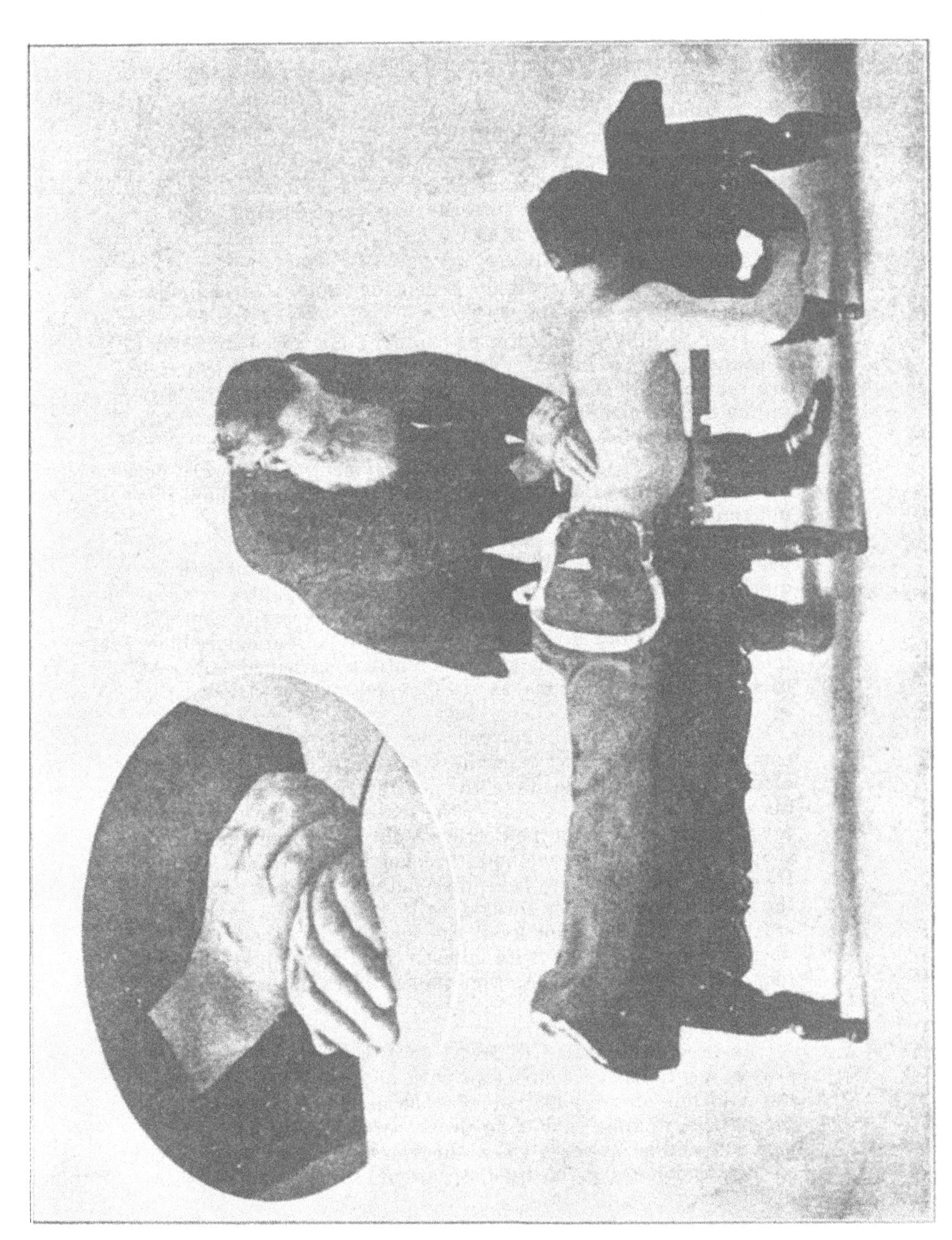

How the Jap got a set-back. See page 908.

the possibility of failure is provided for in the notes, and although a note based on a contingency is void legally, the doctor has reasonable hopes that he will collect them. It should be noted that this plan is seldom offered to a business or professional man, as it would but rarely be accepted, but is largely employed among the uneducated or young men who have not yet been taught to appreciate the import of signing notes or contracts promiscuously.

"The method is as follows:

"In drawing up an ordinary promissory note, a form similar to the following is adopted:

"Four months after date, providing I am cured of Sexual Weakness, Lost Manhood, Bladder and Kidney Disease, which are the result of Masturbation and Sexual Excesses, and providing my Normal Sexual Vigor is completely and satisfactorily restored, I promise to pay to Dr. ————, etc."

"When the specified time arrives payment is promptly demanded, regardless of the condition of the patient. Should he not consider the treatment satisfactory he will naturally refuse to meet the obligation, but after being informed that unless payment is made suit will be brought for collection, his attitude quickly changes, and if the note is not at once paid a compromise is usually effected, whereby the doctor agrees to continue the treatment until a cure is effected, and the patient reduces the note by monthly installments until it is wiped out. At this point their relations as doctor and patient are usually severed.

"Should the patient, however, be obstinate and refuse to compromise or to pay, regardless of the doctor's threats to offer his note for sale, take the matter to court and expose his sexual secrets to the public, the matter is usually dropped, for as a matter of facts the doctor would be injured financially should his despicable methods become known to the public. He may, however, employ some disreputable attorney and annoy the patient with further threats, calling attention to exposure, etc., but if this does not avail the incident is closed, and the doctor squares matters with himself by the thought that he took a chance and lost. As the scheme works out according to the schedule in the large majority of cases, the general average is considered quite satisfactory.

"As previously stated in Example 4, some secret disease is always mentioned in connection with any guarantee that does not omit one of the vital points to be used as a club to bring the patient to time should he prove refractory at the crucial moment, and so in cases when cures are promised in advance of pay, and notes given by the patient, some private disease or secret vice is without exception named as the underlying cause of the patient's condition, and so stated in the note or notes. As masturbation is so universally practiced at some time in life, very few men have the inclination to deny their indulgence to a greater or less extent, or will at least admit that they have freely indulged in sexual excesses. In fact, a considerable portion will feel flattered at the intimation that they have worshipped at the shrine of Venus to excess during their acquaintance with this seductive goddess, hence it is not difficult to convince men that many of their ills are consequental to former indiscretions.

"Example 8. 'Not a cent of pay until cured' is the catchline used in the advertisements of an advertising specialist who has a chain of offices throughout the principal cities of the East.

"In the hope and belief that the doctor is so confident of success that he is willing to wait an indefinite period for his pay, the public is attracted to his office.

"After due inquiry regarding the ailments of the prospective patient, and the latter anxious to obtain the benefit of a system of treatment in which the doctor has sufficient confidence to make so liberal an offer, he is suddenly awakened by something like this:

"Yes, indeed, my dear sir, I am perfectly willing to cure you to your entire satisfaction without one cent of pay until you are ready to admit that you are fully restored to health, but I must have the assurance that you will fulfill your promise to pay when cured, as faithfully as I fulfill my duty toward you, and as you are a stranger to me, you would surely not object to securing some well-known person with whom you are acquainted, or your employer, perhaps, to agree to pay me for my services in case you should not do so.

"This, of course, turns a different light upon the matter, and as the patient is suffering from some secret disease, or some sequel to it, as before detailed, he spurns the suggestion of the doctor in a manner most unmistakable.

"Under these circumstances the doctor naturally feels hurt. He repeats his assurances of skillful treatment and renews his promises of a certain cure, and attempts to lead the patient to think that he sees no objection in seeking for a 'well-known or influential man' to stand sponsor for him.

"During the interview the doctor never fails to mention the dire consequences that neglect of such a condition will surely bring to the unhappy victim, and impresses him with narratives of persons similarly situated, who, untreated, terminated their existence by suicide or in an asylum for the insane.

"As the patient will probably worry more about it than the doctor, the latter having nothing at stake, a compromise will sooner or later be effected, and the cash divided as may be agreed upon, a transaction anticipated by the doctor at the beginning of the interview.

" 'For ways that are dark and tricks that are vain' the dishonest mercenary, advertising fake specialist, has the 'heathen Chinee' denuded to the deep fascia."

"Thus the interview is prolonged, and if the doctor is a good 'case taker' he will land his victim by hook or crook, giving him one of the guarantees previously mentioned, and will receive a certain amount of cash on account.

"The 'not a cent until cured' slogan means nothing. No one ever for a moment considers the doctor's suggestion to secure another to guarantee the payment of the bill, but this catch-line has served to bring many persons into his office for consultation who otherwise would never have given the matter serious consideration.

"Example 9. Some specialists employ a plan somewhat similar to the foregoing in all essential details regarding the importance of treatment and the consequence of neglect, but instead of suggesting another to guarantee payment the doctor agrees to cure the patient for a certain sum, which shall be deposited in bank to their joint account, with the understanding that if the patient is cured he will release the deposit in the doctor's favor, and in case of failure the cash shall revert to the patient.

"As all joint deposits require the consent of both parties before the money can be withdrawn, it can readily be seen that there is room for considerable argument before this is brought about.

"The contract made between patient and doctor always mentions the inevitable private disease, and while the patient may consider himself not benefited in the least, the doctor will claim the exact opposite, and will offer to call into consultation another physician to arbitrate the matter and abide by his decision. This proposition will naturally be rejected by the the patient, and the cash will remain in bank for an indefinite period.

---

During all these years of suffering, acute diseases have run their course, because they were self-limited; chronic cases have continued, for they were incurable. The medical world has treated the effects rather than adjust the causes. Medicine has been a failure, for therapeutics is built upon superstition.

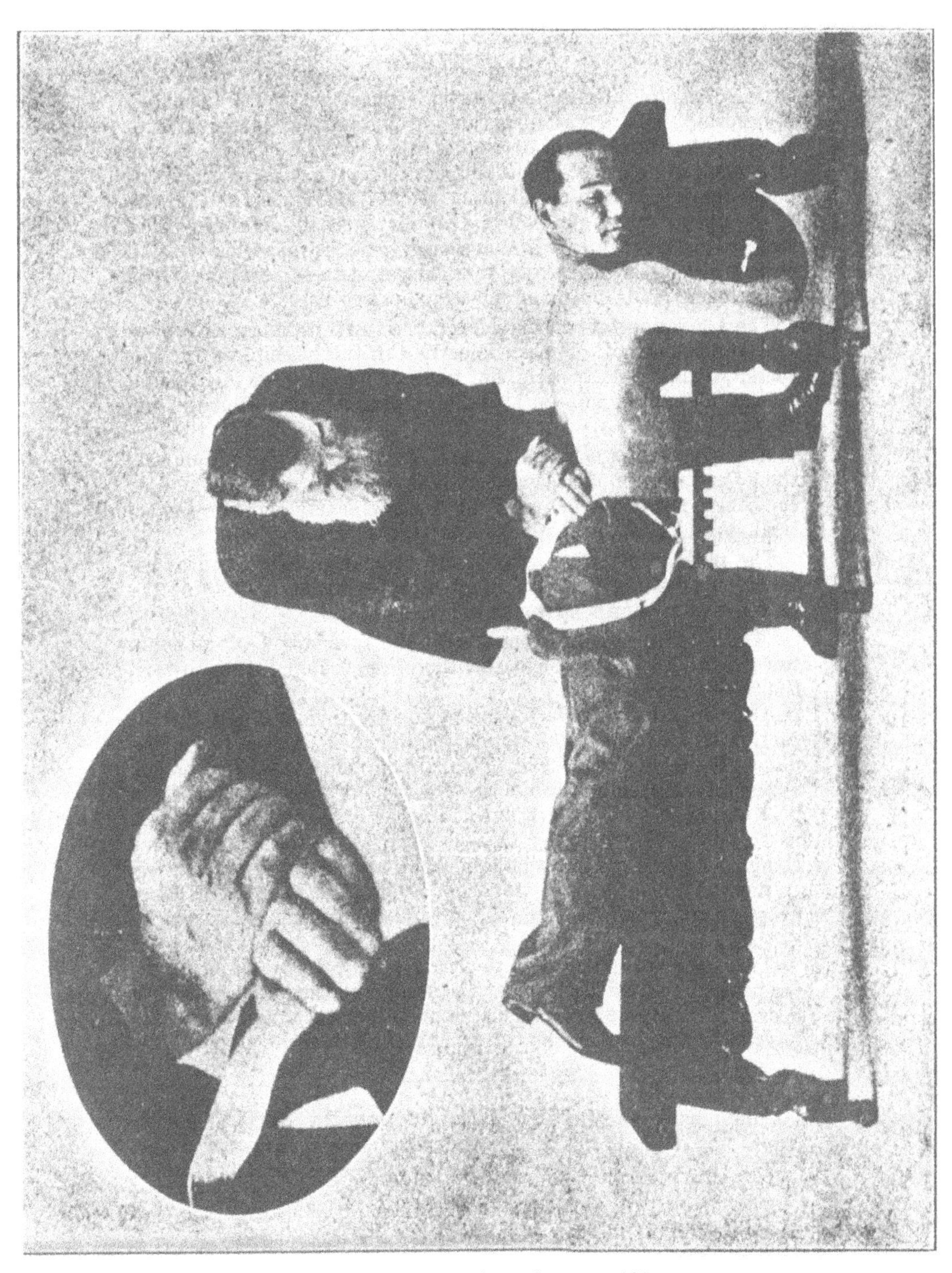

A view of back-setting. See page 908.

## ADJUSTING.

Chiropractic analysis, takes the place of the physician's diagnosis. The art of adjusting is difficult to learn without the personal instruction of a competent teacher. Under my instruction, some get the idea and the knack at once, while a few never learn to make an adjustment. My first instructions are given upon my thighs, while I am in a sitting posture. The first adjustment I ever gave was given chiropractically. All chiropractors look back on that adjustment as being the first adjustment made by using the spinous process.

The Chiropractor should learn to adjust standing on either side of the patient. If this is learned in the beginning, the adjuster will have no trouble, but to one who has always adjusted on one side, that one will find it quite difficult to make the change.

If the vertebra is to be headed, it is immaterial which side the adjuster is on, but where it is to be thrown to one side or the other, the adjuster will find it much easier and more practical to adjust from instead of toward yourself.

The patient should always lie in a prone position and as relaxed as possible, the hands and arms lieing along side of the patient or on thon's buttocks.

The adjuster should stand with the foremost foot pointing toward the head of the patient, the other foot pointing toward the patient.

After locating the vertebrae we desire to move and the direction to be moved, the hands should be placed as shown on pages 899, 903, 907 and 909. The pisiform bone should be placed against the spinous process with sufficient force to hold it in position, then follow with such force as experience has taught us to be capable to move the vertebra as desired. Avoid the common habit of lifting the hand back and forth, up and down, as tho you were trying to get a good swing. I have seen Chiropractors jump up and down several times before giving a thrust.

On page 899 I am represented as giving a dorsal adjustment. On page 903 an adjustment at the second center place, the 12th dorsal. On page 907 an adjustment on a lumbar vertebra. On page 909 as adjusting the 5th lumbar vertebra downward.

---

Compulsory vaccination is upheld only by doctors. They would not do so if the financial interest was withdrawn.

Medical legislation which attempts to decide what particular school of healing is right and which is wrong, is pernicious —worse than wrong.

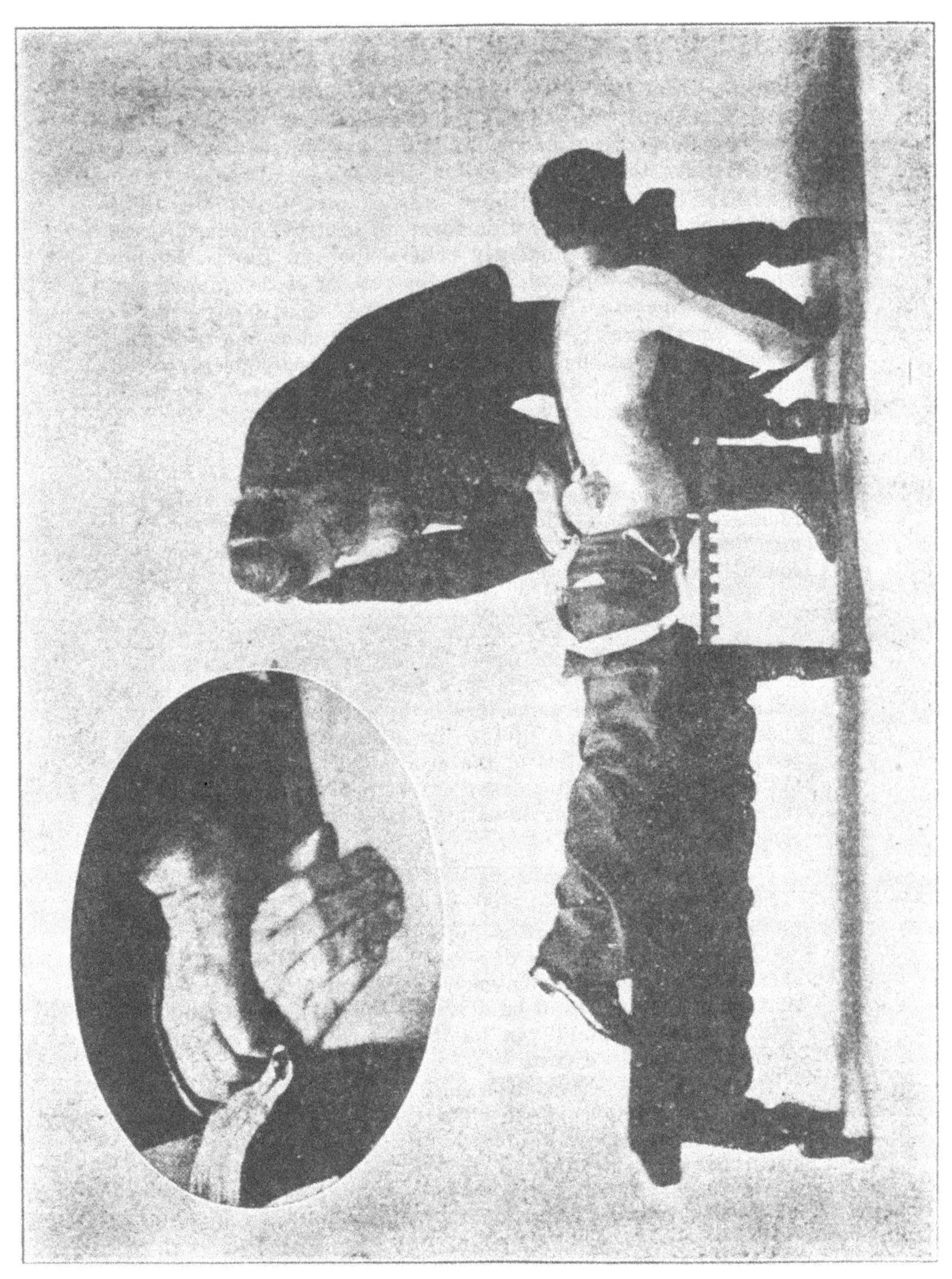

The Jap getting a back-set. See page 908.

## A DOCTOR DENOUNCES APPENDIX CARVERS.

Boston, Oct. 4.—"Operations for appendicitis should be called a criminal operation and as such should be prohibited by law," declares Dr. Charles E. Page, one of the best-known physicians of this city.

"I have been following the records of appendicitis operations ever since the craze for this form of surgery started," says Dr. Page, "and I confidently believe that the day is coming when the people will realize that the cutting of the appendix is a criminal operation.

"As for the widely proclaimed benefits and saving of life by operations to cut the appendix, it seems hardly necessary to cite the long list of deaths following the operation."

---

A conundrum: "Excuse me, I saw your sign 'D. D. Palmer, Founder of Chiropractic.' My brother took a course under the founder of Chiropractic at Davenport, but you are not that man." He could not comprehend how there could be two founders of Chiropractic. An explanation followed.

---

Dr. Copeland, of Ann Arbor, Mich., is reported as saying: "The practice of medicine is a fad, a sport, a chase after scientific facts. The game is won by a careful record of the onset, cause and effects of the disease; by a study of the bacteriological peculiarities of the attack; by a systematic examination of the secretions and excretions and finally, by a radical post mortem examination to confirm the ante-mortem conclusions."

---

Chiropractic education and the adjusting of illiteracy found in Chiropractic literature is the object of this journal. Education is the harmonious development of all our faculties. It continues through life. We may receive much from others, but that which we study out ourselves is the most serviceable.

Chiropractors should put out literature that is becoming—even if it be only a card.

The most derogatory literature is that which is partly copied and partly original. The two kinds do not coalesce; they are incongruous. Some thank us for our friendly criticism. Others as well as the one criticised should be benefited; therefore the Chiropractor Adjuster will continue to adjust all discrepancies we find. We will be pleased to receive Chiropractic literature for inspection.

## PATHOLOGICAL CONDITIONS ALPHABETICALLY ARRANGED.

The following list of diseases is not registered in the index, as it is useless to tabulate them twice.

This book is written upon the same economical plan as that upon which Chiropractic was built, and by the same mind.

In teaching I do not give the number of the vertebra to be adjusted, for several reasons. First, I prefer the student to learn to locate impingements by using Chiropractic principles. Second, while I have given quite a list of illustrative diseases in which the vertebra to be adjusted is mentioned by number, the list is by no means complete. Besides other omissions, it lacks the name and description of about four-fifths of the fevers recognized by pathologists. The new Chiropractic practitioner who wishes to make a great spread by enumerating in a booklet the numerous diseases he treats (adjusts?) can copy this list and then add "and others too numerous to mention."

Third, the practitioner may be called to relieve some pathological condition which I have not mentioned or which is known by some other name than the one given.

Fourth, I have, elsewhere, shown that no two persons are alike either in their osseous, nervous, vascular, muscular or lymphatic makeup. Variations are found so frequently that no definite and reliable rule can be formulated. At times the exception seems to be the rule. For example, headache may be caused by an atlas, 3d cervical, 5th or 12th dorsal subluxation. Therefore there can be no "key" which will unlock all pathological conditions. Although the number of the vertebra usually responsible for each possible pathological condition should be given, cases will arise in which the displaced vertebra will be either one above or below the one mentioned. The practitioner will find it more reliable and expeditious to locate the impingement by the regional method than by the number of the vertebra.

Fifth, regional localization of lesions is specific and educative.

The vertebra herein mentioned as the proper one to be adjusted for each disease given, will be found to be generally reliable, although occasional exceptions will occur. The directions given are based upon the results obtained in a practice of 25 years, beginning in 1885, many of them occurring while practicing magnetic healing. Remember, these adjustments are given for diseases, not for isolated symptoms.

The explanatory remarks that accompany the description of each disease are, of necessity, brief, being only such as seem necessary for instruction. It is presumed that each student or practitioner has an anatomy and dictionary at hand. I advise each reader to make himself or herself familiar with the principles and philosophy of the science so that he or she will be able to make adjustments with accuracy and precision, thereby demonstrating that Chiropractic is a science. Future anatomies will be obliged to designate the origin of functions and point out where pressure may occur to cause impingement upon nerves.

In the following directions the word vertebra is omitted; the reader will understand that it is vertebra, not nerves, that are adjusted, relief being given to the nerves next to, and below, the vertebra adjusted.

**Abscess.**—A localized collection of pus: coagulable lymph due to inflammation. Adjust the vertebra which impinges upon the nerve that reaches the inflamed part. A sensitive, inflamed nerve can be traced, by palpation, from the lesion to the point of its exit from the spinal column. If the offending vertebra is in either the cervical or dorsal region, rack it towards the opposite side; if in the lumbar region, towards the side in which the lesion exists. The 12th dorsal is an exception to this rule; it should be adjusted in the same manner as the lumbar vertebrae. The reason for this difference is given elsewhere. Diseases or abnormal conditions in any part of the body should be adjusted according to this general rule.

**Aching.**—A continuous fixed pain. For a general aching thruout the body, adjust the 6th dorsal.

**Acne**—Pimples: Usually occurring on the face as a result of sexual orgasm induced by friction of the genitals. Adjust the 2d dorsal and advise the patient to cease all lascivious thinking and excitement.

**Acromastitis.**—Inflammation of the nipple. Adjust 3d dorsal.

**Acromegalia.**—Chronic enlargement of the bones and soft parts of the hands, feet and face; also enlarged pituitary body which is attached to the brain by a pedicle. Adjust the 12th dorsal.

**Acromegaly.**—An enlargement of one, two or three extremities; thus one or two toes or fingers may be abnormally enlarged. I have now a patient who, when the 4th dorsal is adjusted in slightly different directions, can feel the sensation in one finger at one time and in a different finger at another time. The reader can see by this that a slightly different pressure on a nerve may affect different nerve fibers of different extremities; a fact not only to be noticed in adjusting, but one also noteworthy on account of its pathological significance.

THE

SCIENCE OF CHIROPRACTIC

---

ITS

PRINCIPLES AND ADJUSTMENTS

by

Dr. D. D. Palmer, Discoverer and Developer of Chiropractic.

and

B. J. Palmer, D. C., Sec., *The P. S. C.*, Davenport, Iowa, U. S. A.

The above is a reproduction of the title page of a book compiled and copyrighted by B. J. Palmer, in 1906. It may be observed that I was given due credit of being the "Discover and Developer of Chiropractic." B. J. is the author of that title page which states that D. D. Palmer and B. J. Palmer were responsible for its make-up and its publication. The contents are nearly all from my pen.

On page 915 I exhibit a copy of the title page of a revised edition of this volume, which contains but little new material. It is dated "1906-1910."

B. J. represents himself therein as being the author of forty of my articles, as being "the fountain head" of all it contains and it was he who performed the many cures mentioned therein; also, it was he who made the discovery that "the body is heat by mental impulse" as given in the first paragraph of which

(Continued on page 915).

**Acroparalysis.**—Paralysis of the extremities. When both arms and legs are debilitated, adjust the 6th dorsal.

**Acroparasthesia.**—Abnormal or perverted sensation in the extremities. Adjust 6th dorsal.

**Actinomycosis.**—A purulent disease of the submaxillary bone. Adjust 4th cervical.

**Addison's Disease.**—Progressive anemia and asthenia ending in death from exhaustion. Adjust 12th dorsal.

**Adipose Tissue, Excessive.**—Adjust 12th dorsal, thereby increasing elimination through the kidneys.

**After-pains.**—Pains after childbirth, caused by the uterus contracting to expel blood-clots. Adjust 1st lumbar.

**Ague.**—See malaria.

**All-gone, Tumble-down Feeling in the Abdomen.**—This sensation is real. The muscles and ligaments are in a relaxed condition; they lack tonicity. Adjust lower dorsal or upper lumbar.

**Allochiria.**—A form of transferred sensation in which an impression in one part of the body is felt in the corresponding part on the other side.

**Alopecia.**—See baldness.

**Alveolar Pyorrhea.**—Receding gums and a purulent discharge at the neck of one or more of the teeth which are usually loose and aching. A result of inflammation. Adjust the 12th dorsal, observing whether one or both kidneys are affected. This can be determined by palpation, following the sensitive nerve from between the 12th dorsal and 1st lumbar to the affected kidney, and adjust accordingly. This fact I learned while I was a magnetic practitioner. Remember that Chiropractic is an outgrowth of the study of magnetic healing.

**Alveolitis.**—Inflammation of the alveolus of a tooth. A suppurative inflammation of the dental nerves which supply the roots of the teeth. Individual teeth may be affected and cause gum boils. Adjust 3d cervical.

**Amaurosis.**—Loss of sight from paralysis or atrophy of the optic nerve or retina. Adjust 4th cervical.

**Amblyopia.**—Dimness of vision. Adjust 4th cervical.

**Amenorrhea.**—Abnormal absence of the menses. Primitive, when they have not appeared at puberty. Secondary, when arrested after they have existed. The absence during the menstrual epoch is pathological; after the menopause and during gestation, physiological.

**Analgesia.**—Insensibility to, or absence of, pain.

**Anasarca.**—An accumulation of serum in the subcutaneous aerolar tissue because of a lack of osmosis.

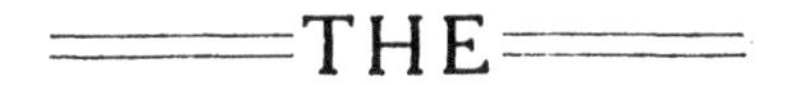


# Science of Chiropractic

—ITS—

## Principles and Philosophies

BY

B. J. PALMER, D. C., Ph. C.

heads my article on page 179 of five lines; then follows my written statement almost verbatim as I wrote it, even mentioning the name of the clinic patient and the date. His statement and mine (which is represented as his) disagreeing materially. All credit is taken unto himself. He has mutilated my writings and misrepresented facts, laying himself liable to the United States courts for a $100 fine for each article of mine appropriated by him, for which see the index for copyright.

On page 917, is a copy of the man and his name whom B. J. said in 1906 was the "discoverer and developer of Chiropractic;" but "the entire book has been torn to pieces. Much has been cut" and mutilated in order to plagarize that which belongs to another. By so doing he has been able to replace principle with principal.

**Anemia.**—A deficiency of blood in a part or the whole of the body. If general, adjust 6th dorsal; if local, adjust accordingly.

**Anesthesia.**—Total or partial loss of sensation. Adjust according to area affected.

**Aneurysm.**—An enlargement produced by rupture or dilatation of the coats of an artery. Venous circulation is obstructed by pressure, preventing the return of arterial blood. Remove the pressure from nerves or veins according to the region obstructed. Remember, there are no two of us formed alike in our vascular makeup; therefore, no set rules can be laid down. See articles on variations of the nervous, vascular, osseous and glandular systems.

**Angina Pectoris.**—A paroxysmal neurosis with intense pain and oppression about the heart, due to inflammation. Adjust 4th cervical.

**Anhidrosis.**—See seborrhea.

**Animal Parasites.**—A parasite, whether internal or external, lives off its host. Scavenger parasites live upon decaying food. Improve digestion by adjusting 5th dorsal, standing on the left and throwing it towards the right shoulder.

**Ankylosis.**—Union of bones forming an articulation, resulting in a stiff joint. It may be cartilaginous, ligamentous, muscular or bony. Chiropractors have to deal with these conditions, more especially in the vertebral column and the toe joints. Daily thrusting against the ankylosed joint will eventually loosen it; a continuation will remove the roughness.

**Anorexia.**—An aversion for food. Adjust the 5th dorsal to the right. Do not forget that the innervating nerves of the stomach emerge on the left of the spinal column and that I was the first person to make such a statement.

**Anosmia.**—Loss, or perversion, of smell. See smell.

**Anthracosis.**—A disease of coal miners. A species of carbuncle on the eyelids and globes of the eye; a carbuncle of any kind; also a chronic disease of the lungs, induced by inhaling coal-dust. Broken-down lung tissue among miners is named black pthisis or coal miners' pthisis. Adjust according to area affected.

**Anthrax.**—See carbuncle.

**Aphasia.**—Partial or complete loss of the use of language by the tongue, ear or pen. Adjust atlas.

**Apoplexy.**—Sudden loss of consciousness and motion. Adjust 6th dorsal.

**Appendicitis.**—Inflammation of the appendix, due to an impingement of the 9th dorsal. Throw the vertebrae towards the right shoulder.

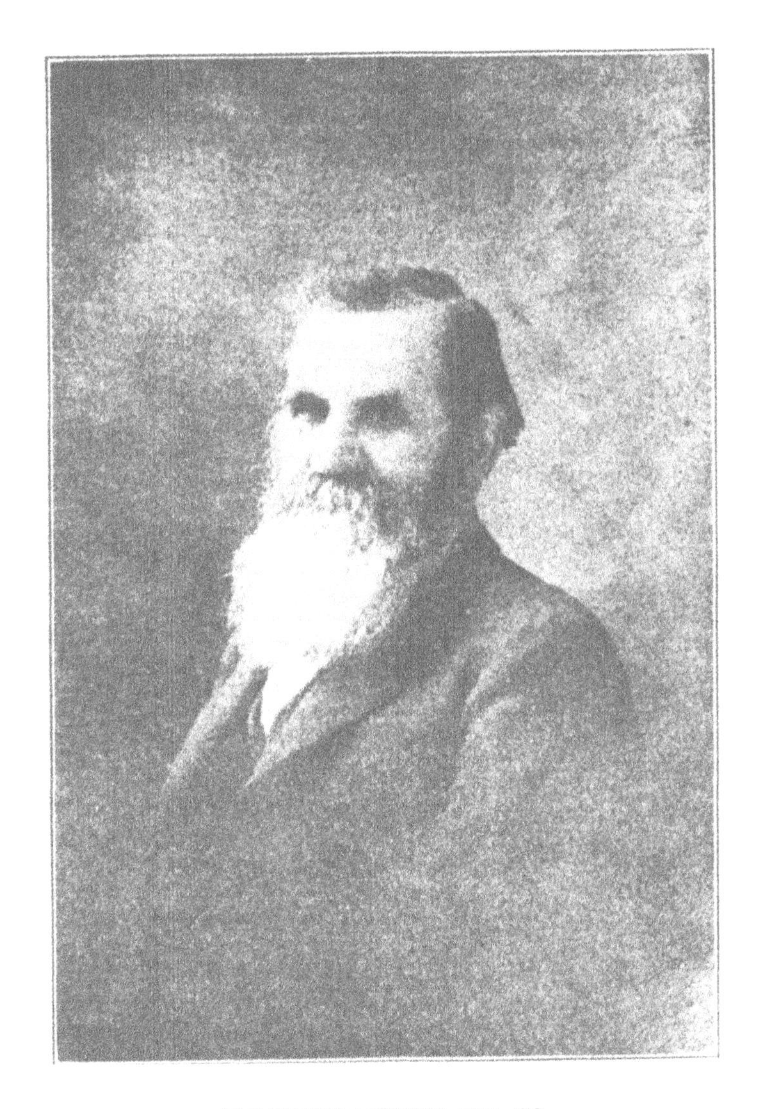

ILLUSTRATION NO. 28.

DR. D. D. PALMER, DISCOVERER AND DEVELOPER OF CHIROPRACTIC.

The above is copied from The Science of Chiropractic, published and copyrighted by B. J. in 1906. It illustrates Dr. D. D. Palmer as the discoverer and developer of Chiropractic.

**Arm, Diseases of.**—Adjust either of 4 lower cervicals or 1st dorsal as may be indicated by palpation.

**Arrest of Development.**—Lack of function. Adjust according to area affected.

**Arteritis Deformans.**—Inflammation of an artery due to atheromatous changes in its walls.

**Arteritis Hyperplastica.**—Inflammation of an artery with new formation of connective tissue.

**Arteritis.**—Inflammation of an artery.

**Arteritis Obliterans.**—Inflammation of an artery leading to obliteration of its calibre by increase of connective tissue.

**Artero-Sclerosis.**—A peculiar change occurring in the small blood vessels thruout the body, consisting of a thickening of the adventitia and intima by a deposit of a hyaline-fibroid material which diminishes the calibre of the vessels, increases the arterial tension, and thus gives rise to the hypertrophy of the heart that is found in this condition.

**Arthralgia.**—Pain in a joint. See gout, arthritis and rheumatism.

**Arthritis.**—See rheumatic arthritis.

**Arthritis Deformans.**—Chronic rheumatic arthritis with resulting deformity from ossification of some parts of the joint and atrophy of others. Excessive heat softens tissue, a subsidence of temperature hardens and ossifies. Thus ankylosis of joints is formed. If general, look to 6th dorsal; if local, remove the pressure according to region.

**Arthropathia.**—Disease of joints. Disseminated, multiple, or insular sclerosis.

**Ascites.**—Dropsy of the abdomen accompanied with scanty urine. Adjust 12th dorsal.

**Assymetry of Face.**—If from congenital wry-neck, see wry-neck.

**Asthma.**—A disease characterized by great difficulty in exhaling. The asthmogenic foci may exist anywhere in the course of the vagus nerve, or the broncho-constrictor fibers of this nerve may lack tone. It is difficult to empty the lungs rather than the filling; the fact is, they are too full of air that has been used. There is a feeling of constriction and suffocation. Because of inflammation, the bronchial membrane is swollen and heavily coated with catarrhal mucous. The bronchial tubes are hypersensitive to fumes, pollen, dust and temperature. Adjust 4th dorsal.

**Atrophy.**—A wasting away or diminution of an organ or part of the body. Look to the area affected and the nerves which ramify the affected part.

**Baldness.**—I have, on two occasions, caused plenty of hair to grow on bald heads, and on two heads have changed gray hair to black by adjusting the 6th dorsal towards the right shoulder.

**Barber's Itch.**—Adjust 5th dorsal.

**Barrenness.**—There may be any one of several causes; chief among them is prolapsus uteri, for which adjust 11th dorsal.

**Bed-Sore.**—A sore produced on any projecting part of the body by prolonged pressure against the bed and by nutritive changes in the paralyzed parts.

**Bell's Paralysis.**—See facial paralysis.

**Bilious Remittent Fever.**—Recognized by vomiting of bile from the stomach. Here are two prominent conditions, fever and the ejection of bile from the duodenum into the stomach. The bile duct is formed by the union of the cystic and hepatic ducts. Jointly it and the duct of the pancreas enter the descending duodenum at from 3 to 4 inches below the pylorus. In this disease there is an inflamed area including the entrance of these two ducts, which wholly or in part closes the orifice. Consequently these juices flow into the stomach. The condition which we name bilious fever—diffused heat—is the result of inflammation—too much heat. Adjust 6th dorsal.

**Blackhead.**—See facial worms.

**Bladder, Diseases of.**—It will be understood that the bladder is a receptacle for the urine; that the quantity and quality is not altogether dependent upon the condition of the bladder. There may be cystitis. Inflammation will cause catarrh of the mucous membrane which lines the internal surface of the bladder or the retention or incontinence of urine. Adjust 1st lumbar.

**Blear Eye.**—Marginal blepharitis. See eyelids, diseases of.

**Bleeder's Disease.**—A popular term for those who are subjects of the hemorrhagic diathesis. See hemophilia.

**Blepharitis Ulcerosa.**—See eyelids, diseases of.

**Boils.**—See furuncle. Local inflammation; necrosis of soft tissue, resulting in purulent secretion. Trace the inflamed, sensitive nerve to the place of its impingement, then adjust to relieve.

**Bones, Variations of.**—As Chiropractors, we account for the change in functional activity of any part or organ by a slight displacement of bone. Is it not a fact that the biostatic relation of size, weight and shape has much to do with functional deviation? Does not the static variation of bones meet with a corresponding change of external form and internal structure? Does not bone variation in shape and structure make a difference in physiological as well as in pathological functional phenomena?

**Brain Fever.**—Excessive heat, here, as elsewhere, softens tissue. Fatty changes take place. Liquefaction, described as white, yellow or red softening, depending upon the amount of blood coloring, occurs in a more or less degree. The brain tissue may soften and become diffluent. Microscopically the softened tissue is seen to consist of more or less fluid, broken down tissue and fragments of nerve fibers. If the patient survives and his temperature becomes subnormal, a process of sclerosis occurs. A branch of each spinal nerve is recurrent, returning thru the intervertebral foramen to innervate the meninges of the spinal cord and brain. Inflammation is too much innervation. By palpation, locate the nerve impinged upon and relieve by adjusting.

**Breast, Diseases of.**—The mammae are liable to suffer from inflammation. They are subject to tumors, carcinoma and sarcoma. A tumor is smooth; a cancer is rough, gnarly, tender and sensitive to the touch. Sensitive nerves can readily be traced from the cancer in the breast to their exit from spine or vice versa. Adjust 4th dorsal.

**Bright's Disease.**—Inflammation of the kidneys. Determine by palpation whether one or both are affected, and adjust, accordingly, at 12th dorsal. See nephritis.

**Bronchitis.**—Inflammation of the bronchial tubes. There is tension—too much tonicity. Adjust 4th dorsal.

**Bronchocele.**—See goitre.

**Bronchorrhea Serosa.**—Serous and purulent expectoration. Adjust at upper thoracic region.

**Bubo.**—An inflamed swelling or tumor in the groin or axilla, usually of venereal origin. Adjust 1st lumbar.

**Bulbar Paralysis.**—A progressive and symmetrical paralysis of the facial muscles about the mouth, including those of the tongue, pharynx and sometimes those of the larynx.

**Bunion.**—An enlargement on the second joint of the big toe, owing to inflammation caused by the displaced bone of the joint pressing on a nerve. Adjust the joint. It may take several adjustments, usually many more than for corns, to afford relief.

**Cachexia.**—Any morbid tendency; depraved nutrition; loss of red corpuscles.

**Calculi, Biliary.**—See gall-stones.

**Calculi, Renal.**—See gravel.

**Calculi, Urinary.**—See gravel.

**Calf of Leg.**—For abscess or cramps, adjust 4th lumbar.

**Camp Fever.**—See typhus fever.

**Cancer.**—For description and location see pathological books. For any kind, interior or exterior, follow sensitive nerves to their origin at the spine and adjust accordingly. Cancers may be absorbed or be decomposed, becoming a liquid inflammatory product. Chiropractors are especially interested in the area they occupy and in localizing the seat of nerve impingements.

**Cancrum Oris.**—See canker.

**Canker of the Mouth.**—Ulceration of the mouth and lips. Adjust 5th dorsal. Throw toward the left shoulder.

**Carbuncle.**—See boils.

**Carcinoma.**—A malignant tumor or cancer. Adjust to correspond to the location.

**Cardialgia.**—See heartburn.

**Carditis.**—See myocarditis.

**Caries.**—Molecular decay; death of bone; disintegration by particles. Caries is usually of the vertebrae and necrosis of the long bones. Adjust according to location.

**Catalepsy.**—Morbid sleep. Adjust atlas to rouse the sleeper.

**Cataract.**—An opacity of the crystalline eye-lens or of its capsule. A white deposit covers the retina. There are many forms. It is a condition caused by a lack of functionating. Stand on the right side and adjust the 6th dorsal toward the left shoulder.

**Catarrh.**—A discharge of mucous from an inflamed mucous membrane. Any hollow organ may become inflamed and its mucous membrane affected with catarrh. A mucous membrane is a delicate layer of tissue which lines all closed cavities of the body. It exudes or secretes certain fluids by a process known as osmosis or dialysis—not circulation. For catarrh of the head look to the cervicals or 6th dorsal; of the throat, 6th dorsal; of the bronchial tubes, 2d dorsal; of the lungs, 3d to 5th dorsal; of the stomach, 5th dorsal; of the bowels, the lower dorsal or upper lumbar; of the bladder, 1st lumbar; of the vagina, 1st lumbar; of the urethra, 1st lumbar.

**Celiac.**—A chronic intestinal disorder in children. The stools are pale, loose, like gruel; bulky, not watery, yeasty, frothy and extremely offensive. It is supposed to be due to a suspension of the pancreatic function.

**Cephalalgia.**—See headache.

**Cephalitis.**—Inflammation of the brain. See brain fever.

**Cephalodynia.**—Rheumatism affecting the occipito-frontanalis muscle, the pain being chiefly experienced in the forehead or occiput, and at all times involving the eyeballs.

**Cerebro-Spinal Meningitis.**—Inflammation of the meninges of the brain or spinal cord. Ascertain which recurrent nerve is impinged upon by palpating close to the exit of the spinal nerves. When you find the recurrent nerve impinged upon, adjust the displaced vertebra next above. This will relieve the pressure from the nerve and allow functions to be performed in a normal manner.

**Change of Life.**—The physiological cessation of menstruation, usually occurring between the forty-fifth and fifty-fifth years. During this period women are liable to many ailments. Adjust according to the region affected, guided by palpation.

**Chicken-breasted.**—A forward projection of the sternum caused by an anterior curvature of the vertebral column or by extreme narrowness of the thorax.

**Chicken Pox.**—A mild form of smallpox. A severe case of chicken pox is smallpox. Adjust 5th cervical for either. I have always been successful in relieving either chicken pox or small pox by one adjustment.

**Child-bed Fever.**—This fever is caused by displacement of an upper lumbar vertebra during child-birth. I have always given relief by one adjustment. In one instance recovery occurred by one adjustment after four physicians had given the patient up.

**Child Crowing.**—Spasm of the glottis. A sudden, partial or complete contraction of the opening.

**Chill.**—A sensation of being cold; an involuntary contraction of the voluntary muscles of the skin. The sensation of being cold, when one has a fever, is deceptive, for the thermometer shows hyperthermia. Adjust the 6th dorsal, unless otherwise indicated.

**Chills and Fever.**—See malaria.

**Chloasma.**—Liver spots; brown patches on the skin; a pigmentation.

**Chlorosis.**—A condition found in adolescent girls from the age of fourteen to twenty-five years, particularly in those who have not menstruated. Adjust 6th dorsal.

**Choking During Deglutition.**—A constriction of the esophagus. Adjust 5th dorsal, throwing vertebra toward left shoulder.

**Cholangitis.**—Obstruction of the bile-duct because of inflammation. See bilious remittent fever.

**Cholera, Asiatic.**—A disease caused by a poison inhaled or taken in the food or drink. The poison affects the nervous system. Adjust 12th dorsal.

**Cholera Infantum.**—A diarrhoea of young children, prevalent in the summer months. Adjust 10th dorsal.

**Cholera Morbus.**—Acute gastro-enteritis with diarrhoea, cramps and vomiting, occurring in summer or autumn. Improper food sets up the inflammation. Remember that an infant's bowels are more sensitive to deleterious food and drink than an adult's. Remember, also that, what may be food for one is poison to another. Adjust 1st or 2d lumbar.

**Chordee.**—Adjust 2d lumbar.

**Chorea.**—When a general affection, adjust 6th dorsal. If local, adjust accordingly.

**Chromatosis.**—See pigmentation.

**Chyle.**—The milk-white fluid absorbed by the lacteals during digestion.

**Chylocele.**—An effusion of chyle into the tunica vaginalis testis.

**Chylorrhea.**—An excessive flow of chyle. Also, a diarrhea characterized by a milky color of the feces.

**Chyluria.**—The passage of milk-colored urine, due to disturbed metabolism.

**Cirrhosis of Liver.**—Degeneration by thickening and atrophy from chronic interstitial inflammation.

**Clap.**—See gonorrhea.

**Clavus.**—See corn.

**Claw-hand.**—A deformity due to contraction of tendons and atrophy of muscles. Muscle contraction, either physiologically or pathologically, is the result of excitation of nerves. If nerves are irritated, over excited, muscles are unduly contracted. If the deformity is of the hands only, adjust 3d cervical and upper thoracic. If of the feet, look to lower lumbar.

**Clubbed Fingers.**—Knobbed deformity of the finger tips, also curvature of the nails. Adjust in upper thoracic.

**Club Foot.**—A deformity of the foot. It is twisted out of normal shape. Adjust 4th lumbar.

**Coccygodinia.**—Pain in the region of the coccyx. This condition is confined, almost exclusively, to women who have given birth to children. Look to the lumbar for the sub-luxation.

**Cold.**—"Catch cold." See coryza.

**Cold Feet.**—Cold, clammy, persistent perspiration of hands and feet denotes kidney trouble. Adjust 12th dorsal.

**Cold in the Head.**—A catarrh of the mucous membrane lining the nasal passages and sinuses, because of inflammation. Adjust 3d cervical.

**Colic.**—An acute pain in the abdomen, at intervals aggravated. Adjust some one of the vertebrae from the 10th dorsal to 2d lumbar; the nerve will be found inflamed and sensitive.

**Colica Hepatica.**—See gall-stone colic.

**Colic, Renal.**—Biliary colic. See calculi.

**Colitis.**—Inflammation of the colon. Adjust 2d lumbar.

**Collapse.**—Extreme depression and prostration from lack of vital force.

**Coma.**—A condition of stupor more than of sleep. A symptom arising in many diseases. A profound sleep symptomatic of brain tissue. Adjust the "hot box"—6th dorsal.

**Comedones.**—See facial worms.

**Compression.**—Impinging on or upon. To encroach or infringe on or upon.

**Concussion.**—A jarring or shaking of an organ.

**Congestion.**—A result of hyperthermia. Congestion may be active, atonic or inflammatory; functional or hypostatic. Disease is either too much or too little functional activity.

**Conjunctivitis.**—See granular eyelids.

**Consumption.**—A wasting disease of the lungs or bowels. Adjust accordingly.

**Convulsions.**—Where to adjust will depend largely upon the cause. If it be from poisons taken into the stomach, adjust 5th dorsal, standing on the left side of patient and throw it toward the right shoulder, as the nerve of innervation for the stomach emerges from the left of the spine.

**Corneitis.**—See keratitis.

**Corns.**—Small hard tumors on feet or toes. Nerves are impinged upon. Remove the pressure by adjusting the displaced bones of the joint. Examine carefully to see which way to adjust the displaced bone.

**Corpulence.**—See obesity.

**Corrosive Sublimate, Poisoning by.**—I have had only one case. The poison was taken with suicidal intent. I adjusted the patient, in the presence of the class, on two different days. The sublimate was taken on three different days, the last being fatal, as I was away. Relief in the first two instances was given instantly. I adjusted the 5th dorsal, throwing it headward, as throat and stomach were both affected.

**Coryza.**—See cold in the head.

**Costiveness.**—A condition in which the stool is dry and hard, lacking the proper amount of liquid. The kidneys are too active, absorbing more than their normal quantity of liquid, thereby depriving the stool tract of the amount due it. Adjust 12th dorsal.

**Cough.**—A sudden noisy expulsion of air from the lungs, produced by an irritation of the throat, bronchial tubes or lungs. It may also arise from a condition of the stomach or spleen. That from the spleen will be recognized by its dryness and unsatisfactory effect. Adjust according to the organ affected.

**Cow Pox.**—See vaccina.

**Coxalgia.**—Hip disease. Adjust lower lumbar.

**Coxitis.**—See coxalgia.

**Cramps, Muscular.**—Spasmodic contraction of muscles. For cramping of the arms, adjust 1st to 3d dorsal; diaphragm, 7th dorsal; of the bowels, one of the last two dorsal or the first two lumbar; of the lower extremities, the 4th lumbar. See spasm.

**Craniomalacia.**—An atrophy of the cranial bones, occurring in infancy, with small conical pits in the bone-substance.

**Craniotabes.**—See craniomalacia.

**Cretinism.**—Premature ossification of the bones, stunted growth, marked deformity thruout more especially noticeable in the head and face; idiocy and mental dullness; dwarfish deformity of the head and body. Adjust 6th dorsal.

**Crossed Hemiplegia.**—See Hemiplegia crossed.

**Cross-eye.**—Lack of co-ordination of the visual axis. Adjust 4th dorsal.

**Croup.**—A disease of childhood. Inflammation of the mucous membrane of the larynx and trachea, which diminishes the caliber of the air passages. Adjust the 5th dorsal toward the left shoulder.

**Curvature, Spinal.**—For kyphosis, lordosis and scoliosis adjust 12th dorsal. See article on rachitis.

**Cyanoses.**—Blueness. Lividity from plethora of the venous system.

**Cystitis.**—Inflammation of the bladder, shown by heat, swelling and painful discharge of urine, tenesmus being present. See bladder.

**Dactylitis.**—Inflammation of a finger or toe. Adjust, for the former, the 4th dorsal, and the latter, the 4th lumbar.

**Dandruff.**—The scurf or scales found upon the scalp in seborrhea, a result of too much heat. Adjust for local inflammation.

**Deafness.**—Catarrh does not cause deafness any more than deafness causes catarrh; they are two different effects from the same impingement. Either of these diseases (deafness and catarrh) may be present without the other. Attributing one disease as the cause of another is an allopathic conception. When deafness is a sequel of measles, adjust the 5th dorsal. When there is a ringing and other noises in the head, look to the atlas; for other causes, examine the cervicals. The first case of deafness ever relieved by the scientific method now known as Chiropractic, has never been equaled. Those who call it "crude Chiropractic" have never done as well. Harvey Lillard, so deaf for 17 years, that he could not hear a watch tick, was relieved nearly 15 years ago. His hearing was restored by two adjustments. That was as scientific as any pseudo "fountain head" can do after years of practice. Only one vertebra was adjusted, the spinous process being used as a lever. The book which "gives the location of the cause of all possible combinations of functions to coincide with all complexed effects," says of deafness, "Nervous, from hardened ear wax."

**Delirium.**—A disturbance of the cerebral functions, characterized by hallucinations; an incoherence of speech and a staggering gait.

**Dengue.**—An acute epidemic fever with pain in the bones, joints and muscles and, at times, a cutaneous eruption. When the conditions are generally distributed over the body, look to 6th dorsal, center place. Adjust the vertebra towards the head. By so doing the pair of nerves emerging at its inferior surface are freed.

**Dental Tophus.**—A collection of hard calcareous matter which forms at the roots of the teeth. Adjust 12th dorsal.

**Dermatitis.**—An inflammation of the skin. The skin is supplied with numerous nerves, the number varying in different parts of the body. Adjust according to area affected.

**Diabetes Mellitus and Diabetes Insipidus.**—Disease is produced and maintained by either excessive or insufficient functional activity. In diabetes and Bright's disease we have two pathological extremes. In the former the amount of urine passed is too copious; in the latter it is too scanty. In diabetis mellitus the urine is saturated, freely, with sugar, and in diabetes insipidus sugar is entirely lacking. Do not forget that the bladder is a receptacle for the urine; that the kidneys secrete what has already transuded (not circulated) thru the system and ready to be thrown out as waste. The kidneys are not responsible for the quantity nor the quality of fluid received. The organs and membranes thru which the serum, chyle and lymph transude should have a normal temperature of 98 to 99 degrees for the proper performance of the function of osmosis. The liver, pancreas, spleen, the intervening membranes and glands are directly concerned in dialysis. When two miscible liquids or solutions are brot into contact a diffusion occurs, the movements of the molecules finally effecting a homogenous mixture. Diffusion of this kind thru a membrane is referred to as dialysis or osmosis. It is not circulation. Urine is the escaped waste that has served its usefulness and is ready to be excreted by this process of osmosis. If dialysis is normally performed the urine is of natural color and composition. Under pathological conditions the composition is modified as seen in diabetes insipidus and diabetes mellitus.

In diabetes of both forms we find an excessive flow of urine, robbing the stool tract of its normal amount of liquid. As a result the stool is dry and hard. Because of abnormal metabolism the urine is heavily saturated with sugar, or entirely free from it and clear as water. In diabetes mellitus we have several conditions due to superheat, viz., drowsiness and coma, boils, caries of the teeth, meningitis, congestion of the brain, enteritis, enlarged liver, and dry, harsh skin. A great variety of lesions, caused by excessive heat, are found after death. These are summed up as faulty metabolism, the result of a superabundant amount of heat, and all of these conditions occur because of an impingement on the sixth pair of nerves which can be relieved by adjusting the 6th dorsal vertebra.

This is a lengthy dissertation to be included in a brief reference to diseased conditions, abnormal functions and morbid tissue, but my pen refused to stop until the thot was fully expressed.

**Diaphragmitis.**—Inflammation of the diaphragm. Adjust 4th dorsal.

**Diarrhea.**—Abnormal frequency and liquidity of fecal discharges. These evacuations may be physiological for the purpose of freeing the body from some poisonous food or drug. Inflammation, excessive heat, may cause a diarrhea which is pathologic. Adjust 2d lumbar with such modifications as are indicated.

**Diffuse Inflammation.**—Fever is but diffused inflammation. Inflammation, spread out, produces different effects from that of localized inflammation. One of the earliest effects of inflammation is an increased exudation of fluid from the vascular vessels. The more severe the inflammation, the more nearly does the fluid approach blood plasma in its composition and tendencies, while, when less severe, it is more like the serous fluid exuded in artificial hyperemia. The tissues of an inflamed part are softer than natural and watery looking. In either case, the component elements are blurred or altogether undistinguishable.

**Dilatation of Stomach.**—See gastritis.

**Dilation of the Heart.**—See aneurism.

**Diphtheria.**—A throat affection caused by a 5th dorsal vertebral impingement against the nerve which innervates the throat. A similar impingement upon this nerve, in early childhood, produces symptoms called croup; in adult life, it is the cause of conditions recognized as bronchitis and quinsy. These different results are due to changes in the structure of the nerve which gradually take place with advancing years. Adjust 5th dorsal for any of these throat affections, standing on the right side and throwing the vertebra in the direction of the left shoulder.

**Dipsomania.**—An uncontrollable desire for spirituous liquors which can be relieved by adjusting the 5th dorsal toward the left shoulder. I have seen some wonderful effects follow a few adjustments.

**Diseases of the Hip-Joint, Knee, Ankle or Foot.**—As a rule adjust the 1st lumbar for hip, 2d for knee, 3d for ankle and the 4th for the foot.

**Dislocation.**—A permanent, abnormal, total or partial displacement from each other of the articular portions of the bones entering into the formation of a joint. Usually a dislocation is traumatic, the result of external violence. When the bones forming a joint are gradually displaced—drawn out of their normal position by nerve tension—the displacement is called a pathological or spontaneous dislocation.

**Dizziness.**—See vertigo.

**Dropsy.**—A writer states "Liquid food (serum) is also absorbed, but by a distinctly separate and complete serous circulation. This is as thoro, as to starting and ending, as the arterial or venous circulation."

"Complete serous circulation." The serum does not circulate; it starts and ends, but does not circulate, does not make a circuit. There is an arterial and venous circulation, but it takes the arteries and veins to make the circuit. The arteries carry the blood outward and the veins inward, but, there are no return channels for the serum. Consequently, there is no circulation of the serum. Chyle, lymph and serum do not circulate, they transude. Serum is produced by osmosis and transudes thru membranes. When transudation is lacking, there is stasis, a condition producing dropsy. Always adjust the 12th dorsal and no other, regardless of the location of the dropsy. Dropsy is water dropped—not excreted.

**Dumbness.**—See stammering.

**Duodenitis.**—Inflammation of the duodenum. Adjust the 12th dorsal, standing on the right side and adjust toward the left shoulder.

**Duodenocholangitis.**—Inflammation of the duodenum and common bile-duct. Inflammation in this region causes the bile to flow into the stomach. Adjust 7th dorsal.

**Dysacousia.**—See deafness.

**Dysentery.**—Mucous, bloody stools from ulceration; inflammation of large intestine and lower ilium. Adjust 2d lumbar.

**Dysmenorrhea.**—Painful menstruation, usually caused by prolapsus uteri. Adjust 2d lumbar.

**Dyspepsia.**—Impairment of the power or the function of digestion. Quite a share of dyspeptics are made so thru fear and humoring; or rather by Educated mind trying to direct Innate concerning a function of which Educated knows but little. Innate knows a thousand times more in regard to digestion than Educated will ever know. Educated has been misguided, but Innate never. If there is something wrong, if the nerves of innervation are impinged upon, why not adjust the 5th dorsal, standing on the left side and throwing it towards the right shoulder?

**Dysphagia.**—Difficulty of swallowing. Adjust 5th dorsal, standing on the right side and adjust to the left.

**Dysphonia.**—A condition of defective voice, hoarseness. Adjust 5th cervical.

**Dyspnea.**—Difficulty, labored breathing. See asthma.

**Dystrophy.**—Imperfect or faulty nourishment.

**Earache.**—Pain in the ear. Adjust 4th cervical.

**Ear Roaring.**—Adjust atlas.

**Ear Wax.**—Hardening of, because of overheat. Adjust 4th cervical.

**Ectropion.**—A turning out of the eyelid. May depend on an ulcer or relaxation of the conjunctiva. Adjust 12th dorsal.

**Eczema.**—Many affections of divers character are grouped under this term. Moist tetter, running scall, with more or less inflammation, appear on various parts of the body. There is often burning or itching. If general, look to center place, the 6th dorsal.

**Edeitis.**—Inflammation of the genital organs. Adjust 1st or 2d lumbar.

**Edema.**—A swelling due to effusion of watery liquid (serum) into connective tissue.

**Edematous.**—See edema.

**Elephantiasis.**—A chronic disease characterized by inflammation and obstruction of the cutaneous and subcutaneous tissues. The legs and external genitals are principally affected. Adjust one of the lumbar.

**Emesis.**—See vomiting.

**Empyema.**—Suppuration in the pleural cavity. Adjust the 3d, 4th or 5th dorsal.

**Emphysema.**—Wind dropsy. Term applied to any tumor filled with air.

**Encephalitis.**—See brain fever.

**Encephalomalacia.**—Softening of the brain; mollities cerebri.

**Encephalomyelitis.**—Encephalitis combined with myelitis, which see.

**Encephalopathy.**—Any disease or symptom of disease referable to disorders of the brain.

**ndarteritis.**—See endoarteritis.

**Endoarteritis.**—Inflammation of the intima, the inner coat of an artery.

**Endocarditis.**—Inflammation of the endocardium, the lining membrane of the heart, usually associated with rheumatism. Adjust 4th dorsal.

**Enteralgia.**—Pain or neuralgia of the intestine. Adjust one of the vertebra from the 7th dorsal to the 2d lumbar.

**Enteritis.**—Inflammation of the bowels. By palpation find the nerve impinged on, between the 10th dorsal and 2d lumbar.

**Enteroptosis.**—A falling down of the bowel from a relaxed condition or decreased tension of the walls of the abdomen.

**Eonosus.**—See morning sickness.

**Eontiasis.**—A bilateral and symmetric hypertrophy of the bones of the face and skull, leading to a lion-like facial expression.

**Epilepsy.**—As a rule adjust atlas. I have found but one exception, and in that case the impingement was at the 6th dorsal, the fibers reaching the brain by way of the ganglionic chain.

**Epiphora.**—See weeping.

**Epiphyseitis.**—Inflammation of an epiphysis or that portion of a bone.

**Epistaxis.**—See nosebleed.

**Epithelioma.**—A malignant tumor of the skin and mucous membrane caused by too much nutritive functioning. Adjust the vertebra impinging upon the nerve which supplies that locality.

**Equinia.**—See glanders.

**Eruption of Teeth.**—See teething.

**Eruptions.**—See eruptive diseases.

**Erysipelas.**—A febrile disease with redness and inflammation of the skin, oftener of the face than elsewhere. It is, as in many cases of fevers, ushered in with a chill, high temperature and a well-defined rash. It is usually associated with other diseases.

**Esophagitis.**—An acute inflammation affecting either the mucous membrane or submucous tissue of the esophagus, or both.

**Ethmoiditis.**—Inflammation of the ethmoid bone, or of the ethmoid sinuses.

**Exanthema.**—See eruptions.

**Exarteritis.**—See exoarteritis.

**Exoarteritis.**—Inflammation of the outer coat of an artery.

**Exophthalmic Goitre.**—Protrusion of the eyeballs accompanied with goitre. The action of the heart is usually violent, giving the patient the sensation of constant palpitation. At times the action of the heart is much increased in force and frequency. Adjust the 5th dorsal, standing on the right side, and throwing the vertebra towards the left shoulder.

**Exostosis.**—A bony growth on the surface of bone. There are physiological and pathological growths of bone. This distinction was made by me years before there was a graduate of Chiropractic. Innate builds osseous growths for the purpose of repair or to prevent further displacement of osseous tissue. A close observer will frequently find in the spinal canal and on the external surface of vertebrae and other bones, intelligently constructed bony abutments and piers designed for special purposes. These are physiological, built with a design and an aim in view. Pathological bone defects include disintegration and growth, necrosis, caries, sarcoma, osteoma, osteosarcoma, osteosarcosis, osteocephaloma and cystosarcoma.

**Eyeball, Involuntary Spasmodic Motion of.**—Pathological lateral vibration. The eyeball vibrates from one side to the other. Adjust 3d cervical.

**Eye, Diseases of.**—The eye does not include the eyelids, nor the eyebrows; only the eyeball. For inflammation or cataract, adjust the 6th dorsal. Throw it toward the left shoulder.

**Eyelids, Diseases of.**—For stys, blear eyes and granulated eyelids, adjust the 12th dorsal.

**Eyelids, Drooping.**—See ptosis palpebra.

**Eyelids Tumefied**—See granular eyelids.

**Facial Hemiatrophy.**—A wasting of the bones and subcutaneous tissue of one-half of the face.

**Facial Hemihypertrophy.**—One-half of the face normal, the other gigantic in growth. Adjust 3d cervical.

**Facial Paralysis.**—Peripheral paralysis of the facial nerve, or more correctly speaking, of some of its fibers, which are impinged upon by a displaced 3d cervical.

**Facial Worms.**—A minute cylinder of inspissated sebum with a blackened tip occupying the sebaceous follicles of the face.

**Fainting.**—A swoon. A sudden failure of heart action, with pallor, coldness of the skin, muscular relaxation and unconsciousness. Adjust 6th dorsal.

**Feet.**—Cold, clammy, sweat. See hands.

**Felon.**—An abscess in the cellular tissue in or around the terminal phalanx of the finger. It may be superficial and confined to the structures about the nails, or deep-seated. In the latter case the periosteum and bone are affected and there is pain, necrosis and metabolic disturbances.

**Female Weakness.**—A condition depending upon atony; usually a prolapsed condition of the generative organs. See all-gone feeling.

**Fever.**—A general elevation of temperature. Adjust 6th thoracic. There are about 100 kinds of fever recognized by pathologists. Age and various conditions cause the difference in symptoms.

Inflammation is produced by traumatic displacement of osseous tissue, wounds or poison. The amount of fever always corresponds to the amount of local inflammation. Fever is diffused inflammation. Displaced osseous tissue impinges on nerves thereby exciting them to greater activity. Poisons excite and irritate nerves which, in turn, cause muscles to contract, drawing vertebra out of alignment. Fevers of the kind mentioned are the result of pathological conditions, since they are caused by the performance of functions in a degree greater than normal. The rise of temperature during the uniting of wounds of osseous tissue is physiological. It is called into existence to make conditions favorable for the creation of callous tissue for fusing the fractured parts. The physiological rise in temperature, even to 102 degrees—a febrile condition—does not cause the patient to suffer from malaise or rarely to become conscious of feeling ill. This physiological rise in temperature is not to be confounded with either pathological or suppurative fever.

The rise of bodily temperature, because of traumatism or poisons, is degenerative; while that from a physiological change is regenerative. In pathologic fever, all the functions of the body are more or less deranged; the tissues of both the osseous and soft parts suffer from morbid processes.

**Fibroid Tumor.**—A tumor composed of fibers. Tumors cause but little inflammation. Their growth is slow. The area affected will determine the location of the vertebra to adjust.

**Fibroma.**—See fibroid.

**Film of Eye.**—See pterygium.

**Fissure, Anal.**—A linear ulcer at the muco-cutaneous junction of the anus and rectum. It causes intense suffering at the time of evacuation. It is caused by inflammation. Adjust the 4th lumbar.

**Fistula.**—An abscess tube which transmits fluid-pus secretions or contents of some organ or body cavity. Make yourself acquainted with regional anatomy.

**Floating Kidney.**—One that is displaced from its normal position, because of a lack of tonicity in its supporting tissue.

**Floating Liver.**—One with abnormal mobility. To restore normal tonicity, adjust 7th dorsal.

**Flux.**—See dysentery.

**Focal Inflammation.**—Inflammation is always focalized; the lesion is definitely circumscribed. Local inflammation, localized excessive heat, diffused to other organs, causes abnormal functions in them also. It is not necessary to adjust for each organ ailing. Adjust the displaced vertebra which caused (not the general fever) but the local lesion.

**Fracture.**—The length of time required for the healing of fractured bones is about two weeks for a broken phalanx, three for a broken rib, five for a forearm, six for the upper arm, seven for the tibia, ten for the thigh, and twelve for the neck of the femur. Healing is more rapid in children and well persons than in those who are weak or advanced in years.

**Fragilitas Ossium.**—Brittleness of the bones, friability in certain diseases. The cause is excessive heat. If the whole body is affected, adjust 6th dorsal; if the affection is local, adjust according to the locality.

**Funnel Chest.**—A peculiar deformity of the chest; usually congenital, the sternum often resting against the vertebral column.

**Furuncle.**—See boil.

**Furunculosis.**—A diseased condition favoring a crop of boils. Locate the nerve which covers that area, trace it to its origin at the spine and adjust.

**Gall Stone Colic.**—Severe abdominal pain caused by the passage of gall-stones through the gall-duct.

**Gall Stones.**—A calculus in the gall bladder. Adjust 7th dorsal.

**Gangrene.**—Local death of a part. When the lifeless part has become black, with no feeling or circulation in it, mortification has set in. Adjust the patient into the hands of another practitioner.

**Gastralgia.**—Pain in the stomach. See cardialgia.

**Gastric Ulcers.**—Ulcers of the stomach, caused by exposure of such parts of its walls as have been deprived of their mucous coating to the gastric juice. Behind all is an inflammatory condition, known as catarrh, which thickens the mucous of the stomach. The loosening of this coating is the cause of the exposure. The pathogenesis of these ulcers has occasioned much dispute among pathologists. Their differences are explained and harmonized by the basic physiologic law, we so often see illustrated, namely, that abnormal functionating and morbid tissue are inseparable conditions that always result from continued excessive heat. To adjust for gastric ulcers, is to adjust for catarrh of the stomach. Adjusting for gastritis will relieve all conditions named. Adjust the 5th dorsal, standing on the left side, for the nerves of stomach innervation emerge from the spinal column on the left. Throw the vertebra toward the right shoulder.

**Gastritis.**—Inflammation of the stomach. It may be acute or chronic, catarrhal, suppurative, plegmonous, or diptheric.

It may be acute gastric inflammation due to the ingestion of poisonous or corrosive substances. Either of the above conditions act on nerves and they in turn on muscles which draw vertebrae out of alignment. The replacing of the 5th dorsal has a remarkable effect of ameliorating the toxic effects. if from poisons, likewise, if from traumatism. Stand on the left side and adjust toward the right shoulder.

**Gastroduodenitis.**—Inflammation of the stomach and duodenum. Adjust 5th dorsal.

**Gastrodynia.**—Pain in the stomach. Adjust 5th dorsal.

**Gastro-enteritis.**—Inflammation of stomach and bowel. Adjust 5th dorsal.

**Gastromalacia.**—Softening of the mucous membrane of the stomach from inflammation.

**Gastroptosis.**—Abnormal downward displacement or sagging of the stomach.

**Genital Organs, Diseases of.**—"Functional or organic derangement." There can be no organic derangement without functional interference. Abnormal functionating, whether excessive or insufficient, constitutes disease; morbid tissue is the result. "Organic derangement" does not imply a morbidity of tissue, a change of structure, altho such may have been intended by the author. Adjust 2d lumbar.

**Gibbosity.**—Angular deformity.

**Gigantism.**—Abnormal overgrowth; excessive size of the whole body; monstrous size and stature. Excessive growth may begin in intra-uterine life. It is the result of an inflamed pituitary body whose function is to secure two substances, a compresser and a depresser, which respectively increases and diminishes the blood pressure. In some diseases the pituitary body undergoes pathological change; in acromegaly it has been found very much enlarged. Where are the fibers which proceed from within the spine and eventually reach the pituitary gland within the cranium?

**Glanders.**—An infectious disease of equine origin.

**Gleet.**—Gleet is a chronic condition, the result of gonorrhea. All chronic stages of any disease follow the acute. Diseases are easily relieved by the Chiropractor while in the acute stage. Gleet is a slight, purulent discharge, not infectious. Adjust 2d lumbar.

**Glossitis.**—Inflammation of the tongue. Adjust 5th dorsal standing on the right side.

**Glossoplegia.**—Paralysis of the tongue, due to injury of, or pressure on, the hypoglossal nerve.

**Glycosuria.**—The presence of grape sugar in the urine. See chyluria.

**Goitre.**—Enlargement of Thyroid Gland. Adjust the 5th dorsal, standing on the right and throwing to left shoulder. Remember, all diseases of the throat are because of injury to the 5th thoracic nerve, on the right side of the spine.

**Gonorrhea.**—A specific inflammation accompanied by a discharge of mucous and pus from the membranes of the urethra in man or woman. The catarrhal discharge is poisonous. It may enter other cavities and affect their membranes. It is credited with producing prostatitis, cystitis, arthritis and salpingitis. I have been successful in adjusting for gonorrhea and gleet. Adjust 2d lumbar.

**Gout.**—One writer says: "If you restore to the patient who suffers with gout normal nerve supply to the stomach and the digestive and eliminative organs, you will remove the condition that permits the diseased condition. Adjustments—The first, fifth and tenth thoracic and fifth lumbar vertebrae."

There is no need of restoring that of which the patient has already too much—energy, heat, nerve supply. I will wager a copy of my book against one of the author of the above quotation, that he has never successfully adjusted a case of gout. I have just relieved a bad case in the big toe by adjusting the 3d lumbar only. There was an impingement upon the lumbar nerve and nowhere else, **why adjust four vertebrae?** Why restrict the patient's diet or drink?

**Granular Eyelids.**—Small, sago-like, inflamed elevations upon the inner surface of the eyelids which causes friction when moving them. Adjust the 12th dorsal, as fibers go from this region to the eyelids.

**Granuloma Fungoides.**—See Mycosis.

**Gravel.**—Urinary calculi, often passed with the urine in the form of granular, sand-like detritus. Adjust 12th dorsal, as the wrong doing is in the kidneys.

**Grave's Disease.**—See exophthalmic goitre.

**Green Sickness.**—See Chlorosis.

**Grippe.**—See influenza.

**Gum Boil.**—Abscess of a gum, caused by inflammation of the maxillary nerve which supplies the roots of the teeth. The abscess burrows an opening thru the alveolar process and lodges the pus under the gum. Adjust 3d cervical to relieve the inflammation.

**Gums, Bleeding.**—Gums bleed because they are inflamed. The blood-vessel walls are softened by excessive heat which allows the blood to ooze thru them.

**Gums, Ulcerated.**—See alveolar pyorrhea.

**Haematuria.**—Blood in the urine; the hemorrhage may be of the kidneys, ureters, bladder, prostate or urethra. If pathologic, not traumatic from poison, but inflammatory, adjust 12th dorsal or 1st lumbar.

**Habit Spasm.**—An acquired movement.

**Hallucination.**—A false sense perception; it is the apprehension of an object or phenomena which exists only in the imagination. These false perceptions of sight, sound, smell, taste or touch have no corresponding external cause, yet they are real to the one deluded. Adjust the atlas to restore normal tonicity, not circulation: this is a nerve disorder, not one of the blood. The impulses and blood will be transmitted in normal amount and manner if the temperature is normal.

**Hands, Sweaty and Clammy.**—Such a condition indicates an abnormal action of the kidneys. Adjust 12th dorsal.

**Hay Asthma.**—See hay fever.

**Hay Fever.**—The main symptoms are periodic attacks of coryza, sneezing, headache, cough and asthma. It is caused by a supersensitive condition of the nasal passages and bronchial tubes. The olfactory nerves are the special nerves of the sense and smell. Each nasal passage is supplied with one nerve which ends in a bulb at the upper end of the nasal concha. From this emerges about twenty branches which form a plexus on the mucous membrane; these are the nerves of sensation. Now, do not forget for one moment, that disease is either too much or not enough functionating. In hay fever, or hay cold, as it is sometimes called, this plexus of the mucous membrane is over-sensitive—over functionating. Adjust the 4th cervical and 4th dorsal as this is a combination of rhinitis and asthma, which see.

**Headache.**—Cephalalgia may be from displacement of atlas, 3d cervical, 5th or 12th dorsal. If in doubt, palpate for sensitive, swollen nerves.

**Heartburn.**—Cardialgia, a burning sensation in the esophagus. Adjust 5th dorsal toward the right shoulder.

**Heat Stroke.**—See sunstroke.

**Hematomyelitis.**—An acute myelitis attended with an effusion of blood into the spinal cord. The inflammation softens the walls of the blood vessels, permitting the blood to seep thru the three coats which compose its walls.

**Hematuria.**—The presence of blood in the urine.

**Hemichorea.**—A form of chorea in which the convulsive movements are confined to one side of the body. The sympathetic, ganglionated chain, the great distributing agency, is only affected in its lateral half.

**Hemicrania.**—Pain confined to one-half of the head; usually intermittent; it may be periodical, one day in the week, or daily, as long as the sun is above the horizon; hence called sun pain.

**Hemiglossitis.**—Inflammation of one-half of the tongue.

**Hemiparaplegia.**—Paralysis of one-half of the lower extremities. Adjust in the lumbar, standing on the well side and adjusting toward the shoulder of the side affected. In the lumbar the axial center is on the line of the articulating processes; whereas, in the dorsal and cervical, it is anterior to the bodies; therefore, the difference of direction in adjusting.

**Hemiplegia.**—Paralysis of one side of the body. Adjust 6th dorsal, standing on the side affected and throw the vertebra toward the opposite shoulder.

**Hemitaxia.**—Lack of ability to co-ordinate the movements of one side of the body.

**Hemitis.**—A certain pathological condition of the blood associated with inflammation. Excess of heat modifies the constituent elements of the fluids of the body.

**Hemophilia.**—An abnormal tendency to spontaneous bleedings and efusions of blood into joints. Where hemorrhages occur, there will be found softening of the blood-vessels from hyperthermia.

**Hemoptysis.**—The spitting of blood; if from the lungs, it is frothy and bright red.

**Hemorrhage.**—Pathological hemorrhage is an escape of blood from vessels because of softening of their walls. Do not forget that blood vessels are covered with a network of nerves; that these may become inflamed, necrosed, softened with hemorrhage—a leakage or exudation—as a result.

**Hemorrhage in Disease.**—Nearly all diseases are of inflammatory origin from the nervous system coming in contact either with poisons or osseous tissue. Therefore, it is not surprising that blood-vessels should discharge their contents thru walls which have been softened and necrosed by inflammations.

**Hemorrhoids.**—An enlarged and varicosed condition of the vessels in the tissues around the anus. The rectum may be piled internally or there may be an eversion of the rectal mucous membrane. Hemorrhoids are caused by an inflamed condition of the rectum and a lack of tonicity in the superior tissue.

**Hepatitis.**—The liver, like other organs inflamed, becomes congested. To relieve the excited, inflamed condition, adjust the 4th dorsal on the right.

**Heredity.**—A law by which structure, mental and physical characteristics and diseases are more or less transmitted from progenitors.

**Hernia.**—A protrusion of a viscus thru an abnormal opening in the wall of the cavity in which it is lodged. Hernia is the result of a lack of tone in the supporting tissue. Locate the impingement causing the pressure and relieve it by adjusting. Inguinal, scrotal, umbilical and femoral are the most common. Adjust according to the area whose supports are weakened.

**Herpes.**—An acute, inflammatory affection of the skin, attended with rigors and fever. The skin or mucous membrane is inflamed in patches and covered with groups of vessicles. Adjust 6th dorsal.

**Hiccough.**—Involuntary contraction of the diaphragm. A symptom of several morbid conditions. A sob is similar to a hiccough. Adjust 4th cervical.

**Hives.**—An itching skin disease. Adjust 6th dorsal.

**Hoarseness.**—Voice hoarse and rough; mucous membrane inflamed. Adjust 5th dorsal, standing on the right side and throw toward the left shoulder. The nerves which supply the throat emerge from the right side of the spinal column.

**Homesickness.**—See nostalgia.

**Hordeolum.**—See sty.

**Housemaid's Knee.**—Inflammation of the bursa in front of the patella, with accumulation of fluid.

**Hydrocele.**—A collection of fluid in the scrotum. Adjust for dropsy, at 12th dorsal.

**Hydrocephalous.**—A disease of childhood. Water on the brain. A fluid effusion within the cranium. Adjust 12th dorsal.

**Hydrophobia.**—Rabies occurs in the dog, wolf, cat and fox, and by them transmitted to other quadrupeds and man. See article on spasm.

**Hydrops.**—See dropsy.

**Hyperesthesia.**—A supersensitive condition of sensibility. It may be of the hearing, taste, smell, the eyes to light, or an abnormal excitability of sexual impulse, touch or oversensitiveness to pain.

**Hyperosmia.**—Excessive acuteness of smell. Adjust 4th dorsal.

**Hyperpyrexia.**—Excessive high fever. Adjust 6th dorsal unless a local inflammatory condition directs otherwise.

**Hypersecretion.**—Excessive secretion—too much functionating. What nerve is at fault and which vertebra to adjust will depend upon the region affected. Instead of "restoring a perfect nerve supply," the surplus should be curtailed.

**Hypertension.**—See hypertonia.

**Hypertonia.**—Excessive tone, tension, or activity.

**Hypertonicity.**—See hypertonia.

**Hypotension.**—Diminished or abnormally low tension.

**Hypertrophy.**—Excessive nutrition. It may be physiological, compensatory or regenerative. When pathological, it is known as hyperplasia. Pathological growths are attended with hyperthemia; whereas, physiological growths have normal temperature. Hypertrophy is an increase in the size of an organ or tissue independent of the general growth of the body. Gigantism is an even growth of all parts.

**Hypochondriasis.**—Probably so named because of some hypochondriacs having felt an uneasy sensation in the hypochondriac region. A species of mental alienation.

**Hysteria.**—A functional disorder, largely from auto-suggestion. A bucket of cold water dashed upon the patient is said to be an effectual adjustment.

**Icterus.**—See jaundice.

**Imbecility.**—Weakness of intellect; nearly allied to idiocy.

**Impotence.**—Lack of reproductive power. Adjust 1st lumbar.

**Impotency.**—See impotence.

**Incontinence.**—Inability to hold the feces or urine. Adjust 2d lumbar.

**Incoordination.**—The inability to produce voluntary movements in proper combination; a lack of harmony between the will and muscular activity.

**Indigestion.**—A lack of, or too much, digestive functionating; in other words, too much or not enough heat for the proper maintenance of metabolism. Adjust 5th dorsal toward the right shoulder.

**Induration.**—See schlerosis.

**Infantile paralysis.**—Use the same principles and judgment in adjusting a child as an adult. Palpation needs much closer work on account of the spines being smaller and the epiphyses not united to the spinous processes. Adjust the 6th dorsal.

**Inflammation.**—Gould defines it as "A condition of nutritive disturbance characterized by hyperemia, with proliferation of the cells of a tissue or organ and attended by one or more of the symptoms of pain, heat, swelling, discoloration and disordered function." Inflammation, excessive heat, causes a pathological process. Nerves irritated cause excessive heat. Extreme inflammation causes caries and necrosis. Inflammation, in any degree, disturbs metabolism. Normal heat insures normal functionating. Inflammation is manifested by disordered functionating and altered structure. It is always destructive and disintegrative.

**Inflammation of Bile Duct.**—This will, usually, be found to be in the duodenum, closing the orifice at the junction of the ducts. The duodenum, from the pylorus of the stomach to the junction mentioned, is comparatively large; in fact, it appears as a part of the stomach. But the lower half of the duodenum is much smaller, so that inflammation in that region closes the orifice and turns the bile into the stomach instead of into the bowels. If this condition is continued, the bile is diffused thruout the whole body. Adjust 6th dorsal.

**Inflammation of Bowels.**—Adjust in the region between the 7th to 12th dorsal.

**Inflammation of Eyes.**—The eye is the organ of vision. The eyelids, brows and lachrymal apparatus are appendages; they are not a part of the eye. For inflammation of the eyeball, adjust the 5th dorsal, standing on the right side, throwing the spinous process toward the left shoulder.

**Inflammation of the Kidneys.**—Adjust the 12th dorsal.

**Inflammation of the Liver.**—The nerves of liver innervation emerge from the right side of the spinal canal: stand on the right side and adjust toward the left shoulder.

**Inflammation of the Uterus.**—Adjust 4th lumbar.

**Influenza.**—Adjust 6th dorsal, as this is a general affection.

**Ingrown Toe Nails.**—Adjust last lumbar.

**Inoculation.**—Operation by which a disease may be artificially communicated by introducing its virus into the body by puncture or a scratch made in the skin, by subcutaneous injection, introduction into the peritoneal cavity. For example, the Jennerian inoculation of vaccination.

**Insanity.**—Adjust atlas or 3d cervical.

**Insolation.**—See sunstroke.

**Insomnia.**—Inability to sleep. Sleeplessness may be from fever, pain or nervous. Adjust to the dorsal to the right shoulder.

**Intermittent Fever.**—The symptoms are those of a decided and completely marked cold stage of concentration, or **contraction**, paleness, collapse, impaired sensibility and coldness, more or less diffused, followed by more or less rigors. After this occurs the hot stage of **expansion**, the heat returning partially and irregularly, at length becoming universal, much above the standard of health, the pulse hard and strong, tongue white, urine high colored, thirst considerable. At last the sweating stage, or stage of termination appears, the moisture usually beginning on the forehead, face and neck, and soon extending universally, heat abates, thirst ceases, the urine throws down a sediment and functions are restored to their normal state. See malaria.

**Intestinal Catarrh.**—A catarrhal inflammation of the mucous membrane of the whole or of any anatomic division of the intestinal tract. It may be acute or chronic, primary or secondary.

**Intestinal Hemorrhage.**—If pathological, accompanied with fever (excessive heat), softening of blood-vessel walls, adjust 2d lumbar.

**Intestinal Obstruction.**—There may be any one of several causes. For temporary relief give an injection of water about 70 degrees. Cool water is a tonic, hot or warm water is weakening.

**Intoxication.**—Poisoning. The symptoms of acute alcoholism range from mild intoxication to an acute delirium or a profound stupor and coma. It begins with a vascular relaxation and of feelings of warmth and exhileration, due to the depressing and paralyzing effects of the alcohol upon the vasomotor tone. The second stage is one of partial functional paralysis of the nerves, marked disturbance of the faculties, muscular incordination and delirious speech. In the third stage of "dead-drunkenness," there are acute coma, stertorious breathing, a bloated and congested face, a slow and full, but weak pulse, a cold and clammy skin and sometimes incontinence of urine and feces. Chronic alcoholism is considered a disease. It is not whether one "cannot" or "will not"; but in which one "cannot will" to resist the desire for alcohol.

**Intussusception.**—The introduction of one part of the intestinal canal into another which serves it as a sort of vagina or sheath; generally the upper part of the small intestine is received into the lower.

**Invagination.**—See Intussusception.

**Iritis.**—Inflammation of the eyes. Unless from direct injury, it will be found associated with syphilis, gonorrhea, rheumatism, gout, tuberculosis, scrofula or small pox. Adjust as indicated by the disease it accompanies.

**Itch.**—Includes various forms of skin diseases. Adjust 6th dorsal where it is general.

**Itching.**—A sensation more annoying than painful. A neurosis of the skin characterized by the single symptom of itching over the entire, or certain regions of, the body. It is due to a functional derangement of the cutaneous nerves.

**Jacob's Ulcer.**—See lupus.

**Jaundice.**—Recognized by the yellowness of the eyes, skin and secretions. It seems to arise from over-secretion and diffusion of bile. Adjust 7th dorsal on the right.

**Keratitis.**—Inflammation of the cornea.

**Keratosis.**—Any one of a large class of skin diseases presenting thickened epidermis or horny growths, as warts and callosities. Consider the location and determine what nerve covers that region.

**Kidney, Amyloid.**—Waxy or lardaceous degeneration of the kidneys. A diffuse nephritis is always present.

**Kyphosis.**—Posterior curvature of the spine.

**Kyphoskoliosis.**—Lateral and posterior curvature of the spine.

**Lacrymation.**—The secretion and discharge of tears. Lacrymation is a profuse secretion of the lachrymal gland which is poured between the globe of the eye and the eyelids to facilitate motion. Irritation causes inflammation which excites the flow of tears; the physiological function becomes pathological. While anatomists tell us that lachrymation is controlled by the lachrymal nerve, a branch from the ophthalmic division of the fifth cranial (the trigeminal, the trifacial) nerve which arises from the pons varolii—an organ situated at the base of the brain, connecting the cerebrum, cerebellum and oblongata—this information is not just what a Chiropractor desires. He wants to know in what region he can find a fiber of the lachrymal nerve, that is, impinged upon at the spinal foramina or elsewhere. This information in anatomies is lacking; they were not gotten up for Chiropractors.

**Lactosuria.**—Urine containing sugar of milk, observed occasionally in pregnant women.

**La Grippe.**—In looking over the symptoms, complications and sequelae, we find catarrhal inflammation of the mucous membrane of the respiratory tract, which includes the nose, larynx and bronchial tubes, accompanied by a mucopurulent discharge. As we might expect, there is fever—**diffused inflammation**—pain in the muscles, prostration. Among the complications are pneumonia, affections of the ear and eye, chills, cough, headache and cardiac oppression. There are three forms, viz., gastroenteritic, nervous and pulmonary. That is, these three regions are liable to be affected with some ingredient that is contaminating and poisonous. Now, what do we as Chiropractors gather from all this? Simply that where we find a general condition, we adjust center place, the 6th dorsal. A displacement at 6th dorsal especially affects the sympathetic ganglionated chain, the great distributing agent.

**Laryngeal Vertigo.**—See child-crowing.

**Laryngismus.**—See child-crowing.

**Laryngitis.**—Inflammation of the larynx. Any mucous membrane, inflamed, produces catarrh, for the reason that heat dries and thickens the mucous which covers all lining membranes. Adjust 5th dorsal; throw to the left.

**Lead Poison.**—A disease largely confined to plumbers. This disease, with general symptoms, calls for adjustment at 6th dorsal. I made a step forward for Chiropractors when I discovered that diseases which are dependent upon general conditions can be relieved by adjusting the 6th dorsal.

**Leontiassis Ossa.**—A variety of elephantisis in which the patient's face resembles that of a lion. This affection is characterized by hyperostosis of the facial and cranial bones.

**Leontiasis Ossium.**—Enormous thickening of the skull also a form of sclerosis of bone, following osteitis, with nodular deposits.

**Leprosy.**—A chronic contagious disease. It is distinguished by tuberculous masses in the muco-cutaneous surfaces, and by nerve changes.

**Leucorrhea.**—A catarrhal discharge from the vagina. Adjust 2d lumbar.

**Leukemia.**—A disease known by a permanent increase in the number of white blood corpuscles and enlargement of the spleen. Adjust 7th dorsal, standing on the left side and adjusting towards the right shoulder as the nerves of innervation arise on the left of the spine.

**Lienteric Diarrhea.**—Frequent, liquid evacuations. The food is only partially digested as a result of great irritation in the intestinal canal. There is increased sensibility and activity—too much functionating.

**Liver, Diseases of.**—Adjust 7th dorsal, on the right.

**Localization, Cerebral.**—The designating of a particular part of the brain as the center, the origination of certain physiological functions.

**Localization, Spinal.**—The specifying of different segments of the spinal cord from which the different functions have their apparent origin.

**Lockjaw.**—See tetanus.

**Locomotor Ataxia.**—Inability to co-ordinate the muscles in walking. When the eyes are closed the body sways. It is difficult to stand upon one foot. The ataxic has difficulty in descending stairs.

**Lordosis.**—Curvature of the vertebral column forward. See chicken-breasted.

**Loss of Memory.**—Look to atlas.

**Lumbago.**—Rheumatism in the lumbar region. Vertebrae wrenched from their normal position in the loins create pain and stiffness. Adjust in the lumbar region, using the bifid table, being careful to so adjust the patient on the tables that the place of adjustment will be midway between the two tables. The tables will need spacing just right, neither too far apart nor too near together. The space between them must be regulated by the height of the patient. To elevate the patient's chest answers the same purpose.

**Lung Fever.**—See pneumonia.

**Lupus.**—An erosive ulcer of the skin with necroses on one side and nodules of granulating tissue on the opposite side. Adjust according to the area affected.

All diseases coexist with an abnormal amount of heat; either subnormal or hyperthermic. A change of bodily temperature from that which is normal accompanies all diseased conditions. In all diseases nerves are too tense or too slack, too firm or too lax, enlarged or lessened in diameter, inflamed or atonic; they lack tonicity, a condition of partial contraction—health tension—which is physiological.

We cannot get away from that basic principle, first given to the world by me, that disease is too much or not enough functionating. If nerves possess normal temperature their functions will be performed naturally and in a normal amount. The reader will observe that, in most instances, the name used to designate the disease from which an organ is suffering, ends with the word itis, a suffix meaning inflammation. Inflammation is but an excited condition of the nervous system. Nerves are only excited by tension. Bones are the only hard substances capable of impinging on nerves, and they only do so when displaced. They are luxated by poisons and traumatism.

**Lymph.**—The fluid in the lymphatic vessels, the product of the liquid portion of the blood thru the walls of the capillaries.

**Lymphadenitis.**—Inflammation of a lymphatic gland.

**Lymphangitis.**—Inflammation of a lymphatic vessel.

**Lymphenteritis.**—Inflammation of the bowels attended with serous infiltration—serum stasis.

**Lympho-Nephritis.**—Inflammation of the serous or outer coat of the kidney.

**Malaria.**—A poisoned condition of the system from the effluvia of decaying vegetation; air-borne emanations poisonous only to human beings. The exciting element which causes malaria. Adjust the 6th dorsal.

**Malarial Fever.**—This disease is associated with an enlarged liver and spleen. The paroxysms may be intermittent, remittent or irregular. They may be daily, alternately, every third day, or twice a day. A paroxysm consists of three stages, each of which may vary in its intensity. The fever is preceded by a chill and followed by porfuse sweating. A cold or chill period is present, in a more or less degree, in injuries which result in fever, during infectious (poison) diseases, at the crisis of some ailment and during the formation of pus. The characteristic lesions are found in the brain, spinal cord, nerves liver, spleen, kidneys and blood. The brain and spinal cord are more or less congested; there may be punctate hemorrhages. The nerves are contracted, swollen and inflamed. The liver shows focal necrosis. The spleen is increased in size, the pulp softened and very dark, transudation is impeded by congested tissue. The kidneys exhibit albuminous degeneration and diffuse nephritis is noticeable. A close inspection of the intestines may show necrosis and bacteria as scavengers. There is diminution of the red corpuscles of the blood. Adjust 4th dorsal.

**Malformation.**—An abnormal development of parts during embryonic life, during the formation period, before quickening. Malformation may consist of variations of growth, excessive or arrested, or of defective union of component embryonic parts, including those embryonal cleavages of parts not ordinarily coalesced. Malformations are the result of functions performed abnormally.

**Mammary Glands.**—See breast.

**Mammitis.**—See mastitis.

**Mania.**—Disorder of the intellect in which there is erroneous judgment or hallucination, which impels to acts of fury; acute mental excitement; fury or frenzy.

**Marie's Disease.**—See acromegaly.

**Mastadenitis.**—Inflammation of the mammary gland.

**Mastitis.**—Inflammation of the breasts. Adjust 4th dorsal.

**Measles.**—A disease which arises from noxious exhalation, deleterious effluvia. Deafness is often a sequela of measles; if so, why not adjust 4th dorsal?

**Meat Poisoning.**—Poisoning by meat which contains ptomain. Various tainted meats, as mince meat, warmed over veal pie, carelessly-kept chicken salad, badly-preserved and canned meats, partly decayed sausages, have caused violent symptoms of poisoning. Diseased raw and partially cooked meat has also been eaten with disastrous results. It should be borne in mind that even prolonged cooking fails to destroy the toxic action of certain ptomains in infected meats; also, that meat which has been cooked and kept under certain conditions may become infected, as well as when it is raw. On the other hand, bad, putrid meat has been known not to cause toxic symptoms. What is food for one may be poison to another.

**Megrim.**—See hemicrania.

**Melano-Carcinoma.**—Cancerous growths that are dark because of congestion.

**Melano-Chlorosis.**—A disease in which the skin has a dark green hue.

**Melanoma.**—Is characterized by a development and growth of black or dark-colored tubercules within the tissues of the viscera.

**Melanosis.**—A dark granular pigment found in the tissues, often associated with malignant growths.

**Melena.**—The evacuation of tar-like stools due to the presence therein of altered, retained blood.

**Meningitis.**—Inflammation of the meninges (membranes) of the brain or cord. The sensitive areas will only be found close to or between the transverse processes. Adjust for some one of the **recurrent** branches of the spinal nerves which return thru the foramina and into the spinal canal to innervate the meninges. See brain fever.

**Meningo-Encephalitis.**—An inflammation of the brain and its membranes. See brain fever.

**Menopause.**—See change of life.

**Menorrhagia.**—Very profuse or excessive menstruation. Adjust 2d lumbar.

**Menstruation, Painful.**—The menstrual flow when deficient or suppressed.

**Mental Depression.**—May arise from any one of several lesions.

**Mercurial Poisoning.**—A form of palsy, the result of mercurial intoxication in those who are exposed to the vapor of mercury. A mercurial tremor noticed among smelters who are exposed to the fumes of mercury. A mercurial rash, an eczematous eruption from the continued use of mercury.

**Mercurial Stomatitis.**—See salivation.

**Meearteritis.**—Inflammation of the middle coat of an artery.

**Mesenteritis.**—Inflammation of the mesentery, a fold of the peritoneum, which serves to hold the organs in position, and to support and convey blood vessels, nerves and lympathics.

**Metamidophenylparamethoxyquinolin** is an antiperiodic and antipyretic drug used instead of quinine. If the cooling period is equal to the length of—look in a medical dictionary and save repetition—it must be effective.

**Metritis.**—Inflammation of the uterus. Adjust 2d lumbar.

**Microcephalous.**—Having an abnormally small head or a small, imperfect cranium. A deficiency in the amount of heat contracts and retards growth. There is less circulation of blood, slower and less dialysis of the chyle, a nutritive fluid extracted by intestinal absorption from food which has been subjected to the action of the digestive organs; a return flow of the lymph, a fluid contained in the lymphatic vessels and thoracic duct; and slower osmosis of the serum, the most watery portion of animal fluids. Who said that the chyle, the lymph or the serous fluid circulated? Owing to the lack of proper osmosis of these fluids there is a lack of nutrition. The diploe is decreased, the functions of bone formation is lessened, consequently the head is smaller. The bones are more compact and less vascular, because of a lower bodily temperature and less circulation of the blood and osmosis of the other fluids.

**Micturition.**—The act of passing urine. For abnormality of this function, adjust the 12th dorsal or 1st lumbar, depending upon whether the cause is in the kidneys or bladder. See urination.

**Migraine.**—See hemicrania.

**Milk Fever.**—A slight elevation of temperature preceding or accompanying the secretion of milk in women recently delivered. It occurs usually about the third day after delivery. Such a rise of temperature is physiological and due to an impulse from Innate.

**Milk, Lack or Excess of.**—Adjust 4th dorsal.

**Milk Leg.**—A painful swelling of the leg, beginning either at the ankle and ascending, or at the groin and extending down the thigh. It is an after-labor disease. Adjust the lumbar when displaced at child-birth.

**Milk-Sickness.**—A peculiar infectious disease, supposed to be caused by certain weeds eaten by milk cows. It formerly prevailed extensively in the Western and South-western States and often with fatal effects. Cultivation and civilization has almost exterminated it.

**Miosis.**—A decrease in the size of an organ; a lessening of existing symptoms.

**Mithridatism.**—Immunity from the effects of poison induced by taking gradually increased doses. Mithridates, the Grecian king, is credited with the fabled story of taking poison so as to be immune against it, as he feared being poisoned by his enemies. See poison.

**Mollities Cerebri.**—Softening of brain tissue. Remember that excessive heat softens tissue and subnormal heat hardens it.

**Mollities Ossium.**—Softening of bones because of excessive heat. Adjust 6th dorsal—the "heat regulator."

**Monoplegia.**—Paralysis limited to a single organ or part, dependent on special lesions of the nervous system caused by lesions of the osseous system, as in glossoplegia—paralysis of the tongue.

**Monstrosities.**—A fetus or being with an unusual development of either superfluous or deficient parts. Abnormal development of growth is made during fetal life after all the parts are formed. A deficiency can only occur during the formative, embryonic period—the first four months—before the time of quickening. Physiological functions form the fetus during the first four months and develop its growth during the last five months. The absence of these functions or their pathologic performance is the cause of maliformations.

**Morning Sickness.**—The nausea of pregnant women, occurring in the early months of gestation; also a term applied to the sympathetic nausea sometimes experienced by the husband during the gestative period. Adjust 5th dorsal.

**Morphine Habit.**—Morpheus was the mythical god of dreams and sleep. Morphine is the principal alkaloid of opium. It is an anodyne, hypnotic and narcotic.

**Morphinism.**—A chronic intoxication, due to the habitual use of morphin.

**Morvan's Disease.**—A disease of the skin with pain, followed by analgesia, first on one side, then on the other. After this there follows a succession of whitlows, usually painless, and necrosis of the phalanges. Atrophy, paresis, contraction of the fingers, loss of sensation of heat or cold may occur. See felon. Adjust 6th dorsal.

**Mother's Marks.**—See nevi.

**Mouth, Diseases of.**—Adjust 5th dorsal, standing on the right side and adjust toward the left shoulder.

**Mumps.**—This infectious disease from poison begins with a chill, which is followed by fever. Impingements on the nervous system excite, contract, draw on muscles. Nerves are affected by traumatism and poisons. The first effect is that of contraction The somatic, cutaneous muscular system responds, giving the patient the sensation of a chill. This disease is characterized by local inflammation of the parotid gland. Diffused inflammation is fever. Adjust 5th dorsal, throwing it toward the left shoulder.

**Mushroom Poisoning.**—Some varieties of mushrooms are edible and some are poisonous.

**Mutism.**—See mutitas.

**Mutitas.**—See dumbness.

**Myalgia.**—Muscular rheumatism; muscular cramps. Neuralgia of the sensory nerves.

**Mycosis.**—An inflammatory, fungoid neoplasm.

**Mydriasis.**—Paralysis of visual accommodation. Usually caused by mydriatic medicines.

**Myelitis.**—Inflammation of the spinal cord. Find the recurrent nerve which is impinged upon and relieve it by adjusting the vertebra which is racked out of its normal position.

**Myosis.**—Contraction of the pupils, usually associated with iritis, which see.

**Myocarditis.**—Inflammation of the muscular structure of the heart; chronic carditis may lead to degeneration of the heart-muscle and induration.

**Myositis.**—Inflammation of muscular tissue. See rheumatism.

**Myositas Ossificans.**—This disease is characterized by the formation of osseous deposits in the muscles. Look to the "hot box," 6th dorsal.

**Myotonia.**—Muscular spasm. Adjust according to locality contracted.

**Myxedema.**—A general nutritional disorder, consequent upon atrophy and loss of function of the thyroid gland and characterized by a myxedematous infiltration of the subcutaneous tissue and a cretinoid cachexia. It is upon the absence of the thyroid secretion that the condition depends. The medical treatment consists of administering thyroid extract to replace the deficiency. The Chiropractor relieves the impingement upon the nerves which innervate this gland; its nerves are derived from the middle and inferior cervical ganglia of the sympathetic and from the inferior and superior laryngeal nerves. The thyroid gland tends to atrophy in old age. Enlargement of the thyroid gland is named goitre. In individuals in which the thyroid gland is absent, the worst form of cretinism is observed. See goitre.

**Nasal Catarrh.**—See coryza and rhinitis.

**Necrobiosis.**—Molecular death of tissue.

**Necrosis.**—Death in mass. Necrosis of bone corresponds to gangrene of the soft tissue.

**Nephritis.**—Inflammation of the kidneys. It occurs in various forms as acute, chronic, desquamative, glomerular, parenchymatous and tubal. Adjust 12th dorsal.

**Nervous Exhaustion.**—See neurasthenia.

**Nervousness.**—A condition of over-excitability of the nervous system, characterized by great unrest, mental and physical.

**Nettle Rash.**—A skin disease attended by severe itching. If general over the body, adjust 6th dorsal.

**Neuralgia.**—An acute, intermitting, throbbing pain, which follows the course of a nerve, due to local pressure. It occurs more frequently in the head and face than in other parts. Remove the pressure and nerve vibration will be normal.

**Neurasthenia.**—Debility and exhaustion of the nervous system. Among the more common symptoms are a lack of energy, disinclination to activity, a sense of fullness of pressure at the top of the head, pain in the back, impaired memory and disturbed sleep.

**Neuritis.**—Inflammation of a nerve, especially of a nerve trunk.

**Neurosis.**—Disordered sensation, volition or abnormal mental manifestation without an evident lesion to account for it.

**Nevi.**—Mother's marks. Here is an unbroken field for Chiropractors. These "mother's marks" are of a great variety. I have relieved some of them.

**Nictitating Spasm.** — A continuous and uncontrolable winking.

**Nodding Spasm.**—A disease of young children. The head and upper part of the body are bowed forward several times in succession, attended with temporary disordered consciousness.

**Non-Union of Bone.**—Adjust to relieve the nerves supplying the injured part. It is not only possible, but occasionally happens, that the accident which causes the fracture also dislocates a vertebra, causing an impingement on the nerves supplying the part to be united. As a result, there is too much or too little reparative callous formed for the proper uniting. Remove the pressure on the reparative nerves so that their functions may be performed normally.

**Nosebleed.—Hemorrhage.**—Hemorrhage from the nose due to softening of the walls of the blood vessels from excessive heat, necrosis.

**Nostalgia.—Home-Sickness.**—This disease may be accompanied with fever and result in death. A few hours at home will relieve the patient.

**Numbness.**—Deficiency of sensation due to pressure on the nerves which go to, and end in, the part affected.

**Obesity.**—An excessive development of fat thruout the body. It may be congenital or occur at any period of life. Fat, considered physiologically, has for its function protection of organs, the maintenance of an even temperature, and the supplying of nutritive material when food is lacking. Fat may be excessive or deficient. To bring the amount to normal, the function which governs water production must be made normally active. This can be accomplished by adjusting the 12th dorsal.

**Oedema.**—See dropsy.

**Oliguresis.**—Morbidly diminished urinary secretion.

**Onychitis.**—Inflammation of a finger or toe nail.

**Oophoritis.**—See ovaritis.

**Oophoromalacia.**—Softening of the ovary.

**Ophthalmia.**—See Ophthalmitis.

**Ophthalmitis.**—An inflammation of the superficial tissues of the eye and especially of the conjunctiva. As a rule adjust the 6th dorsal, standing on the right side, adjusting to the left. There are those who always adjust on one side using the same position of the hands. Such persons, usually, know but little of the art of adjusting.

**Ophthalmoplegia.**—Ophthalmo paralysis; paralysis of one or more of the muscles of the eye.

**Orchitis.**—Inflammation of the testes. Adjust 1st lumbar.

**Organic Disease of the Heart.**—Organic disease is attended with structural change in the organ affected. A functional disease is one of function only, there being no appreciable organic alteration. The latter, if continued for a length of time, will cause the former. One cannot continue to exist without the other, except in those instances in which the functional change in a certain organ causes a corresponding change in a neighboring organ or organs, as is the case with diabetes mellitus. Adjust for either functional or organic diseases of the heart at the 4th dorsal.

**Ostalgia.**—Pain in a bone.

**Osteitis.**—Inflammation of a bone.

**Osteitis Interna.**—Caries, centrally. Condensing or ossifying osteitis, sclerosis ossium. Osteitis fungosa; granular absorbtion. Rarefying osteitis; bone softening. Osteitis, suppurative; inflammation of bone attended with suppuration.

**Osteo-Arthritis.**—Chronic inflammation of the bones forming a joint.

**Osteoma.**—A bony tumor.

**Osteomalacia.**—Softening of bone from excessive heat, which deprives it of its earthly constituents.

**Osteomyelitis.**—Inflammation of the marrow of bone.

**Osteophlebitis.**—Inflammation of the veins of a bone.

**Osteosarcoma.**—A sarcoma of bone. A tumor of bone and flesh.

**Otalgia.**—See earache.

**Otitis.**—Inflammation of the ear.

**Otorrhea.**—A discharge of pus from the auditory canal. Adjust 3d cervical.

**Ovaritis.**—Inflammation of the substance of the ovary. Adjust 2d lumbar.

**Oynchia.**—See ingrown toe nails.

**Ozena.**—A chronic disease of the nose with a fetid discharge. Necrosis, because of inflammation. Adjust 3d cervical.

**Pachymeningitis.**—Inflammation of the dura mater of the brain or spinal cord. Gould says it is usually due to extension from adjacent bone-disease, especially caries; it may be due to syphilis, sunstroke or injuries. Inflammation, hyperthermia, often affects the bone in the form of caries, and the adjoining soft parts by degeneration.

**Pain.**—Distressing or agonizing sensations are due to the irritation of a sensory nerve. It is said to be acute when sharp and violent; twinging, when short and sudden; when more violent, a pang; when like a sharp instrument, pungent; heavy, when it has a sensation of weight; tensive, when it has a feeling of being tense; boring, when there is a grinding, penetrating feeling; lancinating, when shooting; like lightning, when momentary; lacerating, when the part seems to be tearing; burning, when it has a sensation of heat, and throbbing when it beats regularly with the pulse. All kinds of pain are accompanied by irritation, neuritis, hyperthermia, being the result of impingement of nerves.

**Painful Menstruation.**—See menstruation.

**Palpitation of the Heart.**—Adjust 4th dorsal.

**Palsy.**—A form of paralysis. See paralysis agitans.

**Panaris Analgicum.**—A rare disease, marked by a succession of painless felons, usually followed by destruction of the ends of the fingers caused by inflammation. Adjust 4th dorsal.

**Pancreas, Diseases of.**—Adjust 6th dorsal.

**Pancreatitis.**—Inflammation of the pancreas. The pancreas is known in animals as the sweetbread. It lies transversely across the posterior walls of the abdomen. It secretes a limpid, colorless fluid for the digestion of proteids, fats and carbohydrates. Adjust the 7th dorsal, standing on the right side.

**Paralysis.**—A loss of sensation or motion or of both.

**Paralysis Agitans.**—A disease of late life marked by tremor of muscles, weakness, delay in making voluntary motions, festination gait, and excessive perspiration. Adjust 12th dorsal.

**Paraplegia.**—Paralysis of the lower half of the body. It may interfere with micturition and the evacuation of stool. Adjust in the region of 9th dorsal to 3d lumbar.

**Paresthesia.**—An abnormal sensation of burning, pricking, formication, numbness, or of pricking with pins or needles.

**Paronychia.**—Inflammation about the finger nail. It may be phlegmonous and form an abscess. Adjust 4th dorsal.

**Paronchychitis.**—See paronychia.

**Parosmia.**—Smell.

**Parotid Gland, Diseases of.**—See parotitis.

**Parotitis.**—Inflammation of the parotid glands, known as mumps, which see.

**Parulis.**—Alveolar abscess of the gums. See gum boil.

**Pemphigus.**—Vesicular fever. See skin diseases.

**Periarteritis.**—Inflammation of the sheath of an artery.

**Pericarditis.**—Inflammation of the pericardium. The pericardium is a fibro-serous sack which surrounds the heart. Pericarditis is attended with fever, pain in the precordial region, rapid pulse, cough and dyspnea. Adjust 4th dorsal.

**Periostitis.**—Inflammation of the periosteum which covers the surfaces of bones, except at the points of tendinous and ligamentous attachment and on the articular surfaces where cartilage exists.

**Periphalangeal Cellulitis.**—Any phlegmonous tumor of the fingers or toes, especially of the first phalanx. If of both extremities, adjust 6th dorsal; but if of the upper only, the 4th dorsal; if of the feet, the last lumbar.

**Peritonitis.**—Inflammation of the peritoneum. The peritoneum is a serous membrane which lines the abdominal walls surrounding the contained viscera. Adjust in the region of 8th to 12th dorsal.

**Pertussus.**—See whooping cough.

**Pharyngitis.**—Inflammation of the pharynx. It is attended with fever, pain in the throat, especially on swallowing, congestion and dryness of the mucous membrane. Adjust 3d cervical.

**Pharyngocele.**—A sacculated opening in the esophagus in which the food may be retained.

**Phlebehepathitis.** — Inflammation of the portal or hepatic veins. Arteries and veins are well supplied with both medullated and nonmedullated nerve-fibres. The fibres form dense plexuses on the outer surface of the vessels. From thence filaments pass to the middle coat to be distributed almost entirely to its muscular fibres. The circulation of the blood is dependent upon this nervous vascular system. Like all nerves, these may become inflamed by traumatism or by poisons. It is this system of nerves that is influenced, unduly excited, by poisons, and not the blood as usually supposed. The poison of an insect, snake or that from the hypodermic syringe of the physician, acts upon the nervous system. The function of this nervous vascular net-work is to propel the blood. This is done by the intermediary muscular fibres. When these nerves are excited by pressure or poisons they act on the muscular fibres thru contraction. Irritation causes nerves to contract; increased irritation augments the flow of blood.

**Phlebitis.**—Inflammation of a vein; if superficial, it can often be traced by a red line which marks its course.

**Phrenitis.**—Frenzy, delirium, brain fever, encephalitis, violent pyrexia, pain in the head, redness of the face and eyes, intolerance of light and sound, watchfulness and either furious or muttering delirium. Its causes are the same as of those of other inflammations.

**Pigeon-Breast.**—Chicken-breast. A bulging of the sternum; seen in rickety children and mouth-breathers.

**Pigment.**—In biology, a pigment is any organic coloring-matter in the tissues of plants or animals, the coloring matter in the iris, retina, hair and skin are examples.

**Pigmentation.**—Deposition of or, discoloration by, pigment.

**Piles.**—The hemorrhoidal nerves emerge from the sciatic and hypogastric plexuses and cover the rectum with their numerous filaments. The prolapsed bowel may be internal or external to the sphincter ani. Adjust 4th lumbar.

**Pin-Worm.**—Ascaris vermicularis. Seat-worm. Thread-worm. Maw-worm. It is found in the colon and rectum.

**Plantar Neuralgia.**—Neuralgia of the plantar nerve which supplies the superficial and deep muscles of the foot. It is both motor and sensory. Adjust in lower lumbar.

**Plegmasia Alba Dolens.**—See milk leg.

**Pleura, Diseases of.**—Adjust 3d dorsal.

**Pleurisy.**—Inflammation of the pleura with exudation into its cavity and upon its surface of thickened serum from excessive heat. Should be relieved by one adjustment at region from 3d to 5th dorsal.

**Pleuritis.**—See pleurisy.

**Pleuritis Deformans.**—Chronic inflammation with great thickening and induration of the pleura, usually accompanying fibroid pneumonia. See pleurisy.

**Plumbism.**—See lead poisoning.

**Pneumonia.**—Inflammation of the lung. The inflammation when diffused thruout the body is known as lung fever. All fevers are diffused heat from local inflamed tissue. Inflammation is the result of a nerve being unduly excited by pressure. The pressure may be from a vertebra or other bone displaced by an accident or from one drawn out of alignment by the muscular contraction induced by the action, upon the nerves, of some poisonous substance in the system. In either case the nerves become excited, irritated and more or less inflamed. All diseased conditions—the result of either excessive or insufficient performance of functions—exist because of heat modification. Extremes of bodily temperature cause tissue to become morbid, necrosed. Pneumonia should be relieved by one adjustment in the upper dorsal region. In all acute cases, the vertebrae have not yet become illshapened, do not require to be grown back to their normal shape, as do those of long standing.

**Pneumonia, Crossed.**—Croupous pneumonia. Inflammation of the mucous membrane attended with pseudomembranous exudation. The lower lobe on one side, associated with the same disease in the upper lobe of the other side. This double crossed pneumonia necessitates the adjustment of two different vertebrae; one for the higher and one for the lower impingement. Adjustments will be needed from both sides and toward each shoulder. See pneumonia.

**Pneumonia, Double.**—Croupous pneumonia of both lungs. See pneumonia and pneumonia crossed. See poison.

**Pneumonitis.**—Inflammation of the lungs. See pneumonia.

**Poison.**—All diseases are the result of displacement of osseous tissue. Bones are displaced by violence, as by accidents, or by poisons. Those which are traumatic, may be luxated during sleeping or waking hours. Many an M. D. has been called out of his comfortable bed, in the small hours of the night, to see a patient who had retired in usual health, but was awakened by a stitch in the side. The good doctor injected morphine to deaden sensation. If he had known that thon had had a dream, while fully relaxed, and that a sudden movement had slightly displaced a vertebra, causing it to press against a nerve, he would have adjusted the vertebra and relieved the case of pleurisy or pneumonia at once, instead of giving a poisonous drug to paralyze the sensory nerves. There are many diseases which seem not to be the direct result of accidents or poisons, altho violence has occurred. Instead of a traumatic, it may have produced a toxic lesion. I refer to those deleterious substances in the air we breathe, in the food we eat, in the water we drink, the poison on the saloon counter, or that sucked from the tobacco pipe or administered by an M. D. These, just as surely, produce vertebral lesions as those which are traumatic. Lesions caused by poisons can be as readily relieved as those which are traumatic. I have had quite a number of patients who were poisoned from these various sources and have adjusted all with success. Irritant or acrid poisons are those which produce irritation or inflammation. Narcotic poisons are such as produce stupor or delirium. Sedative poisons are those which directly reduce the vital powers.

**Poisoning.**—Tainted canned fish, eels, oysters, mussels, crabs and lobsters are often the cause of poisoning.

**Poliomyelitis.**—Inflammation of the spinal cord. It will be understood by Chiropractors that many diseases of inflammatory origin, caused by an impingement upon spinal nerves, are attributed to the spinal cord by pathologists because they know nothing either of vertebral subluxations or their effects.

**Polypi.**—Polypi are tumors which grow from the mucous membranes of the nose, bladder, rectum and uterus; more rarely in the pharynx, stomach, intestines, bronchial tubes, vagina and meatus auditorius externus. They vary much in size, number, mode of adhesion and structure; for remember, that the nerves of all persons do not functionate alike. Therefore, the same impingement on the same nerve in different persons will cause conditions which will not be the same in every respect.

**Polypi of the Ear.**—Adjust 3d cervical.

**Polypi of the Nose.**—Adjust 4th cervical.

**Polypi of the Rectum.**—Adjust 4th lumbar.

**Polypi of the Uterus.**—Adjust 3d lumbar.

**Polysarcia.**—See obesity.

**Pott's Disease.**—Caries of the spine. This disintegration is caused by continued, excessive heat which, if not arrested, ends in death of the affected part. Pathologists and orthopedists suppose that caries is the cause of spinal curvature. Caries is molecular death of bone, ulceration, rarefaction and absorption, because of excessive heat. I have seen many specimens of spinal curvatures and vertebral caries and I do not believe that either one produces the other. Those curvatures which are supposed to be caused by caries are angular. In all of those I have seen, their position shows that the change of structure was due to traumatic, not pathologic, causes.

**Priapism.**—Constant and distressing erection, with or without voluptuous desires. Adjust 5th lumbar.

**Proctitis.**—Inflammation of the anus and rectum. Adjust 4th lumbar.

**Prolapsus.**—A downward displacement of the bladder, kidney, liver, rectum, spleen, stomach, uterus, uvula and vagina.

**Prolapsus Uteri.**—When this organ is prolapsed it may assume any one of many malpositions which are unimportant to a Chiropractor. This organ or other viscera may become prolapsed from relaxation, loss of tonicity of the supporting tissues. Adjustments at the 4th lumbar will replace the vertebra to its normal position, relieve pressure on nerves and restore normal tone.

**Prostatalgia.**—Pain in the prostate gland.

**Prostatitis.**—Inflammation of the prostate gland. Adjust 3d lumbar.

**Proud Flesh.**—An inflamed, exuberant, fungous, granulated tissue, usually found in wounds and ulcers. Adjust to cover the area and you will be surprised to see how soon the inflammation will subside and the sprouting, fungous growth disappear.

**Prurigo.**—A chronic inflammatory skin disease developing in childhood, with eruptions of pale papules, attended with severe itching. Adjust 6th dorsal.

**Pruritus.**—An important neurosis of the skin. It may cover the entire body or be limited to certain regions. It is attended with itching usually worse at night. Adjust 6th dorsal.

**Psoriasis.**—Scaly tetter; dry scale; one form is named baker's itch and another the washerwoman's scall. Adjust according to area.

**Pterygium.**—A triangular patch of mucous membrane growing on the conjunctiva of the eyeball. Adjust 5th dorsal toward the left shoulder.

**Pthisis.**—Pulmonary pthisis or consumption. Adjust in the upper dorsal. See consumption.

**Ptomain Poison.**—Any one of the active, inanimate septic or toxic substances resulting from processes of decomposition and disintegration of albuminous material. As Ptomains are chiefly developed by puterfaction, they have been termed putrefactive alkaloids. The name cadaveric alkaloids has also been given to them, but this applies, properly, only to those obtained from a dead body. Some of these ptomains are poisonous; the greater number are not. That which may be poison to one may not be to another, as noticed in another place in this book. I have only had one case; it was sudden and severe. Adjustment at 5th thoracic gave instant relief. I threw the vertebra toward the right shoulder.

**Ptosis Palpebra.**—Complete or partial drooping of the upper eyelid. The levator palpebrae superioris is a branch of the infraorbital branch of the facial nerve which originates in the cervical sympathetic. For paralysis of, adjust 3d cervical.

**Ptyalism.**—See salivation.

**Puberty.**—That period of life at which sexual maturity occurs. This is about the age of fourteen years in the male and twelve in the female. At this time there is a change of voice in the male and the menses appear in the female. The menstrual flow is a physiological function which may become pathological by being delayed or by occurring in excess. Adjust 3d lumbar.

**Puerperal Fever.**—An acute febrile affection of women in child-bed. Considered by the medical profession as grave. See child-bed fever.

**Pupil of the Eye, Diseases of.**—Adjust 4th cervical. See eye, diseases of.

**Purpura-Hemorrhagica.**—Hemorrhages may arise from eruptive patches in the skin, forming blood tumors, or they may take place from the mucous surfaces or from the inner surface of the serous cavities.

**Pyelitis.**—Inflammation of the pelvis and chalices of the kidney. It may occur as a complication of scarlatina, typhoid fever, smallpox, purpura and other diseases. The symptoms comprise pain in the lumbar region, pus, and perhaps blood, in the urine, irritability of the bladder and fever. Adjust in the lumbar region.

**Pyemia.**—Is characterized by intermittent fever, with recurrent rigors, profuse sweats, a sweetish odor to the breath, a dry, brown tongue and rapid emaciation. Slight jaundice frequently develops; sometimes, also, a purpuric eruption, the temperature may reach as high as 105 deegrees.

**Pyorrhea Alveolaris.**—Suppurative inflammation of the root membranes of the teeth in connection with the tissue of the gums beneath the mucous membrane. The teeth become loose, the gums recede from the teeth. Hemorrhage is liable to occur because of inflammation. The nerves which carry innervation to the kidneys, also, contain fibres which go to the eyelids and gums. Kidney diseases usually accompany affections of the gums.

**Pyrosis.**—See heart-burn.

**Quinsy.**—Inflammation of the tonsils.

**Rabies.**—See hydrophobia.

**Rachialgia.**—Pain in the back.

**Rachitis.**—See rickets.

**Railway Brain.**—Cerebral and nervous disorders following concussions in railway accidents—similar to railway spine.

**Railroad Spine.**—Traumatic hysteria. Disorders following the concussions experienced in railway accidents.

**Rash.**—An eruption of the skin.

**Relapsing Fever.**—Begins with a chill, then fever, pains in the head, body and limbs. In a week, after a profuse sweating, the symptoms may disappear. But a second, third or fourth attack may follow. Adjust the "hot box," the center place, the 6th dorsal.

**Retinitis.**—Inflammation of the retina, the expansion of the optic nerve. It is usually associated with some other affection showing that a fiber of a sensory nerve reaches the eye and that it is impinged upon.

**Rheumatic Arthritis.**—A form of rheumatism. It. usuallv, comes on with the ordinary symptoms of chills and fever. Adjust 6th dorsal.

**Rheumatic Fever.**—Rheumatism may affect joints, muscles, fibrous or serous structures. Diffused inflammation is fever. Inflammation is always caused by bone pressure on nerves. There you have it. I was the first man to present these facts to the world.

**Rheumatism.**—A disease of the joints and muscles. It is accompanied by fever and inflammatory swelling of the joints. Stiffness, pain and deformity are usual accompaniments.

**Rhinitis.**—Inflammation of the mucous membrane of the nose.

**Rickets.**—A disease of infancy inducing pathological changes in the osseous system. The bones become softened and various deformities are produced. There is always present in such cases a light fever. Remember, that heat above normal softens tissue. Adjust 6th dorsal for general fever.

**Ringing in the Ears.**—Adjust the atlas.

**Ringworm.**—A spreading skin disease, usually circular or in patches, tending to be clear in the center. Any portion of the body is liable to be affected, so the Chiropractor adjusts the 6th dorsal.

**Roseola.**—A skin disease in patches similar in shape to a rose leaf. The eruptions cause itching.

**Rose Rash.**—See roseola.

**Round Worms.**—See worms.

**Rubeola.**—See measles.

**Runround.**—An inflammation at the end of the finger following the circumference of the nail. Adjust 4th dorsal.

**Rupture.**—See hernia.

**Salivation.**—A superabundant secretion of saliva. A pathological condition that may be caused by certain poisons as mercury and pilocarpin.

**Salpingitis.**—Inflammation of the Eustachian or Fallopian tube.

**Salt Rheum.**—A skin disease. See eczema.

**Sarcocele.**—A solid or fleshy tumor of the testicle. Sarcocele is one form of elephantiasis.

**Sarcoma.**—A malignant tumor. Adjust according to location.

**Sausage Poisoning.**—See ptomain poison.

**Scabies.**—See itch.

**Scarlatina.**—See scarlet fever.

**Scarlet Fever.**—An acute, specific, epidemic disease. Its special feature is a scarlet flush which spreads progressively from the face over the body. Acute nephritis and otitis are frequent complications. The fever may be mild or very high.

**Scelorosis Cerebri.**—Hardening of brain tissue. See brain fever.

**Schlerosis.**—Thickening with condensation by calcareous depositions. There is an overgrowth due to hyperthermia followed by deposits of calcareous deposits on account of subnormal temperature.

**Sciatica.**—Neuralgia of the sciatic nerve. This may be confined to the proximal half of the thigh or follow out the entire course of the nerve and its branches. It is most commonly found in adults of middle age. Adjust 4th lumbar.

**Scoliosis.**—A distortion of the spine to one side; lateral curvature.

**Scorbutus.**—See scurvy.

**Scrofula.**—A disease of early life. It is recognized by enlargement of the lymphatic glands and necrosis of bones. Adjust the 6th dorsal.

**Scurvy.**—A disease observed among persons who have been deprived of a wholesome diet for quite a length of time. The gums become spongy and bleed; the skin is indurated in patches; the breath is fetid and there are painful contractions of the muscles. It seems that the food becomes poisonous by being monotonous, thereby poisoning the nervous system. It is attended with weakness and an irregular fever. Adjust 6th dorsal.

**Scybala.**—See costiveness.

**Seborrhea.**—A functional disease (what disease is not functional?) of the sebaceous glands which secretes an excessive amount of sebum, collecting upon the skin as oil or crusts. Adjust 6th dorsal.

**Seminal Emissions.**—Nocturnal, seminal losses. Usually the result of self-abuse and lascivious thinking, after retiring to bed.

**Septicemia.**—Blood (?) poison. It is accompanied by chills, profuse sweating and an irregular, remittent fever. A condition which is understood by pathologists to be induced by the absorption of putrefactive products. Instead of the blood being contaminated, the nerves are irritated and excited.

**Serodermitis.**—An inflammatory skin affection attended with serous effusion.

**Serous Circulation.**—A recent discovery (?) that the serum circulates without making a circuit. The same developer (?) may discover that the blood does not circulate, but goes thru the process of dialysis, osmosis and diffusion.

**Serum.**—The most watery portion of animal fluids, exhaled by serous membranes.

**Sewer Gas.**—The inhalation of sewer gas may act like the gases of putrifactive animal and vegetable matter—a poison.

**Sexual Weakness.**—Adjust 4th lumbar.

**Shaking Palsy.**—See paralysis agitans.

**Shingles.**—See herpes.

**Shock.**—A sudden depression of organic or vital force, occasioned by severe injury or profound emotion. Recovery may be attended by exaltation of the vital processes known as reaction.

**Sick Headache.**—Migraine. A neurosis. Headache accompanied with nausea.

**Singultus.**—See hiccough.

**Skin Diseases.**—As a rule adjust 6th dorsal.

**Sleeplessness.**—See insomnia.

**Smallpox.**—A severe case of chicken pox is smallpox. A disease known by vomiting, lumbar pains, eruption and fever. Adjust 5th cervical.

**Smell.**—Perversion of smell. Adjust 3d dorsal.

**Snake Poison.**—Snake poisons produce rapid and extensive hemorrhagic extravasations, due to softening of the vascular walls, which is due to hyperthermia, which in turn is due to excessive excitation and vibration of the nervous system.

**Sneezing.**—A convulsive motion of the expiratory muscles, carrying with it the mucous which has occasioned the irritation and expulsion.

**Somatic Death.**—The final cessation of all vital activities in the whole body in distinction to localized death, necrosis and gangrene. The molecular death of caries, necrosis and ulceration.

**Sordes.**—The dark, brown, foul matter which collects on the teeth in low fever. It consists of a mixture of food, epithelial matter and microorganisms. The latter are there as scavengers—a blessing, not a disaster.

**Spasm.**—Convulsive contractions of the muscles. See article on spasm.

**Spasm Habit.**—Mimic spasm. A disease of the facial nerve that manifests itself in clonic spasms of the muscles to which this nerve is distributed. The spasm may be general or partial, affecting only the orbicularis palpebrarum. The organic lesions are irritative, the impingement is situated in some portion of the facial motor tract.

**Spina Bifida.**—A congenital defect in the posterior wall of the vertebral canal, with protrusion of its contents in the form of a fluid tumor. This and other congenital imperfections are the result of the abnormal manner in which one or more of the functions of the mother are performed. How necessary, then, that the mother should be normal in all of her tissues and functions.

**Splanchnoptosis.**—A prolapsed condition of the abdominal viscera. See prolapsus.

**Splenitis.**—Inflammation of the spleen, sometimes terminating in suppuration. Adjust 8th dorsal.

**Spondylitis.**—Inflammation of one or more vertebra. See Pott's disease.

**Sprain.**—A sprain is caused by a strain, wrench or a violent twist. It is characterized by swelling, inflammation, soreness and disablement of the joint. Incomplete luxation is looked upon by an M. D. as a sprain.

**Stammering.**—You stammer when you can't think of what you want to say. See stuttering.

**St. Anthony's Fire.**—See erysipelas.

**Stenosis.**—Constriction or narrowing. It may be aortic, cardiac, cicatricial or mitral.

**Stomach, Diseases of.**—Adjust toward the right shoulder, standing on the left side. A student should learn to adjust from either side as an adjustment sometimes can be given with more advantage from one side than upon the other.

**Stomatitis.**—Inflammation of the mouth. Adjust 5th dorsal to the left.

**Stone in the Bladder.**—See gravel.

**Strabismus.**—See cross-eye.

**Strain.**—In pathology, an abnormal tension placed on a part. A strain may cause a sprain. See sprain.

**Struma.**—A scrofulous swelling or tumor. See bronchocele.

**Stuttering.**—An inability to say what you are thinking about. See stammering.

**St. Vitus's Dance.**—See chorea.

**Sty.**—A furuncula; inflammation of the connective tissue of the eyelids, usually at a hair-follicle.

**Summer Complaint.**—A disease of infants and young children, occurring in warm weather. The symptoms are pain, vomiting, purgation, fever and prostration. Adjust 2d lumbar.

**Sunstroke.**—A state supposed to be caused by excessive heat of the sun. There is coma, feebleness of pulse, coldness of skin and diminished temperature. Adjust 6th dorsal.

**Suppuration.**—The formation of pus. The process performed by and because of inflammation, excessive heat, whereby the white blood corpuscles become the distinctive corpuscles of pus and thus form an abscess. The stasis of inflammation is because of the change in tissue, whereby the normal transudation (not circulation) of the blood-serum thru the membranes, tissues and vessel-walls is prevented. The redness of an inflamed surface is owing to the commingling of red corpuscles. The thickened membranes preventing the normal transudation of serum, the blood plasma is transuded and the white corpuscles are retained, in stasis, forming pus. In Chiropractic pathology, the same principles are involved in the formation of catarrh as that of pus. There is only the difference of degree and location.

**Suppurative Fever.**—All suppuration is attended with fever —diffused inflammation.

**Suppurative Tonsilitis.**—See quinsy.

**Sweat, Abnormal.**—As the kidneys, or rather the 12th dorsal nerves, control perspiration, therefore adjust the 12th dorsal, which is impinging upon the nerves whose functionating produces perspiration.

**Sweating Sickness.**—Military fever; profuse sweating with eruption of military vesicles.

**Swooning.**—See faint.

**Sycosis.**—An inflammatory disease which affects the hair follicles of the beard, permanent baldness resulting in long standing cases.

**Syncope.**—See fainting.

**Synovitis.**—Inflammation of the synovial membrane. The place to adjust will depend upon what joint is affected.

**Syphilis.**—A venereal disease. Adjust according to the region affected. There are many affections credited to syphilis of which it is not guilty; the accusation is only an excuse to cover up ignorance and inability to cope with the disease.

**Tabes Dorsalis.**—See locomotor ataxia.

**Talipes.**—A deformity of the feet, either congenital or acquired (?). If its first appearance is at birth, it was acquired during gestation—thru functions of the mother abnormally performed.

**Tapeworm.**—It has an elongated, flattened, ribbon-like, articulated body. It is a scavenger living on decayed food—cannot exist where metabolism is normal. Improve digestion by adjusting the 5th dorsal to the right.

**Tarsalgia.**—Pain in the tarsus; gouty or rheumatic. Adjust 5th lumbar.

**Taste, Abnormal.**—Partial or complete inability to discern the difference in the flavor of soluble bodies by the sense of taste is a pathological condition. The nerves associated with taste are the glossopharyngeal and the lingual branch of the 5th trigeminal.

**Tears, Overflow of.**—See lachrymation.

**Teeth, Diseases of.**—The tissue of the teeth may be too hard. brittle, soft or fragile. They may suffer from decay, caries dentium. Adjust 4th cervical.

**Teething.**—Irritation of the nervous tissue produces fever. Adjust in the dorsal.

**Temperature, Subnormal.**—Due to lack of functional activity. Adjust 6th dorsal. This will correct abnormal metabolism.

**Tenia.**—See tapeworm.

**Terrata.**—The ancients attributed anomalous structures in mankind as warnings and punishments from the Almighty. Under astrology, they made a system of birth horoscopes which explained all abnormalities of mental aberations and tertatology. They claimed that an experience of 470,000 years of observation, all concordant, fully justified their system and that the influence of the stars marked, in an indubitable manner, the fatal law which determined the destiny of each individual toward certain diseases. This was determined by the position of the heavenly bodies at birth. I am sorry to say that a few Chiropractors believe in those ancient mythological myths.

**Tetanus.**—Spasm with rigidity, the result of poison. Which vertebra to adjust will depend upon the nature of the poison and where it enters the body. The adjuster will need to know what nerves are affected.

**Tetter.**—A name for various skin eruptions, such as herpes, eczema and psoriasis. Adjust 6th dorsal.

**Thermic Fever.**—See sunstroke.

**Thread Worm.**—See pin worm.

**Throat, Diseases of.**—Adjust 5th thoracic. Stand on the right side and throw toward the left shoulder.

**Thrush.**—A formation upon the oral mucous surfaces of small, whitish, soft and lightly adherent spots or flakes, tending to coalesce and spread thruout the entire buccal cavity.

**Thyriod Gland.**—See goitre.

**Thyroidenitis.**—Inflammation of the thyroid gland. See goitre.

**Tic Douloureux.**—Neuralgia of the trifacial nerve, involving one or more branches. Adjust 4th cervical.

**Tinnitus.**—Ringing, singing or roaring in the ears. It may be the result of traumatic injuries or the administration of drugs, such as quinin. Adjust atlas.

**Tired.**—To rest one after a hard day's work, adjust the 5th dorsal. The patient will feel rejuvenated and rested at once.

**Tobacco, Desire for.**—The habit may be relieved by adjusting the 5th dorsal; throw to the right.

**Toe Nails, Diseases of.**—Adjust 5th lumbar.

**Tone.**—Normal tension of nerves, muscles or an organ. The basic principle of Chiropractic.

**Tonsilitis.**—See quinsy.

**Toothache.**—Impingement on the 5th cervical nerve may cause neuralgia or toothache. Adjust to relieve.

**Torticollis.**—See wry neck.

**Toxic Inflammation.**—Some poisons irritate (excite) the nervous system, otherwise they would not be poisons. Because of their poisonous nature, physicians use them to irritate, excite, rouse the nervous system to greater activity. A poison either impairs the functions of one or more organs or destroys tissue. Any substance which produces a noxious or fatal effect is a poison, no matter by what avenue it is introduced.

**Toxicodermatitis.**—A disease of the skin due to the action of poisonous substances. The effect is always of an inflammatory character.

**Trachoma.**—See granular eyelids.

**Trance.**—A profound or abnormal sleep, similar to that induced by hypnotism. Apparently it is not due to an organic disease, but it has a cause all the same. Sensibility and consciousness may remain altho volition is absent. Adjust atlas to rouse action of dormant fibers and normal heat diffusion.

**Traulism or traulismus.** — A lisping; the consonants are replaced by b and l.

**Traumatic Inflammation.**—A rise of temperature is not always caused by inflammation. Bone fractures and the healing of wounds are attended with, and require, a rise in temperature. By this means the cells of the injured part are enabled to replace tissue which has been destroyed. This action is physiological. There may be traumatic fever from wounds, which become poisoned by a portion decomposing, or by the introduction of deletereous substances. Inflammation always denotes a condition of pain, heat, swelling, discoloration, disordered function and alteration of tissue.

**Trophoneurosis.**—Local disturbance of nutrition owing to modified trophic action of the nerve supply of the part.

**Tuberculosis.**—There are many cases falsely diagnosed as tuberculosis. This disease is characterized by the presence of tubercles. Any organ or tissue in the body may be affected by tubercles, small, hard, granular bodies, yellowish at the center and bounded by a reddish, vascular zone. The lungs and intestines are more often the seat of tubercles than other parts. Tubercles are growths resulting from inflammation in tissue which functionate excessively, whether from traumatism or poisonous toxins. The result, it is said, whether true or false I do not know, that dairy cattle tested by toxin (poison) may pass inspection but, upon a second trial, they are found to be tuberculous; the poison having made degenerative conditions. Adjust 6th dorsal to relieve impingement caused by the introduced poison. By this means displaced tissue and all functious tissue is returned to normal position; functions (including heat) will be returned to normal.

**Tumors.**—Enlargements due to morbid growth. A cancer is said to be malignant because of its inflamed, angry condition which causes a rapid growth. The diffused inflammation causes abnormal metabolism, "run down condition." A tumor which is not angry has no inflammation to be diffused, therefore is not malignant. Adjust according to the area occupied.

**Typhoid Fever.**—A disease known as abdominal typhus, enteric fever and gastric fever. There is a specific eruption, morbid inflammation and ulceration, enlargement of the spleen and mesenteric glands and catarrhal inflammation of the intestinal mucous membrane. The poison, the cause of this disease, is introduced into the body in food or drink. There is headache, weariness, backache, cough, nosebleed and tenderness in the intestines. The fever increases each day, remitting each afternoon. Why this periodicity in disease?—well, ask someone who knows. Diarrhea is usually a marked symptom, yet the stool movements may be costive. Hemorrhage of the intestines, gums or nose may occur as complications. The heat may cause necrosis, softening of the intestinal walls, so that perforations may occur. There may be well marked symptoms of pleurisy, pneumonia, bronchitis, nephritis, thrombosis of veins, phthisis, pariotitis, etc. These many and varied symptoms, all disturbed functions, are caused by one displaced vertebra, and that one is the 6th dorsal, the central vertebra of the spinal column as well as that of the sympathetic ganglionic chain, the great distributing agent.

The extreme inflammation created at the sixth dorsal by pressure on nerves, whether the pressure is traumatic or toxic, is transmitted thruout the body by diffusion. By its excessive heat it softens tissue, creating all the conditions noticed. And the best of it all is that we, as Chiropractors, by relieving impingements upon nerves, can restore all functions, even that which produces heat, to a normal degree of activity. To me and Chiropractic are the medical and scientific worlds indebted for the discovery of these facts. Adjust the 6th dorsal and no other. This is specific, making of Chiropractic a science.

**Typhus Fever.**—A fever characterized by high temperature, weak but frequent pulse, great prostration and much cerebral disturbance. Adjust 6th dorsal. Chiropractors frequently speak of the 6th dorsal as C. P. (center place), as there are 13 vertebrae above and below the 13th pair of spinal nerves. A displacement of the 6th thoracic seems to cause as many diseases as the rest of the spinal column altogether. There is this special difference, however. The displacement of other vertebrae causes local ailments, whereas the displacement of the one at center place tends to cause general affections. It is from this region that the great splanchnic nerve emerges from the sympathetic ganglionic cord; its exact origin, however, varies in different subjects. This visceral nerve terminates in the semilunar ganglion of the solar plexus.

**Ulcer.**—A sore in the soft parts of the body, the surface of which is granulated. It is kept in a diseased condition by inflammation, excess of heat. If you do not know the vertebra to adjust, locate it by palpation.

**Ulcerated Sore Throat.**—Adjust 5th dorsal, standing on the right side and throw to the left.

**Uraemia.**—A condition presenting such morbid phenomena as mental disturbance, convulsions, coma, headache, nausea, dyspnea and disordered vision. Adjust 6th dorsal.

**Uremic Convulsions.**—These spasms are supposed to be due to suppression, or deficient secretion, of urine. It is recognized by nausea, vomiting, dyspnea, amauroses, headache, vertigo, dimness of vision, coma, hemiplegia, convulsions and urinous odor of the breath and perspiration. The author of the book, Spinal Adjustment, advises to adjust in five places. Carver's Analysis uses five pages in describing this disease and telling what Chiropractors can do with it; however, six inches of one page is blank. The author must consider the condition very abnormal as he uses "abnormalities" twelve times in the first one and one-third pages. He advises "the most careful dieting," but does not say where, when or how to adjust for this ailment. Volume No. IV. of The Science of Chiropractic states: "The condition so known is one of the primary and simple diseases following the lack of normal flow of urine. The name does not express the quantity." This last explanation is not any more enlightening to a Chiropractor than those of the other two advisors. I, the originator and developer of Chiropractic, say, adjust one vertebra, and that one the 12th dorsal. This is the central place between the 6th dorsal and the last vertebral articulation. The diseases arising therefrom, because of an impingement upon the 12th pair of dorsal nerves, are general in their character, but not quite as much so as those caused by an impingement upon the nerves emerging from the central center place.

**Uresis.**—See micturition.

**Urethritis.**—Inflammation of the urethra. Gonorrhea is a common cause. See gleet.

**Uridosis.**—See uraemia.

**Urination, Frequent.**—Gould and Dunglison's dictionaries state that the micturition center which governs the act of micturition is situated in the lumbar region of the spinal cord. If this is so and the act is interfered with by the nerve being impinged upon, why not remove the impingement? This disease may be caused by prostatitis—an inflammation of the prostate gland. The quality of the urine may be of an irritating nature. Adjust 1st lumbar.

**Urination, Stuttering.**—Intermittent urination due to spasm of the bladder. Adjust 1st lumbar.

**Urine, Too Frequent or Too Scanty.**—Adjust 12th dorsal.

**Uteritis.**—Inflammation of the womb. See metritis.

**Uterus, Diseases of.**—Adjust 2d lumbar.

**Uterus, Malpositions of.**—Anteversion, retroversion and procidentia are different abnormal positions of great concern to the medical practitioner because they believe each one requires a different kind of treatment. To a Chiropractor they are of no special concern, because he knows they all originate from a common cause which he can remove. By adjusting the 2d lumbar the supporting nerves, muscles and ligaments acquire their normal tonicity and the uterus its normal position.

**Uticaria.**—See nettle rash.

**Uvulitis.**—Inflammation of the uvula. Adjust 3d cervical.

**Vaccina.**—A disease of the cow. The discovery was made in 1798 that kine-pocks could be transferred to man. Vaccine virus is the poison transferred from one animal or person to another, usually, from a heifer to man. This discovery has met with great favor by physicians and has added to their income, but it has injured their patients. A valuable, wonderful medical discovery, that one or more diseases could be added to and developed in mankind.

**Vaccination.**—A disease produced by inoculation with vaccine virus. Many diseases, however, have been introduced by vaccination and not a few deaths have been caused by it. Adjust 6th dorsal.

**Vaccine Virus.**—Consists of the liquid contained in the vesicle or of the scab resulting from the desiccation of the pustule. If kept in a cool place it will retain its contamination qualities for a week or ten days.

**Vaginitis.**—Inflammation of the vagina. Adjust 3d lumbar.

**Varicella.**—See chicken pox.

**Varicocele.**—Enlargement of the veins of the scrotum and spermatic cord and corresponding veins in the female. Adjust 3d lumbar.

**Varicose Veins.**—Blood vessels, swollen, knotted and tortuous. If of the lower extremities, adjust the lower lumbar. Remember that the flow of blood is controlled by a network of nerves.

**Variola.**—A specific, infectious disease ushered in with severe febrile symptoms and followed by a papular eruption spreading over all parts of the body. Adjust 5th cervical. See smallpox.

**Vasculitis.**—Inflammation of blood vessels. Yes, the walls of arteries and veins are supplied with numerous smaller arteries and veins and medullated and non-medullated nerve-fibers. These nerve-fibers form dense plexuses on the outer surface of the vessels from which filaments pass to the middle coat to be distributed almost entirely to its muscular fibers. Thus blood vessels are supplied with arteries, veins, muscles and lymphatics, and, like other tissue, are liable to become inflamed when the fibers ramifying their structure are impinged upon directly by traumatism, indirectly by poison or auto-mental-intoxication.

**Vertebra, Ill-Shaped.**—Displaced vertebra, racked from their normal position, become set in their new location. Their articulations are immovable and they soon change their shape to conform to their new position, thus becoming ill-shaped. Before they can be permanently replaced. they must be reshaped, made suitable by growth, for their normal position.

**Vertiginous.**—Affected with vertigo; giddy; dizzy; swimming of the head. Look to atlas. Adjust by using the phalangeal joint of the small finger as a knuckle, striking the posterior arch midway between the tubercle and the lateral mass, so as to drive it toward the attachment of the transverse ligament of the opposite side.

**Vertigo.**—See vertiginous.

**Vomiting.**—The forcible, convulsive ejection of the contents of the stomach, duodenum, or intestines thru the mouth. When the matter from either of the last two organs is ejected, it is called stercoraceous or fecal vomiting. There being an intestinal obstruction, the intestinal semi-fluid contents are returned upwards by reflex peristalsis. Such cases are rare. I had one patient who was relieved, in a few days, by adjusting one of the lower dorsal.

**Vomiting During Pregnancy.**—Adjust 5th dorsal.

**Vomitus.**—Vomiting is the effect of an irritation of the gastric nerves causing a reflex action for the expulsion of the contents of the stomach. The diaphragm and abdominal muscles assist in the effort.

**Vulvitis.**—Inflammaton of the vulva. Adjust 3d lumbar.

**Weeping.**—See lachrymation.

**Whites.**—See leucorrhea.

**Whitlow.**—An inflammation of the fingers or toes, generally of the last phalanx, terminating, usually, in suppuration. The inflammation may occur in any portion between the skin and the bone. The term is usually applied to a felon or inflammation of the periosteal structure of the bone. If affected in both fingers and toes, adjust 6th dorsal; if of the fingers only, adjust 4th dorsal; if of the toes only, adjust in the lumbar region.

**Whooping Cough.**—A violent convulsive cough ending with a sonorous whoop. Adjust 4th dorsal.

**Womb, Diseases of.**—Adjust 2d lumbar.

**Worms.**—Worms are scavengers. Improve digestion. Scavengers live upon decaying food. If metabolism is perfect, the stomach, with normal digestion, will dispose of the worms; even tapeworms. Adjust 5th lumbar to the right.

**Wry Neck.**—A contraction of the cervical muscles resulting in an abnormal position of the head; also, an unsymmetrical shape of the face and cranium. See article on wry neck. Adjust 3d cervical.

---

## CONSTIPATION.

E. H. Laughlin says: Constipation is the cause of a large per cent. of diseases.

A distinction should be made between constipation (infrequency of stool) and costiveness (dryness and hardness of the feces). The former is usually caused by paralysis of some portion of the bowel, lack of muscular action. This lesion should be located and the impinged nerve relieved so that normal innervation may be resumed.

In costiveness, where the stool is dry and hard and expelled with difficulty, the cause is too much action of the kidneys. Too much water is passed by the urinary organs, depriving the stool tract of its proper moisture. In all such cases, correct the abnormal action of the kidneys.

---

Cheerfulness makes love of life, and love of life is half of health. On the contrary, sadness and discouragement hasten old age.

---

Learn to digest that which you take in mentally, make it of value, soak it in your system, make it a part of yourself, develop your intellect and body by its addition. Absorb it into your brain, use it as an instrument, an equipment to your mind.

---

The school inspectors (medical) of Portland report an unusually large number of cases of pediculosus capitis. More than one hundred pupils were found to be suffering from this annoying ailment.

---

Slates have been banished from the schools of Sacramento as disease-breeders. The longer we live the more we wonder that any pupil of the old red schoolhouse of a past generation lived to tell the tale of his or her school days.

## TONE.

Tone is the foundation upon which, as a basic principle, I built my science. From tone originates all the principles which constitute the science and philosophy of Chiropractic.

Tone is the elasticity and renitency of tissue which responds to compression.

Renitency is the state or quality of being renitent. The renitency of tissue is the inherent quality of life, the ability to resist pressure. In biology it is the condition resulting from elastic force acting against an impulse. The elastic force of nerves furnishes the momentum of impulses. This innate quality of springing back, recovering its normal size, shape and position is known as tone. Hence, we have nerve tone, muscle tone, arterial tone, etc., meaning the ability of those tissues to assume, return to their normal position, size and shape after being acted upon by pressure.

It is a self-evident fact that any change in tissue other than that of normal tension, produces disease, tone being the product of elasticity and renitency.

The distinctive character of tone is due to tension. Tension is the condition of being stretched, drawn tight, strained to stiffness. Gaseous tension is the elasticity of gas, its tendency to expand. Electric tension is its tendency to overcome resistence. Arterial tension is the strain on an artery at full pulse. Intraoccular tension is the pressure of the fluids of the eye against its envelopes produced by the continual renewal of the fluids within the interior of the eye. Intravenous tension is the strain from the flow of blood upon the coats of a vein. Muscular tension is the condition of moderated contraction produced by stretching a muscle.

Life consists in the renitency and the elasticity of tissue; its response to impulses; these constitute intelligent action, life guided by intelligence, the soul, the symphysis which unites spirit and body.

Accurate measurements of tension is made by means of instruments called tonometers. For all practical purposes it is estimated by palpation with the fingers. In registering tension, its varying degrees from normal, it is noted by using the minus or plus sign prefixed to numeral figures; the normal tension (tn) of tone being the standard.

---

A Portland mixup. The cuts of five doctors and their ads occupy a right hand lower corner of a newspaper. There are three Chinese, one "Men cured, pay when satisfied," and the fifth under a plug hat says "Chiropractic nerve specialist. Curing without drugs is my business; to get cured, that's your business. For constipation and dizziness is the herald of the undertaking business."

As I am closing this volume I am pleased to see in the November number of The Chiropractor, 1910, the following from A. P. Davis. "The would-be opposer of Chiropractic expresses himself in such a manner as to manifest profound ignorance of what Chiropractic Science is, and seems to be 'talking thru his coat sleeve' or beating the air." In order to write intelligently about any question one must know something about the question.

"As to using other than Chiropractic in adjusting patients, I would say that I do not mix it with any other treatment, although I am in a position to have to teach other methods—simply because the college demands it. I do not even mix them—'One thing at a time' is all that is taught or practiced by your humble servant."

Dr. Davis visited me twice in Portland, the last was in March, 1910, during which he was quite interested to learn more of my science, as shown by the following.

Portland, Oregon, March 11, 1910.

"Having attended four lectures of Dr. D. D. Palmer on specific adjusting; I note with satisfaction the elimination of superfluous adjustments as given by many Chiropractors.

"Dr. Palmer determines where the conditions causing disease are to be found, and where, if properly adjusted will accomplish the desired result.

"If his book contains a review of some writers, as per sample I have seen, it will be of the greatest possible interest and value, as well as to establish a reliable standard for all future Chiropractic practitioners—or adjusters. It will be Chiropractic up-to-date and worthy a place—the first place, so far as Chiropractic is concerned—in the library of every Chiropractor.

"Very respectfully, "DR. A. P. DAVIS."

Dr. Davis writes me from Pittsburg, Pa., under date of October 19, 1910, saying:

"My Dear Friend and Doctor: Your book is the book I want, the book that is needed as a Chiropractor instructor. I am pleased to learn that you are making it worthy, giving it the very best effort of your life—making it replete with the cream, the ripest experience of your long and ardent studies. It will be just what the world needs along the line of scientific adjustment. I hope to get great good and much new and useful information out of your book. I have no words with which I can fully express my appreciation of your most wonderful science. I shall never be remiss in my efforts to advance the science of Chiropractic, and praise for its discovery. I am anxiously awaiting its completion, its reception and perusal."

## WHAT WE SHOULD KNOW.

We should know that a light pressure on a nerve excites, irritates the filaments which it contains; that a heavy pressure closes the nerve tubes. That either too much or not enough functionating is disease. That to have health, pressure must be removed from the nerves, thereby allowing Innate to perform its functions in a normal manner.

We should know that the heating of the body, normally or abnormally, is a function; that fever is but excessive heat caused by nerve tension; that if the pressure causing the various kinds of fever is removed, normal heat will be restored in from 5 to 15 minutes. It is not necessary for a Chiropractor to wait until the fever is fully developed before he aborts it.

We should know that pimples, boils, ulcers, tumors and cancers are due to nerve pressure, causing too much action and heat; which articulation is out of alignment, making an unnatural projection, pressing against a nerve, causing irritation, excessive heat, over-action, an over-supply of nutrition; also that, to remove the impingement by replacing the exposed projection, is to reinstate Innate, so that all functions may be performed in a normal manner.

We should know how to trace affected nerves in the living subject rather than in the cadaver. We should aim to benefit the patient rather than the undertaker. We should know that boils, ulcers, tumors and rheumatism are not the result of bad blood, or "an abnormal condition of the kidneys."

We should know that by being specific we learn what nerve is impinged upon, what vertebrae is displaced and how to adjust it; that to adjust haphazardly, here and there, anywhere up and down the spine, every other vertebra today and the intervening ones tomorrow, so as to drive the disease down and out of the spine is far from Chiropractic; that to give each vertebra the same movement is not scientific, is not using Chiropractic as a science; that to adjust all displacements in the same manner is not perfecting it towards a higher development; that a vertebra that is not displaced cannot be adjusted, replaced; that to jump onto vertebrae which are in alignment, is not only useless, showing ignorance on the part of the practitioner, but is dangerous, for we are liable to displace vertebrae and cause disease.

We should know that gastritis, cancer of the stomach, cardialgia, gastrodynia, acute inflammation caused by corrosives taken for suicidal intent, alcoholism, tobacco habits, stomach worms, including tape worms, dyspepsia, indigestion, ulcers and dilatation of the stomach, are because of a sub-luxation at S. P.; that not to know upon which side of the spine the nerves of stomach innervation emerge betrays ignorance of anatomy; that being unable to make the precise movement to relieve the impingements which cause these diseases, displays ignorance of the art; that to be proficient and make our work efficacious, we should know that the nerves emerging from S. P. on the right, go to the throat, mouth and head; that an impingement of that bundle of fibers cause such diseases as croup, diphtheria, goitre, quinsy, mumps, cancers of the mouth, throat and thyroid gland, catarrh of the throat, pharyngitis, some headaches, inflammation of the eye-ball and cataracts.

---

McFarland says: "Fatty infiltration is the assumption and retention of fats by the cells. It is a common physiologic phenomena and becomes pathologic only when it occurs in unusual tissues or in excessive degree."

Physiologic functions become pathologic when functions are performed in a degree either too great or too little, Therefore, we use the term pathologic physiology, meaning abnormal functions.

---

"Like the representatives of all schools of the healing art, the Osteopath recognizes the strength of the evidence in favor of germs being the cause of many disases."

Therein is one great difference between Osteopathy and Chiropractic. The Allopaths and Osteopaths hold that germs are the exciting cause of many diseases; whereas, the Chiropractors do not believe that germs are the cause of any disease.

The Osteopath and the Allopath use antidotes for poisons. The Chiropractor adjusts certain vertebrae for certain poisons, be they slow or active.

"The Osteopath, instead of giving drugs to reduce fever, stimulates the action of the sweat glands and excretory organs to throw off the poison which causes the temperature and other symptoms."

The Chiropractor does not use drugs, neither does he stimulate organs to reduce fever.

The Osteopath and the Allopath believe poisons to be the cause of fevers. The Chiropractor finds bone pressure on nerves the direct cause; however, these bones may have been drawn out of alignment by poisons. He, therefore, removes the impingement.

"The Osteopath uses the natural fluids and forces of the body as healing agents." The Chiropractor removes pressure from nerves so that functions may be performed in a natural manner.

## D. D. PALMER WAS THE FIRST

Chiropractor.
To use nerve tracing.
To write upon Innate.
To define Chiropractic
To use the name Innate.
To write upon Chiropractic.
To edit a Chiropractic journal.
To add the cumulative function.
To give a Chiropractic adjustment.
To teach the Science of Chiropractic.
To state that action is intelligent life.
To found a Chiropractic school—the P. S. C.
To discover that the body is heated by nerves.
To assert that molecular action produces animal heat.
To harmonize the scope and action of the two intellects.
To state that nerve irritation increases molecular action.
To affirm that life depends upon the condition of nerves.
To assert that disease is too much or not enough functionating.
To declare that vertebrae out of alignment impinge upon nerves.
To affirm that nerves are impinged upon; not squeezed or pinched.
To define disease and its cause as understood by Chiropractors.
To insist that spirit, soul, mind and body are four different, distinct entities.
To locate the Center Place and the Second Center Place of the spinal column.
To determine that the normal rate of nerve vibration is about 200 a minute.
To prove that the degree of animal heat is determined by the firmness of nerve tissue.
To state that there are four functions — vital, vegetative, intellectual and consumative.
To state that 95 per cent of diseases are caused by displaced vertebrae; the remainder by luxations of other joints.
To ascertain that functions are created by impulses which are modified by the force or momentum received from nerve vibration.
To determine that nerve tension, the condition of being tense, strained, stretched to stiffness, is the cause of all diseases; that normal tone is health.
To state that poisons act on nerves and that by their action on muscles, vertebrae are drawn out of alignment, and that antidotal drugs or poisons may replace vertebrae.

To state that excessive heat softens nerve tissue, thereby lessening vibration and the consequent heat until the temperature of the patient becomes normal, or in some cases even subnormal.
To declare that the degree of heat determines the quality of tissue which, in turn, determines the degree or extent of functional activity, and that either excessive or deficient functional activity is disease.

---

Brain power is estimated by the way you use it.

---

Why not learn to adjust displacements and help the disabled?

---

Chiropractic is a science just so far as it is specific.

---

The only failure a man should fear, is the failure to do his best.

---

Disease is either a lessening or an exaggeration of functionating.

---

Ponderable matter can be weighed on scales; imponderable cannot.

---

The man who practices Chiropractic is a Chiropractor. He who practices music is a musician.

---

Pathological phenomena are variations of physiological processes—modification of functions, structure and position.

---

Chiropractic rays of light are causing ignorance and superstition to varnish as surely as the rising sun chases away the midnight darkness.

---

We recognize only five senses, if we had eight we would know more. The future will see more senses developed and unknown forces utilized.

---

There is a vast difference between treating effects and adjusting the cause. We have been accustomed to the former; the latter was discovered fifteen years ago and is gradually being developed into a science.

---

A Chiropractor is not a therapeutist; he is not interested in discovering nor in applying remedies. To be versed in therapeutics would be to be skilled in the use and application of remedies. Chiropractors do not use remedies.

"Chiropractic is the most scientific and practical system of locating and adjusting by hand the cause of diseases, or reestablishing and maintaining perfect health of mind and body of patient."

The above infers that there are other systems which are scientific and practical, and that Chiropractic is not fully scientific and practical, but the most so. I would say, Chiropractic is scientific and practical. Avoid stuffing a sentence, trying to say too much. Let the other fellow report his system.

To establish is to make stable, to secure firmly, to make permanent. To "reestablish perfect health of mind and body," is self-evident that it was not previously established, was not stable, or permanent. To "re-establish" would be to place the patient in the same unstable, not permanent, condition. If anything is established, it cannot be reestablished.

A patient is one who is ill, under the care of a doctor. A patient "maintaining perfect health of mind and body" would not be a patient.

"The Chiropractor recognizes life as the normal expression by the tissue and organs of the body."

An organ is a part or structure, in an animal or plant, adapted for the performance of some specific function. Every part of the body has a special function. Organs are composed of tissue. There is no tissue that does not constitute a part or all of an organ. In the above sentence "tissues and organs" mean one and the same—one of the terms being superfluous.

"Life is the normal expression."

Functions performed in a normal or abnormal manner is life. That is all there is of disease: life—action—performed in an unusual degree—more or less than normal.

"Functional impulses which are created by innate (inborn) intelligence in the brain."

Impulses are not functional, they do not perform any regular functions. Organs perform functions. Impulses order, direct, prompt, cause action of organs.

"The Chiropractor recognizes in each system a disease."

A system is an aggregation of many things methodically arranged, united by some form of regular interaction or interdependence. In biology, those organs collectively which are of the same or similar tissue or which especially contribute toward one of the more important, complex, vital functions. We have the absorbent system, the adifose system, the alimentary system, the vascular system, the cerebro-spinal system, the system of transudation, the dentinal system, the dermoid system, the esthesiodic system, the glandular system, the Haversian system, the lymphatic system, the muscular system, the nervous system, the projection system, the sympathetic system and the cranial nerve system. Does the writer of the above mean to say that in each of these systems he recognizes a disease? If so which one? If not, in what other system does he recognize a disease?

"The Chiropractor traces disease directly to its cause, which is an interference to the normal transmission of current between the brain and the tissues and organs diseased."

"The cause of disease is an interference to the normal transmission of current."

There is no current action nor such a thing as a current in the body. The blood circulates, it flows, but it has no current. The current is the swiftest part of a stream. We have aerial currents and ocean currents, but no body currents. I presume the author used "current" as a synonym for impulse; if so, they have no correlation. They have an entirely different meaning, are not interchangeable. An impulse does not flow, has no current.

"Interference" is not known in physiology. Circulation, transudation, vibration, tension and action, may be increased or diminished, but not interfered with. No obstacle can be placed, so as to interfere, interpose, hinder, impede or retard the nerve channels so as to obstruct the transmission of impulses. The transmission, rate of travel of impulses may be increased or decreased, and their momentum modified, but not obstructed or interfered with.

"Between the brain and the tissues and organs diseased."

The brain is tissue and an organ, as much so, as any portion of the body. The brain may be diseased. Considering these facts, please reread "Between the brain and the tissues and organs diseased."

"This interference to current is produced by partially displaced vertebrae."

There being no such a thing as a "current" in the body, it cannot be interfered with. Interference and current are not physiological terms.

"Vertebrae pressing upon and impinging nerves."

An impingement, and pressing upon, are one and the same thing. Nerves are impinged upon by displaced vertebrae.

"Remember we do not treat the effect of disease, but we adjust the cause."

Why not say, "We do not treat disease or its symptoms; we adjust causes."

---

"This school has practically revolutionized and developed the science of Chiropractic." So much so that Chiropractic as a science and philosophy is hardly recognizable as such in that school.

The various answers received to my question, "What is the basic principle of Chiropractic," has not surprised me, as Chiropractors have always talked (the plural) basic principles. By far the larger number have no answer. Of those who attempted to answer, give several principles, none of which are the basic the fundamental principle, the one from which all other Chiropractic principles are derived, the one upon which the science of Chiropractic is founded, the one upon which health depends. When I refer to the basis of the science, I do not mean the art, nor its philosophy.

One D. C. thinks the cycle, the basic principle upon which the science is based. A cycle is a complete course, returning into itself, restoring the original state. Another says, "The principle of locating different diseases by subluxated vertebrae impinge nerves, diverging from spinal cord thru intervertebral foramina—causing either too much or not enough function." And still another thinks "the Chiropractic **thrust is entitled** to the distinction of being the **corner stone of the basic principle** of Chiropractic."

The thrust belongs to the art, not the science. Science relates to something to be known, or to that which is to be done. I did not ask what was **entitled** to be known as the basic principle, but what is the basic principle upon which I builded the science (not art or its philosophy) of Chiropractic. Neither did I ask for **the corner stone of the** basic **(base)** principle. I want to know what constitutes the base, the fundamental principle upon which I built the science.

---

"The Chiropractor, the truthful exponent of Chiropractic unadulterated."

Articles are adulterated to increase their weight or bulk, or to improve their flavor or change their appearance, that they may imitate another article of higher grade or different kind.

Can the science, art or philosophy of Chiropractic be increased in weight, or bulk by the addition of an inferior article? Can you think of any substance which would change the color or improve the appearance of Chiropractic in any way, if so please give us the method and percentage of the combination. Why all this buncome of "pure unadulterated?" The honest man does not need to be prating his honesty before the observing public. It is the thief who cries "thief, thief" in order to divert attention. To refer to a science, art, or philosophy being adulterated, is to infer that it is debased as an article or substance by adding an ingredient of inferior value.

## INJURED BRAKEMAN RECOVERS MIND, BUT DOCTORS TAKE THE $16,000 DAMAGES.

Terre Haute, Ind., Jan. 5.—John Sudbrink, who has been insane since he was injured two years ago when working as a brakeman on the Big Four, has been restored to sanity by an operation on the skull, only to be told that the $16,000 damages granted by the court had been used by the medical men in treatment of his case.

---

Among all fine arts, one of the finest is that of painting the cheeks with health.—Ruskin.

---

To study functions without Innate—the controller—is like studying creation without a creator.

---

A lesion is the **cause** of functional derangement, abnormal position of tissue or diseased substance.

---

Antonyms, words of opposite meaning are: health, robustness, soundness, strength, sturdiness and vigor.

---

One would think Chiropractic a contortionist when observing the variety of tables, the position of the operator and the many movements used by Chiropractors.

---

"External injuries from falls, jars or bruises," do not cause subluxations. Injuries do not cause displacements. A sudden jar or fall unexpected may cause displacement of vertebrae, but bruises never.

---

Chiropractors are not interested in discovering medical remedies for the curing or healing of diseases. They repair. adjust, fix, replace displaced bones of the skeletal frame which are impinging upon sensitive nerves.

---

A D. O. wants to know how we can give corrective treatment for spinal lesions when the patient is flat on his back with typhoid.

**Turn him over**—to a Chiropractor, of course.

---

Chiropractic is specific; in saying this, I do not refer to those who know but little of it as a science. Osteopathy in its practice of contraction, relaxation, extension, rotation and counter-extension is neither specific nor direct.

## SURGEONS LIABLE FOR BIG DAMAGES.

St. Louis, Aug. 18, 1909.—Surgeons who overlook instruments and appliances and sew them up in a patient are liable for damages, according to a decision of the United States Court of Appeals for the Southern District of Iowa, presented yesterday in the case of Russell Johnson, of Lockridge, Ia., against Dr. Charles E. Ruth, formerly of Keokuk, Ia. This decision sustained the decision of the Federal Court of Appeals and gave Johnson a judgment for $20,000.

The petition states that Johnson was operated on, at Keokuk, Ia., for appendicitis, March 30, 1907. The wound failed to heal and caused much pain. A second operation revealed that a piece of gauze 24 inches long and 9 inches wide had been left in the wound.

---

Roses Fragrant, Roses Rare, Roses, Roses, Everywhere.

---

"The articular surfaces of the bones are very richly supplied with sensory nerves."

---

A Chiropractor's card reads, "The Chiropractor recognizes in each symptom a disease."

Chiropractors, as well as physicians, recognize a group of symptoms which occur together as constituting a disease. Certain symptoms taken collectively, represent a distinct form of disease. Each symptom does not make a disease.

---

Many booklets have been written on Chiropractic. Some of them I have criticised, I hope, for the benefit of the student.

Of books, the first was a compilation of my own writings—"The Science of Chiropractic, by Palmer." I seriously objected to its publication, as I felt that I did not then know enough of the science to write a book. Several volumes have been added by B. J., my son, which are not worth the paper they have worse than wasted, because of their erroneous teaching. Langworthy and Smith put out a book in two volumes, under the title of "Modernized Chiropractic," which I have not seen. Neuropathy, by Davis—"Chiropractic, really what we call Neuropathy," and Chiropractic Analysis, by Carver, have nothing in them that is really Chiropractic. Spinal Adjustment, by Gregory, contains much that is Chiropractic and some that is not. And now there is one by the discoverer and founder of the science and art of Chiropractic. I hope it will be judiciously criticised in the same spirit that I have criticised others.

Carbuncle coffee and concentrated lies.

---

Do right, fear no man, be a law unto yourself.

---

He that listens to reason is a man of the highest type.

---

Truth is stranger than fiction because less frequently told.

---

Truth and honesty are twins; reason is their guardian angel.

---

The new is not always true; the true is not always new; a trite saying.

---

Chiropractic is founded upon different principles than those of medicine.

---

Relieving human suffering and diffusing universal knowledge is humanitarian.

---

The most wonderful study of mankind is man. The grandest and greatest science is Chiropractic.

---

The practitioner and patient are often surprised at quick recoveries when causes are adjusted.

---

This book is written for those who are thinkers; those who do not know it all. Readers of this class will peruse it from cover to cover.

---

The osteopath accepts all of allopathy except that of drugs. Of late, many are accepting the science of pharmacology. Chiropractors assent to nothing that is allopathic.

---

In all conditions, make the adjustment (move the vertebra) with as little force and as few movements as possible. Remember that every move creates some inflammation. The quicker the move, the less force required.

Worship truth and justice—you need no other God.

---

I claim to be the first person to adjust vertebrae by hand, using the spinous and transverse processes as levers. I developed the art known as adjusting, and formulated the science of Chiropractic, and developed its philosophy.

---

The Chiropractors and Spinologists of a certain school get out their cards with "Dr. U. C. Blank, D. C." It is a sign of egotism to place both Dr. and the letters of your degree to your name. Some think it not good taste to use either, but one is permissible.

---

"They contended that if it is **mis**placed at all it must be entirely dislocated." "Spinal tissues strained and **mis**placed."

Bones and organs are **dis**placed when moved from their normal location. We **mis**place an article when we place it where it should not be. We **dis**place, put out of place, bones by accident. We **mis**place our confidence.

---

"The stretcher. Invaluable to Osteopaths, Chiropractors, Mechano-therapists, and Physical Culturists, because it provides a means for securing complete spinal extension permitting freedom of blood and nerve flow to diseased and debilitated parts."

The Chiropractor recognies the flow of blood and serum, but deny that nerves flow. Diseased parts may be debilitated or exhibit too much energy. Chiropractors do not need a stretcher for spinal extension to assist them to replace displaced bones.

---

"Flow of mental impulses."

To flow is a type of motion characteristic of fluids, that is, of liquids, gasses and viscous solids. A viscous solid is one distinguished by viscosity, having the quality of being adhesive, sticky, ropy, or glutinous consistency. Impulses do not flow as a liquid, transudate or circulate as a fluid, or become softened sufficiently to run as a viscous solid. Rivers flow from lakes, tears flow from the eyes, and the menstrual flow is periodical. Motor impulses are of the mental, the sensory are not. Impulses are not liquid, therefore, do not flow. Light, heat, sound and impulse are transmitted by vibration—molecular action—they do not flow. Vital force is inherent, consequently, does not flow.

Science is a collection of demonstrated facts.

---

Those who love their fellowmen serve their Creator.

---

Song birds are vegetarians; carnivorous birds are croakers.

---

A waste of money—a ten-dollar hat on ten cents' worth of brains.

---

He can never know any deep joy who can laugh at the sorrows of another.

---

Don't try to get well by two systems at once; it is unfair to both systems and to yourself.

---

"Dr. Blank, Chiropractor and masseur. Chiropractic removes the cause of disease." If so, why use massage?

---

Chiropractic is fascinating and remunerative it is founded on osteological and neurological facts, which are demonstrable.

---

Our readers will find mental Chiropractic food, which will require intellectual digestion whether they be laymen or practitioners.

---

We have to take the nervous system as we find it, and not as we might like to have it. Innate Intelligence has so formed it as best suited for its environments.

---

"The regular physician treats symptoms, whereas the osteopath treats the lesion causing the symptoms." Chiropractors do not "treat symptoms" or "lesions."

---

Every Chiropractic school is a college and every "Chiropractic college is superior in every respect to that of any other college of Chiropractic." Each and every school has the greatest teachers.

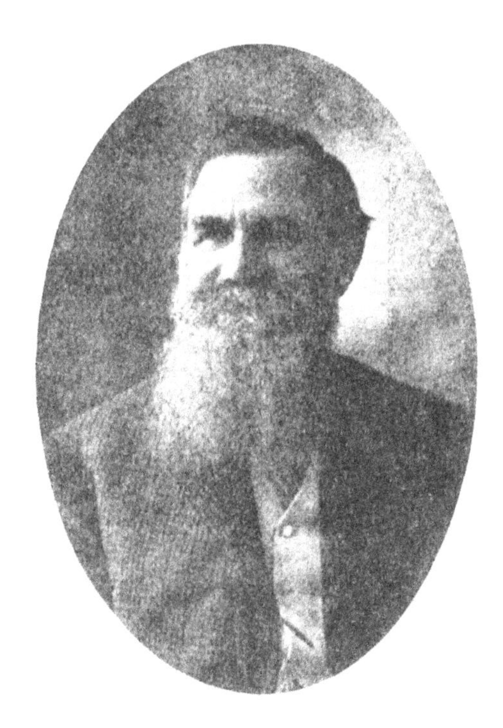

## HE DID HIS BEST.

When I am dead, if men can say,
**I helped the world** upon its way;
With all my faults of word and deed
**Mankind did have some** little **need**
For what I've done—then in my grave
No greater honor shall I crave.

If they can say—if they but can—
**"He did his best, he played the man,**
**His ways were straight; his soul was clean;**
His failings not unkind nor mean.
**He loved his fellow man and tried**
**To help him"**—I'll be satisfied.

But when I'm gone, if **only one**
Will weep because my life is gone
And feel the world is somewhat bare
Because I am no longer there—
Call me a knave, my life misspent—
No matter. **I shall be content.**

# INDEX.

## POEMS.



## CUTS.

# INDEX.

Printed in the USA
CPSIA information can be obtained
at www.ICGtesting.com
LVHW020936201023
761400LV00010B/6